HEALTHCARE TECHNOLOGIES SERIES 42

Smart Health Technologies for the COVID-19 Pandemic

IET Book Series on e-Health Technologies

Book Series Editor: Professor Joel J.P.C. Rodrigues, College of Computer Science and Technology, China University of Petroleum (East China), Qingdao, China; Senac Faculty of Ceará, Fortaleza-CE, Brazil and Instituto de Telecomunicações, Portugal

Book Series Advisor: Professor Pranjal Chandra, School of Biochemical Engineering, Indian Institute of Technology (BHU), Varanasi, India

While the demographic shifts in populations display significant socio-economic challenges, they trigger opportunities for innovations in e-Health, m-Health, precision and personalized medicine, robotics, sensing, the Internet of things, cloud computing, big data, software defined networks, and network function virtualization. Their integration is however associated with many technological, ethical, legal, social, and security issues. This book series aims to disseminate recent advances for e-health technologies to improve healthcare and people's wellbeing.

Could you be our next author?

Topics considered include intelligent e-Health systems, electronic health records, ICT-enabled personal health systems, mobile and cloud computing for e-Health, health monitoring, precision and personalized health, robotics for e-Health, security and privacy in e-Health, ambient assisted living, telemedicine, big data and IoT for e-Health, and more.

Proposals for coherently integrated international multi-authored edited or co-authored handbooks and research monographs will be considered for this book series. Each proposal will be reviewed by the book Series Editor with additional external reviews from independent reviewers.

To download our proposal form or find out more information about publishing with us, please visit https://www.theiet.org/publishing/publishing-with-iet-books/.

Please email your completed book proposal for the IET Book Series on e-Health Technologies to: Amber Thomas at athomas@theiet.org or author_support@theiet.org.

The Institution of Engineering and Technology

Smart Health Technologies for the COVID-19 Pandemic

Internet of medical things perspectives

Edited by
Chinmay Chakraborty and Joel J.P.C. Rodrigues

The Institution of Engineering and Technology

Published by The Institution of Engineering and Technology, London, United Kingdom

The Institution of Engineering and Technology is registered as a Charity in England & Wales (no. 211014) and Scotland (no. SC038698).

First published 2022

The Institution of Engineering and Technology
Michael Faraday House
Six Hills Way, Stevenage
Herts, SG1 2AY, United Kingdom

www.theiet.org

British Library Cataloguing in Publication Data
A catalogue record for this product is available from the British Library

ISBN 978-1-83953-518-5 (hardback)
ISBN 978-1-83953-519-2 (PDF)

Typeset in India by MPS Limited

Contents

About the editors

Chinmay Chakraborty, Birla Institute of Technology, India

Chinmay Chakraborty has published more than 70 conference presentations, journal papers, book chapters and books. He has served on the Editorial Boards of more than ten journals, including Future Internet Journal (Wiley), Internet Technology Letters (Springer), and Advances in Smart Healthcare Technologies (CRC Press) and the organizing committees of numerous IEEE international conferences.

Joel J.P.C. Rodrigues, College of Computer Science and Technology, China University of Petroleum (East China), Qingdao, China; Senac Faculty of Ceará, Fortaleza-CE, Brazil and Instituto de Telecomunicações, Portugal

Joel J.P.C. Rodrigues is an Highly Cited Researcher has published over 1,000 papers in refereed international journals and conferences, 3 books, 2 patents, and 1 ITU-T Recommendation. He is the editor-in-chief of the *International Journal of E-Health and Medical Communications* and an editorial board member of several high-reputed journals. He has chaired many international conferences, including IEEE ICC, IEEE GLOBECOM, IEEE HEALTHCOM, and IEEE LatinCom. He has received several Outstanding Leadership and Outstanding Service Awards by IEEE Communications Society. He is a member of the Internet Society, a senior member ACM, and a Fellow of AAIA and IEEE.

Preface

Intelligent health technologies are in the revolution phase due to recent developments in sensor technology, wearables, edge computing, the Internet of Things, and enabling wireless communication protocols, creating value-based care delivery in terms of outcome monitoring, therapeutic and preventive interventions. This book focuses the COVID-19 monitoring and analysis using intelligent e-healthcare systems. The innovative solutions might include (but are not limited to) detection and treatment methods for COVID-19, strategies to find suspected patients, contact tracing of infected patients, intelligent strategies to predict future pandemic or epidemic outbreaks, informatics-based policies to contain such mass infectious outbreaks, ensuring the safety of patients, careers, and the public, information exchange, and knowledge sharing.

This book will include reviews and original works on the COVID-19 in terms of e-healthcare, telemedicine, other medical technology, life support systems, fast detection, and diagnoses, developed technologies and innovative solutions, bioinformatics, datasets, apps for diagnosis, solutions for monitoring, and control of the spread of COVID-19, among various other topics. The book focuses on recent advances in the Internet of Medical Things in smart advanced healthcare technologies. Intelligent advanced healthcare informatics plays a vital role in this crucial time. The objective of the book is to present innovative technological solutions utilizing informatics to deal with various COVID-19 outbreak issues. This book covers comprehensive studies from healthcare informatics, biomedical engineering, artificial intelligence, big data, blockchain, and data mining with a prime focus on the COVID-19 pandemic.

At last, we would like to extend our sincere thanks to authors from industry, academia, and policy expertise to complete this work for aspiring researchers in this domain. We are confident that this book would play a key role in providing readers a comprehensive view of COVID-19 health informatics and developments around it and can be used as a learning resource for various examinations, which deal with cutting-edge technologies.

Book organisation

The book consists of 16 chapters in the field of COVID-19 healthcare systems. A summary of each chapter is presented in the following.

Chapter 1: Internet of Things (IoT) and blockchain-based solutions to confront COVID-19 pandemic

In this demanding period, the applications of the latest technologies to prevent the spread of the virus are critical. Among various technologies, the Internet of Things (IoT) and blockchain are being used in several solutions starting from contact tracing to forecasting. Blockchain-based solutions are also being used during the ongoing pandemic in various aspects for secure contact tracing, data handling, and preventing data fabrication. In this chapter, IoT and blockchain technology are discussed briefly while describing their core elements. Then, the latest solutions were presented based on these technologies in different aspects of COVID-19 pandemic prevention. These solutions mainly focus on using these technologies for remote patient monitoring, secure data handling, and telemedicine.

Chapter 2: Application of big data and computational intelligence in fighting COVID-19 epidemic

Big data is driving the digital revolution in an increasingly knowledge-driven, healthcare-innovation-driven, and connected society. The combination of computational intelligence (CI) and big data analytics (BDA) has developed methods that make accessing and processing vast amounts of data easier and less demanding on human expert. This chapter reviews the applicability and importance of big data and CI methods to data produced from the countless ubiquitously connected healthcare devices that produced entrenched and distributed information handling capabilities in fighting the COVID-19 outbreak. The use of CI in BDA has resulted in a knowledge-based system that transformed big data into big knowledge with new approaches and visions to provide people with better understanding and information-driven results.

Chapter 3: Cloud-based IoMT for early COVID-19 diagnosis and monitoring

This chapter introduces an effective scheme for the diagnosis and tracking of patients with COVID-19 based on symptoms. The concept behind the proposed approach is to use an IoT-based system to handle the real-time symptom data from patients to diagnose coronavirus cases early. The proposed framework must learn automatically about the origin of the virus by monitoring and analyzing necessary data. The health status of patients is determined in this model by predicting critical situations and examining physiological data received from smart medical IoT devices, ensuring that patients' personal information is kept private. Based on current advancements, the suggested model is thought to be suitable for delivering an appropriate remote patient monitoring model with accurate data in cloud-based IoT systems.

Chapter 4: Assessment analysis of COVID-19 on the global economics and trades

In light of the epidemic's context, this chapter gives a critical evaluation of the inventory of the pandemic's bad and positive influences in a different section. This advocates for a complete overhaul of the global economic development paradigm, which is based on a linear economy system that leverages profiteering and energy-guzzling industrial processes. The utilization of publicly accessible data, as found on Yahoo Finance, the International Monetary Fund, and John Hopkins COVID-19 map, and regression models were used to carry out the goal of this study. This study will aid those with government-level decision-making, business-stage strategic thinking, and capital-market investment to better comprehend the current state of affairs and use the model for forecasting.

Chapter 5: Early diagnosis and remote monitoring using cloud-based IoMT for COVID-19

Hence, it is essential to detect the disease at an early stage and ensure that the transmission of the virus is curbed, in turn, saving the lives of many other people. With the advancements and developments in the information technology field, it is possible to diagnose infectious diseases like the current COVID-19 pandemic at an early stage and give proper treatment to the infected. In this chapter, various IoTs that are being used to track the patients' health and provide them the necessary care and treatment even in remote locations have been discussed. Also, machine learning and deep learning for early diagnosis and remote monitoring have been discussed. An experimental case study using COVIDX dataset has been discussed along with the results. Comprehensive experiments have been carried out with varying CT sizes of CT images and an average accuracy of above 80% has been achieved.

Chapter 6: Blockchain technology for secure COVID-19 pandemic data handling

The decentralized and immutability features of blockchain have facilitated the rapid development of the beyond 5G wireless services for health-related data sharing and processing. However, the adoption of blockchain technology in medical data handling is still in its infancy, and the need for a rigorous study in this domain cannot be overemphasized. This chapter first highlights the recent developments in blockchain technology and its applications in the medical data-handling space. Further to this, the chapter examines the potential benefits, key challenges, and prospects in blockchain technology. Additionally, the chapter proposes highlighting the recent blockchain-related research efforts within the healthcare domain, especially as it relates to the dreaded COVID-19 pandemic. The chapter also discusses how blockchain would be applied to healthcare data-handling practices to build trust with automated provenance tracking and accountable credential verification. Finally, practical COVID-19 pandemic data were analyzed and presented to motivate the chapter further.

Chapter 7: Social-distancing technologies for COVID-19

Social divides have a role in illness prevention. As a result, Thailand is focusing on adopting different technologies to assist us in managing the gap and support everyone's ability to work. Adopting this technology has resulted in it being the

New Normal in use as a substitute for older systems. This chapter offers a template analysis of stakeholder interviews conducted with the aid of technology to accomplish social distancing, which is divided into three categories: educational, public health, and social distancing, as well as manufacturing employees. A software usage pattern has been developed due to data analysis utilizing content analysis to help create social distancing for job planning and everyday use. It can also be used to plan future smart cities.

Chapter 8: Social health protection in touristic destinations during COVID-19

This chapter gives a proposal for a software solution that would significantly improve the control and registration of infected persons. The straightforward use of the proposed software solution aims to prevent the spread of the virus by tourists. The proposed software system should enable better control of COVID-19 positive individuals, while on the other hand should support the improvement of traveling conditions and allow the tourism sector to work for people who are not virus-positive. The system will allow us to check vaccination or home isolation status of individuals, and based on the results, approve or deny reservations. The edge/cloud architecture will provide data availability, and at the same time data access control.

Chapter 9: Analysis of Artificial Intelligence and Internet of Things in biomedical imaging and sequential data for COVID-19

In this chapter, the authors surveyed various array-based sequence data analyses and biomedical imaging along with their integrated studies for different tissue-specific dreadful diseases (such as cancer). The integrated studies of biomedical imaging and array-based data analysis for the same set of patients (samples) has been discussed that covered the problem of combinatorial gene signature detection as well as disease subtype image classifications while specific multimodal data from a well-known data repository (e.g., TCGA, ICGC) had been provided. This chapter covers the maximum area of biomedical imaging as well as array-based sequence data analysis along with the contribution of AI and ML to build a smart healthcare system and provide a new dimension to the interested biomedical researchers.

Chapter 10: Review of medical imaging with machine learning and deep learning-based approaches for COVID-19

Early detection of COVID-19 is inevitable as it helps in seeking early medical intervention and to minimize community spread. COVID-19 can be diagnosed with the help of gold standard RT-PCR tests, quick antigen and antibody tests supplemented with CT scan, and X-ray imaging. Considering the increase in the number of cases worldwide, there is a need for economical and viable ways to detect COVID-19. Medical imaging and analytic tools that use machine learning and deep learning algorithms can enhance the diagnosis and prediction of COVID-19. There are many effective and proven image recognition techniques in deep learning like Convolutional Neural networks and Transfer learning that can be used to design very promising applications for COVID-19 detection. They enhance these models using advanced image segmentation and edge detection techniques. The authors have been reviewed the impact of the COVID-19 pandemic on the global community, the need for reliable, quick, and economical ways to detect it.

Chapter 11: Machine-based drug design to inhibit SARS-CoV-2 virus

Due to the lack of animal and human trials data, the process is still complicating and causing more death worldwide. The keen analysis of the amino acid sequences in the coronavirus-19 infection-causing proteins will give very important information about the virus transformation and replication cycle. The amino acid sequences and their active sites provided in the 3D crystalline structure of M-pro (PDB ID; 6LU7) afford valuable data to the researchers about the type of inhibitors that corresponds to the severe acute respiratory syndrome (SARS)-coronavirus-2 (SARS-CoV-2) inhibition. Compared to all other deadly viruses like flu, HIV, and SARS, novel coronavirus SARS-CoV-2 shows superior binding affinity over a human transmembrane protein christened angiotensin-converting enzyme 2, found in human lungs. Since the coronavirusid-19 infection spread more vigorously, the traditional RT-PCR test will need more time for infection confirmation, so machine-based imaging studies like MRI, CT, and X-ray are needed.

Chapter 12: Stress detection for cognitive rehabilitation in COVID-19 scenario

This chapter highlights the mobile phone exposure to people increased at least 2-fold way, so games have been used as stimuli for detecting how our brain becomes overburdened with increased exposure. After the data acquisition from 14 channels of an electroencephalogram, the activated regions were identified. Features were extracted from the most activated ten electrode channels using discrete wavelet transform. To reduce the dimensions of the feature space for enhancing the performance, principal component analysis was used. The mental state classification was performed using a support vector machine based on the detected stress. The proposed system has outperformed the existing ones for its effectiveness and efficiency in a broad application area of cognitive rehabilitation. Classification accuracy was obtained as 92.79% and different other metrics proved that the combination of channel selection, feature extraction, and classification methods in our proposed approach has outperformed the others.

Chapter 13: Arduino-based robot for purification of COVID-19 using far UVC light

The proposed work elaborates on the necessity of sterilization, especially during the COVID-19 period. In this chapter, we will discuss the development and construction of an "Arduino-based robot for the purification of COVID-19 using far

UVC light". The objective of the current work is to discuss various inventions made during the pandemic scenario and to contribute to the battle against COVID-19 propagation. Authors have developed a UV-based sterilization method that uses single-wavelength far-UVC light produced by filtered exclaims to selectively inactivate microorganisms while causing no biological damage to exposed cells and tissues. The robot can also be used as a vacuum cleaner, eliminating the need for and expense of cleaning by humans.

Chapter 14: Effect of COVID-19 pandemic on waste management system and infection control

Personal protective equipment has become a very vital element to guard against exposure of any infectious materials. It is usually used in healthcare or hospital settings during any outbreak. These enormous challenges are with all stakeholders for avoiding spread through waste. Among all the issues created by COVID-19, the problem that will create a major mess is, not handling biomedical waste properly. If the spreading needs to be controlled, it requires strict monitoring of the complete cycle starting from the point of generation. However, due to the invaluable service of the waste management sector only, it is possible to avoid the spread of the COVID-19 and to ensure that the weird tons of waste will not be gathered, which increases health risks and the spread of disease.

Chapter 15: Natural adjunctive therapies options other than COVID-19 antiviral therapies

The COVID-19 pandemic is the largest health problem worldwide. Unfortunately, the lack of an effective and clear treatment causes it to be a major health problem. There are currently no effective antiviral drugs or vaccines. The symptoms and course of the disease differ individually. Most of these nutrients also have been demonstrated to be useful in the treatment of COVID-19. The importance of such dietary elements in immunity and their particular consequences in COVID-19 patients are discussed in this review.

Chapter 16: Risk assessment and spread of COVID-19

The word risk assessment refers to the procedure of identifying, evaluating the factors that cause harm to the environment and living beings. It also involves making decisions on how to put an end to it. This chapter discussed the steps taken to assess the risk and stop the spread of pandemics like COVID-19. Prevention is always better than cure. The chapter presented an analysis of prevention using prediction techniques. Using sentiment analysis in machine learning, weighted density ensembles, forecasting models, and risk assessment can be done. Further, a bot named SAUCHA is proposed for automatic sanitization.

Chinmay Chakraborty
Joel J.P.C. Rodrigues

Chapter 1

Internet of Things (IoT) and blockchain-based solutions to confront COVID-19 pandemic

Abu Hasnat Md Rhydwan[1], Md Mashrur Sakib Choyon[1], A.S.M. Mehedi Hasan Sad[1], Kazi Ahmed Asif Fuad[1], Kawshik Shikder[1], Chowdhury Akram Hossain[1] and M. Shamim Kaiser[2]

Abstract

COVID-19 pandemic, an unprecedented event that has severely affected every aspect of human civilization. From the beginning of the pandemic, the contagious nature of this virus resulted in its rapid transmission throughout the world. As a result, worldwide health organizations and governments are facing tremendous pressure to deal with the affected populations. In this demanding period, the applications of the latest technologies to prevent the spread of the virus are critical. Among various technologies, the Internet of Things (IoT) and blockchain are being used in several solutions starting from contact tracing to forecasting. The use of IoT technologies has proved to be highly effective in such a state of the pandemic. Conducting real-time health monitoring on patients or suspected cases of COVID-19, tracking medications, detecting any new suspected cases, diagnosing patients from a distance, etc. have become exclusively possible with the use of IoT technologies in this COVID-19 pandemic. On the other hand, the blockchain technology that became popular with the increase of different cryptocurrencies has seen its applications almost everywhere. The technology uses a decentralized system instead of a single point of contact, proving to be more secure than existing solutions. Blockchain-based solutions are also being used during the ongoing pandemic in various aspects for secure contact tracing, data handling, and preventing data fabrication. In this chapter, IoT and blockchain technology are discussed briefly while describing their core elements. Then, the latest solutions were presented based on these technologies in different aspects of COVID-19 pandemic prevention. These solutions mainly focus on using these technologies for remote patient

[1]Department of Electrical and Electronic Engineering, American International University-Bangladesh, Dhaka, Bangladesh

[2]Institute of Information Technology, Jahangirnagar University, Savar, Dhaka, Bangladesh

monitoring, secure data handling, and telemedicine. Finally, challenges of using these technologies were discussed, and possible solutions were recommended to improve their efficacy in the future.

Keywords: COVID-19; IoT; Blockchain; Contact tracing; Telemedicine; Smart Healthcare; Smart system; Health monitoring

1.1 Introduction

"Coronavirus Disease 2019" that is mostly known as "COVID-19" is mainly a highly infectious disease caused by the SARS-CoV-2 virus, otherwise known as the coronavirus. This virus infects the respiratory system in the human body. The common symptoms of the disease are cold, fever, fatigue, dry coughs, headache, loss of appetite, smell, etc. There are also some cases found where the infected human body showed no symptoms while some others showed severe symptoms like high fever, shortness of breath, difficulties in breathing, pneumonia, etc. The virus has spread so rapidly toward the end of 2019 throughout the whole world that the World Health Organization (WHO) had declared it a "pandemic" [1]. Until the first week of May 2021, the disease has infected over 153,738,171 people throughout the whole world while claiming the lives of 3,217,281 people [2]. Modern technologies throughout the entire world have given a chance to confront the infectious disease. The rapid spread of the disease required the development and use of technological resources at a dire speed. The advanced technologies have given healthcare professionals and patients a great advantage to confront this sudden pandemic situation.

Among many advanced technologies, the Internet of Things (IoT) and the blockchain technologies have provided some of the fascinating features that marked significant contributions in the health sector and fought against COVID-19. Maintaining physical distance is a crucial aspect of treating a COVID-19 patient; it has become rather difficult for healthcare professionals to provide service to the patients in such a situation. However, IoT technologies have enabled health monitoring systems to provide service to the patients remotely, detect possible cases, deliver logistics, disinfect areas, and carry out telemedicine services for patients [3]. The IoT technologies enable a continuous interaction between devices and physical surroundings or any subject. Among many operations, healthcare service, public safety monitoring, and environmental monitoring are some of the commonly used areas where IoT technologies are leaving huge impacts. Amidst the COVID-19 pandemic, the IoT technologies significantly impact the healthcare service by maintaining medical data, patients' history, patients monitoring, emergency response, and telemedicine service. Because of the rapid and devastating spread of COVID-19 worldwide, countries and their economic activities have remarkably ceased. However, IoT technologies can play a crucial part in mitigating a large portion of these issues by helping carrying out these activities while minimizing the spread of the virus.

On the other hand, due to the increasing pressure because of the ongoing pandemic, healthcare system of many countries faced catastrophe. The number of diagnoses of other diseases was significantly reduced [4]. Data management in hospitals and federal repositories has faced unforeseen situations and tremendous risks of data breaching. As a result, a new challenge has arrived to ensure the privacy of the database in the healthcare sector. Blockchain technology can provide significant advantages in this aspect and can maintain privacy in the healthcare sector, especially when combined with IoT [5]. This technology is being used to increase medical system security and ensure feasible data sharing [6]. It has also seen its application in electronic medical records (EMRs), pharmaceutical supply chain, and health insurance claim [7]. In addition to that, blockchain-based solutions are also effective against other recent issues by maintaining the efficacy of contact tracing, data sharing, Internet of Medical Things (IoMT), and preventing data breaching [8].

In this chapter, different aspects of IoT and blockchain technologies that are being used throughout the world to confront COVID-19 were discussed briefly. The chapter gives an overall idea of how these technologies are making significant contributions in this pandemic by facilitating in different sectors like healthcare, telemedicine, logistics delivery, surveillance, data management, data privacy, supply chain, securing database, etc. Multiple recent works have also reviewed the application of these technologies in different aspects of COVID-19 [9–13]. However, these works have focused on a single technology and excluded some latest applications that simultaneously use both technologies. Hence, it is necessary to survey applications of both IoT and blockchain technology, and through this chapter, we tried to cover the existing research gap. Key contributions of this chapter are as follows:

- We provided an overview of the main components of IoT and blockchain technology.
- We reviewed the latest IoT and blockchain-based solutions that can be effective against the COVID-19 and future pandemic scenarios.
- We discussed the significant limitations and challenges of IoT and blockchain technology and provided deliverables to solve these issues to ensure their efficient usage.

The rest of this chapter is organized as follows: Section 1.2 contains the description of these two technologies and their components. Then, Sections 1.3 and 1.4 describe various latest developments of IoT and blockchain-based technology to reduce the effect of the COVID-19. Then, Section 1.5 addresses various issues of these technologies, discusses their solutions, and provides recommendations for their effective implementation. Section 1.6 summarizes the significant findings of the survey, and finally, Section 1.7 summarizes this study and addresses the future development of these technologies.

1.2 Internet of Things (IoT) and blockchain overview

This section contains an overview of IoT and blockchain technology.

1.2.1 Internet of Things

The IoT has brought significant advancement in the technological sectors and engineering throughout the entire world. The IoT is mainly a network of different embedded entities or objects such as sensors, devices, and databases, and all these are connected through the Internet. IoT applications basically consist of three crucial steps. These are data collection, data transmission, and data management. At the first step, the data is collected by the IoT devices from the targeted environment or subject utilizing any sensors or devices. Later, these data are transmitted to other devices, computational units, or data-processing units. Finally, these data are sorted for thorough analysis, management, extracting meaning or value, making predictions and decisions. The IoT has enabled access to low-cost technologies, more effortless connectivity of different entities through the Internet, access through cloud computing platforms, and push the boundaries with machine learning and analytics along with artificial intelligence applications [14]. IoT applications are being explored and deployed in numerous sectors (e.g., enterprises, industries, healthcare, retails, governments) [15,16]. Therefore, IoT plays a tremendous role in developing smart cities, smart grids, smart healthcare, smart homes, etc. An estimation suggests that by the year 2025, the number of IoT connections will cross over 75 billion worldwide [17]. That means the total number of IoT-connected devices would be more than six times that of the total world population of humankind. Due to the sudden surge of COVID-19 infections, maintaining physical distance among humans has become crucial [18]. As a result, the usual flow of many sectors like healthcare, business, deliveries has become challenging to maintain. However, IoT applications have given a great chance to mitigate such issues and offer faster solutions to these sectors. One of the most highly benefited sectors by IoT is the healthcare sector. The IoMT is also playing an important role in the healthcare sector in the COVID-19 pandemic [19–21]. Researchers worldwide have given great effort to work on different projects and applications to confront the COVID-19 [22–24]. In addition, many tech companies also made significant contributions in manufacturing some of the advanced technologies to confront the coronavirus pandemic. As a result, there has been a significant growth of technological applications in both research sectors and industrial sectors to confront the COVID-19 pandemic.

1.2.1.1 Major IoT components

This section will provide an overview of the different vital components of IoT. Figure 1.1 shows the summary of these components.

Things or devices: The most primary requirement for the implementation of any IoT application is the devices. Every IoT application has its physical entity, and necessary devices or sensors consist of that entity. The devices continuously collect the data from the environment or any subject and transfer those data to the next layer or gateway [14]. IoT applications' device entities may consist of various sensors ranging from micro smart sensors to large industrial machinery.

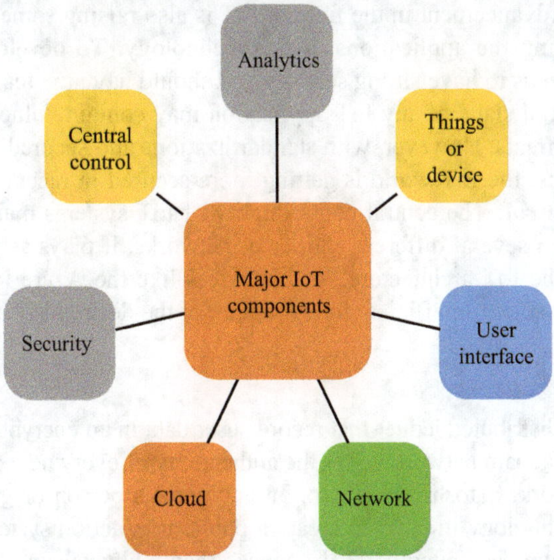

Figure 1.1 Components of IoT

User interface: The user interface or UI is the visible entity of an IoT application that the users see and provide actions or commands to the application. In recent times, most IoT applications consist of well-designed UIs that are attractive and user-friendly. Any IoT-based UI design must have proper hardware constraints along with the software design. In their work, Toyama and Hirayama presented some rules and methods in designing such UI for IoT systems [25].

Cloud: The IoT cloud entity is a high-performing sophisticated network of servers that receives and sends data between the device end and the user end. The cloud entity is also responsible for preserving data and conducting accurate data analysis. The cloud also processes the machine learning algorithms and other user commands or programs. The advanced and highly distributed cloud network architecture of IoT applications facilitates promising aspects to design, host, manage, and optimize more futuristic IoT applications with less power consumption and more security [26].

Analytics: In IoT applications, analytics play a crucial role in managing and improving the entire system architecture. Upon receiving analog data from the device end, the analytics entity carries out a thorough interpretation, analysis and provides possible solutions based on the analysis to improve the system. Real-time intelligent analytics allow system designers or engineers to find any irregularities and prevent them [27].

Network: Any IoT application must be connected to a good network or Internet. The device end is controlled by the Internet and maintains the overall communications between all entities of the system architecture. To develop a smart city with different IoT applications, it is vital to establish a secure and robust network platform for these applications to rely on [28].

Security: Advancement in the field of IoT is also raising some severe security concerns regarding the applications of this technology. To develop any efficient IoT system, it needs to have strong security and should have the feature to maintain privacy. The initial stage of any IoT application may contain vulnerabilities to fall prone to cyber threats. However, with standardizations and secured development of these applications, the IoT world is getting more secured in recent times [29–31].

Central control: The central control entity of IoT systems maintains two-way data traffic within several different entities or networks. It plays as the central controlling unit in the IoT architecture. With services like the Azure IoT Central, any developer can establish an efficient infrastructure of the desired IoT application [32].

1.2.2 Blockchain

Blockchain is a distributed ledger that records user data in an encrypted manner [33]. Peers of the blockchain network verify the authenticity of every new block within the blockchain network. Satoshi Nakamoto, an anonymous person or group of people, invented this technology in 2008 to create a public transaction system for the cryptocurrency known as bitcoin [34]. Since then, blockchain has become a trustable solution for digital transactions due to its decentralized structure and immutability [35]. Apart from cryptocurrency transactions, blockchain has been widely used in other applications, including energy trading, healthcare, supply chain, and video games, as shown in Figure 1.2. The continuous growth of blockchain use cases can be observed from a recent report that shows that the worldwide blockchain market is likely to reach USD 39.7 billion by 2025 from USD 3.0 billion in 2020 [36].

1.2.2.1 Blockchain components

This section will give a brief idea about different parts of blockchain technology.

Block: Every blockchain network contains numerous blocks chained next to one another. Each of these blocks includes similar components: block header, timestamp, Merkle root hash, nonce, previous block hash. These blocks are immutable, and new blocks require permission from previous blocks within the blockchain [37]. Thereby, attackers cannot easily add their block to the blockchain without authorization from others. As shown in Figure 1.3, the blocks are stacked on top of each other and grow like a chain until the final block is added [37]. The initial block of this chain is known as the "genesis block."

Hash algorithm: A function that transforms an input of any length into an encrypted output of a fixed length using a mathematical function is known as the hash function [38]. This ensures that security as decrypting fixed-length output without knowing the input length is a complex and time-consuming operation.

Header: A block header is used to identify a particular block on an entire blockchain. Every block has a unique header, and they are used for documentation and efficient task recording. They contain three separate sets of block metadata, including version number, previous block hash, Merkle root, timestamp, and difficulty target. Information like previous block hash and Merkle root are used to navigate specific bytes within the blockchain easily.

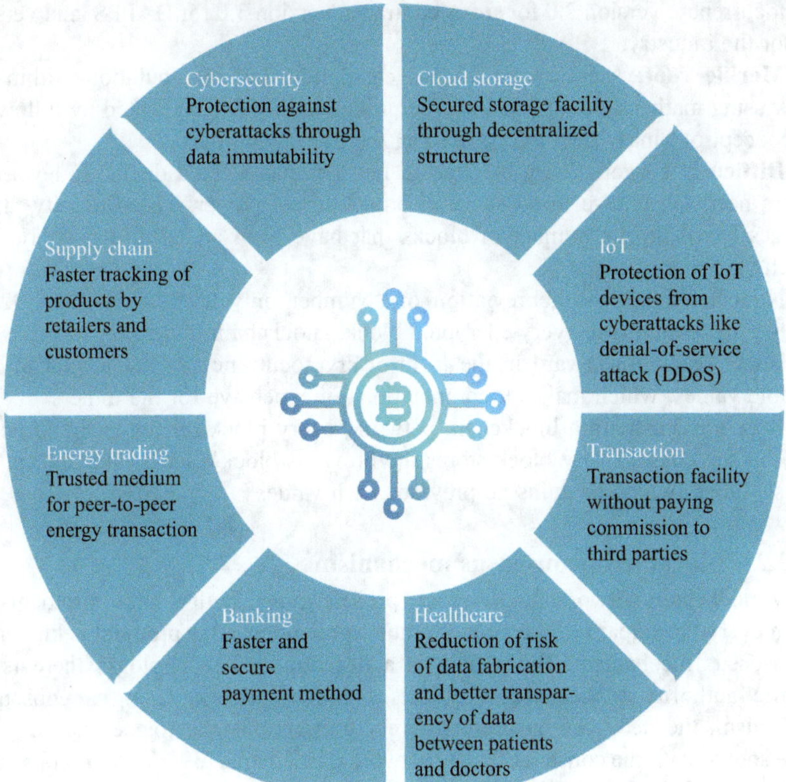

Figure 1.2 Current applications of blockchain technology

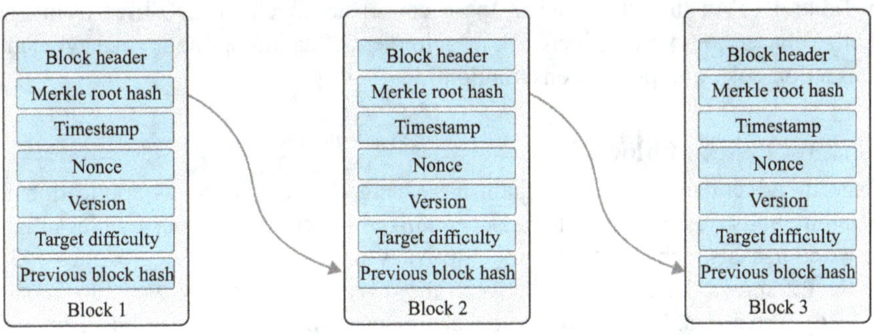

Figure 1.3 Blockchain structure

Timestamp: Timestamp is used to prove the approval time of a block. It also helps block authentication.

Version: The version number helps to track the changes throughout the protocol. There are various versions based on their applications. Version 1.0 is used for cryptocurrency, version 2.0 for smart contracts, version 3.0 for DAPPS, and version 4.0 for the industry.

Merkle root: Merkle root checks corruption and manipulation within the block using mathematical formulas. The unique hash value is created by following the concept of binary tree and combining the transaction data.

Difficulty target: Every blockchain network has a fixed difficulty level that miners need to achieve through their computational power. The difficulty target changes based on the number of blocks that have been added to a network in a specific amount of time.

Nonce: Nonce, the abbreviation of "Number only used once," is a 32-bit number that contains in every encrypted block. Blockchain miners try to solve this number to receive a reward in the form of cryptocurrency. It has a total of 232 possible values, which makes it computationally expensive for the miners.

Previous hash: In a blockchain network, every block relates to the previous block of the chain. Every block stores the previous block's hash value except the genesis block, which contains no previous hash value.

1.2.2.2 Blockchain consensus mechanism

Every blockchain network follows some predetermined fault-tolerant protocols, to which every participant of the network must agree upon. This protocol is known as a consensus mechanism. Blockchain is a decentralized technology; there is no specific authority to set necessary acts for the network. Using a consensus mechanism, the networks ensure that every transaction takes place from a legitimate source with the consent of other network participants [39]. Various consensus mechanisms have been emerged in recent times based on the application of blockchain networks. Among these, proof of work (PoW), proof of stake (PoS), delegated proof of stake (DPoS), practical byzantine fault tolerance (PBFT), and ripple are being used the most. A comparison between these mechanisms is shown in Table 1.1. As the table shows, these consensus mechanisms differ from one another based on various network requirements, including node management, transaction cost, and power consumption [38,40–42].

1.2.2.3 Types of blockchain

Since its advent in 2008, blockchain has changed a lot due to its application in different industries. As a result, the decentralized structure of the earlier blockchain network has also changed into more privacy-preserving and secure ones [43]. Table 1.2 shows the difference between three types of primarily used blockchain [43–46]. Private and consortium blockchain seems more viable for business purposes due to factors like transaction speed, privacy, and ownership. However, these two blockchain deviates from the fundamental quality that makes blockchain special—decentralization. But they also eliminate the scalability, power, and transaction issues of the public blockchain network. A hybrid between public and private blockchain, which is known as a consortium or federated blockchain, can offer the perfect spot by offering the benefits of both of them [46].

Table 1.1 Comparison between various blockchain consensus mechanisms

Property	PoW	PoS	DPoS	PBFT	Ripple
Node management	Open	Both	Open	Permissioned	Open
Transaction rate	Low	High	Medium	High	High
Power consumption	Large	Less	Less	Negligible	Negligible
Scalability	Good	Good	Good	Bad	Good
Storage consumption	High	High	Medium	High	Medium
Transaction cost	High	High	Medium	Low	Low
Adversary tolerated power	≤25% of computational power	<51% of stake	<51% faulty replicas	<33% Voting power	<20% of defective nodes
Application	Public	Public	Public	Permissioned	Permissioned

Table 1.2 Difference between various types of blockchain

Property	Blockchain type		
	Public	**Private**	**Consortium**
Network	Decentralized	Partially decentralized	Hybrid
Privacy	Open	Permissioned	Permissioned
Ownership	Open	Single entity	Multiple entities
Consensus mechanism	PoS/PoW	Voting	Voting
Transaction speed	Slow	Fast	Fast
Decentralization	Completely decentralized	Less decentralized	Less decentralized

1.3 IoT technologies to confront COVID-19

In recent times, applications developed with IoT and IoMT technologies have become significantly popular among many sectors, and security measures like the blockchain, edge computing, and fog computing, available for these applications make them more efficient [39]. The rapid developments made in the IoMT have made healthcare professionals realize the sector's vast potential [47]. Figure 1.4 shows the summary of IoT-based solutions in different sectors against the COVID-19 pandemic. As shown in Figure 1.4, IoT technologies have given great advantages in several sectors to confront the COVID-19 pandemic.

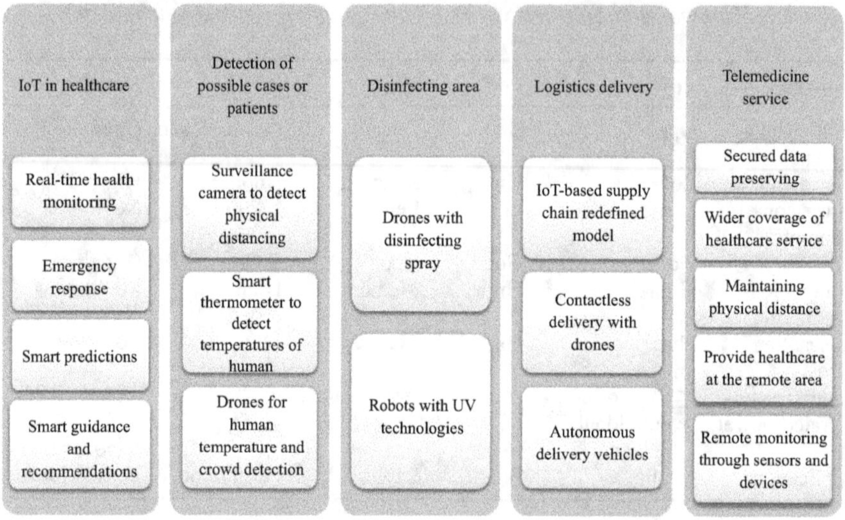

Figure 1.4 IoT solutions in various aspects of COVID-19

1.3.1 Health monitoring systems

IoT-based technologies and other technologies related to IoT have proven to be significantly helpful and efficient in the battle against the COVID-19 pandemic. These technologies can provide real-time health monitoring data, physical exercise checks, blood pressure, disease condition, and many other data of the human body that prove to be extremely valuable in fighting the coronavirus [48]. The use of IoT has increased the smartness of healthcare by efficiently collecting data from numerous sources. This has resulted in prompt and more accurate health monitoring and can also be beneficial for COVID-19 monitoring [49]. An operating system for information kiosks was developed in [50] that can monitor users' health in real time by using different sensors and presenting those data on the kiosk screen, which can be beneficial for crowded locations. Choyon *et al.* developed an IoT-based health monitoring system that combines real-time monitoring facilities through hardware and COVID-19 prediction programs through a machine learning algorithm [51]. The researchers developed the hardware device with a Raspberry Pi microcontroller, Arduino Uno, and other necessary sensors to monitor patient's health. On the other hand, the machine learning algorithm carries out its analysis on a cloud-based server where the data collected from the device is sent and stored. The system can predict the possibility of coronavirus present in a patient's body by analyzing the collected data from the symptoms. The developed device can also deliver guidance from healthcare professionals to monitor the state of a patient's health from a distance. In addition, in an emergency, the response team can quickly take actions based on the data provided by the device and mitigate the damage.

Other wearable devices like Fitbit or Apple Watch used for regular health fitness tracking have also shown some promising features that could be used to sense early signs of COVID-19 symptoms [52]. Similarly, another successful gadget that made an essential contribution against COVID-19 is the WHOOP strap. A study was conducted with the WHOOP strap on 271 people between the age of 25–50 years. All these people experienced symptoms like that of SARS-CoV-2, but 81 individuals were tested positive for the virus in later days. The study consisted of building a dataset collected by the WHOOP strap and training a novel algorithm using those data. Later, the developed model monitored the raspatory rate of the individuals and successfully detected 20% of the people 2 days before the symptom commencement and 80% of the people on the third day [53].

In another work in [54], an IoMT system was developed that utilizes deep learning for identifying different types of health-related issues caused by COVID-19. The system generates reports based on the analysis that can be used for medical care. Bai *et al.* researched the IoT-based nCapp technology to diagnose COVID-19 at an earlier stage [55]. Based on the collected data, the diagnosis automatically labels the patient's case as confirmed, suspected, or suspicious of the coronavirus infection. The nCapp intelligent assisted management can play a crucial role in treating the infected patients through various instructions based on data analysis collected from the patient's body. A health monitoring model was developed based on the Business Process Management paradigm, where the main focus was to increase the empowerment of the patients and healthcare professionals [56]. The architecture of the model was developed with the help of health monitoring devices and environmental sensors. Together with the connection of the web system, an efficient IoT technology was developed for the model that could fulfill the purpose. The patients could monitor their state of health and contribute to their health routine by deciding what to do and when to do it. Lomotey *et al.* developed a "Petri Nets" service model that focuses on wearable IoT-based device data management [57]. The proposed model by the authors has resulted in high scalability of the IoT architecture, transparency of medical IoT data, and distributed health information system threats. In [58], an IoT-based smart system was developed for monitoring the health of patients. The patients can use the system through a mobile application, and it gives the patients the freedom to monitor their health from home by themselves and also enables them to send necessary health reports to the doctors through the system. Furthermore, the doctors can provide necessary health guidance to the patients through the system as well. The system was proven to be quite helpful for elderly people or people living independently at home. In [59], an IoT-based health monitoring system was developed utilizing three core parts: IoT node, mobile app, and machine learning tools. The developed system also utilizes a radio frequency method to alert the user to maintain physical distance in both indoor and outdoor environments. In another work, Li *et al.* designed a health monitoring system that could analyze the breathing sound in real-time and detect any wheeze in the breathing [60]. As the lungs are one of the most commonly affected parts of the human body due to the coronavirus, such a system could prove highly useful for healthcare professionals in detecting any blockage created in the lungs by the virus.

In another work, de Morais Barroca Filho *et al.* proposed an efficient IoT-based healthcare platform where patients in critical conditions can be monitored remotely [61]. The researchers, in this case, utilized wearable and unobtrusive sensors to monitor patients in ICUs.

1.3.2 Tracking and detecting possible patients

IoT-based smart thermometer developed by a health technology company called Kinsa from the United States has a significant advantage in detecting people with high body temperature [62]. The service can be used on a massive scale and detect potential hotspots of COVID-19 affected areas. In terms of COVID-19 surveillance, various advanced methods are now being used in different parts of the world. In [63], a novel IoT-based occupancy system was developed that enables the facility to detect the level of occupancy in any area such as buildings, public space, classroom, office room, and transportations. The developed system is also secured with the blockchain while containing a decentralized traceability. The developed system does not record any unauthorized personal data, and therefore it is also proven to be secured while maintaining privacy. In China, drones called "MicroMultiCopter," manufactured by the Shenzhen company, carry out surveillance to detect any crowds, detect body temperature, ensure mask-wearing by the civilians, etc. In addition, drones are also being used for contactless products or medicine delivery in various places [64]. In Madrid of Spain, drones are also being used for delivering important COVID-19-related guidelines or emergency announcements to the citizens from the authority [65]. In Australia, the University of South Australia developed an advanced drone associated with a Canadian company called Dragonfly Inc. The drone could carry out surveillance on a large area while detecting humans with infectious diseases. The drone could detect the temperature of the human body and use image processing to detect heart rate [65]. Since maintaining the physical distance from one person to another is vital in fighting against COVID-19, the IoT technologies with the combination of computer vision (OpenCV) and deep learning can be of great help to law enforcement agencies in maintaining it [66]. The surveillance camera placed around the corner of streets can monitor the movement of the people and thus detect whether people are maintaining or violating physical distance among them during the COVID-19 pandemic. As per the developed algorithm, the system detects those who maintain a safe physical distance from others and mark them with an identifying-colored box on the footage (e.g., green box). On the other hand, those who do not maintain a safe physical distance are marked with another colored box on the footage (e.g., red box). The local law enforcement agency gets notified of the activity as well to take specific measures if required.

In another work, Abdulrazaq *et al.* developed an IoT-based novel smart helmet that could detect possible COVID-19-affected people from the thermal image taken by the camera mounted with the helmet [67]. The device has a great promise to be fruitful in detecting suspected cases in the public or hospitals. The device detects any suspected case with higher body temperature, and it sends a notification to the paired mobile, any other device, or database with the captured face image and GPS location. Based on the received information, the healthcare professionals or any other concerned party can take necessary actions. Similarly, IoT-based smart glasses were developed to fulfill the same purpose [68]. In [69], the researchers aimed to design an IoT-based global platform to confront COVID-19 through monitoring and tracking the suspected cases. The system utilizes a virtual IoT node to determine the suspected cases. The system was also designed to ensure the privacy and authenticity of information providers. The information providers are given with individual secret keys to ensure the authenticity and privacy of data. Garg *et al.* reviewed different contact tracing models, and later on, they presented a novel contact tracing model that proved to be scalable and can also maintain the patient's privacy [70]. The developed model utilizes IoT and blockchain technologies that can maintain a greater efficiency in contact tracing of COVID-19 cases while also considering moving objects with the help of RFID transceivers. In [71], a privacy-preserving IoT model was presented that can efficiently identify a large number of infection contacts while preserving the individual's privacy with the help of blockchain. In another work, Tedeschi *et al.* developed IoT-based contact tracing architecture that could preserve privacy while being configured to support several models ranging from centralized to decentralized [72]. Furthermore, to impose strict lockdown on any COVID-19 hotspot area, an IoT-based three-layered decentralized biometric face detection framework was designed in [73], where the authors built a deep learning framework. The framework showed significantly better results when compared with other existing state-of-the-art architecture.

1.3.3 Disinfecting area

IoT-based robots are also proving to be quite helpful during the COVID-19 pandemic. Robots are deployed in many advanced countries to disinfect areas, detect affected patients, carry out contactless delivery, and other diagnosis or screening purposes. The new generation robots of macro- to microscale also enable more significant advantages to navigate or sterilize high-risk areas [74]. A USA-based company called Xenex manufactures Germ-Zapping robots that use UV lights to destroy any kinds of germs quite efficiently [75]. The company has reported attaining colossal success and demand in various countries worldwide like Italy, Singapore, Japan, and South Korea to fight against coronavirus. Another robotic company from Denmark called the UVD Robots had developed a highly effective remote-controlled robot that uses powerful UV light to disinfect the surface. The UV light focuses on destroying the DNA of the viruses or bacteria directly. Each robot advances 3 m every minute while disinfecting the area with the UV. The company has already produced robots in many hospitals in different parts of the world like Asia, Europe, and the United States [76]. Furthermore, drones enable quite an advantage in disinfecting any public area as well. China, Indonesia, Chile, Spain, and many other European countries use drones to disinfect public areas amidst coronavirus pandemic [77].

1.3.4 Telemedicine

The telemedicine service has seen a significant surge in usage throughout the world, especially in this COVID-19 pandemic. The demand for medical counseling has been higher than before while maintaining social distance was an essential condition to abide by. In such a circumstance, telemedicine service proves to be a great help in delivering medical services to the patients to a certain extent. The doctors or healthcare professionals provide their expert guidance to the patients through telemedicine service through telecommunications equipment with the minimum facility of audio and video [78]. In some cases, necessary sensors or biomedical devices that can collect patients' biological data are also installed [79]. As a result, the demand for telemedicine services has gone up significantly in the COVID-19 pandemic [80]. The healthcare professionals could examine the patients' data from their mobiles or desktops and provide necessary instructions to the patients or medical staff taking care of the patient [81]. With the help of telemedicine service, the massive pressure of providing medical service by the hospital staff got lifted, along with the risk of coronavirus emanation was reduced. In the United States, the George Washington University hospital and Rush University Medical Center utilized telemedicine services to provide medical consultation to their patients during the pandemic [82,83]. These hospitals arranged one-to-one video calls and webinars to provide medical consultations. The German-made WAS vehicles are equipped with advanced IoT technologies that can enable medical staff to monitor a patient's health remotely [84]. Therefore, the emergency vehicle can provide healthcare support even on the move to the hospital. The 5G technologies combined with IoT and other related technologies can also influence carrying out swift telemedicine service [85,86]. Such a highly advanced technology could perform critical actions like surgeries on patients through robotic devices while being controlled by the doctors remotely.

1.3.5 Logistics delivery

The use of autonomous vehicles has also been quite promising in logistics delivery without the risk of human exposure to the coronavirus [87]. These autonomous vehicles have been quite successful after being deployed in several parts of the United States and China. Končar *et al.* analyzed the setbacks of digitalized business processes and the fast-moving consumer goods supply chain based on IoT technologies [88]. The authors carried out the research during the COVID-19 pandemic and identified some of the lackings that usually occur due to human errors or capabilities. The authors proposed that the traditional business models and supply chain should be changed with the help of intelligent systems and IoT technologies to regain stability, especially during a pandemic like COVID-19.

1.4 Blockchain technologies to confront COVID-19

Blockchain-based technologies are being used everywhere to improve the current technologies of pandemic handling. Most of these applications are related to security improvement, which is a massive issue in the current scenario. Figure 1.5

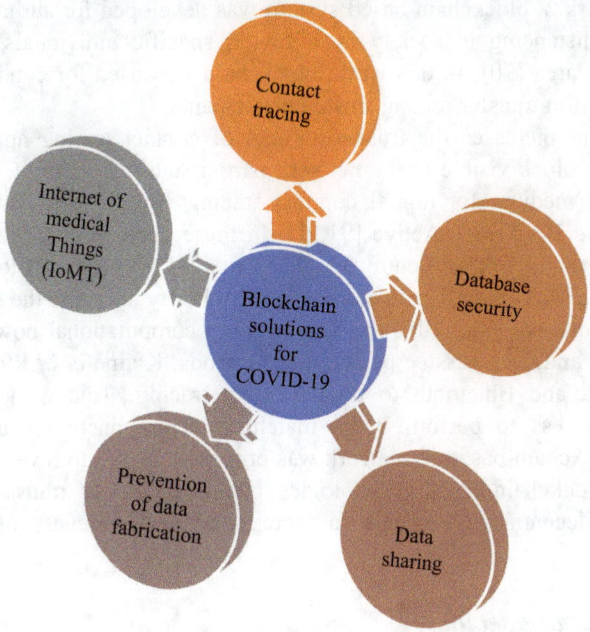

Figure 1.5 Use of blockchain technologies in various perspectives of COVID-19

shows different perspectives of blockchain-based solutions against COVID-19. This section will highlight the recent developments in these sectors.

1.4.1 Contact tracing

From the initial stage of the COVID-19 pandemic, the governments of different countries depended on contact tracing to reduce the spread of the virus. However, some obstacles are reducing the efficiency of this method: (1) patient information stored in centralized databases is prone to tampering. (2) Existing infection tracing systems consisting of location-based contact tracing and individual contact tracing cannot track infections from different dimensions [89]. While location-based tracking provides information within a given area without information on the movement of the infection, individual tracing focuses on person-to-person tracking without any data on the area where the infection takes place. To solve these issues, third-party servers are required to check contact and sending alerts. Furthermore, in [90], a contact information and risk notification sharing system was designed using smart contracts and Bluetooth that can eradicate this issue by recording the visited location of the users and providing the option to update their infection status. The system can also update infection status and estimate the probability of being infected based on the user's visited places. In another contract tracing solution, a public blockchain network is used as a distributed public ledger to allow the user to securely register, upload and query their contact list in the blockchain network [69].

In another work, a blockchain-based system was developed for authorities to promote social distancing in society by allowing specific individuals to visit any location in an area [70]. In this work, blockchain was used for conducting privileged information transfer among trusted participants.

Blockchain increases the trustworthiness of contact tracing applications by keeping every block visible to the network participants. As a result, it has turned into a trusted medium for digital contract tracings (DCT) applications such as BeepTrace and BeepTrace-Active [91,92]. In these applications, blockchain was used as the primary infrastructure for DCT. In [91], the use of blockchain was proposed to work as a bridge between user and authority to secure the user's ID and location information. While this application faces computational power and complexity issues and uses passive positioning methods, Klaine *et al.* [92] used geographical data and Bluetooth to track contact tracing. This work also allows tamper-free access to perform local matching, which increases user privacy. Finally, a blockchain-based framework was proposed in [93] to investigate the use of various blockchain-based technologies like peer-to-peer transactions, timestamps, and decentralized storage to increase the effectiveness of COVID-19 detection.

1.4.2 Database security

One of the core strengths of blockchain networks is their ability to decentralize information, which removes existing technologies like database and cloud, which has a single point of failure [94]. In [95], the authors proposed blockchain technology for data storage and management in hospitals to securely store patient data and track affected patients. Blockchain ensures the digitalization of data and enables more accessible access to everyone, which eventually leads to the detection of more potential cases. To ensure that, Manoj *et al.* [96] developed a unique incentive-based approach to prevent information tampering within a database. Many recent works focused on developing a secured database for storing patient information. Choudhury *et al.* proposed the use of blockchain for secure record-keeping of different personal information like age and medical records to ensure anonymity [97]. The data within the records would be available on a read-only basis to the stakeholders (state health centers, government, hospitals). In another work, a smart contract-based Ethereum blockchain was developed to prepare digital medical passports for COVID-19 test takers. The work has reduced the response time of healthcare facilities for the users and reduced the extent of fabricated information [98]. Similarly, Resiere *et al.* implemented medical cooperation in the Caribbean using blockchain technology to protect patient data, ensure facilities like patient referral, and establish new payment standards [99].

1.4.3 Information sharing

COVID-19 pandemic has also significantly raised the necessity of gathering the latest and reliable data related to the virus spread. Blockchain has the ability to do that as this technology allows to verify data easily using the distributed ledger and peer-to-peer networking facility [70,100]. Many recent platforms are also using this technology to record patient information with high-security symptoms, location, and medical records. The WHO has also launched a blockchain-based platform called MiPasa that allows private information sharing between its users, health organizations, and authorities. The platform also has a self-reporting feature using which the users can report their infection with public health organizations with precise locations [101]. In another work, a blockchain-based framework was developed for exchanging health information [102]. The framework also allows the patients to control their medical information and to preserve personal autonomy. Also, in [103], a decentralized healthcare system was developed using blockchain technology to encourage patients to safely share their medical information with health organizations while retaining complete control of their data privacy. The framework has the potential to solve many existing challenges of the conventional healthcare system by offering data protection, less operating cost, and easier access to data. A blockchain-based method was built to ameliorate data transmission and improve the reliability of physiological information [104]. The method protects recorded data from node manipulation threats and enables secure information sharing between multiple parties.

1.4.4 Prevention of data fabrication

Access to uncorrupted datasets is one of the critical requirements while researching various diseases, including COVID-19. However, storing the data in a conventional database can result in tampering. In addition, cases of medical data fraud are also rising in recent days [105]. For instance, the result of a recent report on the frontline workers of Pakistan shows that data falsification by the vaccinators is a typical case [106]. In this regard, blockchain can help with its decentralized structure and other features like a smart contract. Several recent literature studies have focused on the necessity of good data for prediction on the pandemic spread and prevention and raised the question of the quality of existing database management systems [95,107]. The tracking system presented in [107] addressed the data manipulation issue and removed the single-point failure issue. In another work, an incentive-based technology was introduced using blockchain technology to prevent tampering in COVID-19 test results [96]. Similarly, in [108], the possibility of causing panic in public during the pandemic due to tampered data was discussed. The authors also investigate the possibility of poor scientific results due to working with falsified data. The work of Ramachandran and Kantarcioglu showcases a blockchain-based data provenance system that can store encrypted data and can trigger smart contracts in the case of any sort of data fabrication [109]. A blockchain-based framework was proposed in [110] to increase the security of EMRs. The framework also uses a credit score system to ensure the credibility of authorities who enters data into the blockchain. Finally, in [111], a Merkle-tree-based approach was followed to protect the integrity of EMR while removing complex features of blockchain like mining. This method can be extremely useful of pandemic data handling due to the simple approach followed in that work.

1.4.5 Internet of Medical Things

There have been numerous recent applications of the IoMT in healthcare due to the advances in sensors and medical devices. This technology also has massive potential in pandemic handling. However, IoMT has also faced some privacy concerns due to the vulnerabilities of the biomedical sensors. These sensors are often resource-limited and prone to wiretapping, malware, and word attacks [112]. Blockchain can improve this issue by improving authentication, and access control on various layers of blockchain enables IoMT. Dai *et al.* presented a blockchain-enabled IoMT solution and discussed the privacy concerns of IoMT devices [113]. In another work, the combination of IoMT application and blockchain was illustrated for efficient patient data analysis [114]. A remote patient monitoring system was proposed in [115] that uses blockchain to overcome the security concerns of IoT devices. In [116], the authors proposed a blockchain system using the Ethereum platform where IoMT devices can be used in carrying out telemedical laboratory examinations. The system was proven to be efficient in both time and cost. Another work in [117] introduced IoT device monitoring architecture with the help of a private blockchain. This architecture can detect changes to the IoT device architecture and can ensure a feasible and secure management of IoT device in large networks.

Our results show that such a system is possible, and the blockchain can secure the dissemination of configuration changes to IoT devices. The key novelty of our solution is a distributed management of configuration files of IoT devices in enterprise networks utilizing blockchain technology.

Telemedicine, a technology that enables features like remote patient monitoring, diagnosis, and treatment at a lower cost, is highly effective in the current situation [118]. As COVID-19 is a highly contagious virus, it is highly challenging for frontline workers to aid patients while keeping themselves safe. Various IoMT devices like wearable devices and advanced sensors are a crucial part of telemedicine throughout the years. However, this technology is also prone to cyberattacks and data breaching [119]. There are many recent works where blockchain was used to make the IoMT devices more secure for their effective use with telemedicine. In [120], a blockchain-based framework was proposed that uses blockchain technology to improve the security and efficiency of telemedicine services. In another work in [121], an attribute-based encryption scheme was presented that can ensure higher efficiency for on-demand medical services in telemedicine system.

1.5 Challenges, solutions, and deliverables

In this section, different challenges that obstruct the development of IoT and blockchain applications are mentioned. Furthermore, some practical solutions and recommendations to mitigate these issues are also briefly discussed.

1.5.1 Challenges of IoT and blockchain technology

With any technology, there are always some issues and challenges that need to be mitigated. In the case of IoT applications, the devices are prone and vulnerable to cyberattacks. Cyberattacks on IoMT applications can cause severe damage to patients' lives as some of these applications mount devices directly to the patient's body. Furthermore, IoT applications are closely related to some sensitive data of the subjects. In terms of IoMT, there is a considerable amount of data consisting of patients' information. Therefore, the sensitive data and privacy of people using these IoT-based applications are vulnerable to cyberattacks. Some of these attacks may even result in the identity theft of patients. IoT applications are vulnerable to various types of cyberattacks such as botnets attack [122], DoS attack [123], DDoS attack [124], and Eavesdropping attack [125]. Clark *et al.* showed how botnets attack could even lead to physical damage to human patients [126]. The authors also elaborated how IoMT devices may cause psychological damage to patients due to being surrounded by machines and devices instead of human beings. There are also some concerns regarding IoT technologies by the user communities. People are concerned by the possibility that robots might take over their jobs in the coming days, resulting in trust issues on these applications [127]. There are also concerns regarding the accuracy of sophisticated IoMT applications. Furthermore, the lack of standardization of IoT technologies has put a massive concern among users, developers, researchers, and engineers [128]. Therefore, to implement and confront a pandemic-like COVID-19 with IoT-based solutions more efficiently, these issues must be addressed and resolved [20].

In the case of blockchain, there are still some issues and challenges that need to be addressed before implementing the technology against COVID-19. Due to the increasing number of transactions, the traffic data becomes bulky, and it affects the creation of a new block due to the time interval set by the blockchain networks. Another issue is the processing speed of primarily used blockchain platforms as they process very few transactions per second and not suitable for processing millions of real-time transactions. High computational power usage is another huge caveat for implementing blockchain-based platforms. In the case of PoW, to add a block in the blockchain, a user has to solve a problem that requires enormous computational power. Therefore, it would not be suitable for resource-limited cities. Moreover, blockchain is still pretty complex, and it will require time before people get used to the technology [129]. Lastly, even though blockchain removes most of the security problems of conventional databases and cloud, it is prone to various cyberattacks such as Sybil attack, eclipse attack, 51% attack, DDoS attack, long-range attack, and P + epsilon attack [37]. The attacker can take over the entire blockchain network through these attacks and significantly slow down the operation.

1.5.2 Possible solutions and deliverables

Worldwide, researchers are working to mitigate the cybersecurity issues of IoT devices. In [130], the researchers proposed an Anomaly detection system that was developed using a random Forest machine-learning algorithm. The proposed system has the ability to find compromised IoT devices in a distributed Fog Nodes. In another work, researchers utilized IoT HoneyNets in order to generate distractions for the attackers from their desired targets and to mitigate cyberattacks [131]. Recent works also focused on the psychological attacks suffered by humans due to leakage of their personal data through IoT devices, and to mitigate those issues, and various frameworks were developed [132,133]. On the contrary, recent attacks on blockchain have raised the question of the immutable nature of the blockchain network. To prevent future cyberattacks, numerous recent works have focused on mitigating those attacks, including mitigating pool hopping attacks, false data injection attacks, and 51% attacks [37,134,135]. A parallel PoW network was proposed in [104] instead of solo mining to increase the processing speed of transactions in the blockchain network. The proposed method can also improve the scalability issue of blockchain. In another work, various versions of blockchain were reviewed to find the optimal versions that require less computational power [136].

Without resolving the crucial issues of IoT applications, the public acceptance of these services will not increase significantly. First, the data of these applications must be adequately encrypted. Without proper encryptions, the systems might fall under cyberattacks, and they might also get beyond recovery. Also, the privacy of personal data of any patient, subject, or human must be ensured in these applications. Since some of the attacks might occur through phishing, the people associated with the system should be trained appropriately and raise their technical knowledge or awareness. Also, the staff in charge of maintaining these applications should be specialized to have sufficient knowledge in maintaining, safeguarding, securing, and developing the systems. Increasing the trust and awareness of users or patients about IoT applications is another aspect that needs to be ensured. In the end, standardizations of these IoT applications should be ensured to have efficient implementations of these applications.

To effectively use the blockchain-based solutions against COVID-19, specific steps are required to be taken. Network latency of the blockchain network needs to be improved to handle extensive data, and a suitable blockchain platform is required to use based on the application to handle large transactions. Besides, security issues need to be prioritized to increase user trust in such applications. To do that, available latest technologies should be implemented against various cyberattacks. Finally, energy consumption issues need to be handled to ensure the large-scale use of blockchain-based platforms.

1.6 Key findings and discussion

In this section, the key findings from the conducted survey have been mentioned, and these applications' strengths and limitations have been discussed.

As shown in Table 1.3, IoT-based applications have made a huge impact on ensuring contactless and remote healthcare monitoring. During the ongoing pandemic or such future events, these applications can reduce the damage significantly. In addition to that, these applications are primarily user-friendly and cost-efficient. Therefore, it can be used in almost every area. However, these applications are prone to different security threats that can mitigate their efficient usage. On the other hand, blockchain has ensured a secure and trusted environment

Table 1.3 Key findings from reviewed IoT and blockchain-based solutions

Technology	Applications	Strengths	Limitations	References
Internet of Things (IoT)	• Health monitoring systems • Tracking and detecting possible patients • Disinfecting area • Telemedicine • Logistics delivery	• Enables healthcare service remotely without any physical contacts • Broader coverage of service • Quicker response in emergencies • Real-time monitoring • Safe and clean environment • Always available rooms for improving or adding features • User-friendly • Low-cost projects	• Requires specific knowledge and training to maintain • Less security could lead to becoming vulnerable to cyber-threats • Maintenance and checking required	[41–81]
Blockchain	• Contact tracing • Database security • Information sharing • Prevention of data fabrication • IoMT	• Increased security over traditional databases • Trusted platform for COVID-19 application development • Rise of trustability among users • Improvement of remove healthcare monitoring	• Lack of user awareness of the technology • Slower performance in comparison to cloud-based services • High computational power usage • Not suitable for resource-limited cities	[82–114]

for application development despite being a comparatively new technology. Blockchain-based solutions are secure and can ensure trustability during among users. Nevertheless, these applications use substantial computational power and can be inappropriate for small cities.

1.7 Conclusion and future scopes

In this study, different applications of IoT and blockchain-based technologies that can be effective against the COVID-19 pandemic were presented. In this demanding time, these solutions can help to slow down the spread of the virus. The study includes a brief investigation of different core components of these technologies to understand their potential in the health sector. It was found that while IoT-based solutions can solve issues like patient detection, health monitoring, and telemedicine, blockchain-based applications can be used to ensure a privacy-preserving environment. However, these technologies have some caveats requiring consideration and should be solved before their widespread use for pandemic handling. The future scopes for these technologies are enormous as applications of both technologies are expanding rapidly. Systematic development of these applications can significantly improve their efficiency and trustability in the future. In addition, with efficient implementations and resolving some of the drawbacks of these technologies, confronting any pandemic like COVID-19 or a similar difficult situation can be more effective.

References

[1] Harvard Health Publishing. *COVID-19 Basics* [online]. 2021. Available from: https://www.health.harvard.edu/diseases-and- conditions/covid-19-basics [Accessed May 2021].

[2] WHO. *Coronavirus disease (COVID-19) pandemic* [online]. 2021. Available from: https://www.who.int/emergencies/diseases/novel-coronavirus-2019 [Accessed May 2021].

[3] Pittaway, D. *The Use of IoT During COVID-19* [online]. 2020. Available from: https://www.iotforall.com/use-of-iotduring-covid-19 [Accessed May 2021].

[4] Dinmohamed, A.G., Visser, O., Verhoeven, R.H., *et al.*: 'Fewer Cancer Diagnoses During the COVID-19 Epidemic in The Netherlands' *The Lancet Oncology*, 2020, **21**(6), pp. 750–751.

[5] Liang, X., Zhao, J., Shetty, S. and Li, D.: 'Towards Data Assurance and Resilience in IoT Using Blockchain', in '*MILCOM 2017–2017 IEEE Military Communications Conference (MILCOM)*', (2017), pp. 261–266.

[6] McGhin, T., Choo, K.-K.R., Liu, C.Z. and He, D.: 'Blockchain in Healthcare Applications: Research Challenges and Opportunities' *Journal of Network and Computer Applications*, 2019, **135**, pp. 62–75.

[7] Agbo, C.C., Mahmoud, Q.H. and Eklund, J.M.: 'Blockchain Technology in Healthcare: A Systematic Review' *Healthcare*, 2019, **7**(2), p. 56.

[8] Kaiser, M.S., Mahmud, M., Noor, M.B.T., *et al.*: 'iWorksafe: Towards Healthy Workplaces During COVID-19 with an Intelligent Phealth App for Industrial Settings' *IEEE Access*, 2021, **9**, pp. 13814–13828.

[9] Nasajpour, M., Pouriyeh, S., Parizi, R.M., Dorodchi, M., Valero, M. and Arabnia, H.R.: 'Internet of Things for Current COVID-19 and Future Pandemics: An Exploratory Study' *Journal of Healthcare Informatics Research*, 2020, **4**(4), pp. 325–364.

[10] Javaid, M. and Khan, I.H.: 'Internet of Things (IoT) Enabled Healthcare Helps to Take the Challenges of COVID-19 Pandemic' *Journal of Oral Biology and Craniofacial Research*, 2021, **11**(2), pp. 209–214.

[11] Ndiaye, M., Oyewobi, S.S., Abu-Mahfouz, A.M., Hancke, G.P., Kurien, A.M. and Djouani, K.: 'IoT in the Wake of COVID-19: A Survey on Contributions, Challenges and Evolution' *IEEE Access*, 2020, **8**, pp. 186821–186839.

[12] Nguyen, D.C., Ding M., Pathirana P.N., and Seneviratne A. 'Blockchain and AI-based solutions to combat coronavirus (COVID-19)-like epidemics: A survey' *IEEE Access*. 2021, 9, pp. 95730–95753.

[13] Sharma, A., Bahl, S., Bagha, A.K., Javaid, M., Shukla, D.K. and Haleem, A.: 'Blockchain Technology and Its Applications to Combat COVID-19 Pandemic' *Research on Biomedical Engineering*, 2020, pp. 1–8.

[14] Oracle. *What is the Internet of Things (IoT)?* [online]. 2021. Available from: https://www.oracle.com/internet-ofthings/what-is-iot/ [Accessed May 2021].

[15] Reshetchenko, D. *Top Five Sectors of IoT: Use Cases and Security* [online]. 2018. Available from: https://dzone.com/articles/5-sectors-which-use-the-iot-efficiently- but-what-a [Accessed May 2021].

[16] Naeem, M.R.H., Gawhar, S., Adib, M.B.H., Sakib, S.A., Ahmed, A. and Chisty, N.A.: 'An IoT Based Smart Irrigation System', in '*2021 2nd International Conference on Robotics, Electrical and Signal Processing Techniques (ICREST)*', (2021), pp. 243–247.

[17] Cisco. *Internet of Things (IoT) – The Future of IoT Miniguide: The Burgeoning IoT Market Continues* [online]. 2021. Available from: https://www.cisco.com/c/en/us/solutions/internet-of-things/future-of-iot.html [Accessed May 2021].

[18] Satu, M.S., Rahman, M.K., Rony, M.A., *et al.*: 'COVID-19: Update, Forecast and Assistant – An Interactive Web Portal to Provide Real-Time Information and Forecast COVID-19 Cases in Bangladesh', in '*2021 International Conference on Information and Communication Technology for Sustainable Development (ICICT4SD)*', (2021), pp. 456–460.

[19] Asif-Ur-Rahman, M., Afsana, F., Mahmud, M., *et al.*: 'Toward a Heterogeneous Mist, Fog, and Cloud-Based Framework for the Internet of Healthcare Things' *IEEE Internet of Things Journal*, 2019, **6**(3), pp. 4049–4062.

[20] Farhin, F., Kaiser, M.S., and Mahmud, M. 'Towards secured service provisioning for the internet of healthcare things', in *2020 IEEE 14th International Conference on Application of Information and Communication Technologies (AICT)* 2020 Oct 7 (pp. 1–6). IEEE.

[21] Farhin, F., Kaiser, M.S. and Mahmud, M.: 'Secured Smart Healthcare System: Blockchain and Bayesian Inference Based Approach', in Kaiser, M. S., Bandyopadhyay, A., Mahmud, M., and Ray, K. (Eds.): '*Proceedings of International Conference on Trends in Computational and Cognitive Engineering*', (Springer, Berlin, 2021), pp. 455–465.

[22] Kaiser, M.S., Zenia, N., Tabassum, F., *et al.*: '6G Access Network for Intelligent Internet of Healthcare Things: Opportunity, Challenges, and Research Directions', in Kaiser, M.S., Bandyopadhyay, A., Mahmud, M., and Ray, K. (Eds.): '*Proceedings of International Conference on Trends in Computational and Cognitive Engineering*', (Springer, Berlin, 2021), pp. 317–328.

[23] Kaiser, M.S., Al Mamun, S., Mahmud, M. and Tania, M.H.: 'Healthcare Robots to Combat COVID-19', in Santosh, K.C., and Joshi, A. (Eds.): '*COVID-19: Prediction, Decision-Making, and Its Impacts*', (Springer, Berlin, 2021), pp. 83–97.

[24] Mahmud, M. and Kaiser, M.S.: 'Machine Learning in Fighting Pandemics: A COVID-19 Case Study', in Santosh, K.C., and Joshi, A. (Eds.): '*COVID-19: Prediction, Decision-Making, and Its Impacts*', (Springer, Berlin, 2021), pp. 77–81.

[25] Toyama, S. and Hirayama, M.: 'User Interface Design Method Considering UI Device in Internet of Things System', in '*2018 6th International Conference on Future Internet of Things and Cloud Workshops (FiCloudW)*', (2018), pp. 1–6.

[26] Barcelo, M., Correa, A., Llorca, J., Tulino, A.M., Vicario, J.L. and Morell, A.: 'IoT-Cloud Service Optimization in Next Generation Smart Environments' *IEEE Journal on Selected Areas in Communications*, 2016, **34**(12), pp. 4077–4090.

[27] Levy, E. *IoT Analytics: Challenges, Applications, and Innovations* [online]. 2019. Available from: http://www.upsolver.com/blog/iot-analytics-challenges- applications-innovations [Accessed May 2021].

[28] Valerio, P.: 'Is the IoT a Tech Bubble for Cities?: With More Cities Joining the Smart City Revolution and Investing in Sensors and Other IoT Devices, the Risk of a New Tech Bubble Is Rising' *IEEE Consumer Electronics Magazine*, 2016, **5**(1), pp. 61–62.

[29] Bhuyan, H.K., Chakraborty, C., Pani, S.K. and Ravi, V.: 'Feature and Subfeature Selection for Classification Using Correlation Coefficient and Fuzzy Model' *IEEE Transactions on Engineering Management*, 2021, pp. 1–15.

[30] Dhawan, S., Chakraborty, C., Frnda, J., Gupta, R., Rana, A.K. and Pani, S.K.: 'SSII: Secured and High-Quality Steganography Using Intelligent Hybrid Optimization Algorithms for IoT' *IEEE Access*, 2021, **9**, pp. 87563–87578.

[31] Frustaci, M., Pace, P., Aloi, G. and Fortino, G.: 'Evaluating Critical Security Issues of the IoT World: Present and Future Challenges' *IEEE Internet of Things Journal*, 2018, **5**(4), pp. 2483–2495.

[32] Dominicbetts. *What is Azure IoT Central* [online]. 2021. Available from: https://docs.microsoft.com/en-us/azure/iot- central/core/overview-iot-central [Accessed May 2021].

[33] Nofer, M., Gomber, P., Hinz, O. and Schiereck, D.: 'Blockchain' *Business & Information Systems Engineering*, 2017, **59**(3), pp. 183–187.

[34] Zheng, Z., Xie, S., Dai, H., Chen, X. and Wang, H.: 'An Overview of Blockchain Technology: Architecture, Consensus, and Future Trends', in '*2017 IEEE International Congress on Big Data (BigData Congress)*', (2017), pp. 557–564.

[35] Chowdhury, S.M.H.M., Jahan, F., Sara, S.M. and Nandi, D.: 'Secured Blockchain Based Decentralised Internet: A Proposed New Internet', in '*Proceedings of the International Conference on Computing Advancements*', (Association for Computing Machinery, New York, 2020), pp. 1–7.

[36] MarketsandMarkets. *Blockchain Market by Component (Platform and Services), Provider (Application, Middleware, and Infrastructure), Type (Private, Public, and Hybrid), Organization Size, Application Area (BFSI, Government, IT & Telecom), and Region – Global Forecast to 2025* [online]. 2020. Available from: https://www.marketsandmarkets.com/Market-Reports/blockchain- technology-market-90100890.html [Accessed May 2021].

[37] Sayeed, S. and Marco-Gisbert, H.: 'Assessing Blockchain Consensus and Security Mechanisms Against the 51% Attack' *Applied Sciences*, 2019, **9**(9), p. 1788.

[38] Onik, M.M.H., Aich, S., Yang, J., Kim, C.-S. and Kim, H.-C.: 'Chapter 8 – Blockchain in Healthcare: Challenges and Solutions', in Dey, N., Das, H., Naik, B., and Behera, H.S. (Eds.): '*Big Data Analytics for Intelligent Healthcare Management*', (Academic Press, New York, 2019), pp. 197–226.

[39] Hassija, V., Chamola, V., Saxena, V., Jain, D., Goyal, P. and Sikdar, B.: 'A Survey on IoT Security: Application Areas, Security Threats, and Solution Architectures' *IEEE Access*, 2019, **7**, pp. 82721–82743.

[40] Yang, J., Onik, M.M.H., Lee, N.-Y., Ahmed, M. and Kim, C.-S.: 'Proof-of-Familiarity: A Privacy-Preserved Blockchain Scheme for Collaborative Medical Decision-Making' *Applied Sciences*, 2019, **9**(7), p. 1370.

[41] Zhang, S. and Lee, J.-H.: 'Analysis of the Main Consensus Protocols of Blockchain' *ICT Express*, 2020, **6**(2), pp. 93–97.

[42] Kaur, M., Khan, M.Z., Gupta, S., Noorwali, A., Chakraborty, C. and Pani, S. K.: 'MBCP: Performance Analysis of Large Scale Mainstream Blockchain Consensus Protocols' *IEEE Access*, 2021, **9**, pp. 80931–80944.

[43] Niranjanamurthy, M., Nithya, B.N. and Jagannatha, S.: 'Analysis of Blockchain Technology: Pros, Cons and SWOT' *Cluster Computing*, 2019, **22**(6), pp. 14743–14757.

[44] Choi, S. and, Lee, J.-H.: 'Blockchain-Based Distributed Firmware Update Architecture for IoT Devices' *IEEE Access*, 2020, **8**, pp. 37518–37525.

[45] Czachorowski, K., Solesvik, M. and Kondratenko, Y.: 'The Application of Blockchain Technology in the Maritime Industry', in Kharchenko, V., Kondratenko, Y., and Kacprzyk, J. (Eds.): '*Green IT Engineering: Social, Business and Industrial Applications*', (Springer International Publishing, Berlin, 2019), pp. 561–577.

[46] Rhydwan, A.H.M., Choyon, M.M.S., Iftekhar, M.N., Hasan Sad, A.M. and Nandi, D.: 'Smart Grid Implementation With Consortium Blockchain: A Proposed Model for Bangladesh', in '*2020 Emerging Technology in Computing, Communication and Electronics (ETCCE)*', (2020), pp. 1–6.

[47] Rodrigues, J.J.P.C., Segundo, D.B.D.R., Junqueira, H.A., *et al.*: 'Enabling Technologies for the Internet of Health Things' *IEEE Access*, 2018, **6**, pp. 13129–13141.

[48] Ye, J.: 'The Role of Health Technology and Informatics in a Global Public Health Emergency: Practices and Implications From the COVID-19 Pandemic' *JMIR Medical Informatics*, 2020, **8**(7), p. e19866.

[49] Faria, T.H., Shamim Kaiser, M., Hossian, C.A., Mahmud, M., Al Mamun, S. and Chakraborty, C.: 'Smart City Technologies for Next Generation

Healthcare', in Chakraborty, C., Lin, J.C.-W., and Alazab, M. (Eds.): *'Data-Driven Mining, Learning and Analytics for Secured Smart Cities: Trends and Advances*', (Springer International Publishing, Berlin, 2021), pp. 253–274.

[50] Sad, A.S.M.M.H., Choyon, M.M.S., Rhydwan, A.H.M., Shikder, K. and Hossain, C.A.: 'Nekray: A Linux Kernel-Based Customized Operating System for Information Kiosk' *IJERTCS*, 2021, **12**(3), pp. 49–68.

[51] Choyon, M.M.S., Rahman, M., Kabir, M.M. and Mridha, M.F.: 'IoT Based Health Monitoring Automated Predictive System to Confront COVID-19', in '*2020 IEEE 17th International Conference on Smart Communities: Improving Quality of Life Using ICT, IoT and AI (HONET)*', (2020), pp. 189–193.

[52] Michalska, A.: 'Could Your Fitbit or Apple Watch Detect Early COVID-19 Symptoms?' *Reuters*, 2020.

[53] Miller, D.J., Capodilupo, J.V., Lastella, M., *et al.*: 'Analyzing Changes in Respiratory Rate to Predict The Risk of COVID-19 Infection' *medRxiv*, 2020, 2020.06.18.20131417.

[54] Rahman, M.A. and Hossain, M.S.: 'An Internet of Medical Things-Enabled Edge Computing Framework for Tackling COVID-19' *IEEE Internet of Things Journal*, 2021, **8**, pp. 15847–15854.

[55] Bai, L., Yang, D., Wang, X., *et al.*: ''Chinese Experts' Consensus on the Internet of Things-Aided Diagnosis and Treatment of Coronavirus Disease 2019 (COVID-19)' *Clinical eHealth*, 2020, **3**, pp. 7–15.

[56] Ruiz-Fernández, D., Marcos-Jorquera, D., Gilart-Iglesias, V., Vives-Boix, V. and Ramírez-Navarro, J.: 'Empowerment of Patients With Hypertension through BPM, IoT and Remote Sensing' *Sensors*, 2017, **17**(10), p. 2273.

[57] Lomotey, R.K., Pry, J. and Sriramoju, S.: 'Wearable IoT Data Stream Traceability in a Distributed Health Information System' *Pervasive and Mobile Computing*, 2017, **40**, pp. 692–707.

[58] Taiwo, O. and Ezugwu, A.E.: 'Smart Healthcare Support for Remote Patient Monitoring During Covid-19 Quarantine' *Informatics in Medicine Unlocked*, 2020, **20**, p. 100428.

[59] Vedaei, S.S., Fotovvat, A., Mohebbian, M.R., *et al.*: 'COVID-SAFE: An IoT-Based System for Automated Health Monitoring and Surveillance in Post-Pandemic Life' *IEEE Access*, 2020, **8**, pp. 188538–188551.

[60] Li, S.-H., Lin, B.-S., Tsai, C.-H., Yang, C.-T. and Lin, B.-S.: 'Design of Wearable Breathing Sound Monitoring System for Real-Time Wheeze Detection' *Sensors (Basel)*, 2017, **17**(1).

[61] de Morais Barroca Filho, I., Aquino, G., Malaquias, R.S., Girão, G. and Melo, S.R.M.: 'An IoT-Based Healthcare Platform for Patients in ICU Beds During the COVID-19 Outbreak' *IEEE Access*, 2021, **9**, pp. 27262–27277.

[62] Winn, Z. *Real-Time Data for a Better Response to Disease Outbreaks* [online]. 2020. Available from: https://news. mit.edu/2020/kinsa-health-0821 [Accessed April 2021].

[63] Fernández-Caramés, T.M., Froiz-Míguez, I. and Fraga-Lamas, P.: 'An IoT and Blockchain Based System for Monitoring and Tracking Real-Time

Occupancy for COVID-19 Public Safety' *Engineering Proceedings*, 2020, **2**(1), p. 67.

[64] Marr, B. *Robots And Drones Are Now Used To Fight COVID-19* [online]. 2020. Available from: https:// www.forbes.com/sites/bernardmarr/2020/03/18/how-robots-and- drones-arehelping-to-fight-coronavirus/ [Accessed April 2021].

[65] Gascueña, D. *Drones to Stop the COVID-19 Epidemic* [online]. 2020. Available from: https://www.bbva.com/en/drones-to-stop-the-covid-19-epidemic/ [Accessed April 2021].

[66] Rosebrock, A. *OpenCV Social Distancing Detector* [online]. 2020. Available from: https://www.pyimagesearch.com/2020/06/01/opencv-social-distancing-detector/ [Accessed April 2021].

[67] Abdulrazaq, M., Zuhriyah, H., Al-Zubaidi, S., Karim, S., Ramli, R. and Yusuf, E.: 'NOVEL COVID-19 Detection And Diagnosis System Using IoT Based Smart Helmet' *International Journal of Psychosocial Rehabilitation*, 2020, **24**, pp. 2296–2303.

[68] Abdulrazaq, M., Istiqomah, N., Zuhriyah, H., *et al.*: '2019 Novel Coronavirus Disease (Covid-19): Detection and Diagnosis System Using IoT Based Smart Glasses' 2020, **29**.

[69] Jung, Y. and Agulto, R.: 'A Public Platform for Virtual IoT-Based Monitoring and Tracking of COVID-19' *Electronics*, 2021, **10**(1), p. 12.

[70] Garg, C., Bansal, A. and Padappayil, R.P.: 'COVID-19: Prolonged Social Distancing Implementation Strategy Using Blockchain-Based Movement Passes' *Journal of Medical Systems*, 2020, **44**(9), p. 165.

[71] Garg, L., Chukwu, E., Nasser, N., Chakraborty, C. and Garg, G.: 'Anonymity Preserving IoT-Based COVID-19 and Other Infectious Disease Contact Tracing Model' *IEEE Access*, 2020, **8**, pp. 159402–159414.

[72] Tedeschi, P., Bakiras, S. and Di Pietro, R.: 'IoTrace: A Flexible, Efficient, and Privacy-Preserving IoT-enabled Architecture for Contact Tracing' *arXiv:2007.11928 [cs]*, 2021.

[73] Kolhar, M., Al-Turjman, F., Alameen, A. and Abualhaj, M.M.: 'A Three Layered Decentralized IoT Biometric Architecture for City Lockdown During COVID-19 Outbreak' *IEEE Access*, 2020, **8**, pp. 163608–163617.

[74] Yang, G.-Z., J. Nelson, B., Murphy, R.R., *et al.*: 'Combating COVID-19—The Role of Robotics in Managing Public Health and Infectious Diseases' *Science Robotics*, 2020, **5**(40), p. eabb5589.

[75] Xenex. *Xenex LightStrike Robot – Destroy Deadly Pathogens and Deactivate SARS-CoV-2* [Online]. 2021. Available from: https://xenex.com/ [Accessed April 2021].

[76] Ackerman, E. *Autonomous Robots Are Helping Kill Coronavirus in Hospitals* [online]. 2020. Available from: https://spectrum.ieee.org/automaton/robotics/medical-robots/autonomous-robots-are-helping-kill-coronavirus-in-hospitals [Accessed April 2021].

[77] Sharma, M. *How Drones Are Being Used to Combat COVID-19* [online]. 2020. Available from: https://www.geospatialworld.net/blogs/how-drones-are-being-used- to-combat-covid19/ [Accessed April 2021].

[78] Hossain, C., Mohamed, M.A., Zishan, M., Ahasan, R. and Sharun, S.: 'Awareness on e-Health Among Undergraduate Students in Bangladesh' *Indian Journal of Public Health Research & Development*, 2019, **10**, p. 636.

[79] Medicaaid. *Telemedicine* [online]. 2020. Available from: https://www.medicaid.gov/medicaid/benefits/ telemedicine/index.html [Accessed April 2021].

[80] Matsos, S. *In Fight Against Coronavirus, Telemedicine Ramps Up at Johns Hopkins* [online]. 2020. Available from: https://www.hopkinsmedicine.org/coronavirus/articles/telemedicine.html [Accessed April 2021].

[81] Athena, P., Rumsfeld, J.S. and Wessler, J.D.: 'Telehealth Is Having a Moment' *Journal of the American College of Cardiology*, 2020, **75**(23), pp. 2989–2991.

[82] Gilgore, S. *GWU Hospital tackles COVID-19 with new testing site, telemedicine and outreach on D.C.'s east side* [online]. 2020. Available from: https://www.bizjournals.com/washington/news/2020/04/08/gwu- hospital-tackles-covid-19-with-new-testing.html [Accessed April 2021].

[83] Shah, M. *Industry Voices—How Rush University Medical Center's Virtual Investments Became Central to Its COVID-19 Response* [online]. Available from: https://www. fiercehealthcare.com/hospitals-health-systems/industry-voices- how-rushuniversity-system-for-health-s-virtual [Accessed April 2021].

[84] WAS. *WAS ambulance and special vehicles of the WAS brand* [online]. 2021. Available from: https://www.was- vehicles.com/en/home.html [Accessed April 2021].

[85] Hossain, C., Zishan, M. and Ahasan, R.: 'A Review on the Security Issues of Telemedicine Network' *IJIREEICE*, 2014, pp. 2183–218.

[86] Siriwardhana, Y., De Alwis, C., Gür, G., Ylianttila, M. and Liyanage, M.: 'The Fight Against the COVID-19 Pandemic with 5G Technologies' *IEEE Engineering Management Review*, 2020, **48**(3), pp. 72–84.

[87] Dawkins, T. *How COVID-19 Could Open the Door for Driverless* [online]. 2020. Available from: https://www.weforum.org/agenda/2020/04/how-covid-19-could-open-the-door-for-driverless-deliveries/ [Accessed April 2021].

[88] Končar, J., Grubor, A., Marić, R., Vučenović, S. and Vukmirović, G.: 'Setbacks to IoT Implementation in the Function of FMCG Supply Chain Sustainability During COVID-19 Pandemic' *Sustainability*, 2020, **12**(18), p. 7391.

[89] Rivest, R.L., Weitzner, D.J., Ivers, L.C., Soibelman, I. and Zissman, M.A.: 'PACT: Private Automated Contact Tracing' 2020, p. 3.

[90] Song, J., Gu, T., Feng, X., Ge, Y. and Mohapatra, P.: 'Blockchain Meets COVID-19: A Framework for Contact Information Sharing and Risk Notification System' *arXiv preprint arXiv:2007.10529*, 2020.

[91] Xu, H., Zhang, L., Onireti, O., Fang, Y., Buchanan, W.J. and Imran, M.A.: 'BeepTrace: Blockchain-Enabled Privacy-Preserving Contact Tracing for COVID-19 Pandemic and Beyond' *IEEE Internet of Things Journal*, 2020, **8**, pp. 3915–3929.

[92] Klaine, P.V., Zhang, L., Zhou, B., Sun, Y., Xu, H. and Imran, M.: 'Privacy-Preserving Contact Tracing and Public Risk Assessment Using Blockchain for COVID-19 Pandemic' *IEEE Internet of Things Magazine*, 2020, **3**(3), pp. 58–63.

[93] Torky, M. and Hassanien, A.E.: 'COVID-19 Blockchain Framework: Innovative Approach' *arXiv preprint arXiv:2004.06081*, 2020.

[94] Gupta, A, Chinmay, C. and Gupta, B: 'Secure Transmission of EEG Data Using Watermarking Algorithm for the Detection of Epileptical Seizures' *Traitement du Signal*, 2021, **38**(2), pp. 473–479, https://doi.org/10.18280/ts.380227.

[95] Azim, A., Islam, M.N. and Spranger, P.E.: 'Blockchain and Novel Coronavirus: Towards Preventing COVID-19 and Future Pandemics' *Iberoamerican Journal of Medicine*, 2020, **2**(3), pp. 215–218.

[96] Manoj, M., Srivastava, G., Somayaji, S.R.K., Gadekallu, T.R., Maddikunta, P.K.R. and Bhattacharya, S.: 'An Incentive Based Approach for COVID-19 Planning Using Blockchain Technology', in '*2020 IEEE Globecom Workshops (GC Wkshps)*', (2020), pp. 1–6.

[97] Choudhury, H., Goswami, B. and Gurung, S.K.: 'CovidChain: An Anonymity Preserving Blockchain Based Framework for Protection Against Covid-19' *ArXiv*, 2020.

[98] Hasan, H.R., Salah, K., Jayaraman, R., *et al.*: 'Blockchain-Based Solution for COVID-19 Digital Medical Passports and Immunity Certificates' *IEEE Access*, 2020, **8**, pp. 222093–222108.

[99] Resiere, D., Resiere, D. and Kallel, H.: 'Implementation of Medical and Scientific Cooperation in the Caribbean Using Blockchain Technology in Coronavirus (Covid-19) Pandemics' *Journal of Medical Systems*, 2020, **44**(7).

[100] Rab, S., Javaid, M., Haleem, A. and Vaishya, R.: 'Face Masks Are New Normal After COVID-19 Pandemic' *Diabetes & Metabolic Syndrome: Clinical Research & Reviews*, 2020, **14**(6), pp. 1617–1619.

[101] Ahir, S., Telavane, D. and Thomas, R.: 'The Impact of Artificial Intelligence, Blockchain, Big Data and Evolving Technologies in Coronavirus Disease – 2019 (COVID-19) Curtailment', in '*2020 International Conference on Smart Electronics and Communication (ICOSEC)*', (2020), pp. 113–120.

[102] Christodoulou, K., Christodoulou, P., Zinonos, Z., Carayannis, E.G. and Chatzichristofis, S.A.: 'Health Information Exchange With Blockchain amid Covid-19-like Pandemics', in '*2020 16th International Conference on Distributed Computing in Sensor Systems (DCOSS)*', (2020), pp. 412–417.

[103] Khatoon, A. *Use of Blockchain Technology to Curb Novel Coronavirus Disease (COVID-19) Transmission*. Preprints 2020, 2020050117 (doi: 10.20944/preprints202005.0117.v1).

[104] Alam T. 'Internet of things and blockchain-based framework for Coronavirus (COVID-19) disease'. Available at SSRN: http://dx.doi.org/10.2139/ssrn.3660503.

[105] Herland, M., Khoshgoftaar, T.M. and Bauder, R.A.: 'Big Data Fraud Detection Using Multiple Medicare Data Sources' *Journal of Big Data*, 2018, **5**(1), p. 29.

[106] Batool, A., Toyama, K., Veinot, T., Fatima, B. and Naseem, M.: 'Detecting Data Falsification by Front-line Development Workers: A Case Study of Vaccination in Pakistan', in '*Proceedings of the 2021 CHI Conference on Human Factors in Computing Systems*', (Association for Computing Machinery, New York, 2021), pp. 1–14.

[107] Marbouh, D., Abbasi, T., Maasmi, F., *et al.*: 'Blockchain for COVID-19: Review, Opportunities, and a Trusted Tracking System' *Arabian Journal for Science and Engineering*, 2020, **45**(12), pp. 9895–9911.

[108] Ahmad, R.W., Salah, K., Jayaraman, R., Yaqoob, I., Ellahham, S., and Omar, M. 'Blockchain and COVID-19 pandemic: Applications and challenges', *IEEE TechRxiv*. 2020 Sep 17.

[109] Ramachandran, A. and Kantarcioglu, M.: 'SmartProvenance: A Distributed, Blockchain Based DataProvenance System', in '*Proceedings of the Eighth ACM Conference on Data and Application Security and Privacy*', (Association for Computing Machinery, New York, 2018), pp. 35–42.

[110] Siva Rama Krishnan, S., Manoj, M.K., Gadekallu, T.R., *et al.*: 'A Blockchain-Based Credibility Scoring Framework for Electronic Medical Records', in '*2020 IEEE Globecom Workshops (GC Wkshps)*', (2020), pp. 1–6.

[111] Sharma, B., Sekharan, C.N. and Zuo, F.: 'Merkle-Tree Based Approach for Ensuring Integrity of Electronic Medical Records', in '*2018 9th IEEE Annual Ubiquitous Computing, Electronics Mobile Communication Conference (UEMCON)*', (2018), pp. 983–987.

[112] Boudagdigue, C., Benslimane, A., Kobbane, A. and Liu, J.: 'Trust Management in Industrial Internet of Things' *IEEE Transactions on Information Forensics and Security*, 2020, **15**, pp. 3667–3682.

[113] Dai, H.-N., Imran, M. and Haider, N.: 'Blockchain-Enabled Internet of Medical Things to Combat COVID-19' *IEEE Internet of Things Magazine*, 2020, **3**(3), pp. 52–57.

[114] Aileni, R.M. and Suciu, G., 2020. 'IoMT: A blockchain perspective', *in Decentralised Internet of Things* (pp. 199–215). Springer, Cham.

[115] Srivastava, G., Crichigno, J. and Dhar, S.: 'A Light and Secure Healthcare Blockchain for IoT Medical Devices', in '*2019 IEEE Canadian Conference of Electrical and Computer Engineering (CCECE)*', (2019), pp. 1–5.

[116] Celesti, A., Ruggeri, A., Fazio, M., Galletta, A., Villari, M. and Romano, A.: 'Blockchain-Based Healthcare Workflow for Tele-Medical Laboratory in Federated Hospital IoT Clouds' *Sensors*, 2020, **20**(9), p. 2590.

[117] Košťál, K., Helebrandt, P., Belluš, M., Ries, M. and Kotuliak, I.: 'Management and Monitoring of IoT Devices Using Blockchain' *Sensors*, 2019, **19**(4), p. 856.

[118] Ahmad, R.W., Salah, K., Jayaraman, R., Yaqoob, I., Ellahham, S. and Omar, M.: 'The Role of Blockchain Technology in Telehealth and Telemedicine' *International Journal of Medical Informatics*, 2021, **148**, p. 104399.

[119] Kim, D., Choi, J. and Han, K.: 'Risk Management-Based Security Evaluation Model for Telemedicine Systems' *BMC Medical Informatics and Decision Making*, 2020, **20**(1), p. 106.

[120] Kordestani, H., Barkaoui, K. and Zahran, W.: 'HapiChain: A Blockchain-Based Framework for Patient-Centric Telemedicine', in '*2020 IEEE 8th International Conference on Serious Games and Applications for Health (SeGAH)*', (2020), pp. 1–6.

[121] Guo, R., Shi, H., Zheng, D., Jing, C., Zhuang, C. and Wang, Z.: 'Flexible and Efficient Blockchain-Based ABE Scheme With Multi-Authority for Medical on Demand in Telemedicine System' *IEEE Access*, 2019, **7**, pp. 88012–88025.

[122] Tzagkarakis, C., Petroulakis, N. and Ioannidis, S.: 'Botnet Attack Detection at the IoT Edge Based on Sparse Representation', in '*2019 Global IoT Summit (GIoTS)*', (2019), pp. 1–6.

[123] De Rango, F., Tropea, M. and Fazio, P.: 'Mitigating DoS Attacks in IoT EDGE Layer to Preserve QoS Topics and Nodes' Energy', in '*IEEE INFOCOM 2020 – IEEE Conference on Computer Communications Workshops (INFOCOM WKSHPS)*', (2020), pp. 842–847.

[124] Luo, X., Yan, Q., Wang, M. and Huang, W.: 'Using MTD and SDN-Based Honeypots to Defend DDoS Attacks in IoT', in '*2019 Computing, Communications and IoT Applications (ComComAp)*', (2019), pp. 392–395.

[125] Liu, G., Quan, W., Cheng, N., *et al.*: 'Softwarized IoT Network Immunity Against Eavesdropping With Programmable Data Planes' *IEEE Internet of Things Journal*, 2021, **8**(8), pp. 6578–6590.

[126] Clark, G.W., Doran, M.V. and Andel, T.R.: 'Cybersecurity issues in robotics', in '*2017 IEEE Conference on Cognitive and Computational Aspects of Situation Management (CogSIMA)*', (2017), pp. 1–5.

[127] Taylor, C. *Robots Could Take Over 20 Million Jobs by 2030, Study Claims* [online]. 2019. Available https://www.cnbc.com/2019/06/26/robots-could-take-over-20- million-jobs-by-2030-study-claims.html [Accessed May 2021].

[128] 'IoT Standardization and Implementation Challenges – IEEE Internet of Things', https://iot.ieee.org/newsletter/july-2016/iot-standardization-and-implementation-challenges.html, accessed May 2021.

[129] Mbunge, E., Akinnuwesi, B., Fashoto, S.G., Metfula, A.S. and Mashwama, P.: 'A Critical Review of Emerging Technologies for Tackling COVID-19 Pandemic' *Human Behavior and Emerging Technologies*, 2021, **3**(1), pp. 25–39.

[130] Alrashdi, I., Alqazzaz, A., Aloufi, E., Alharthi, R., Zohdy, M. and Ming, H.: 'AD-IoT: Anomaly Detection of IoT Cyberattacks in Smart City Using Machine Learning', in '*2019 IEEE 9th Annual Computing and Communication Workshop and Conference (CCWC)*', (2019), pp. 0305–0310.

[131] Zarca, A.M., Bernabe, J.B., Skarmeta, A. and Alcaraz Calero, J.M.: 'Virtual IoT HoneyNets to Mitigate Cyberattacks in SDN/NFV-Enabled IoT Networks' *IEEE Journal on Selected Areas in Communications*, 2020, **38**(6), pp. 1262–1277.

[132] Park, M., Oh, H. and Lee, K.: 'Security Risk Measurement for Information Leakage in IoT-Based Smart Homes from a Situational Awareness Perspective' *Sensors*, 2019, **19**(9), p. 2148.

[133] Sharma, M., Samriti and Singh, G.: 'Need and Design of Smart and Secure Energy-Efficient IoT-Based Healthcare Framework', in Mittal, M., Tanwar, S., Agarwal, B., and Goyal, L.M. (Eds.): '*Energy Conservation for IoT Devices: Concepts, Paradigms and Solutions*', (Springer, Berlin, 2019), pp. 259–281.

[134] Ghiasi, M., Dehghani, M., Niknam, T., Kavousi-Fard, A., Siano, P. and Alhelou, H.H.: 'Cyber-Attack Detection and Cyber-Security Enhancement in Smart DC-Microgrid Based on Blockchain Technology and Hilbert Huang Transform' *IEEE Access*, 2021, **9**, pp. 29429–29440.

[135] Singh, S.K., Salim, M.M., Cho, M., Cha, J., Pan, Y. and Park, J.H.: 'Smart Contract-Based Pool Hopping Attack Prevention for Blockchain Networks' *Symmetry*, 2019, **11**(7), p. 941.

[136] Salimitari, M., Chatterjee, M. and Fallah, Y.P.: 'A Survey on Consensus Methods in Blockchain for Resource-Constrained IoT Networks' *Internet of Things*, 2020, **11**, p. 100212.

Chapter 2

Application of big data and computational intelligence in fighting COVID-19 epidemic

Joseph Bamidele Awotunde[1], *Chinmay Chakraborty*[2] and *Gbemisola Janet Ajamu*[3]

Abstract

The current epidemic called coronavirus (COVID-19) is wreaking havoc on society, humanity, and causing economic difficulties around the world. Many techniques have been attempted to manage and contain the COVID-19 outbreak; however, many governments remain powerless to combat and contain the virus. Big data is driving the digital revolution in an increasingly knowledge-driven, healthcare-innovation-driven, and connected society. The combination of computational intelligence (CI) and big data analytics (BDAs) has developed methods that make accessing and processing vast amounts of data easier and less demanding on human expert. Hence, in combating the outbreak, big data and CI can be applied since the use of both technologies empowered BDA and yielded imaginable results in combating infectious diseases globally. Therefore, this chapter reviews the applicability and importance of big data and CI methods to data produced from the countless of ubiquitously connected healthcare devices that produced entrenched and distributed information handling capabilities in fighting COVID-19 outbreak. The use of CI in BDAs has resulted in knowledge-based system that transformed big data into big knowledge with new approaches and visions in order to provide people with better understanding and information-driven results. There have been tremendous positive results using IoT-based capture data with BDA and CI models for monitoring, diagnosis, and prediction of COVID-19 outbreak. The huge amount of data can be managed using CI and BDA by developing models that will reduce the spread of any infectious diseases to monitoring, tracking and in the production of drugs and vaccines for the treatment of the any outbreak globally.

[1]Department of Computer Science, University of Ilorin, Ilorin, Nigeria
[2]Department of Electronics and Communication Engineering, Birla Institute of Technology, Ranchi, India
[3]Department Agricultural Extension and Rural Development, Landmark University, Omu-Aran, Nigeria

Keywords: Big disease diagnosis and prediction; COVID-19 outbreak; Healthcare system; Big data analytics; Computational intelligence; Big data; Diseases diagnosis

2.1 Introduction

The coronavirus (COVID-19) epidemic outbreak, which began in Wuhan, China in December 2019, has already spread around the globe. According to the WHO, in 213 countries/regions of the world as at 10:35 AM CEST, there were 199,203,664 COVID-19 cases worldwide as of August 2, 2021, with 4,244,184 global deaths [1]. Although there have been new vaccine provided for citizens around the world, but the drugs are not enough considering the population globally, and the fear of side effects have made many to reject the vaccine available. Hence, there is need for a better way of managing this pandemic globally. Also, the community-based control strategies adopted globally have not proved useful to curtail the outbreak [2,3].

The cause of COVID-19 has globally affected almost the aspect of human activities because it is highly contagious. Every nation adopts the system of containment, monitoring, and lockdown to be able to curtail the spread of the outbreak by isolating those that have infected the communities in order for them not to spread the pandemic within the community further. Patients with the virus may have modest symptoms like sneezing, sore throat, and fever or major symptoms that can lead to death like heart failure and pneumonia [3]. COVID-19 is the coronavirus induced by the SARS-CoV-2 transmittable condition. Thanks to recent advances in analytical techniques brought about by information and communication technologies (ICTs), big data analytics (BDAs), and computational intelligence (CI) can be used to manage the enormous and unprecedented volume of data generated by medical data. These huge data can be used to monitor patients' in real time, giving daily reports of the situation of any outbreak, tracking of the pandemic, daily situation briefings, and public updates. According to a recent assessment, about 86.60% of all patients infected so far are susceptible to the COVID-19 pandemic given a median age of around 47 years [4].

In this larger proclivity outbreak, men are taking the lead, while studies have not found a substantial gender difference [5]. The primary carrier of COVID-19 outbreak is through human-to-human transmission having aerosols, respiratory aspirates, droplets, feces, and direct exposure all being classified as carriers by China's National Health Commission [6]. Although there is no substantial proof of infrequent instances of SARS-CoV-2 being transmitted vertically, it has been shown that this could be a route for COVID-19 to spread [7].

The various integrations of devices in healthcare sectors have generated big data, and the advancement of CI in the processes of this huge data has achieved significant success in several infectious diseases like influenzas [8], SARS [9], and MERS [10]. The CI models have been used to predict and diagnose various infectious diseases, thus, help in dealing with their several challenges. This has result to the development of various CI systems for fighting COVID-19 outbreak. The CI system plays a crucial role for combating COVID-19 pandemic by building robust system used to diagnose, monitor, forecast, and develop COVID-19 vaccine. The application of CI would require various types of CI models like computational modeling, artificial intelligence (AI), data analytics, and particularly machine learning, a powerful subfield of CI. The integration of various devices with CI mechanisms in developing different applications would require various models to be able to fight any infectious diseases. Researchers have made efforts to develop systems and applications using CI models for the fight against COVID-19 outbreak.

The use of CI and analytical methodologies to predict unpredictable or foreseeable results is known as predictive analysis [10,11]. It answers the question, "What's the next step?" It also uses historical and current data to forecast future behaviors, patterns, and activities. To make a better prediction model, automated CI and statistical analysis with quantitative questions play prominent role [11]. Predictive models must be built by experts for forecasting in predictive analytics [11]. The CI is a catch-all term for a variety of information and control tools. The generated data from IoT-based wearable devices will be worthless without the use of CI models to generate useful insight that can be useful for both physician and the patients. Wearable app creators are gradually integrating CI engines into wearable medical apps for this purpose. Furthermore, the integration of CI models has really helped in the development of a better healthcare system connected to various IoT devices, smartphones, and wearable sensors to collect data that will improve the understanding of patient problems by the physicians [12,13].

The recent technological development with innovations in data sciences has facilitated the gathering of a huge amount of data, especially in healthcare systems, thus termed big data, and clouding has been the warehouses where such huge data can be safely stored [14,15]. Researchers must broaden researches beyond the standard surveillance model in order to make an efficient use of the captured data. The research should be based on the models that will make use of huge data to generate various results that are focusing on treatment-oriented healthcare systems by narrowing the BDA to diagnose, track, monitor, and treat various diseases. As a result, big data can be used in the heterogeneous population for various purposes to reflect the needs of each sector for a better decision-making [16]. This necessities speedy research that can make use of modern computing technologies to process the huge data gathered in healthcare systems and make use appropriate tools to lessen their implantation complexity [17]. Big data generated in healthcare systems can be used for proper diagnosis and treatment of patients with given accurate results.

The mutual collaboration in healthcare industries has resulted in the collection of a huge amount of data from various sources [18]. This collaboration has brought medical workers from various departments to achieve a common goal of reducing medical cost, and errors as a result inaccuracy in medical diagnosis. A huge amount of data generated from each section of the hospitals from various departments like nurses, pathologists, radiologists, and laboratory technologists is used. In addition to deliver high-quality and standardized healthcare services, data is obtained from a variety of sources by various stakeholders, which can be used for monitoring, prediction, diagnosis, and treatment of various diseases.

As a result, sophisticated technologies such as virtualization and cloud computing can be used in the healthcare system to process large amounts of data efficiently. These make the healthcare system as big data-generated industries, which have been developed in recent years. Meanwhile, advancements in ICT have resulted in the development of huge data from various sources in recent years. Big data is altering every element of human life in the twenty-first century, including biology and medicine [19]. The introduction of electronic medical records to replace the paper medical records transformed the healthcare systems into big data-generated sectors and resulted into massive data explosion [20]. Thus, it helps to make evidence-based decisions that ultimately improve patient diagnosis, monitoring, and treatments by doctors, policy-makers, and the epidemiologists [21]. Big data has been an imperative force that must be properly utilized and grasped but not only a modern reality for biomedical scientists in the pursuit of new knowledge [22].

As a result, this chapter addresses how CI and big data could be used to handle and combat COVID-19 pandemic by improving traditional public health ways to regulate, monitor, and detect infected people, hence reducing the health impact of the outbreak. The chapter is arranged as follows: Section 2.2 presents the applications of CI in modern days in helping the reduction of COVID-19 outbreak. Section 2.3 presents applications of BDAs during this pandemic. Section 2.4 discusses the problems and challenges of using CI and BDA in fighting the infectious outbreak. Section 2.5 presents the practical applications of CI during COVID-19 pandemic for the classification of the disease and finally the conclusion is presented in Section 2.6.

2.2 Applicability of computational intelligence in combating COVID-19 pandemic

The technological innovations have really helped the healthcare professionals all through this truculence health challenges to monitor the spread of COVID-19 pandemic. CI with enabled BDAs can be used for real-time monitoring of infected patients and helped to classify high-risk patients, which has helped to promptly monitor the spread of this pandemic. Based on thorough examination, CI can use to predict mortality risk by the physicians. Through mass screening, medical support, warnings, and suggestions about how to manage diseases, CI enabled with BDAs aids in the fight against epidemics [23,24]. As a dependable medical procedure, this innovation can be used to produce drugs and vaccines to treat infected patients and be used to report the performance of these intervention programs.

In 1994, Bezdek formally defined that CI [25,26] has a computationally intelligent system if it deals with data at basic level like in the case of image pixels and does not use prior information that have been generated. Pattern recognition is one of such examples of such computational intelligent system that did not use prior information to generate result using CI model. AI is one of the branches of CI according to Bezdek's description. In the real sense, both AI and CI target the realization of general intelligence in real-world models. The authors in [27] explained the distinction in both AI and CI by suggesting that hard computing technologies are made of the former, whereas soft computing technologies are made of the latter.

We may therefore assume that there are two forms of machine intelligence: (1) CI, defined by the hard-computing principle, and (2) AI developed by the soft-computing theory. Compared to hard-computing-based CI, the advantages of the soft-computing concept allow AI to adapt to several different conditions. The hard computing models are built using Boolean logic that is based on true or false values. The main challenge of this method is that it cannot be interpreted easily in natural language problems. The ambiguous cases are fully taken care of with soft computing models using fuzzy logic. One patented feature of CI is this form of logic that approximated the human brain through the aggregation of data into partial facts [27].

CI focuses on problems that, in theory, only individuals and animals can solve and require intellect. It is a branch of computer science without operational computational algorithms, which involve only intelligence to study and solve any challenges. It studies problems for which no operational computational algorithms exist. The CI allows the addition of new ideas through time and serves as patronage of other existing algorithms like AI [27–29]. The use of CI methods has resulted in a higher level of focus in the research community. Machine learning algorithms, as stated in a number of recent studies, provide superior detection accuracy when compared to various data classification techniques [30]. Due to its suitability in precaution programming, the model achieved and resulted in great prediction models. The accuracy of forecasting can vary depending on the approaches used by various research systems. As a result, identifying equipment capable of providing extremely accurate diagnosis and tracking for the outbreaks and outbursts are critical. CI approaches are the most effective policymaking strategies for dealing with real-world and systemic issues. The goal is to see how different CI techniques perform when it comes to categorizing COVID-19 samples. The performance of CI techniques has been evaluated using a variety of categorization performance abilities. The following are five regularly used CI models: artificial neural network (ANN) for classification, *K*-nearest neighbor, support vector machine (SVM), linear regression, and multilayer perceptron.

In the classification of diabetes proteins, machine learning has already been used as an instance in biological sector [31,32], and in the prediction of diabetes and heart disease [33]. The ANN, fuzzy logic, *K*-mean, SVM are some of the best classifiers used in this reaction [34]. The fuzzy logic classifier approach is an alternate form of CI methodology that scholars have used to categorize COVID-19 situations [35]. In [35], the authors propose a classification model for calculating and projecting the occurrences of COVID-19 outbreak for a period of 10 days based on previously documented cases in China. The suggested framework is an enriched adaptive neuro-fuzzy inference system (ANFIS) with flower pollination algorithm using the Salp swarm algorithm model. The rate of misclassified instances with contradiction was used to measure the accuracy of their studies, and by using other performance metrics like determination coefficient (R^2), computational time, MAPE, and RMSRE, and perform reasonably better than the existing methods. Furthermore, the suggested methodology makes use of two independent datasets of weekly influenza cases reported in two countries, namely the United States and China. The outcomes revealed much better performance.

In order to properly predict COVID-19 outbreak, various models have been developed to extract information from several biomedical datasets by several researchers. In [36], the authors proposed an ANFIS to evaluate and model time-series difficulties, and it has had a lot of success in recent applications. It has the ability to evaluate nonlinearity in time series data and incorporates features from various algorithms like fuzzy logic, random forest, SVM, and ANN among others. It has been utilized in a variety of prediction applications. In systematic tasks such as thinking, identifying, and accomplishing challenging tasks, CI has the ability to duplicate human intelligence utilizing both computer hardware and software. Because individual intelligence is multidimensional, CI may accomplish tasks such as knowledge representation, language understanding, and intellectual acquisition.

To date, the use of CI approaches to detect new behavior and identify future potential has yielded positive outcomes in a variety of commercial and tourism situations. Recent current methods, such as machine learning and ANN algorithms, have demonstrated promising results in the extraction of nonlinear dynamic patterns from a large dataset. The monitor of rodent reservoirs of zoonotic diseases recently using CI methods within a disease-related framework has been proved useful and provided accuracy results [37]. Extended-spectrum-lactamase-producing species [38], as well as tuberculosis (TB) and gonorrhea outbreaks [39] have been predicted. It is difficult to predict how people will react to infectious diseases. However, with the availability of big data and the introduction of CI approaches, dangerous diseases have been gradually compared to population behavior. Data science and psychosocial informatics have been in use for the prediction of the pandemic in recent time using huge data generated from IoT-based systems [40,41]. In this era of COVID-19 outbreak, search engine data was used to correlate infection control epidemics with digital activity trends (such as Google Trend). To actively monitor the effects of COVID-19 outbreak [42], CI technologies have been used as an analytic tool to improve our ability to actively track social interactions and accurately forecast the spread.

CI is a cutting-edge technology that helps in combating COVID-19 outbreak globally and reduces the spread of the pandemic by monitoring the infected patients. This advancement aids in the improved scanning, monitoring, and forecasting of existing and potential patients. The most important aspect of CI is to identify and diagnose the infection as soon as possible. A CI can be used to make medicines and vaccines, as well as to relieve medical workers stress. The major two types of CI algorithms are supervised and unsupervised learning, and the method incorporating a feature from the training samples through learning. ANN, random forest, SVM, decision tree, naïve Bayes, ANN, bootstrap aggregating, and AdaBoost are examples of supervised learning [43].

All these methods could be useful in determining diagnosis accuracy and prescribing appropriate COVID-19 treatment for infected patients. Predictive results from these methodologies, in particular, might be utilized to inform authorities and the public ahead of time and offer appropriate models and strategies. Unsupervised learning methodologies like principal component analysis (PCA) help scientists to pinpoint some of the primary causes of COVID-19 outbreak within a geographical area [44]. Unsupervised learning like as *K*-means may be used to categorize COVID-19 victims and identify questionable cases, allowing scientists to focus on these medical conditions. Latent Dirichlet Allocation one of the leading models can also be used for feature selection from medical data. Deep learning models have recently been used in medical sectors in areas like prediction, social network filtering, diagnosis, and computational biology and are thought to be excellent tools for assessing infectious diseases. CI can quickly examine aberrant symptoms and other "obvious indications" and inform patients and medical personnel [45,46]. It allows for faster and more cost-effective policymaking. It tends to assist in the establishment of new therapy and monitoring of the outbreak instances through useful strategies. CI aids in the diagnosis of highly contagious cases using modern medical technologies like automated medical scanners, computed tomography (CT), and magnetic resonance imaging.

CI will provide critical information that will help reduce the risk of this outbreak through the use of background knowledge. It could be used to predict possible outbreak sites, disease propagation, and the need for locations and healthcare providers during the pandemic. CI is important for the future detection of infections and illnesses by using previously trained data over data available at numerous periods. It outlines the characteristics, causes, and conditions that have caused infection to spread. In the future, this will be a promising strategy for combating additional epidemics and infectious diseases. It can be used to take preventative measures and to treat a variety of ailments. CI has the potential to make healthcare more transparent and responsive in the future.

CI will develop a sophisticated system to track and forecast the outbreak's spread automatically [34,35,47]. A genetic algorithm could also be developed to erase the infection's esthetic traits. It has the ability to deliver daily alerts to patients as well as enhanced COVID-19 pandemic follow-up options. CI can readily detect the virus's amount of transmission by distinguishing pieces and "hot areas," as well as track and monitor the persons' interactions. It has the ability to anticipate how the disease will progress in the future and whether it will return. The social media with other broadcasting channels can be used to monitor and predict the spread of and pandemic based on existing data, as well as the outbreak's dangers and the number of infected cases with the nature of fatalities in a particular location. CI will aid in the identification of the most affected places, citizens, and communities, as well as the implementation of effective solutions.

CI can be utilized for drug screening based on existing COVID-19 dataset. It is suitable for the production and development of pharmaceuticals. This discovery allows for real-time drug screening, whereas normal screening takes a considerable time, resulting in substantially better results than a person could accomplish [48]. It can be used to find effective vaccine for the treatment of the outbreak globally, and a valuable method for classification and prediction of pandemic and speedy production of vaccines [49]. CI speeds up the manufacture of vaccines and medicines, and it is also useful in clinical trials while vaccines are being developed.

Healthcare workers are overworked as a result of the increase in the spread of the outbreak and increase in number of infected cases; thus the workload of these workers can be reduced using CI models [50–52]. This model can be used for earlier diagnosis, monitoring, prediction, management for better decision-making and provides level playground for both health professionals and their students [53,54]. CI has the potential to have a significant impact on clinical outcomes as well as address additional future issues, easing the burden on clinicians.

2.3 Big data and analytics in battling COVID-19 outbreak

Big data has impacted all areas of people's lives in the twenty-first century, particularly the healthcare industries, which include genetics and medicine [19,55]. The use of electronic health records (EHR) that replace the paper health reports has resulted in data growth [56]. To take evidence-based actions, big data provides incentive and insight for specialist, epidemiologists, and physicians, which resulted in patient safety [57]. In the present era, numerous technologies such as IoT devices and sensors contribute significantly to the tremendous expansion of big data. Current developments in computation, storage, and connection of various devices have resulted in massive datasets. This extracted useful information from the big data generated from the connected devices are used for the benefits of government, industry, science, and society.

The adoption of various IoT-based devices and sensors has increased the number of data collected and yields a huge amount of healthcare [58]. These sensors and devices will be used to generate over 847 zettabytes (ZB) of data by 2021 based on Cisco recent report [59,60]. Conventional methods cannot process, collect, or regulate this kind of data. Hence, the analysis of such data requires BDAs for huge datasets with various kinds of data [61]. In order to identify hidden patterns, latent relationships, market dynamics, consumer demands, and other critical business information BDA are very necessary [62]. The ability to scrutinize this data can assist a company in dealing with significant information that could have a negative influence on the organization [63].

Hence, BDA's main purpose is to help industrial organizations improve their data interpretation and, as a result, make better and more informed judgments. BDA enables research and specialists to examine such data that is normally not possible to analyze using traditional approaches [62]. BDA is a technique that transforms structure and unstructured data into a more intelligible one for investigative purposes. These computational approaches' algorithms must recognize shapes, patterns, and relationships in data across several time horizons [64]. The results of the findings from BDA are presented using tables, three-dimensional maps, and charts to aid decision-making.

The process of big data implementation becomes difficult in some application due to the problem of scalability in the operation of some of these systems, and the data is sophisticated in core operations of these systems [65]. The critical issues in big data analysis are to obtain meaningful information from huge data that will necessitate flexible investigative procedures and methods to report timely results. Since the conventional techniques are not suitable for big data processes compared with BDA in gain, an insight into the big data is predicted for meaningful results [66]. As a result, to accommodate parallel data processing, all-encompassing networks and modern technologies are required. Furthermore, complex data streams from various data sources have several arrangements required analytics models to get better and understandable results from such data [67]. As a result, the existing processing models are not efficient based on the problem of inefficiency arise during computing processes [68]. Figure 2.1 depicts the framework for big data–enabled CI for COVID-19 outbreak.

Although only a few programs can manage big data volumes in a short processing period, customers receive input and advice from BDA systems in a long time [69]. The best of the best systems, on the other hand, cope with huge amounts of data and data complexity using a complicated trial-and-error process [70]. One of the big data graphic analytics is the investigative data examination used to process large datasets collected from an earth structural model [71]. Because the volume of big data is so large, traditional database management applications cannot be used to collect and analyze it. Modern warehouse databases, like as Apache Hadoop, provide the resolution by allowing for the analysis of distributed data.

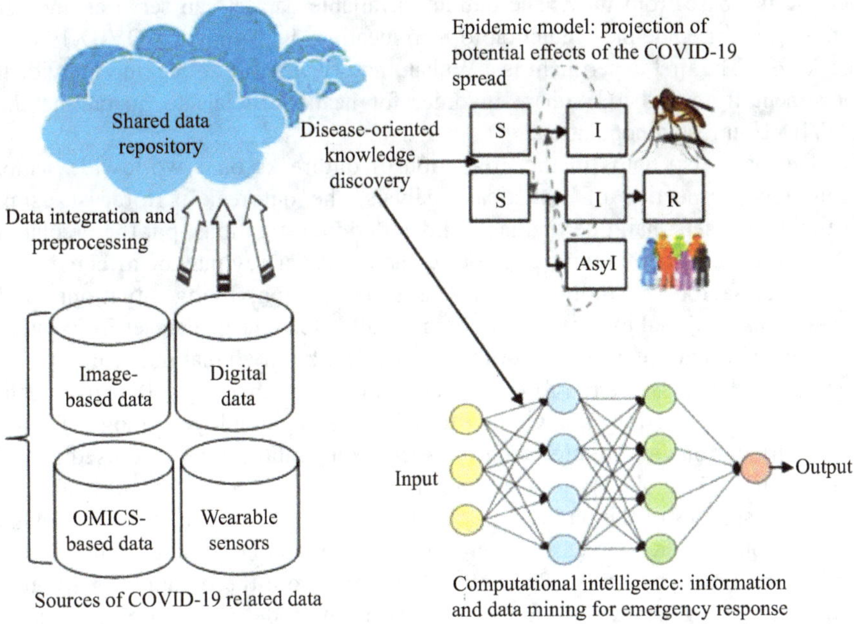

Figure 2.1 COVID-19 pandemic: an integrated big data conceptual model

In the fight against COVID-19 outbreak, big data has played significant roles and shown to be a powerful tool in this direction [72,73]. Big data in combination with BDA have shown to be very useful and creating an intriguing possibilities for fighting this outbreak. The use of these concepts can aid monitoring the spread of this pandemic and is useful in the areas of treatment, vaccine development, monitoring on infected patient, among others [74]. For example, combining coronavirus data streams with AI-based models can be used to create simulation models for epidemic estimation. This will allow health officials to follow the coronavirus's progress and better plan for preventive measures [75]. Big data models, with its ability to aggregate data and use enormous volumes of data for early detection, further boost the potential COVID-19 disease prediction. Large-scale COVID-19 studies can also be used with BDA using data from real-world sources like infected patients to build high-reliability, robust treatment strategies [76,77]. The healthcare providers will have a better understanding of the virus' progression using the BDA for the huge data processing and allow them to respond more effectively to various diagnoses and therapies.

In the control and monitoring of COVID-19 outbreak, big data plays a critical role because of its ability to provide a huge amount of data for predicting outbreaks. Like the case in [78] study, using the big data records from the outbreak in Italy used to assess the likelihood for outbreaks is critical for the formulation of efficient disease management efforts. Rather than utilizing a basic and deterministic human-transmission-based model, the scientists built more sophisticated models that may appropriately define pandemic dynamics utilizing data provided by the civil defense database from Italy. The publicly available dataset can serve as another data source for epidemic prediction to map localities with similar COVID-19 outbreak [79]. The first experiment is a Wuhan inquiry targeted at tracking individual movement from and to Wuhan, in order for health officials to quarantine the COVID-19-infected population.

Big data also helps in the prediction of outbreaks on a worldwide scale. From the perspective of statistical analysis, the outbreak is forecast using available datasets that, due to a lack of detailed investigations, put the precision of the fit for accurate prediction under question. Accuracy may be affected by a variety of factors, including illness cases, population, living situations, and ecosystems. Inspired by this, researchers in [80] used a large dataset from many locations and nations to estimate the pandemic like in China and Korea using logistic model to assess the forecasts' credibility. Another study [81] used data generated from South Korea, China, Italy, and Iran by employed Google Trends to acquire coronavirus-related data. Five environmental regions are used as the data textual: (1) globally, to ascertain the global interest of the outbreak; (2) China the sources of the outbreak; (3) South Korea; (4) Italy; and (5) Iran. This aggregation of data sources will help visualize the pattern of the outbreak and predict the future outbreak. The outbreak reports from these countries are also gathered and evaluated using a data optimization model targeted at accurately predicting everyday cases of coronavirus infection as well as potentially long-term epidemic forecasts [82].

In [83], datasets collected from confirmed, death, and recovered cases of all countries from the John Hopkins University repository were used for prediction model using ML algorithm. The research was for short-term intervals of 2 weeks in India. The proposed data analytic can be extended to create larger model for long-term prediction to estimate the outbreak theoretically. Meanwhile, the American large-scale datasets were used for the purpose of prediction in the United States using data analytical approach for a proper investigation of the outbreak [84]. The main aim of the analysis is to improve the accuracy of the future estimation for any likely pandemic-like coronaviruses, and fitting the prediction errors in order to refine the model.

Big data has been used in the monitoring of COVID-19 spread in order to help the healthcare sectors and government to successfully manage the spread of the pandemic [75,85]. This has also been used to facilitate the tracking of the COVID-19 distribution with a variety of newly emerging solutions. For example, the study in [86] proposed the use of BDA model to track the pandemic spread from the huge generated data from the outbreak. The China National Health Commission provided a large dataset of 854,424 flight travelers that flew from Wuhan Airport with 55 airlines to various parts of the 49 cities in China between December 2019 and January 2020. Using predicted factors such as the local inhabitants and air travelers to measure the variance of recorded cases in China cities, a multiple linear model is constructed. More precisely, the authors used a Spearman correlation analysis with the number of 49 reported cases from Wuhan using travelers' traffic for a period of time. The results of the finding have shown a high correlation between the population and the infection cases within the cities in China. In [87], the Geographic Information Systems (GIS) was used with big data for spatial analysis to promote heterogeneous data integration from healthcare data tools like the data from the patients, patients, clinical laboratories, and the public.

Jin *et al.* [88] provided a detailed guide with valuable methods for the treatment and diagnosis of COVID-19. The techniques of the guiding principle, biological aspects, disease prevention, diagnosis, and COVID-19 disease care are all included in this document. From the 11,500 people tested by Zhongnan Hospital of Wuhan University as a pilot trial, 276 were discovered as potentially infected casualties, with 170 being diagnosed. A huge set of dataset has been investigated using clinical tests, including CT/X-ray imaging, CT/X-ray imaging in response to pathogen detection in the respiratory tract, and manifestations to hematological analysis.

The development of vaccine is very paramount in the prevention of individuals from the burden of infectious diseases and pandemic. In the identification of better vaccine for the treatment of COVID-19 outbreak, big data plays prominent roles. The use of this huge data within this short time has really helped in the production of suitable vaccine for COVID-19 outbreak globally. The use of GISAID database in the work of [89] has aided in the removing residues amino acids. The goal of research is to find effective opportunities for the growth of vaccines and medications to combat the COVID-19 pandemic. Another vaccine research initiative by [90] compares the spike proteins in SARS-CoV, MERS-CoV, and SARS-CoV-2 with other coronavirus strains in four humans previously isolated. This research will aid in the essential screening of the SARS-CoV-2 spike sequence and structure, which could aid in the development of an effective vaccine.

In the production of drugs manufacturing models to battle COVID-19 pandemic, big data has played prominent roles. For instance, [91] proposed a molecular docking-based solution for drug research in fighting COVID-19 outbreak. The first screening involved more than 2,500 small molecules and was validated through the use of Glide molecular docking software in the FDA-approved drug database. In the experiment, 15 of the 25 verified medicines exhibited considerable inhibitory properties. The drug formulation toward COVID-19 is triggered by the inhibitory incremental change and chronic inflammation. In addition, the authors in [92] used big data to develop a drug repositioning strategy to combat the COVID-19 epidemic. For the development of COVID-19 vaccines, the authors use ML to incorporate both the information graph and the literature.

In addition, reverse vaccinology and immunological computer science can be employed to produce vaccines for the global COVID-19 outbreak [93]. The National Center for Biotechnology Information's online database selected SARS-CoV-2 strain to analyze various entries while Immune Epitope Database online epitope was utilized for B-cell and T-cell prediction. To classify the possible vaccine constructions from the produced dataset, a number of procedures may be required, including immunogenicity, genotoxicity, and biophysical features of products. The National Center for Biotechnology Knowledge for Promoting the Manufacture of Vaccines [94] has also acquired a large dataset. Different peptides have been suggested for the two-step production of a new COVID-19 vaccine. To begin, the entire genome of COVID-19 was examined using a comparative genomic method to identify the most likely antigenic target.

2.4 The limitations of using big data and computational intelligence to fight the COVID-19 pandemic

COVID-19 and other infectious illnesses have the potential to benefit from CI. In contrast, the benefits of AI interventions will take time to manifest because AI systems are still in their infancy [95]. In its study of the use of CI toward COVID-19, the authors in [96] stated that just a few of the CI programs studied are operationally mature at this moment. For efficient prediction, CI needs a large amount of data; however, in a circumstance when the data is scarce, the model's overall performance will be limited. To train CI and AI models, there are (yet) insufficient public data and open datasets relevant to the COVID-19 pandemic. Other potential obstacles include non-adjustment procedures, big data arrogance, a torrent of scientific results, and external data that must be swapped for a better CI model.

After the outbreak is gone, the key concerns are issues of data protection for the general public to ensure that the data collected is not used for other purposes by policy-makers, and the degradation is not pushed back in the fight against the COVID-19 pandemic. Though coronavirus diseases could be practically eradicated, as predicted by the authors in [97], some data-hungry governments may claim that biometric tracking techniques must be kept in place in order to prepare for another pandemic outbreak, or second wave of COVID-19-related diseases, as we have seen in India and other Asian nations. An instance of another outbreak of Ebola in the central region of Africa requires the emerging of using modern tracking mechanisms to be put in place for any emergency. CI-based radiological innovation has been considerably adopted by several Chinese clinics, and the promise of CI-based models' complete adoption magically reappears. Radiologists have highlighted concerns about a dearth of data for training CI-based models, and the bulk of the outbreak samples accessible from country medical institutes does not include sample preference. The use of CT scans and X-rays has the tendency to escalate infection and contaminate the instruments.

The use of crowded social platforms, big data hubris, and outlier data are still not reliable and valid due to a lack of evidence, and technological challenges in COVID-19 outbreak forecasting [98]. CI techniques are not used in the bulk of monitoring and forecasting frameworks currently in use. Rather, most analysts consider SIR models, which are epidemiologically validated models. The use of immunological SIR model for instance has been adopted by Robert Koch Institute in Berlin that includes government controls like curfews, sterilization, and social disassociating advice. This approach was created in China to demonstrate that isolation might lower the rate of incidence below the catastrophic value [99]. Table 2.1 summarizes the CI issues in the COVID-19 epidemic.

Table 2.1 Computational intelligence limitations

S. no.	Issues in the use of CI	Explanations
1	It necessitates competent monitoring	It is devoid of any further details, such as a person, to depict the exact outcome. It necessitates meticulous data collection and monitoring; alternatively, professionals and physicians will be unable to produce accurate results
2	Not allowing for creative thought	Only exact data will provide adequate enactment. Human critical judgment is not taken into consideration employing the model, which cannot fit the COVID-19 definition of innovative thinking as a human being does. This model does not give room for latest decisions to be made in the absence of data
3	It only learns from the facts it is given	CI always works with the information provided by the patient. The information gathered is used to create a precise COVID-19 diagnosis and forecast
4	Important for the AI algorithm's treatment	The approximation used by CI model is a drawback in the accuracy percentage, a critical measure for proper care and more so. Predictions could include whether a CI's function is absolute or if more data and training are necessary over time
5	Does not comprehend the human feeling	CI methods to decision-making do not take into consideration human emotions, reasoning, or motivations. CI's models do exactly what they are intended to do

The present pandemic has brought serious challenges because it can spread quickly with human interaction and among people traveling internationally; thus there is total ban on inter-traveling among several nations [100,101]. Due to these, foreign visitors are forced to supply their full details like personal information, travel history, reason for their visiting, and place of residence, and most importantly there is imposed quarantine restriction globally [102]. The Chinese media secretly published visitors secret information is an example of such cases; this explains that the importance of visitor information can cause dispute-of-law in any nation. (1) The important and distinct definitions of right to personal data have been clearly defined by the EU, United States, and China; (2) the growth to centralized approach to relevant laws by these three nations points to the fact that healthcare privacy law is to be a contractual law; and (3) the de-Americanization is aggressively advocated for and has important data privacy laws. This added to how international information regulation is being applied or the patterns and methods of administration of the privacy data laws [1,70].

In the making of CI-based model and BDA, the lack of standard datasets poses a significant challenge for their use in combating the COVID-19 pandemic. Various CI models using huge datasets have been discussed in this literature, but none have been assessed using the same dataset. Thus, to draw conclusion becomes difficult due to the use of two datasets with different quantities of samples for COVID-19 outbreak prediction and detection. In comparison, the majority of datasets in the literature were created as a result of individual efforts, such as when writers acquire information on the Internet then combine them to form their own dataset and test the methods they suggest. Healthcare organization like WHO and CDC plays important roles in resolving this issue as well as the governments, and large since they have accessed to high-quality and massive datasets. Medical data like X-ray and CT scans can be obtained from hospitals, reports from self-diagnosis applications, satellite data, and personal information.

The CORD-19 dataset is being managed by various collaborators with the original owner Georgetown Security Center like Microsoft Research, Chan Zuckerberg Initiative, Allen Institute for AI, and National Institutes of Health [103]. Also, in China, Alibaba DAMO Academy has partnered with various hospitals to create AI-based models for COVID-19 case prediction and identification, and more than 5,000 instances of COVID-19 have been reported, and hospitals are responsible for delivering CT scans. As recorded in [104] thanks to its remarkable performance, this device has been used by more than 20 hospitals in China: 96% accuracy in just 20 s. Data scientists encounter numerous challenges when working with big data. One challenge is compiling, integrating, and storing big data derived from various sources [64,65]. Another vital problem is the administration and application of this generated data in healthcare systems. To maximize the effectiveness of big data in utilization in medical case required the use of a reliable BDA like CI model to facilitate the perception of a dependable data. BDA is built on the foundation of good data management.

The utilization of huge data generated from the use of various techniques like sensors, devices, and patients' symptoms using healthcare internal infrastructure is another difficulty in generating a reliable result from huge data [16]. The majority of the time, analyzing data generated within businesses, is insufficient. We need to take it a step further by linking both internal and external data together to get relevant information and knowledge. Third-party sources, market swings, weather forecasts and traffic problems, social network data, client feedback, and resident input are all examples of external data. The principle of participatory and incremental learning is being applied in big data and analytics. They address a range of difficulties that arise during data learning like resource constraints and data accessibility challenges, thus, resulted in obtaining useful information for a better decision-making in healthcare system. When iterative learning is applied to data, it leads to a faster way of predicting new data streams. When the drift notion is unavailable, the incremental algorithm is strongly suggested. On the other hand, using ensemble techniques to produce reliable results with a big drift notion is highly suggested.

Another key issue is analogical thinking, which is intrinsically unreliable when it comes to disease predictions. In big data and CI, there is always an underlying assumption that their applications in various fields create complicated simulation models that sidestep the need to acquire fundamental epidemiological details. Nonetheless, a trustworthy fact on the scenario counts and the biotic processes that underlie a pandemic for evolving COVID-19 outbreaks, let alone the behavioral reactions of infected individuals, is still lacking, making it harder to alter or comprehend precise complicated prototypes on spatiotemporal scales relevant to decision-making. Due to the requirement for versatile modules that enable quick reactions in light of the high degree of controversy surrounding emergency situations, it is hoped that the most effective systems would stay basic [105]. According to epidemiological studies, simple models are easier to be understood, expressed, and interpreted than complex one, especially in healthcare system [106].

A lack of a clear message risks two undesirable outcomes since most politicians lack in-depth modeling experience. Thinking that without skepticism and options, the technique would be misguided, or ignoring and there is no proof that we must control epidemics as effectively and feasible. During epidemics, choices must be taken rapidly and piecemeal, and erroneous data models may be effective tools for doing so. In light of the aforementioned challenges, computational power of CI model can be utilized to steadily improve the power of big data in healthcare system. These will provide genuine bravery for improved monitoring and bring about some beneficial prediction systems [107,108].

The use of BDA and CI models with information-sharing platforms is being used to protect personal data security and privacy [109]. Rapid data transmission and communication among geographically distributed responder teams are enabled via an Internet connection. Methodologically, effective modeling solutions that incorporate diverse predictions to reduce uncertainty are being created [110]. An innovative, collaborative approach has emerged in response to the outbreak of COVID-19 across academic organizations: for example, using Twitter and other channels to communicate, assess, and openly debate the consequences of new research as it emerges. Ironically, during a crisis, controlling the misinformation that is already circulating on social media is likely to become one of the most pressing problems for restricting the epidemic.

These technologies will remain dislocated and unworkable unless the aforementioned issues are rectified. It appears that all three problems may be aided by directing the majority of funds and knowledge to the communities most vulnerable to epidemics. Methodologically, effective modeling solutions that incorporate diverse predictions to reduce uncertainty are being created. Using modern big data technologies, nimble, distributed groups of people will be required to cover the systematic and functional components of the epidemic response. To complement and explain the restricted availability of socio-geographical data needed to track the progress of significant forecasts. The methods can be used to forecast the current pandemic so that the policy-makers can plan ahead of another similar outbreak or epidemic of this kind. The combination of both BDA and CI models can be troublesome if the available data for modeling is very small since CI model depends meanly on a huge amount of data to be able to diagnosed, predicted, and classifier efficiently and properly.

The fulfillment of these methods in healthcare systems significantly depends on serious investment on training, development of relevant models that can be used to tackle any infectious diseases. Furthermore, there should constant release of fund to fill the critical gap in analytics process, especially in the developing nation. The social media sites, X-ray images, scanning images, phones recordings among others can be a source of generating big data in medical systems with public available data [111], and their text or video can be used in a variety of ways. In the context of COVID-19 outbreak, big data can inform of generated information about the epidemic locations, medical records, infected case history, scanned and X-ray images among others. Big data and analytics have been proving useful in fighting against COVID-19 pandemic [73].

2.5 The practical case of using computational intelligence in fighting COVID-19 pandemic

Data collection and synthesis on the CXR images of COVID-19 dataset are used for the study. The conversion of RGB image into grayscale images was done using image-processing techniques. The feature textual descriptor was performed using a histogram of oriented gradient (HOG) [112,113], and PCA was used for feature selection [114]. The suggested methodology for identifying and classifying COVID-19 includes a train test split of the data, as well as performance evaluation. The proposed model was used for the classification of frontal CXR pictures into COVID-19 infected, and pulmonary tuberculosis (PTB) disorders. Figure 2.2 depicts a four-phased approach.

The dataset from frontal CXR image was used in the chapter for the purpose of classifiers of the dataset into COVID-19 and PTB illness and was obtained from [115] with the sample sizes of 527, 406, and 394 for COVID-19, NORMAL, and PTB, respectively. The feature extraction approach is used to remove linguistic information from the dataset because it is an image (HOG). These lungs were employed in the data categorization experiment. There are presently 1,327 frontal CXR pictures in the collection, separated into three classification classes. The test

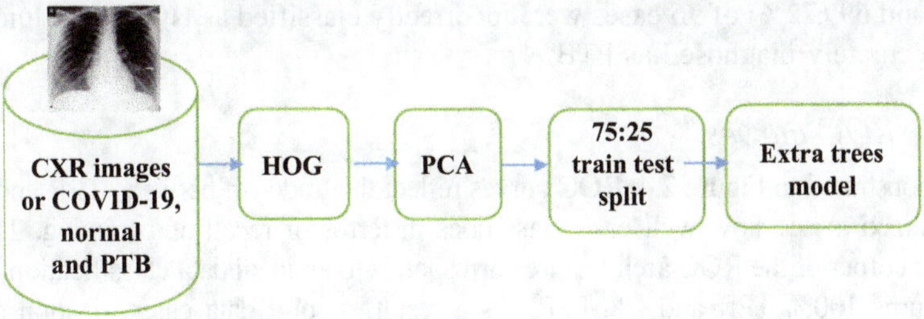

Figure 2.2 The workflow of the framework

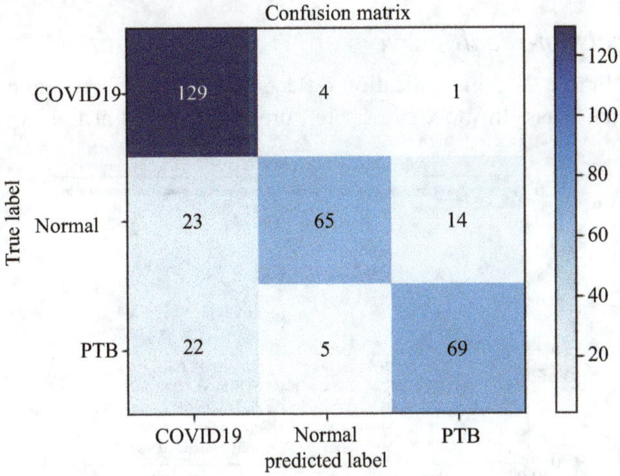

Figure 2.3 Confusion matrix for ET model

result was based on the split set, which represents 25% of the entire dataset because the dataset was split. This experiment was done out on a Windows computer operating systems running on an Intel Core i3-4200 CPU at 2.50–2.70 GHz and 4 GB RAM, with R-programming language for executing the programming code. The Extra Trees algorithm yielded a result of 79.22% accuracy, 81.00% precision, 79.00% recall, and 79.02% $F1$-score. The best features from the generated HOG features were chosen using the PCA technique, resulting in a better outcome.

2.5.1 Confusion matrix

The performance of each class is depicted in the confusion matrix in Figure 2.3. Out of 134 cases of COVID-19 disease, 129 (96%) were accurately recognized as COVID-19 disease, 4 (3%) as NORMAL, and 1 (1%) as PTB disease. In the case of NORMAL lungs, 65 (64%) of the 102 cases were accurately classified as NORMAL, 23 (23%) as COVID-19, and 14 (14%) as PTB. Furthermore, 22 (23%) of PTB patients were improperly classified as COVID-19, 5 (5%) as NORMAL lungs, and 69 (72%) of 96 cases were incorrectly classified as NORMAL lungs but were accurately diagnosed as PTB.

2.5.2 ROC curves

As demonstrated in Figure 2.4, ROC curves reflect the trade-off between TPR and FPR. It is utilized to see how well each class does in terms of recall and training. The top leftmost corner of the ROC architecture corresponds to an ideal data classification model that returns 100% TPR and 0% FPR. As a result, a solid data categorization should produce a point in the ROC layout's upper left corner [113]. The ROC values are all close to one, suggesting exceptional classification performance. The COVID-19 ROC value for Class is 95.02%, NORMAL is 92.24%, and PTB is 90%.

2.5.3 Precision-recall curve

As shown in Figure 2.5, this indication reflects the trade-off between precision and recalls for each class. In most cases, high precision comes at the expense of low

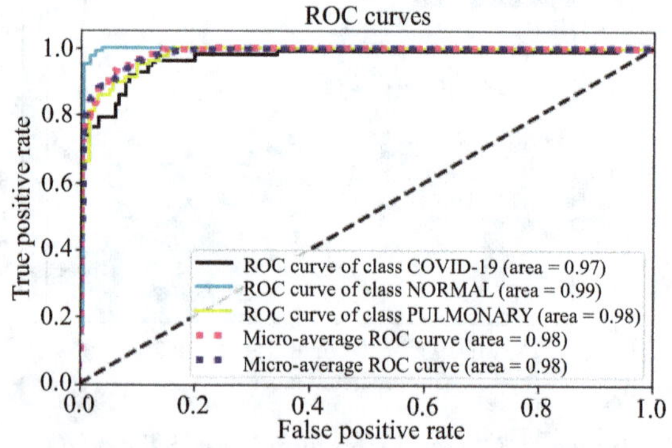

Figure 2.4 ROC curve for ET model

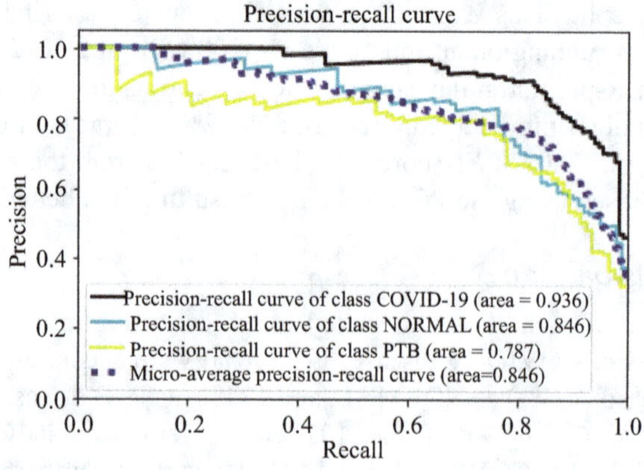

Figure 2.5 ET model precision-recall curve (PRC)

recall, or vice versa. A good data categorization model should be able to keep both precision and recall high [113]. Class has a COVID-19 PRC value of 0.936, NORMAL of 0.846, and PTB of 0.787.

2.6 Conclusion

COVID-19 is a one-of-a-kind coronavirus from the pneumonia family. It is vital to have a reliable method for detecting COVID-19 in infected patients, and CI has proven to be effective. This chapter looked at various recent COVID-19 control strategies that used CI. The majority of the studies we looked at focused on COVID-19 pandemic diagnosis, prediction, and monitoring, as well as image classification with CXR images and CTs for COVID-19 outbreak. While the bulk of the recent studies employed either machine learning/deep learning to extract and choose features, a handful of them combined the two approaches by using ML to extract and select features and DL for classification and prediction. There has been effort to improve the accuracy of CI algorithms, there are still CI-based diagnostic methods that yield positive results, but still there is no readymade answer in this direction. The system developed using CI models has been proved useful in monitoring, diagnosis, and prediction of COVID-19 outbreak in developed nations. The model works on the provided data that is related to COVID-19 signs and symptoms. The models that this has improved have seriously helped physicians in dealing with infected patients and the control of the spread of COVID-19 pandemic globally. This helps in early diagnosis of COVID-19 patients, vaccine development, and the monitoring of isolated patients. Therefore, the use of BDA and CI algorithms has really help in the diagnosis, prediction, classification, and treatment during this outbreak. Though the use of BDA and CI models has not be fully integrated to really combat infectious diseases, its use can never be overemphasized and played substantial role in the development of vaccines for the treatment of any infectious disease. The findings of this chapter show that BDA and CI algorithms place prominent roles in fighting COVID-19 pandemic globally, and their direct application can reduce the spread of this pandemic within nations.

References

[1] Lukman, A. F., Benedicta, A., Awotunde, J. B., *et al.* (2022). Robust statistical modeling of COVID-19 prevalence in African epicentres. *Studies in Systems, Decision and Control*, 366, 315–358.

[2] Dunford, D., Dale, B., Stylianou, N. L., Ahmed, M. and Arenas, IdlT, (2020). Coronavirus: the world in lockdown in maps and charts. *BBC News* (available at https://www.bbc.com/news/world-52103747).

[3] Awotunde, J. B., Jimoh, R. G., AbdulRaheem, M., Oladipo, I. D., Folorunso, S. O. and Ajamu, G. J. (2022). IoT-based wearable body sensor network for COVID-19 pandemic. In *Advances in Data Science and Intelligent Data Communication Technologies for COVID-19* (pp. 253–275). Cham: Springer.

[4] Guan, W. J., Ni, Z. Y., Hu, Y., *et al.* (2020). Clinical characteristics of coronavirus disease in 2019 in China. *New England Journal of Medicine*, 382(18), 1708–1720.

[5] Roy, S. and Chakraborty, C. (2021). Panic buying situation during COVID-19 global pandemic. *Journal of Information Technology Management*, 13(2), 231–244.

[6] Garg, L., Chakraborty, C., Mahmoudi, S. and Sohmen, V. S. (2021). Healthcare informatics for fighting COVID-19 and future pandemics. In *EAI/Springer Innovations in Communication and Computing*. Springer Nature. ISBN: 978-3-030-72751-2.

[7] Shelke, Y. and Chakraborty, C. (2020). Augmented reality and virtual reality transforming spinal imaging landscape: a feasibility study. *IEEE Computer Graphics and Applications*, 41(3), 124–138.

[8] Jang, S., Lee, S., Choi, S. M., Seo, J., Choi, H. and Yoon, T. (2016). Comparison between SARS CoV and MERS CoV using apriori algorithm, decision tree, SVM. In *MATEC Web of Conferences* (Vol. 49, p. 08001). EDP Sciences.

[9] Awotunde, J. B., Folorunso, S. O., Bhoi, A. K., Adebayo, P. O. and Ijaz, M. F. (2021). Disease diagnosis system for IoT-Based wearable body sensors with machine learning algorithm. In *Hybrid Artificial Intelligence and IoT in Healthcare* (pp. 201–222). Singapore: Springer.

[10] Brown, D. E., Abbasi, A. and Lau, R. Y. (2015). Predictive analytics: predictive modeling at the micro level. *IEEE Intelligent Systems*, 30(3), 6–8.

[11] Chakraborty, C. and Abougreen, A. N. (2021). Intelligent internet of things and advanced machine learning techniques for COVID-19. *EAI Endorsed Transactions on Pervasive Health and Technology*, 7(26), e1.

[12] Ahmed, M. B., Boudhir, A. A., Santos, D., El Aroussi, M. and Karas, İ. R. (Eds.). (2020). Innovations in smart cities application. In *The Proceedings of the 4th International Conference on Smart City Applications* (3rd ed.). Springer Nature.

[13] Rodgers, W. (2020). *Artificial Intelligence in a Throughput Model: Some Major Algorithms*. CRC Press.

[14] Priyanka, K. and Kulennavar, N. (2014). A survey on big data analytics in health care. *International Journal of Computer Science and Information Technologies*, 5(4), 5865–5868.

[15] Kruse, C. S., Goswamy, R., Raval, Y. J. and Marawi, S. (2016). Challenges and opportunities of big data in health care: a systematic review. *JMIR Medical Informatics*, 4(4), e38.

[16] Oussous, A., Benjelloun, F. Z., Lahcen, A. A. and Belfkih, S. (2018). Big data technologies: a survey. *Journal of King Saud University-Computer and Information Sciences*, 30(4), 431–448.

[17] Olaronke, I. and Oluwaseun, O. (2016, December). Big data in healthcare: prospects, challenges and resolutions. In *2016 Future Technologies Conference (FTC)* (pp. 1152–1157). IEEE.

[18] Dai, H. N., Wang, H., Xu, G., Wan, J. and Imran, M. (2020). Big data analytics for manufacturing Internet of Things: opportunities, challenges and enabling technologies. *Enterprise Information Systems*, 14(9–10), 1279–1303.

[19] Hulsen, T., Jamuar, S. S., Moody, A., *et al.* (2019). From big data to precision medicine. *Frontiers in Medicine*, 6, 34.

[20] Austin, C. and Kusumoto, F. (2016). The application of Big Data in medicine: current implications and future directions. *Journal of Interventional Cardiac Electrophysiology*, 47(1), 51–59.

[21] Galetsi, P., Katsaliaki, K. and Kumar, S. (2019). Values, challenges and future directions of big data analytics in healthcare: a systematic review. *Social Science & Medicine*, 241, 112533.

[22] Lacroix, P. (2019). Big data privacy and ethical challenges. In *Big Data, Big Challenges: A Healthcare Perspective* (pp. 101–111). Springer, Cham.

[23] Hu, Z., Ge, Q., Jin, L. and Xiong, M. (2020). Artificial intelligence forecasting of COVID-19 in China. arXiv preprint arXiv:2002.07112.

[24] Bai, H. X., Hsieh, B., Xiong, Z., *et al.* (2020). Performance of radiologists in differentiating COVID-19 from viral pneumonia on chest CT. *Radiology*.

[25] Zurada, J. M., Marks, R. J. and Robinson, C. J. (1994). *Computational Intelligence Imitating Life* (No. CONF-940699). Institute of Electrical and Electronics Engineers, Inc., New York, NY.

[26] Siddique, N. and Adeli, H. (2013). *Computational Intelligence: Synergies of Fuzzy Logic, Neural Networks and Evolutionary Computing*. John Wiley & Sons.

[27] Awotunde, J. B., Matiluko, O. E. and Fatai, O. W. (2014). Medical diagnosis system using fuzzy logic. *African Journal of Computing & ICT*, 7(2), 99–106.

[28] Ayo, F. E., Folorunso, S. O., Abayomi-Alli, A. A., Adekunle, A. O. and Awotunde, J. B. (2020). Network intrusion detection based on deep learning model optimized with rule-based hybrid feature selection. *Information Security Journal*, 29(6), 267–283.

[29] Ayo, F. E., Ogundokun, R. O., Awotunde, J. B., Adebiyi, M. O. and Adeniyi, A. E. (2020). Severe acne skin disease: a fuzzy-based method for diagnosis. In *Lecture Notes in Computer Science (including subseries Lecture Notes in Artificial Intelligence and Lecture Notes in Bioinformatics)* (Vol. 12254 LNCS, pp. 320–334). Cham: Springer.

[30] Oladele, T. O., Ogundokun, R. O., Awotunde, J. B., Adebiyi, M. O. and Adeniyi, J. K. (2020). Severe acne skin disease: a fuzzy-based method for diagnosis. In *Lecture Notes in Computer Science (including subseries Lecture Notes in Artificial Intelligence and Lecture Notes in Bioinformatics)* (Vol. 12254 LNCS, pp. 428–441). Cham: Springer.

[31] Kurd, Z., Kelly, T. and Austin, J. (2007). Developing artificial neural networks for safety-critical systems. *Neural Computing and Applications*, 16(1), 11–19.

[32] Berglund, E. and Sitte, J. (2006). The parameterless self-organizing map algorithm. *IEEE Transactions on Neural Networks*, 17(2), 305–316.

[33] Oladipo, I. D., Babatunde, A. O., Awotunde, J. B. and Abdulraheem, M. (2021). An improved hybridization in the diagnosis of diabetes mellitus using selected computational intelligence. In *Communications in Computer and Information Science* (Vol. 1350, pp. 272–285).

[34] Awotunde, J. B., Ayo, F. E., Jimoh, R. G., *et al.* (2020). Prediction and classification of diabetes mellitus using genomic data. In *Intelligent IoT Systems in Personalized Health Care* (pp. 235–292). London: Academic Press.

[35] Al-Qaness, M. A., Ewees, A. A., Fan, H. and Abd El Aziz, M. (2020). Optimization method for forecasting confirmed cases of COVID-19 in China. *Journal of Clinical Medicine*, 9(3), 674.

[36] Jang, J. S. (1993). ANFIS: adaptive-network-based fuzzy inference system. *IEEE Transactions on Systems, Man, and Cybernetics*, 23(3), 665–685.

[37] Han, B. A., Schmidt, J. P., Bowden, S. E. and Drake, J. M. (2015). Rodent reservoirs of future zoonotic diseases. *Proceedings of the National Academy of Sciences of the United States of America*, 112(22), 7039–7044.

[38] Goodman, K. E., Lessler, J., Cosgrove, S. E., *et al.* (2016). A clinical decision tree to predict whether a bacteremic patient is infected with an extended-spectrum β-lactamase-producing organism. *Clinical Infectious Diseases*, 63(7), 896–903.

[39] Wong, Z. S., Zhou, J. and Zhang, Q. (2019). Artificial intelligence for infectious disease big data analytics. *Infection, Disease & Health*, 24(1), 44–48.

[40] Mahroum, N., Adawi, M., Sharif, K., *et al.* (2018). Public reaction to Chikungunya outbreaks in Italy—insights from an extensive novel data streams-based structural equation modeling analysis. *PLoS One*, 13(5), e0197337.

[41] Bragazzi, N. L., Alicino, C., Trucchi, C., *et al.* (2017). Global reaction to the recent outbreaks of Zika virus: insights from a big data analysis. *PLoS One*, 12(9), e0185263.

[42] Sujata, D., Chinmay, C., Sourav, K. G. and Subhendu, K. P. (2021). Intelligent computing on time-series data analysis and prediction of COVID-19 pandemics, *Pattern Recognition Letters*, 151, 69–75, https://doi.org/10.1016/j.patrec.2021.07.027.

[43] Folorunso, S. O., Awotunde, J. B., Ayo, F. E., and Abdullah, K. K. A. (2021). RADIoT: the unifying framework for IoT, radiomics and deep learning modeling. In *Hybrid Artificial Intelligence and IoT in Healthcare* (p. 109–128). Singapore: Springer.

[44] Wang, Y., Fan, Y., Bhatt, P. and Davatzikos, C. (2010). High-dimensional pattern regression using machine learning: from medical images to continuous clinical variables. *NeuroImage*, 50(4), 1519–1535.

[45] Ai, T., Yang, Z., Hou, H., *et al.* (2020). Correlation of chest CT and RT-PCR testing for coronavirus disease 2019 (COVID-19) in China: a report of 1014 cases. *Radiology*, 296, E32–E40.

[46] Luo, H., Tang, Q. L., Shang, Y. X., *et al.* (2020). Can Chinese medicine be used for prevention of corona virus disease 2019 (COVID-19)? A review of historical classics, research evidence and current prevention programs. *Chinese Journal of Integrative Medicine*, 1–8.

[47] Muhammad, L. J., Algehyne, E. A., Usman, S. S., Ahmad, A., Chakraborty, C. and Mohammed, I. A. (2021). Supervised machine learning models for prediction of COVID-19 infection using epidemiology dataset. *SN Computer Science*, 2(1), 1–13.

[48] Haleem, A., Vaishya, R., Javaid, M. and Khan, I. H. (2020). Artificial intelligence (AI) applications in orthopaedics: an innovative technology to embrace. *Journal of Clinical Orthopaedics & Trauma*, 11, S80–S81.

[49] Bobdey, S. and Ray, S. (2020). Going viral – Covid-19 impact assessment: a perspective beyond clinical practice. *Journal of Marine Medical Society*, 22(1), 9.

[50] Gozes, O., Frid-Adar, M., Greenspan, H., *et al.* (2020). Rapid AI development cycle for the coronavirus (COVID-19) pandemic: initial results for automated detection & patient monitoring using deep learning CT image analysis. arXiv preprint arXiv:2003.05037.

[51] Pirouz, B., Shaffiee Haghshenas, S., Shaffiee Haghshenas, S. and Piro, P. (2020). Investigating a serious challenge in the sustainable development process: analysis of confirmed cases of COVID-19 (new type of coronavirus) through a binary classification using artificial intelligence and regression analysis. *Sustainability*, 12(6), 2427.

[52] Smeulders, A. W. and Van Ginneken, A. M. (1989). An analysis of pathology knowledge and decision making for the development of artificial intelligence-based consulting systems. *Analytical and Quantitative Cytology and Histology*, 11(3), 154–165.

[53] Hussain, A. and do Vale Moreira, N. C. (2020). Clinical considerations for patients with diabetes in times of COVID-19 pandemic. *Diabetes & Metabolic Syndrome*, 14(4), 451.

[54] Gupta, R., Ghosh, A., Singh, A. K. and Misra, A. (2020). Clinical considerations for patients with diabetes in times of COVID-19 epidemic. *Diabetes & Metabolic Syndrome*, 14(3), 211.

[55] Riba, M., Sala, C., Toniolo, D. and Tonon, G. (2019). Big data in medicine, the present and hopefully the future. *Frontiers in Medicine*, 6, 263.

[56] Dinh-Le, C., Chuang, R., Chokshi, S. and Mann, D. (2019). Wearable health technology and electronic health record integration: scoping review and future directions. *JMIR mHealth and uHealth*, 7(9), e12861.

[57] McCue, M. E. and McCoy, A. M. (2017). The scope of big data in one medicine: unprecedented opportunities and challenges. *Frontiers in Veterinary Science*, 4, 194.

[58] Tariq, N., Asim, M., Al-Obeidat, F., *et al.* (2019). The security of big data in fog-enabled IoT applications including blockchain: a survey. *Sensors*, 19(8), 1788.

[59] Adeniyi, E. A., Ogundokun, R. O. and Awotunde, J. B. (2021). IoMT-based wearable body sensors network healthcare monitoring system. In *IoT in Healthcare and Ambient Assisted Living* (pp. 103–121). Springer, Singapore.

[60] Hofdijk, J., Séroussi, B., Lovis, C., Sieverink, F., Ehrler, F. and Ugon, A. (2016). Transforming healthcare with the Internet of Things. In *Proceedings of the EFMI Special Topic Conference*.

[61] Mital, R., Coughlin, J. and Canaday, M. (2015). Using big data technologies and analytics to predict sensor anomalies. In *AMOS* (p. 84).

[62] Berman, E., Felter, J. H. and Shapiro, J. N. (2020). *Small Wars, Big Data: The Information Revolution in Modern Conflict*. Princeton University Press.

[63] Raghupathi, W. and Raghupathi, V. (2014). Big data analytics in healthcare: promise and potential. *Health Information Science and Systems*, 2(1), 3.

[64] Teijeiro, D., Pardo, X. C., González, P., Banga, J. R. and Doallo, R. (2018). Towards cloud-based parallel metaheuristics: a case study in computational biology with differential evolution and spark. *The International Journal of High Performance Computing Applications*, 32(5), 693–705.

[65] Candela, L., Castelli, D. and Pagano, P. (2012). Managing big data through hybrid data infrastructures. *ERCIM News*, 89, 37–38.

[66] Marjani, M., Nasaruddin, F., Gani, A., *et al.* (2017). Big IoT data analytics: architecture, opportunities, and open research challenges. *IEEE Access*, 5, 5247–5261.

[67] Assuncao, M. D., Calheiros, R. N., Bianchi, S., Netto, M. A. and Buyya, R. (2013). Big data computing and clouds: challenges, solutions, and future directions. arXiv preprint arXiv:1312.4722, 10.

[68] Hashem, I. A. T., Yaqoob, I., Anuar, N. B., Mokhtar, S., Gani, A. and Khan, S. U. (2015). The rise of "big data" on cloud computing: review and open research issues. *Information Systems*, 47, 98–115.

[69] Singh, D. and Reddy, C. K. (2015). A survey on platforms for big data analytics. *Journal of Big Data*, 2(1), 8.

[70] Awotunde, J. B., Folorunso, S. O., Jimoh, R. G., Adeniyi, E. A., Abiodun, K. M. and Ajamu, G. J. (2021). Application of artificial intelligence for COVID-19 epidemic: an exploratory study, opportunities, challenges, and future prospects. In *Artificial Intelligence for COVID-19* (pp. 47–61). Springer, Cham.

[71] Steed, C. A., Ricciuto, D. M., Shipman, G., *et al.* (2013). Big data visual analytics for exploratory earth system simulation analysis. *Computers & Geosciences*, 61, 71–82.

[72] Chae, S., Kwon, S. and Lee, D. (2018). Predicting infectious disease using deep learning and big data. *International Journal of Environmental Research and Public Health*, 15(8), 1596.

[73] Bansal, S., Chowell, G., Simonsen, L., Vespignani, A. and Viboud, C. (2016). Big data for infectious disease surveillance and modeling. *The Journal of Infectious Diseases*, 214(Suppl. 4), S375–S379.

[74] Eisenstein, M. (2018). Infection forecasts powered by big data. *Nature*, 555(7695).

[75] Buckee, C. (2020). Improving epidemic surveillance and response: big data is dead, long live big data. *The Lancet Digital Health*, 2(5), e218–e220.

[76] Awotunde, J. B., Jimoh, R. G., Oladipo, I. D., Abdulraheem, M., Jimoh, T. B. and Ajamu, G. J. (2021). Big data and data analytics for an enhanced COVID-19 epidemic management. In *Artificial Intelligence for COVID-19* (pp. 11–29). Springer, Cham.

[77] Kent, J. (2020). Understanding the COVID-19 pandemic as a big data analytics issue. Erişim Tarihi, 11, 2020.

[78] Giordano, G., Blanchini, F., Bruno, R., *et al.* (2020). A SIDARTHE model of COVID-19 epidemic in Italy. arXiv preprint arXiv:2003.09861.

[79] Chen, B., Shi, M., Ni, X., *et al.* (2020). Visual data analysis and simulation prediction for COVID-19. arXiv preprint arXiv:2002.07096.

[80] Tátrai, D. and Várallyay, Z. (2020). COVID-19 epidemic outcome predictions based on logistic fitting and estimation of its reliability. arXiv preprint arXiv:2003.14160.

[81] Strzelecki, A. (2020). The second worldwide wave of interest in coronavirus since the COVID-19 outbreaks in South Korea, Italy and Iran: a Google Trends study. arXiv preprint arXiv:2003.10998.

[82] Long, Y. S., Zhai, Z. M., Han, L. L., *et al.* (2020). Quantitative assessment of the role of undocumented infection in the 2019 novel coronavirus (COVID-19) pandemic. arXiv preprint arXiv:2003.12028.

[83] Mahajan, A., Sivadas, N. A. and Solanki, R. (2020). An epidemic model SIPHERD and its application for prediction of the spread of COVID-19 infection in India. *Chaos, Solitons & Fractals*, 140, 110156.

[84] Heroy, S. (2020). Metropolitan-scale COVID-19 outbreaks: how similar are they? arXiv preprint arXiv:2004.01248.

[85] Awotunde, J. B., Ogundokun, R. O., Adeniyi, A. E., Abiodun, K. M., and Ajamu, G. J. (2022). Application of mathematical modelling approach in COVID-19 transmission and interventions strategies. *Studies in Systems, Decision and Control*, 366, 283–314.

[86] Zhao, X., Liu, X. and Li, X. (2020). Tracking the spread of novel coronavirus (2019-nCoV) based on big data. medRxiv.

[87] Zhou, C., Su, F., Pei, T., *et al.* (2020). COVID-19: challenges to GIS with big data. *Geography and Sustainability*, 1, 77–87.

[88] Jin, Y. H., Cai, L., Cheng, Z. S., *et al.* (2020). A rapid advice guideline for the diagnosis and treatment of 2019 novel coronavirus (2019-nCoV) infected pneumonia (standard version). *Military Medical Research*, 7(1), 4.

[89] Ahmed, S. F., Quadeer, A. A. and McKay, M. R. (2020). Preliminary identification of potential vaccine targets for the COVID-19 coronavirus (SARS-CoV-2) based on SARS-CoV immunological studies. *Viruses*, 12(3), 254.

[90] Banerjee, A., Santra, D. and Maiti, S. (2020). Energetics based epitope screening in SARS CoV-2 (COVID 19) spike glycoprotein by immuno-informatic analysis aiming to a suitable vaccine development. bioRxiv.

[91] Ganasegeran, K. and Abdulrahman, S. A. (2020). Artificial intelligence applications in tracking health behaviors during disease epidemics. In *Human Behaviour Analysis Using Intelligent Systems* (pp. 141–155). Springer, Cham.

[92] Ge, Y., Tian, T., Huang, S., *et al.* (2020). A data-driven drug repositioning framework discovered a potential therapeutic agent targeting COVID-19. bioRxiv.

[93] Enayatkhani, M., Hasaniazad, M., Faezi, S., *et al.* (2020). Reverse vaccinology approach to design a novel multi-epitope vaccine candidate against

COVID-19: an in silico study. *Journal of Biomolecular Structure and Dynamics*, 39, 2857–2872.

[94] Koirala, A., Joo, Y. J., Khatami, A., Chiu, C. and Britton, P. N. (2020). Vaccines for COVID-19: the current state of play. *Paediatric Respiratory Reviews*, 35, 43–49.

[95] Petropoulos, G. (2020). Artificial intelligence in the fight against COVID-19. *Bruegel* (23 March).

[96] Bullock, J., Pham, K. H., Lam, C. S. N. and Luengo-Oroz, M. (2020). Mapping the landscape of artificial intelligence applications against COVID-19. arXiv preprint arXiv:2003.11336.

[97] Harari, Y. N. (2020). The world after coronavirus. *Financial Times*, 20.

[98] Naudé, W. (2020). Artificial intelligence against COVID-19: an early review.

[99] Maier, B. F. and Brockmann, D. (2020). Effective containment explains subexponential growth in recent confirmed COVID-19 cases in China. *Science*, 368(6492), 742–746.

[100] Huang, J. J. (2020). COVID-19 and applicable law to transnational personal data: trends and dynamics. *Sydney Law School Research Paper, (20/23)*.

[101] Chen, B. (2014). Historical foundations of choice of law in fiduciary obligations. *Journal of Private International Law*, 10(2), 171–203.

[102] Douglas, M. (2018). Characterisation of breach of confidence as a privacy tort in private international law. *UNSWLJ*, 41, 490.

[103] Alzahrani, N. M. (2020). COVID-19 pandemic: an overview of machine and deep learning methods for analysis of digital media texts. *Research in Computing Science*, 149(5), 179–189.

[104] "How DAMO academy's AI system detects coronavirus cases," (2020). [Online]. Available: https://www.alizila.com/how-damo-academys-ai-system-detects-coronavirus-cases/.

[105] Viboud, C., Sun, K., Gaffey, R., *et al.* (2018). The RAPIDD Ebola forecasting challenge: synthesis and lessons learnt. *Epidemics*, 22, 13–21.

[106] Kahn, R., Mahmud, A. S., Schroeder, A., *et al.* (2019). Rapid forecasting of cholera risk in Mozambique: translational challenges and opportunities. *Prehospital and Disaster Medicine*, 34(5), 557–562.

[107] Armstrong, G. L., MacCannell, D. R., Taylor, J., *et al.* (2019). Pathogen genomics in public health. *New England Journal of Medicine*, 381(26), 2569–2580.

[108] Schiavo, R., May Leung, M. and Brown, M. (2014). Communicating risk and promoting disease mitigation measures in epidemics and emerging disease settings. *Pathogens and Global Health*, 108(2), 76–94.

[109] De-Montjoye, Y. A., Gambs, S., Blondel, V., *et al.* (2018). On the privacy-conscientious use of mobile phone data. *Scientific Data*, 5(1), 1–6.

[110] Ray, E. L. and Reich, N. G. (2018). Prediction of infectious disease epidemics via weighted density ensembles. *PLoS Computational Biology*, 14(2), e1005910.

[111] Cottle, M., Hoover, W., Kanwal, S., Kohn, M., Strome, T. and Treister, N. (2013). *Transforming Health Care Through Big Data Strategies for Leveraging Big Data in the Health Care Industry*. Institute for Health Technology Transformation, http://ihealthtran. com/big-data-in-healthcare.

[112] Hotelling, H. (1933). Analysis of a complex of statistical variables into principal components. *Journal of Educational Psychology*, 24(6), 417.

[113] Folorunso, S. O., Awotunde, J. B., Adeboye, N. O. and Matiluko, O. E. (2022). Data classification model for COVID-19 pandemic. In *Advances in Data Science and Intelligent Data Communication Technologies for COVID-19* (pp. 93–118). Cham: Springer.

[114] Dalal, N. and Triggs, B. (2005, June). Histograms of oriented gradients for human detection. In *2005 IEEE Computer Society Conference on Computer Vision and Pattern Recognition (CVPR'05)* (Vol. 1, pp. 886–893). IEEE.

[115] Cohen, J. P., Morrison, P., Dao, L., Roth, K., Duong, T. Q. and Ghassemi, M. (2020). Covid-19 image data collection: prospective predictions are the future. arXiv preprint arXiv:2006.11988.

Chapter 3

Cloud-based IoMT for early COVID-19 diagnosis and monitoring

G. Boopathi Raja[1], T. Sathya[1], V. Gowrishankar[1] and M. Parimala Devi[1]

Abstract

COVID-19 has been posing a threat to survival from the second half of 2019. Each country in the world must fight against the COVID-19 pandemic with caution. Many researchers around the world have developed many vaccines, but some of them are found to be effective. This chapter introduces an effective scheme for the diagnosis and tracking of patients with COVID-19 based on symptoms. The concept behind the proposed approach is to use an Internet of Things (IoT)-based system to handle the real-time symptom data from patients in order to diagnose coronavirus cases early. Additionally, the framework has the ability to track the medical records of those who have healed from the COVID-19 disease. The proposed framework must learn automatically about the origin of the virus by monitoring and analyzing necessary data. Because of the significant and rapid rise in the number of patients after the COVID-19 pandemic, it is crucial to focus an eye on patients' health before any new disease or infection occurs. IoT security has recently become a serious concern and a hard problem. For researchers, transferring the large amount of collected healthcare information data of patients who do not want their personal healthcare details shared has remained a difficult task. The health status of patients is determined in this model by predicting critical situations and examining physiological data received from smart medical IoT devices, ensuring that patients' personal information is kept private. Based on current advancements, the suggested model is thought to be suitable for delivering an appropriate remote patient monitoring model with accurate data in cloud-based IoT systems.

Keywords: COVID-19; Early diagnosis; Internet of Medical Things (IoMT); Disease prediction; Real-time health tracking

[1]Department of Electronics and Communication Engineering, Velalar College of Engineering and Technology, Erode, India

3.1 Introduction

As of May 27, 2021, more than 168 million COVID-19 confirmed cases had been recorded worldwide since its detection in late December 2019, with a daily rise of about 5%. More than 95,000 people have died as a result of these incidents, representing a 4.2% mortality rate. The World Health Organisation classified this unique coronavirus as a pandemic on March 11, 2020. Unfortunately, there is no effective therapy or vaccination available at this time. The production of an effective vaccine was done, and it had taken over a year, especially because the identification of the existence of the virus is a challenging task. However, the production of the number of vaccines to the entire population worldwide is not sufficient due to a lack of resources [1].

Coronaviruses are a broad category of viruses with a wide range of characteristics. Some of these make sick people with colds. Others infect animals such as cattle, camels, and bats. The first human coronavirus was found in the year 1965. It was the cause of a common cold. During the decade, researchers uncovered a set of identical human and animal viruses with crown-like appearances [2].

Seven coronaviruses are capable of infecting humans. In 2002, the deadly SARS virus was identified in southern China and rapidly spread to 28 other countries. More than 8,000 persons had been affected by July 2003, with 774 of them dying. Only four additional cases were reported in a minor epidemic in 2004. Fever, headaches, and respiratory problems such as coughing and breathing problem are all symptoms of the coronavirus [3].

In 2012, MERS was discovered for the first time in Saudi Arabia. Nearly 2,500 cases are found among the people who stay in or visited the Middle East recently. The coronavirus, though less contagious than SARS, is more deadly, having killed 858 people. It involves respiratory problems similar to a regular cold, but it can also lead to renal failure.

Currently, the only method in the world for dealing with this coronavirus is to use social isolation, hand washing, and face masks to limit its spread. By allowing for early identification and tracking of new outbreaks, technology, on the other hand, could be able to help limit the disease's spread. These approaches require cloud, big data, and fog capabilities, as well as the handling of information collected via remote monitoring to track the real-time health status of the patients located at long distances, teleHealth, m-Health [4]. This research presents an effective approach for the diagnosis and tracking of COVID-19 patients that uses wearable sensor technology to capture real-time symptom data.

The summary of this chapter is discussed as follows. Section 3.2 elaborates the symptoms of COVID-19, possible diagnostic methodologies, therapeutic techniques, suitable vaccination along the important happenings worldwide as a COVID-19 timeline. The existing works along with the requirements are described under Section 3.3. Section 3.4 introduces the methodology and architecture of the proposed framework along with a flow diagram. Section 3.5 describes the implementation of the proposed framework cloud-based IoMT system for early COVID-19 diagnosis and monitoring. Section 3.6 demonstrates the results and discussion with suitable illustrations.

3.2 Overview about COVID-19 treatments

3.2.1 Symptoms

COVID-19 has a wide range of impacts on different people. The majority of sick people will have minor to severe symptoms and will heal without needing to go to the hospital. Patients having COVID-19 have a different range of problems ranging from mild to moderate pain and sometimes up to life-threatening sickness. COVID-19 has a wide range of impacts on different people. The majority of sick people will have minor to severe symptoms and will survive without requiring even going to the hospital. Symptoms include nausea or vomiting, severe diarrhea, and a new lack of taste or odor [5].

Fever, dry cough, and fatigue are the most common symptoms in COVID patients. Any of the less common symptoms are aches and pains, indigestion, fever, loss of color in fingers, lack of taste or odor, a rash on the scalp, conjunctivitis, and sore throat. COVID-19 symptoms include tiredness, difficulties in movement, and shortness of breath or difficulty in breathing, chest pain, and loss of speech.

Patients who are experiencing severe symptoms require prompt medical intervention. Mild symptoms should be managed at home by otherwise healthy people. When a patient is infected with the virus, signs usually start after 5–6 days, although it can take up to 14 days.

COVID-19 illness is more likely to have major symptoms in the elderly and those with severe chronic medical problems such as heart disease or diabetes.

Patients experiencing problems in breathing, persistent discomfort or pain in the chest, gray, pale or blue-colored skin, lips, or nail beds, depending on skin tone, and an inability to wake or stay awake should seek immediate medical assistance.

3.2.2 Methodologies in COVID-19 diagnosis

SARS-CoV-2 can currently be diagnosed using one of two methods: detection of the antibody produced after infection or detection of viral RNA. The most prevalent methods for detecting SARS-CoV-2 viral RNA are polymerase chain reaction (PCR) and nucleic acid hybridization. Viral antibodies or antigens can be detected using ELISA and other immunological and serological methods [6]. The identification of the virus in its active state is accomplished by determining the virus's RNA, while serological assays aid in identifying people whose immune systems have already formed antibodies to combat the infection.

- Amplification techniques
  - Isothermal nucleic acid amplification
  - RT-PCR (reverse transcription-PCR)
- Immunological assays
- SARS-CoV-2 diagnosis using newly discovered technology

For the time being, the most widely used procedures for diagnosing COVID-19 are RT-PCR and immunological testing. These procedures, however, necessitate the use of qualified staff. Furthermore, the findings of PCR might take up to a few days to get. Antibodies and recombinant proteins are required for immunological tests. As a result, there is a tendency toward developing new SARS-CoV-2 diagnostic procedures that are quicker, less expensive, and more reliable.

The findings of RT-PCR can be received in a few hours and have good sensitivity and specificity. In addition to lung samples, saliva, blood, urine, and stools, it may identify viral DNA. However, there are significant disadvantages to RT-PCR, including the requirement for a costly thermocycler and experienced employees to execute the experiment and interpret the data. Furthermore, benchmark validation is critical for the validity of the data, as false-negative findings might occur as a result of sample deterioration, sample collection quality and time, and inefficiency of some test kits. The sensitivity and specificity of LAMP techniques are equivalent to those of RT-PCR. Some kits, on the other hand, have reduced sensitivity. It can be done for about half an hour with a crude sample, allowing them to be used in POC testing. SARS CoV-2 detection has also been created using the CRISPR approach, which has great sensitivity and specificity. It takes 1 h to complete and can be used with the lateral flow assay [7]. For LAMP and CRISPR, a costly thermocycler is not required. A lateral flow assay is a simple approach that may be used by nonprofessionals to produce findings in 15 min in blood or serum samples. Storage, shipping, and sample collection do not affect antibodies. Its disadvantage is that it takes a long time to manufacture antibodies. Although ELISA is simple to use, it cannot be utilized for early detection like the lateral flow test. It can, however, be used to test the immunity of healthcare workers and to investigate herd immunity.

3.2.3 Treatment approaches

The number of medicinal options available to treat COVID-19 is continually increasing and developing. Clinicians, patients and their representatives, and health system management are highly encouraged to study the COVID-19 Treatment Guidelines issued by the National Institutes of Health frequently, according to the CDC [8].

Infection prevention and control methods, as well as supportive care, such as supplementary oxygen and mechanical ventilator support, are being used in the treatment of COVID-19. In some cases during the treatment of COVID-19, the FDA has been permitted to use authorized remdesivir (Veklury) based on the health status of the patient [7,9].

Early and effective treatment of any disease can assist forestall the advancement of the disease to a more serious condition, especially in individuals who are at high risk of disease progression and severe illness, while also minimizing the load on healthcare systems. Under the EUA, a variety of new treatments (such as monoclonal antibodies) are accessible for early outpatient therapy. Outpatients with a high risk of illness progression are undergoing trials to see if these treatments are successful.

3.2.4 *Available vaccine*

As of December 2020, there are over 200 COVID-19 vaccine candidates under development. At this time, at least 52 candidate vaccinations are being tested in humans. Several more are in phase I/II right now and will go to phase III in coming months [9].

A significant number of people are typically tested before a vaccination candidate is shown to be both safe and efficacious. Around 7 out of every 100 vaccines tested in the lab and on laboratory animals will be approved for human clinical trials. Only one out of every five vaccines tested in clinical trials is successful. When a large number of vaccinations are being developed and tested, the chances of one or more successful vaccines proving to be safe and effective for specific population rises.

Vaccination can be designed in one of three ways. They differ in whether they use the entire bacterium or virus, just the bits that activate the immune system, or just the genetic data that direct the production of specific proteins rather than the entire virus.

1. The whole-microbe approach
2. Viral vector vaccine
3. The subunit approach

3.2.4.1 The whole-microbe approach

Inactivated vaccine

The initial stage in creating a vaccine is to use chemicals, heat, or radiation to neutralize or eliminate the infectious virus, or a virus that is genetically identical to it. This method employs technology that has been shown to function in humans, such as flu and polio vaccinations, and pharmaceuticals may be mass produced at a low cost.

However, expensive equipment is necessary to adequately develop the virus or bacteria, and the procedure might take a long time. Two or three treatments are nearly always necessary.

Live-attenuated vaccine

A virus that seems to be alive and has been diluted, or one that is highly close, is used in a live-attenuated vaccine. Rubella, mumps, and measles vaccinations, as well as chickenpox and shingles vaccinations, fall under this category. This process is equivalent to the production of neutralizing antibodies and may be done in huge quantities. People with weakened immune systems, on the other hand, may not be able to benefit from such vaccinations.

3.2.4.2 Viral vector vaccine

This type of immunization uses a harmless virus to transfer specific proteins from the germ of interest to trigger an immune response without causing sickness. The protein is subsequently transported into the body by the virus, which functions as a carrier for it. The protein is the catalyst for the immune response. The ebola vaccines are being manufactured quickly since it is a viral genome vaccine.

3.2.4.3 The subunit approach

Only the fragments of a virus or bacterium that the immune system needs to detect are used in a subunit vaccination. It does not have a harmless virus as a vector, and it does not contain the full microbe. Proteins or carbohydrates might be used as subunits. The majority of vaccinations on the pediatric immunization schedule are subunit vaccinations that protect against illnesses, including diphtheria, tetanus, whooping cough, and meningococcal meningitis.

The genetic approach (nucleic acid vaccine)

A nucleic acid vaccine, unlike all other vaccinations that employ the complete organism or sections of it, employs simply a piece of genetic material that offers instructions for certain proteins, instead of the complete bacteria. In the form of mRNA or DNA, a nucleic acid vaccine gives the cells particular instructions to build the protein that the immune system needs to detect and respond to.

The nucleic acid method is a novel technique for vaccine development. None had gone through the whole licensing procedure for use in people before the COVID-19 pandemic; however, certain DNA vaccines, particularly those for specific tumors, were in human testing. As a result of the pandemic, investigation in this area has increased, and many COVID-19 mRNA vaccines have been granted emergency use authorization, allowing them to be delivered to people who are not in clinical trials.

3.2.5 COVID-19 timeline

Table 3.1 describes the important highlights that have been happened from December 2019 in the Wuhan city of China to date around the world [10,11].

3.3 Related work

3.3.1 Lightweight block encryption–based secure health monitoring system for data management

Akhbarifar *et al.* have suggested the encrypted secure customized healthcare approach in a cloud-based Internet of Things (IoT) context. As a result, the major purpose of this study is to develop a credible health monitoring model for an early detection of HD (heart disorders), HTN (hypertension), and HCLS (hypercholesterolemia) by forecasting the critical patient's state utilizing the procedures as follows [12]:

1. Medical IoT devices collect biological data from patients for remote medical monitoring.
2. Using a suggested lightweight block encryption approach to safeguard medical IoT data and ensure the security and confidentiality of patient medical data.
3. Using the cloud to transfer encrypted data for disease prediction.
4. Detecting unexpected variations in blood cholesterol levels in patients and predicting the HCLS.

Table 3.1 COVID-19 timeline

December 31, 2019	The Wuhan Municipal Health Commission has confirmed a cluster of pneumonia cases in Hubei Province, China. A new coronavirus was later discovered
January 4, 2020	A group of pneumonia cases was reported by the WHO on social networking sites in Wuhan, Hubei province, although no deaths were reported
January 12, 2020	COVID-19's genetic sequence was published by China
January 13, 2020	The first occurrence of COVID-19 outside of China was confirmed in Thailand
January 20 and 21, 2020	A short field visit to Wuhan was performed by WHO specialists from the China and Western Pacific regional offices
February 3, 2020	The International Community's Strategic Preparedness and Response Plan, published by the WHO, would help in the security of countries with poor health systems
February 11 and 12, 2020	Over 400 experts and key contributors from across the world attended a COVID-19 Research and Innovation Forum, which featured lectures by experts from CDC
March 19, 2020	• All incoming international flights banned in India • Export of masks, ventilators and certain medications are banned by Indian government
March 20, 2020	• WHO delivered 1.5 Million Lab test kits to many countries • The largest single increase of the corona virus outbreak recorded 627 deaths in Italy
March 22–25, 2020	• Global corona virus cases doubled and recorded 330,000 cases • WHO declared the "pandemic is accelerating" • Almost one-third of world population is affected by corona virus lockdown • "There will be a shortage of medical supplies" announced by WHO
April 2, 2020	Global corona virus cases recorded the one million; mortality exceeds 50,000
April 8, 2020	Global corona virus cases surpass 1.5 million
April 22, 2020	First trials for a corona virus vaccine are approved by Germany
May 3, 2020	The total number of fatalities in the United States was 65,464 people
May 7, 2020	The UN reports that the corona virus has affected 14 million people. The mortality rate in the United States has reached 1 lakh
May 28, 2020	Latin America accounted for about 40% of COVID-19 mortality worldwide
June 11, 2020	In July, the Biotech company Moderna began the last phase of a testing for a corona virus vaccine on 30,000 people
June 23, 2020	The region's first vaccination trial has begun in South Africa. At the same time, the number of people who have died as a result of the corona virus in Latin America has reached 1 lakh
June 24, 2020	India reports over 15,000 and it was the highest single-day rise new corona virus infections
July 2, 2020	In spite of corona virus cases surpass 600,000 and 17,834 deaths, India announces reopening measures
July 16, 2020	India records 1 million corona virus cases. The corona virus outbreak rises in rural areas of the country

(Continues)

Table 3.1 (Continued)

August 1, 2020	More than 57,000 new victims were reported in India
August 13, 2020	COVID-19 cases have increased by over 67,000 in India. It appears that this is the largest daily rise since the epidemic began
August 15, 2020	Russia starts production of vaccine: Sputnik V COVID-19
September 4, 2020	India has reached 83,000 new positive victims
September 5, 2020	India currently has 90,000 daily cases, overtaking Brazil as the country with the second-highest number of cases
October 12, 2020	After a volunteer experience an unexpected illness, Johnson & Johnson suspends its COVID-19 vaccination trials
October 29, 2020	COVID-19 cases have reached 8 million in India
November 20, 2020	• The world passes 50 million corona virus cases • Preliminary data suggest that Pfizer and BioNTech's vaccine is more than 94% effective
December 21, 2020	According to the WHO, the UK variety of SARS-CoV-2 looks to be more contagious, although vaccinations are unlikely to be affected
December 23, 2020	The first 1 million COVID-19 vaccinations are given out in the United States
February 4, 2021	• COVID-19-related fatalities in the United States have exceeded 450,000, while COVID-19-related fatalities in Spain have crossed 60,000 • Johnson & Johnson has requested emergency use permission for its COVID-19 vaccine from the FDA • The vaccine developed by Oxford-AstraZeneca is effective against the United Kingdom corona virus strain
March 4, 2021	• India's Covaxin COVID-19 vaccine was found to be around 80% effective in a new study • Germany approves AstraZeneca's COVID-19 vaccine
March 12, 2021	The vaccine developed by Johnson & Johnson has been approved by the WHO for emergency use
April 20, 2021	According to the WHO, worldwide COVID-19 cases have risen for the seventh week in a row. The number of people who have died as a result of the coronavirus has exceeded 3 million worldwide
May 1, 2021	In a single day, India becomes the first country to report over 4 lakh cases
May 28, 2021	• Globally, the total confirmed cases of COVID-19 have reached over 169,021,000, with more than 3,511,000 deaths and over 118,593,000 recoveries • The total number of COVID-19 cases has crossed 30 million in South Asia • India is the most heavily affected country in Asia, but neighboring countries such as Nepal, Bangladesh, and Pakistan are also suffering from the disease

5. Detecting HD in the event of an HTN diagnostic test and predicting HTN risk and severities.
6. Providing the medical teams with the disease prediction process's analytical results.

This secure health-monitoring approach is separated into four elements, as explained next.

3.3.1.1 IoT network and data collection

This section contains medical IoT sensors, network devices, and tools for detecting and collecting physiological data from patients. The patient's vital signs, such as heart rate, blood pressure, blood cholesterol, and other essential biological data, are acquired via the body area network by sensors implanted on the patient's clothing or body. A security requirement for secure IoT data has been included because medical IoT sensor network devices are more vulnerable to security attacks than conventional network devices [13,14]. The IoT data are secured using a lightweight block encryption approach before being sent to the clouds with the obtained medical data.

3.3.1.2 Communication service provider

This section is in charge of sending the medical data collected from the patients to the cloud storage [15]. This component must offer confidential sharing for transmission to cloud servers as part of a distributed data storage framework.

3.3.1.3 Distributed data storage

This section stores the medical data that have been transmitted by medical IoT sensors. Also included in the distributed data storage component is the provisioning and delivery of services to the interested users, which include doctors and healthcare professionals. These capabilities might be incorporated into a facility that uses data-mining techniques to estimate the probability of illness. The suggested safe health-monitoring model takes into account a combination of three categories of associated illnesses, including hypertension, hypercholesterolemia, and a heart condition.

3.3.1.4 Healthcare provider

Doctors, hospitals, and emergency responders make up this section. Doctors can use the forwarded diagnosis results to double-check and confirm them before making necessary medical recommendations to patients.

3.3.2 Smart diagnostic/therapeutic framework for COVID-19 patients

The COVID-19 monitoring unit is used to identify suspected people who have primary symptoms. The clinical data of individuals with mild symptoms who might be in a self-quarantine/home environment with few difficulties are tracked utilizing cloud technology. While obtaining those data, the government's safety rules are followed. The adoption of this supporting and tracking system creates a peaceful situation for COVID-19 patients' families and friends [16,17].

These systems also assist the health workers in providing medications whenever required. It aids healthcare providers in not just monitoring patient information but also storing it for future investigation. Patients' essential information is continually recorded without being contacted. This system has a minimum of four primary sensors to update patient's data regularly. This information is updated on mobile phones for monitoring purposes.

Monitor respiration rate, temperature, and pulse of a patient are a major concern and hence the data acquired by the signal conditioning unit could be connected to mobile phones of the patients. The system monitors COVID-19 patients in real time rapidly. The efficiency of the monitoring system has improved by the data collected from the sensors, which are saved in the cloud also in a regular period. This system not only helps the suspected COVID-19 patients but also helps healthcare providers to monitor many patients in remote places.

3.3.3 IoT-based framework for collecting real-time symptom data using machine learning algorithms

The research was carried to explore if machine learning techniques might be used to swiftly detect (or predict) likely COVID-19 diseases [18–21]. The remaining sections of this section go through the experimental setup as well as the results that are presented and discussed.

3.3.3.1 Dataset

The COVID-19 Open Research Collection (CORD-19) repository has made a collection of 14,251 validated COVID-19 cases available. The data in each case comprises a variety of data types. Travel history to suspect regions, symptoms, and contacts with potentially infected people were all investigated. However, for many of the occurrences listed in the database, part of this information was incomplete. Furthermore, the data was not adequately formatted for machine learning algorithms to work with.

3.3.3.2 Data preprocessing

To make it easier for machine learning, the data was preprocessed and formatted. We gathered all of the instances that had recorded symptoms. A total of 80 symptoms emerged as a result of this. Many of these symptoms, however, were determined to be interchangeable. As a result, there were just 20 symptoms left. This ad hoc merging of identical symptoms was done by two medical practitioners. For example, the terms "anorexia" and "lack of appetite" were combined.

The relative relevance of these 20 symptoms was also assessed in prior research. The important key parameters for feature selections have been listed as follows: correlation analysis, interquartile range, intraclass distance, spectral score, information score, and variance-based feature weighting. The variance-based feature weighting method is one, in which, it not only rates the symptoms but also gives each one a weighted significance rating. Cough, sore throat, fever, fatigue, and shortness of breath were discovered to be the most critical five symptoms (ranked from most essential to least significant).

This study employs the five most essential symptoms based on the findings of the previous study. There were also two new features added: contact and live. The first attribute (touch) specifies if the person has previously been known to have come into contact with a potentially confirmed person. The second characteristic (live) indicates whether the person resided, traveled to, or passed through a contaminated location. As a result, a 14,767-data-record preprocessed dataset was produced. There were 854 COVID-19 cases whose records had been confirmed and 622 COVID-19 cases whose records had not been confirmed.

3.3.3.3 Predictive model

The preprocessed data was utilized to develop a prediction model for our classification method in this study. The goal of this model is to forecast how likely a person is to become infected with COVID-19.

This might have been accomplished using a variety of learning techniques (i.e. classifiers). These classifiers can be divided into several groups. The classifiers are divided into six groups by WEKA Software, which we employed in this study:

1. Lazy classifiers, such *K*-nearest neighbors (*K*-NN).
2. Meta classifiers, such neural networks.
3. Function-based classifiers, such as support vector machines (SVMs).
4. Tree-based classifiers, such as decision stump.
5. Bayes-based classifiers, such as naïve Bayes.
6. Rule-based classifiers, such as Decision Tables, ZeroR, and OneR.

All these algorithms were conducted on the dataset using WEKA Software. For each of the eight algorithms, the default parameter values were utilized. The eight algorithms are described briefly in the following:

Support vector machine (SVM). SVM trains the hyperplane that divides the instances from each class while also increasing the distance between the data instances and the hyperplane, given a collection of labeled training examples. The learned hyperplane is then applied to every new test object to assign a class label.

Artificial neural network (ANN). The learning process tries to recreate what happens in the human brain when it comes to learning. To do this, edges connect many layers of nodes. Numerical weights are used to represent the edges linking the nodes. Each node's output is calculated as the weighted sum of its inputs.

The ANN learns the statistical weights that identify the instances for every class consist of a set of labeled training images (each case corresponds to either the positive or negative class). Each test case is then assigned a class label using the trained model. The outputs of the last layer are presented to a threshold to determine the label with this test instance.

Naïve Bayes. Naïve Bayes is one of the supervised learning approaches. A probabilistic technique is used in the learning process. The model parameters are computed using the Bayes theorem.

Naïve Bayes creates several parameter values, such as the likelihood of every class label occurring, given a collection of labeled training data (each case corresponds to either the positive or negative class). Following that, each test case is assigned a class label based on these variables. This is done by estimating the likelihood of the test instance being matched to each of the possible attribute values. The label of that test case is determined by the largest value among these probabilities.

***K*-Nearest neighbors (*K*-NN).** It belongs to supervised learning. The process of learning moves at a slow pace. There is no model creation.

K-NN calculates the similarities among a given test instance along with all the training instances for a specific set of labeled training examples (each case corresponds to either the positive or negative class). The test instance's class label is then assigned (or predicted) using these distances. The class names of the *K* training samples closest to the test sample are combined to achieve this.

Decision table. Another example of a supervised learning approach is the decision table. In this technique, it generates a decision table from a set of labeled training cases to calculate a classifier (each case corresponds to either the positive or negative class). The table is made up of a series of criteria and actions. It is said to be complete when it assesses all combination cases for the criteria and provides appropriate steps with each of them.

Decision stump. This technique belongs to supervised learning. In this technique, it creates a decision tree for only one input feature to find a model from a group of labeled training instances. Alternatively, it makes a forecast for each test instance based just on one sample attribute. Each component is selected by calculating the entropy of all features across all training samples and choosing the one with the highest accuracy.

Zero rule (ZeroR). These types of algorithms fall under the category of supervised learning. Based on the group of labeled training cases, this algorithm defines a classifier using just the target feature (i.e. class) and neglecting most of the other features. It belongs to the basic classification approach. The majority class is assigned to any new test instance. It is usually utilized as a starting point for determining baseline performance.

One rule (OneR). Another technique that falls under supervised learning is OneR. This technique generates one rule for every feature in the dataset from a set of labeled training instances (each case corresponds to either the positive or negative class). After that, the one with the smallest overall error is selected.

3.4 Proposed methodology

The concept behind the suggested technique is to gather real-time symptom data from patients using an artificial intelligence (AI)-based framework to identify coronavirus infections in the early stages. Furthermore, the AI-based framework can track the medical records of people who have recovered from the COVID-19 disease. By obtaining and evaluating relevant information, the proposed approach must automatically learn about the COVID-19 spreading mechanism. The system's five major components are diagnostic data collection and sharing, quarantine/isolation center, predictive analytics center, health specialists, and cloud infrastructure. Both AI-based smart medical devices and IoT have altered health-monitoring services by allowing patients' health conditions to be tracked and operated remotely at any time and from any location. Because of the significant and rapid rise in the number of patients after the COVID-19 pandemic, it is crucial to focus on patients' health before any serious symptoms occur.

3.4.1 Architecture of proposed IoT framework

This chapter explains the IoT-based proposed architecture for real-time monitoring and identification (or prediction) of COVID-19-infected persons. This framework might aid in improving the treatment process for reported cases and gaining a better knowledge of the nature of the COVID-19 illness.

The architecture of the suggested IoT-based framework is shown in Figure 3.1. It is consists of five major elements as follows:

- Collection and upload of symptom data using smart medical IoT device along with Google assistant.
- A center for quarantine and isolation for COVID-19 patients.
- A data analysis center—a place where people may go to get their data analyzed.
- A way to connect with doctors using IoT health management.
- The cloud infrastructure connects them all.

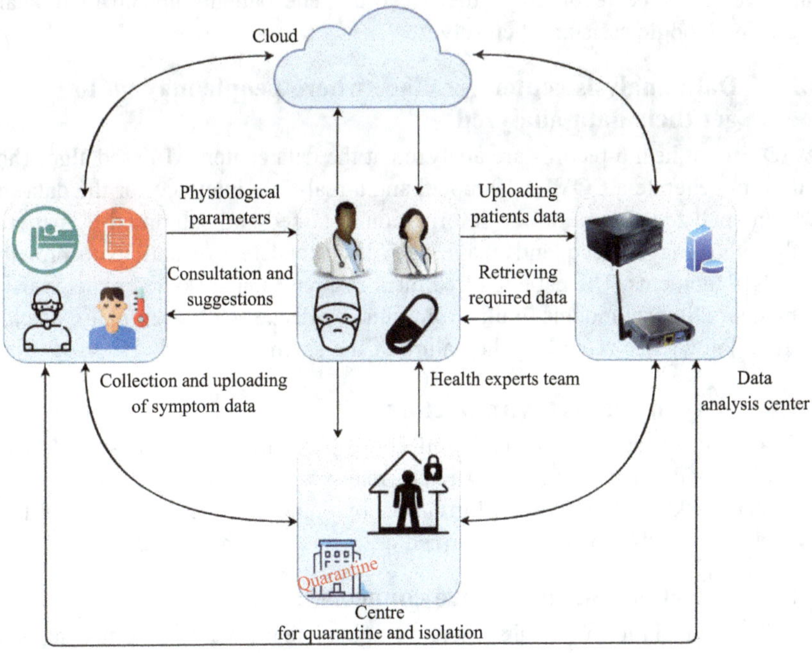

Figure 3.1 Architecture of proposed AI-based framework

3.4.1.1 Collection and upload of symptom data

The objective of this component is to use Smart IoT wearable sensor devices along with Google assistant to record real-time symptom reports from the patient's body. Based on an actual COVID-19 patient dataset, we determined the most significant COVID-19 symptoms in a previous study. Sore throat, fatigue, cough, fever, and shortness of breath were among the symptoms noted.

These major symptoms can be detected using biosensors IC modules in the IoT device. Shortness of breath, for example, may be detected using oxygen-based sensors. Fever may be detected using temperature-based sensors. Fatigue may be detected using both heart-rate and motion-based sensors. The image-based categorization can be used to detect a sore throat. Audio-based sensors combined with acoustic and aerodynamic models could detect and classify cough.

Other pertinent information, such as contact and travel history from the previous few weeks, may be obtained on the move using the Aarogya Setu app.

3.4.1.2 Center for quarantine and isolation

People who have been isolated or confined in a medical facility provide information to this component. These documents include both medical and nonmedical data. Each record contains data information with the previously mentioned symptoms for health data, and each record also includes nontechnical data such as travel and contact history over the previous 3–4 weeks, gender, age, chronic diseases, genetic problems, and any other medical history. Each patient's treatment reaction would eventually be recorded in their records. The patients update their health status using Google assistant themselves.

3.4.1.3 Data analysis center—a place where people may go to get their data analyzed

COVID patient health records are analyzed at the data center. AI-based algorithms are used to generate a COVID-19 model and a real-time interface for the data that has been analyzed. Based on the information obtained and submitted by patients, the algorithm may subsequently have been used to detect or anticipate probable COVID-19 incidents. The patient's treatment response may also be predicted using the model. Disease models built from this evidence will eventually disclose important knowledge regarding the nature of the sickness.

3.4.1.4 Way to connect with doctors

Physicians will focus on any potential infections that our suggested AI-based identification/prediction model advises inspired by real symptom data. Physicians should be able to act quickly to these verified instances by doing any necessary medical tests. This makes it possible to isolate confirmed cases and treat them properly.

3.4.1.5 The cloud infrastructure connects them all

The IoT cloud platform permits users to upload real-time symptom data, keep medical records, share prediction findings, engage with specialist recommendations, and save data.

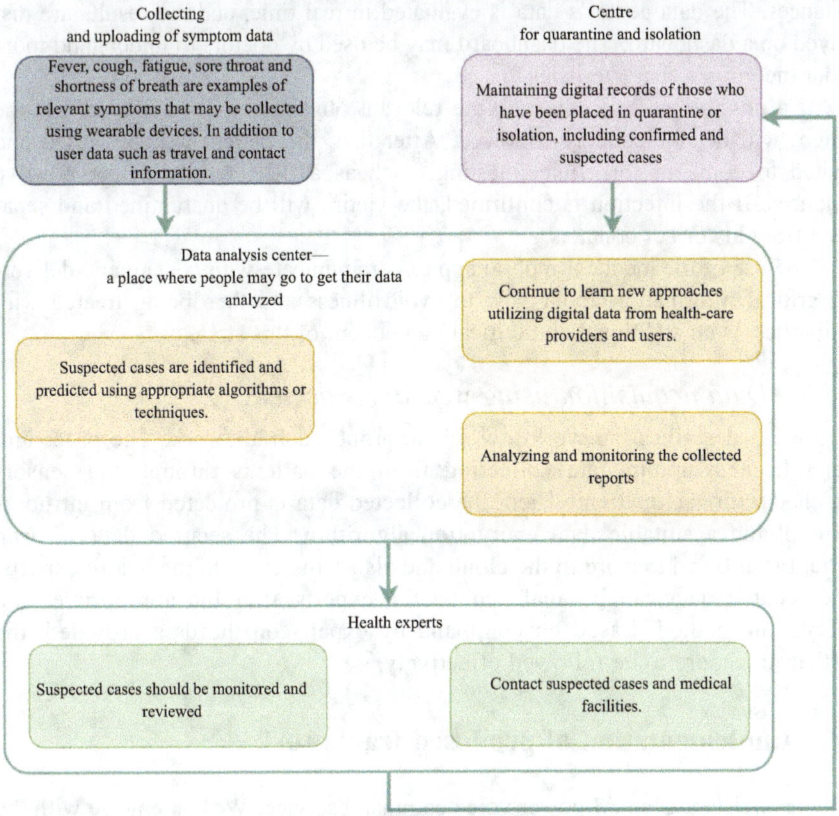

Figure 3.2 Stages of proposed framework

The scenario of the framework (or process) is depicted in Figure 3.2, which may be summarized as follows.

The system uses smart biowearable sensors to collect noninvasive real-time user symptom data. Cough, sore throat, fatigue, fever, and shortness of breath are the symptoms again. Furthermore, the user enters information regarding living in (or traveling to) contaminated locations, as well as probable interaction with COVID-19-affected people, using a mobile application. Regularly, the quarantine/isolation center delivers statistics on isolated and confined patients who are held there. That information is analogous to the real-time information obtained from patients.

Using Google assistant, the collected symptom data is sent to the cloud data analysis center. Regularly, the smart biowearable sensor sends data to the health-care center for data analysis. The data analysis center is home to AI algorithms that update their models daily using data from the research center. Based on each user's real-time symptom data, the AI classifiers are then used to identify possible instances. The data center's data is evaluated in real time, and the results are displayed on a dashboard. The dashboard may be used by doctors to understand more about the virus's characteristics.

If a possible case is detected, the relevant physician will be alerted and the patient will be immediately followed. After that, the patient will be called and invited to come in for clinical testing, such as a PCR test to detect positive instances. If the infection is confirmed, the victim will be quarantined and separated from his or her contacts.

The use of the identical mobile app to communicate with consumers, delivering critical information about how to avoid illness and then being treated with antibiotics, is an additional and critical component of this strategy.

3.4.2 Data acquisition using wearables devices

Figure 3.3 describes the workflow of the proposed framework. The procedure starts from symptom data collecting from the patients through the sensors attached with each patient. Then, the collected data is protected from intruders by applying a suitable data encryption algorithm. The secured data of each patient is allowed to store in the cloud and also transferred to the health experts. The secured data can be analyzed by the experts after the appropriate data decryption method. Based on command by experts on the data provided, the further procedure to be followed effectively.

3.5 Implementation of proposed framework

Google Assistant is an AI power voice command service. We can engage with the Google Assistant by speaking to it, and it can search the Internet, plan events, set alarms, and operate appliances, among other things. This service can be accessed by smart IoT biosensor devices. The Google Assistant conveys the patient illness status to Health management systems. For this research Adafruit, IoT cloud server is used as data analysis [22].

Figure 3.4 describes the implementation of the proposed framework to obtain early diagnosis and provide suitable treatment for COVID-19 patients using Google Assistant and Adafruit IoT cloud server. In this, framework IFTTT (If This Then That)-based web service is used to interface Google Assistant with the cloud platform. Sensor-based setup is attached with each patient who is enabled by a smartphone. The health status of each patient is continuously tracked through Google Assistant by experts/doctors who are placed at the remote location. The Google Assistant may be handled by patients or family members. IFTTT is a free web-based tool that allows users to construct applets, which are chains of basic conditional statements. Changes in other online services, such as Gmail, Facebook, Telegram, Instagram, or Pinterest, might trigger an applet service [23].

Figure 3.5 shows the initial setup in the IFTTT web service. All the patients are categorized into three groups. They are patients with critical conditions,

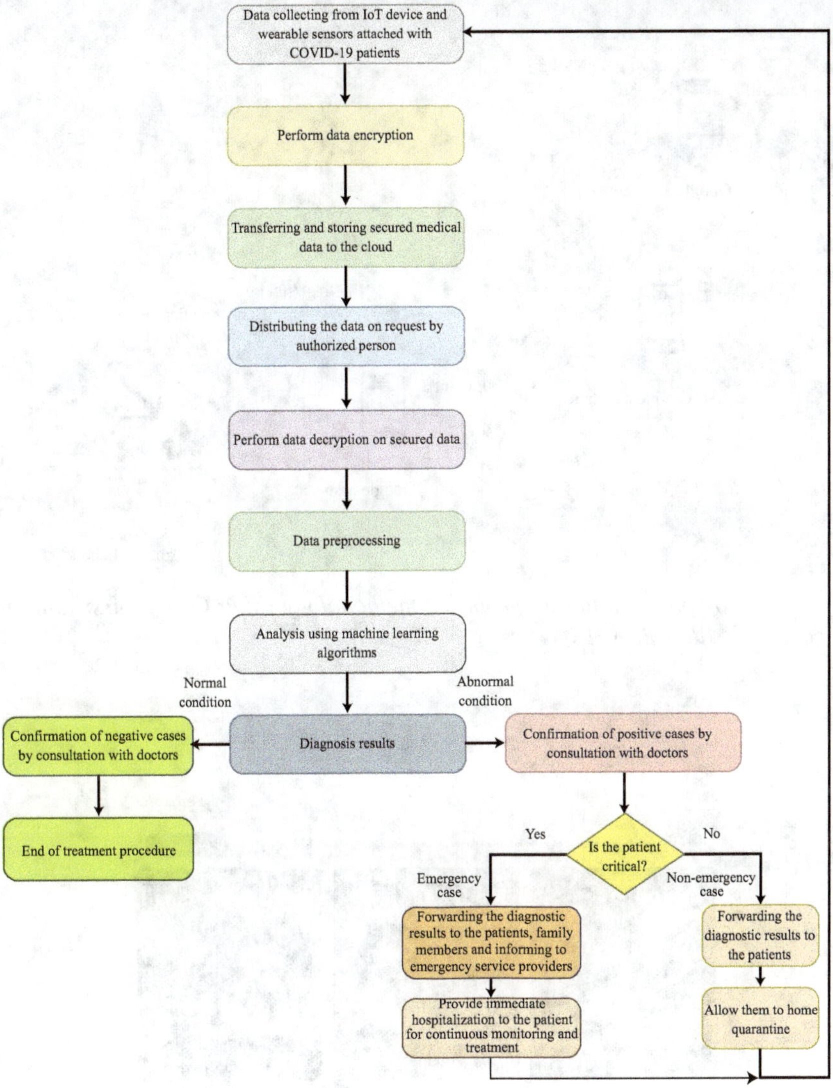

Figure 3.3 Flowchart of proposed framework

patients with normal symptoms (moderate), and patients with light symptoms or no symptoms. Based on suggestions provided by experts, the keywords associated with each symptom are grouped in each category.

Based on the command provided by the patient through the Google Assistant, this setup automatically maps that patient to the corresponding patient group. Through this, doctors can be able to give treatment on a priority basis.

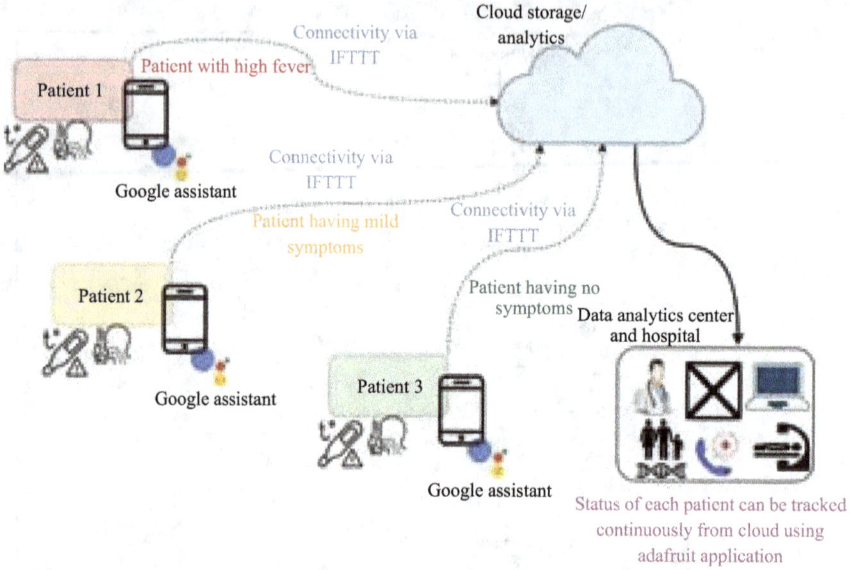

Figure 3.4 Implementation of proposed methodology using Google Assistant and Adafruit API

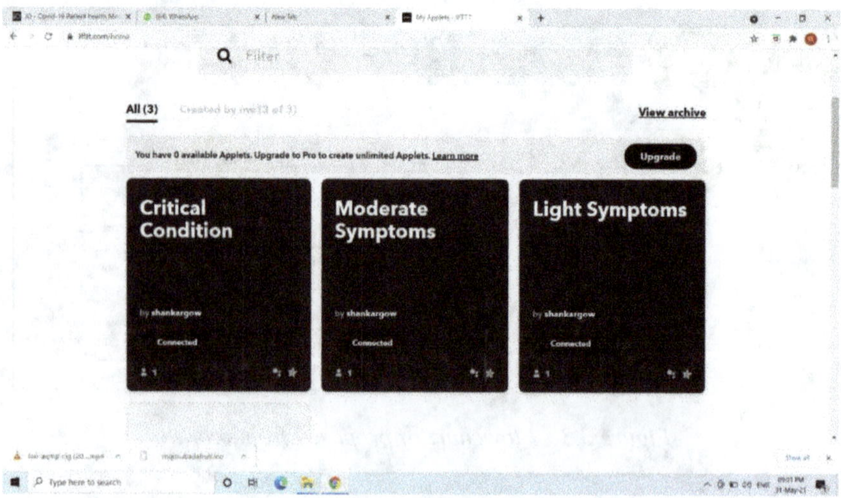

Figure 3.5 Initial setup with IFTTT

3.6 Results and discussion

COVID-19 has a wide range of impacts on different people. The majority of sick people will have minor to severe symptoms and will survive without requiring even going to the hospital. Symptoms include nausea or vomiting, severe diarrhea, and a new lack of taste, tiredness, difficulties in movement, and shortness of breath or difficulty in breathing, chest pain, and loss of speech.

Figure 3.6 shows Google Assistant response for a person having cough symptoms. Based on symptoms (cough) provided, the immediate response will be provided to the patient. Figure 3.7 shows a Google Assistant response for a person having no symptoms.

Patients who are experiencing severe symptoms require prompt medical intervention. Mild symptoms should be managed at home by otherwise healthy people. When a patient is infected with the virus, signs usually start after 5–6 days, although it can take up to 14 days. COVID-19 illness is more likely to have major symptoms in the elderly and those with severe chronic medical problems such as heart disease or diabetes.

Figure 3.8 shows Google Assistant response for a person having fever and Figure 3.9 shows Google Assistant response for a person having severe fever. Based on the status provided, immediate actions will be taken.

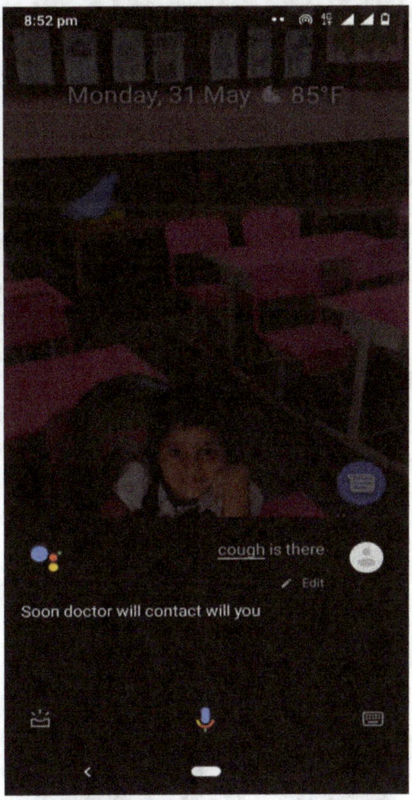

Figure 3.6 Google Assistant response for person having cough symptoms

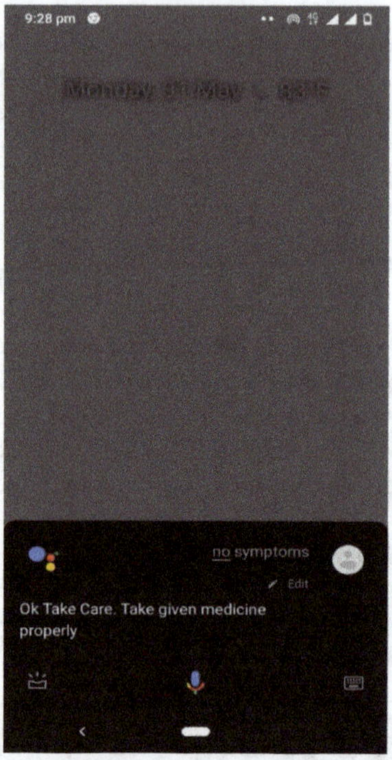

Figure 3.7   Google Assistant response for person having no symptoms

Figure 3.8   Google Assistant response for patient having fever

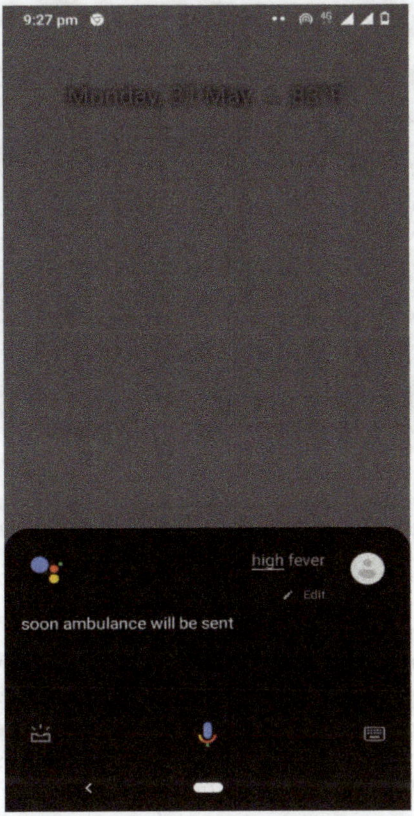

Figure 3.9 Google Assistant response for patient having high fever symptoms

Figure 3.10 illustrates that the cumulative reports of all the patients under treatment are listed along with time. This report is continuously tracked and analyzed by health experts for further decisions.

3.7 Conclusion and future scopes

Due to the increasing elderly population and persons suffering from life-threatening chronic conditions, as well as the high expenses of care for all of these patients, the rising demand for the health-monitoring framework required for the patients at remote places has become a prime requirement in the present scenario in terms of the coronavirus (novel COVID-19) pandemic. Real-time monitoring and analysis of a patient's health status can show crucial and abnormal circumstances, which can aid in the early detection of any potentially fatal ailment. Advanced technologies along with cloud resources and medical IoT devices are critical in the development of digital remote health-monitoring systems.

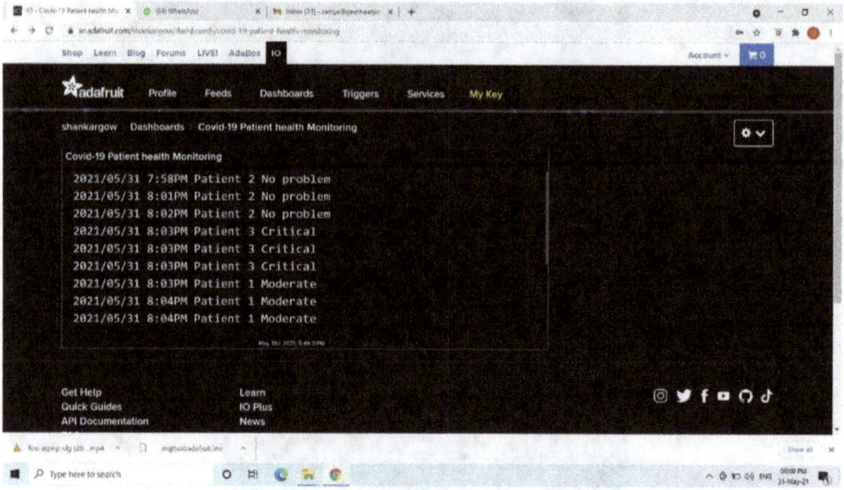

Figure 3.10 Cumulative reports of all the patients through Adafruit API

The healthcare services provided by the proposed framework can be extended for providing treatment to various diseases to reduce the transportation cost, rental expenses, and waiting period. Based on the need, the consultation will be provided to the patients at right time with reasonable expenses. The various experts may interact for each case and provide valuable suggestions as well as recommendations for each healthcare service provider in an effective manner.

References

[1] Parimaladevi M., Sathya T., Gowrishankar V., Boopathi Raja G. and Nithya S. An Efficient Control Strategy for Prevention and Identification of COVID-19 Pandemic Disease. In: Tripathi S. L., Dhir K., Ghai D., Patil S. (eds) *Health Informatics and Technological Solutions for Coronavirus (COVID-19)*. (CRC Press, 2021). https://doi.org/10.1201/9781003161066.

[2] Coronavirus History: https://www.webmd.com/lung/coronavirus-history.

[3] COVID-19: A History of Coronavirus: https://www.labmanager.com/lab-health-and-safety/covid-19-a-history-of-coronavirus-22021.

[4] Kamta N. M. and Chinmay C. A Novel Approach Toward Enhancing the Quality of Life in Smart Cities using Clouds and IoT-Based Technologies. In: *Digital Twin Technologies and Smart Cities, Internet of Things (Technology, Communications and Computing)*, pp. 19–35. (Springer, 2019). https://doi.org/10.1007/978-3-030-18732-3_2.

[5] Symptoms of COVID-19. https://www.cdc.gov/coronavirus/2019-ncov/symptoms-testing/symptoms.html.

[6] Sheikhzadeh E., Eissa S., Ismail A. and Zourob M. Diagnostic Techniques for COVID-19 and New Developments. *Talanta*, 220, 121392, 2020. https://doi.org/10.1016/j.talanta.2020.121392.

[7] Alpdagtas S., Ilhan E., Uysal E., Sengor M., Ustundag C. B. and Gunduz O. Evaluation of Current Diagnostic Methods for COVID-19, *APL Bioengineering*, 4, 041506, 2020. https://doi.org/10.1063/5.0021554.

[8] Information for Clinicians on Investigational Therapeutics for Patients with COVID-19. https://www.cdc.gov/coronavirus/2019-ncov/hcp/therapeutic-options.html.

[9] Lalit G., Emeka C., Nasser N., Chinmay C. and Garg G. Anonymity Preserving IoT-based COVID-19 and Other Infectious Disease Contact Tracing Model, *IEEE Access*, 8, 159402–159414, 2020. 10.1109/ACCESS.2020.3020513, ISSN: 2169-3536.

[10] Archived: WHO Timeline – COVID-19. https://www.who.int/news/item/27-04-2020-who-timeline—covid-19.

[11] Timeline of the Corona virus: https://www.thinkglobalhealth.org/article/updated-timeline-coronavirus.

[12] Akhbarifar S., Javadi H. H. S., Rahmani A. M. *et al.* A Secure Remote Health Monitoring Model for Early Disease Diagnosis in Cloud-Based IoT Environment, *Personal and Ubiquitous Computing*, 2020. https://doi.org/10.1007/s00779-020-01475-3.

[13] Cinay D., Brian L. D and Chinmay C. Generative Design Methodology for Internet of Medical Things (IoMT)-based Wearable Biomedical Devices, *International Congress on Human-Computer Interaction, Optimization and Robotic Applications (HORA'21)*, 1–4, 2021, 10.1109/HORA52670.2021.9461370.

[14] Amit K., Chinmay C. and Wilson J. Intelligent Healthcare Data Segregation using Fog Computing with Internet of Things and Machine Learning, *International Journal of Engineering Systems Modelling and Simulation*, 12 (2/3), 2021, 10.1504/IJESMS.2021.10036745.

[15] Amit K., Chinmay C., Wilson J., Kishor A., Chakraborty C. and Jeberson W. A Novel Fog Computing Approach for Minimization of Latency in Healthcare Using Machine Learning, *International Journal of Interactive Multimedia and Artificial Intelligence*, 1–11, 2020. http://dx.doi.org/10.9781/ijimai.2020.12.004.

[16] Parimala Devi M., Raja G. B., Gowrishankar V. and Sathya T. IoMT-Based Smart Diagnostic/Therapeutic Kit for Pandemic Patients. In: Chakraborty C., Banerjee A., Garg L., Rodrigues J. J. P. C. (eds) *Internet of Medical Things for Smart Healthcare. Studies in Big Data*, vol 80. (Springer, Singapore, 2020). https://doi.org/10.1007/978-981-15-8097-0_6.

[17] Boopathi Raja G., Sathya T., Ragavi P. and Parimaladevi M. Remote Based Wireless Framework for Diagnosing Covid-19 using Internet of Things, *International Journal of Advanced Research in Computer and Communication Engineering*, 10(5), 80–83, 2021. https://doi.org/10.17148/IJARCCE.2021.10514.

[18] Otoom M., Otoum N., Alzubaidi M. A., Etoom Y. and Banihani R. An IoT-based Framework for Early Identification and Monitoring of COVID-19 Cases, *Biomedical Signal Processing and Control*, 62, 102149, 2020. https://doi.org/10.1016/j.bspc.2020.102149.
[19] Chinmay C. and Arij N. A. Intelligent Internet of Things and Advanced Machine Learning Techniques for COVID-19, *EAI Endorsed Transactions on Pervasive Health and Technology*, 1–14, 2021. http://dx.doi.org/10.4108/eai.28-1-2021.168505.
[20] Muhammad L. J., Ebrahem A. A., Sani S. U., Abdulkadir A., Chinmay C. and Mohammed I. A. Supervised Machine Learning Models for Prediction of COVID-19 Infection using Epidemiology Dataset, *SN Computer Science*, 2(11), 1–13, 2021. https://doi.org/10.1007/s42979-020-00394-7.
[21] Sukanya R. and Chinmay C. Panic Buying Situation During COVID-19 Global Pandemic, *Journal of Information Technology Management*, 13(2), 231–44, 2021, DOI:10.22059/jitm.2021.80625.
[22] Adafruit IO website: https://io.adafruit.com.
[23] If This Then That (IFTTT) website: https://ifttt.com/.

Chapter 4

Assessment analysis of COVID-19 on the global economics and trades

Hemanta Kumar Bhuyan[1] *and Chinmay Chakraborty*[2]

Abstract

The worldwide epidemic known as COVID-19 is being labeled a worldwide pandemic on the earlier of 2020, the globe has still not recovered. Cases rapidly spread from China; leading world governments to take extensive infection control measures to several cases and restrict the virus's global transmission rate. However, these controls have undermined the contemporary world economy's main supporting pillars of global commerce and collaboration. In light of the epidemic's context, this chapter critically evaluates the inventory of the pandemic's bad and positive influences in different sections. This advocates for a complete overhaul of the global economic development paradigm based on a linear economy system that leverages profiteering and energy-guzzling industrial processes.

Due to the worldwide breakout of the pandemic COVID-19, the world's political, social, economic, religious, and financial systems have all been thrown into total disarray. As of April 2020, an estimated 4.7 million individuals have been tested, and the illness has resulted in a confirmed infection count of around 2.7 million individuals, with 182,740 deaths attributed to the virus. More than 80 nations have forced companies to shut, locked borders to nations in transition, quarantined their people, and shuttered schools for around 1.5 billion school-age children. A total global economic collapse is inevitable because of the world's largest economies of different countries. The global financial markets have been battered, and tax income sources have crashed into a bottomless pit even more worrisome. Infection is substantially affecting global economic growth. It is anticipated that if the present growth rate continues, the virus might outpace world economic growth by almost 2.0% per month. If the global economic slump is deep and extensive, global commerce might decline from 13% to 32%. It will be years before the full impact of the outbreak is revealed. It looks into the correlation between COVID-19 and the development of the national economy and the stock

[1]Department of Information Technology, Vignan's Foundation for Science, Technology, & Research, Guntur, India
[2]Department of Electronics and Communication Engineering, BIT Mesra, Ranchi, India

market in order to prove how well the COVID-19 economic growth prediction is linked with the gross domestic product. The utilization of publicly accessible data, as found on Yahoo Finance, the International Monetary Fund, John Hopkins COVID-19 map, and regression models was used to carry out the goal of this study. COVID-19 is used to measure the economic effect, and the stock market serves as a proxy for economic variability to test whether or not the forecast is reliable. In the aim that the model can make predictions about two quarters out, it is supposed to provide explanations for changes in the quarter ahead. This study will aid those with government-level decision-making, business-stage strategic thinking, and capital-market investment to better comprehend the current state of affairs and use the model for forecasting.

Keywords: COVID-19; Financial systems; Regression model; Gross domestic products; Product revenue; World economy growth

4.1 Introduction

The World Health Organization (WHO) proclaimed the new coronavirus (COVID-19) a pandemic, the world came to attention to a severe issue [1,2]. The virus quickly spread worldwide, first to Japan, South Korea, Europe, and the United States. In preparation for the official pandemic proclamation, early this year, substantial economic signs showed that the globe was leaning in the direction of an unparalleled watershed in human history if not of our time [3]. Many specialists within the professional cadres of various industries have made warnings of a global financial disaster. Expert commentary had predicted an escalating disease crisis but, by all accounts, the growing chaos brought by the pandemic was more than what was expected. Based on the number of deceased individuals, the virus has spread over 800,000 [4]. As a result, livelihoods have been interrupted for millions of people. At the time of writing, a global recession is looming [5]. Countries worldwide undertook strict steps to combat the epidemic while also trying to minimize the number of cases. These included obligatory national lockdowns and border closures.

The pillars on which these tactics have destroyed contemporary economies rest. The financial consequences of this epidemic are still being calculated as of now. Data is in constant motion, government policies often shift, and the virus that kills its victims spreads from country to country, interrupting manufacturing, introducing supply networks to dysfunction, and destabilizing financial markets [6]. Overall, the increasing data indicates that we are at a time when the earth's sustainability has to be reconsidered. At the same time, though, inevitable accidental environmental and ecological consequences have resulted from governmental policies. Going ahead, it is now possible to imagine a significant shift to human biological and physical activity on Earth [7]. But according to [5], noted by these authors, our investment in global integration and economic growth is no longer feasible for stable development. A possible answer to the quest for numerous economic, environmental, and financial goals is implementing the financial system.

On the one hand, these packages concentrate on accelerating the existing economic status quo. On the other hand, they are dedicated to building a more sustainable low-carbon economy. This chapter urges for the recalibration and rethink of the current global economic growth model, which is predicated on a linear economy system and uses industrial methods that need excessive use of natural resources and the pursuit of profit before the environment. Both future resilience and competitiveness are made possible by this plan and the belief that future unintentional that emerged during the corona virus calamity may be effectively utilized or frozen to supply openings for both long-term strength and the future.

4.2 Backgrounds

A problem statement cannot be developed when an effective literature review is not completed, and a literature review illustrates a paradox [8,9]. Additionally, doing a literature search is critical in pinpointing numerous research questions. A search and evaluation of the current literature is used to get around this problem. Adopting the previous conceptual framework was utilized to build empirical work that presents research derives. Based on the framework, the present research employed theory to undertake an in-depth review.

Given that it utilizes the critical literature review (CLR) methodology, the chapter explores the issue under research, critically assessing, synthesizing, and articulating pertinent materials to help provide new theoretical frameworks and viewpoints from several disciplines [10]. The problem CLR has when it comes to subjectivity is amplified by Grant and Booth [11]. They contend that because of the emphasis on stringent literature selection in systematic literature review (SLR), an SLR might help to improve the issue. While the study does focus on a particular part of the pandemic, it looks at the effects of COVID-19 on the global economy and ecosystems and the benefits of circular economy (CE) initiatives. To achieve this aim, the author believes that a CLR method is the best choice. It enables for a diverse variety of theoretical viewpoints and opinions from other sources to be included [10].

In light of this, the chapter in this collection includes archived data of newspaper stories, government policy documents, experts' interviews, expert opinions, and reports that were pertinent to COVID-19 and the notion of CE. After reviewing the search results, both theoretical and empirical models were developed and then utilized to build the CLR. A specific impact analysis was carried out for the study, using the $I = P \times A \times T$ model, where I is impact defined through population size (P), per capita affluence (A), and technology (T) maintaining and consuming unit-wise.

It was then explored whether the role of CE as a vehicle for a productive variance of COVID-19 can continue to exist in the post-COVID-19 world. These exploratory activities were then completed with observable reflections based on cumulative data of CEs after COVID-19.

4.3 Social impacts on finance

The least amount of time for an epidemic causes stress on the healthcare system, and hardship on the economy is few months. In other words, the long-held view that any sort of infectious illness epidemic is a significant source of localized economic troubles is still correct [12–14]. History is replete with instances of endemics, plagues, and pandemics, all of which represent significant outbreaks. In many cases, this increased the likelihood of states collapsing, healthcare facilities swamped, social unrest, and creating an economic dislocation that affected other sectors. Near the beginning months of the COVID-19 pandemic, it has become apparent that all-natural, incidental, or purposeful risks to global health and the international economy now represent an unquantifiable risk.

Pandemics have been occurring at a higher frequency during the last 100 years, according to [15]. Some sources suggest a petite with numerous records of epidemics of infectious diseases, which comprise the Black Death [16], the Justinian plague [17], the Spanish flu [18], HIV/AIDS [19], SARS [20], Ebola [21], and dengue [22]. This outbreak's potency fluctuates from outbreak to outbreak. Because of this, their impact on the economy differs in various retroactive evaluations [11]. As an example, in 2013–14, while the Ebola virus was ravaging West Africa, it cost the countries involved $53 billion [23].

Today's environment is vastly different from that of previous epidemics. It is not feasible to make direct parallels between the present the socioeconomic crisis of COVID-19 and earlier global pandemics, since several aspects have changed in the last few decades [23] with distinguishing characteristics. Yet, historical lessons from prior epidemics remain valuable, even though the modern world is quite different from what was prevalent in the past [24]. Thus, the CEs strategy in Figure 4.1 shows different historical consequences of COVID-19.

These include reasons such as the fact that the globe is increasingly interconnected because of globalization and technology improvements, which means that the worldwide pandemic known as COVID-19 is a serious concern [25–29]. Science, health, and engineering have all seen dramatic improvements throughout the years. Air travel was hindered during the previous pandemics because of the small number of passengers. There is no longer the case since travel has expanded significantly worldwide. Due to low-interest rates, there is a surplus of goods, but demand and supply are balanced at record lows [23]. Even more critically, the nations experiencing a major impact from the present epidemic are not only lower middle income nations but also the global manufacturing and supply-chain powerhouse nations. The optimization model can use to analyze for the supply chain as [30,31]. Based on the previous issues, the evaluation of the effects of COVID-19 is mentioned in the next section.

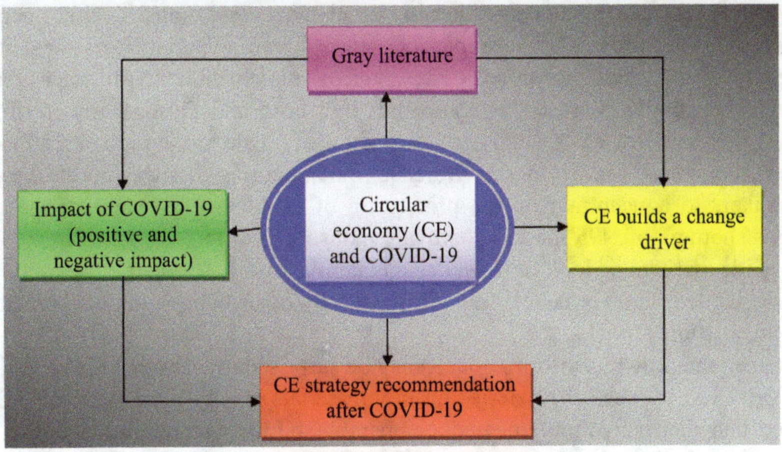

Figure 4.1 The circular economy for COVID-19

4.4 Framework for the international financial system, bionetworks, and maintainability on pandemic

4.4.1 Assessment strategy constructions to fight COVID-19

The various nations have implemented different methods and policies to address COVID-19 at different epidemic stages when resources were at a premium. Even though 65% of global production and exports are done in nations such as China, the United States, Korea, Japan, France, Italy, and the United Kingdom, these nations were most hurt by COVID-19 [32]. Due to the inadequacy of hospitals to respond to situations requiring medical equipment, there has been a focus on acquiring tools such as personal protective equipment (PPE) and ventilators [33]. We have got to design frameworks that maximize their utilization alongside bed areas when it comes to ventilators. Additionally, many businesses have also been negatively impacted, including mining businesses that have been adversely impacted by changes in process and international commodity worth. The features of data can be considered [34–36].

COVID-19 causes panic purchasing because of national and individual degrees of uncertainty, as detailed in future sections. The shortcomings of the traditional supply-chain paradigm have been laid bare in each of these cases. They were concerned about whether the framework would deal with crucial goods when they were necessary. Following are the worldwide finance repercussions of COVID-19, along with further discussion on the situation: global production, export, and import volume.

4.4.2 Macro-finance impacts

One difficulty that the healthcare business faces is that best practices, such as the JIT macroeconomic framework used in the USA (e.g. stockpile critical medical equipment), do not financially incentivize the accumulation of vital medical equipment. This proved to be expensive since governments such as the United Kingdom, India, and the United States had to implement extreme measures to secure their supply chain to let companies like Ford and Dyson compete in the market for ventilator design and manufacturing [37]. Due to the high costs and the critical scarcity of ventilators, the Defense Manufacturing Act was invoked to get automakers to concentrate on the production of ventilators. Because of the continuous shortage of N95 masks, pharmacy industry of different country joined the worldwide market and look for lower cost equipment [38]. The state of scarcity was that the United States was accused of "piracy" by other nations in Asia's medical equipment supply stocks.

Given the previous information, it may be surprised to learn that China and the EU waived or reduced their duties on raw materials and PPE, respectively. Both France and Germany implemented comparable blinkered policies, and the EU enforced limitations on the exporting of PPEs, placing a lot of nations that had previously depended on the exporting of PPEs in jeopardy [39]. Logistics problems and the misallocation of important equipment may cause an increase in the transparency and traceability of emerging technologies like blockchain, RFID, and Internet of Things (IoT). Technology alone will never solve our future problems, which need cooperation and scenario planning to supplement it. To help states avoid incurring federal competition, the EU put a procurement framework for member states to reduce competition amongst themselves.

On the other hand, in the United States, where state governments had complained that federal involvement with orders had the potential to stifle competition, a ventilator exchange program was established. Realization creates openings for manufacturing localization, which comes with the repercussions of developments in ecological and communal maintainability [32]. It is shown in the instance of N95 masks, which skyrocketed in popularity enough that both private and commercial flights employed air freight services to provide them instead of using standard shipping containers [40].

To sum up the findings presented in upcoming parts, there was a notable decrease in emissions associated with conventional shipping, but at the same time, a rise in the use of air shipping because of customers' and suppliers' desperation and hurry. In any case, many nations worldwide have had to reevaluate their international prices as a consequence of COVID-19 epidemic reality. This is because a pandemic in the early 1990s, COVID-19, and several eastern European and Mediterranean nations have all led to a greater appreciation of national interests and protectionism. The graph in Figure 4.2 shows the worldwide sell overseas for each nation, compared to China's share of the equivalent sell overseas (*x*-axis and *y*-axis). The ideal chart for each product has a huge circle that is located in the upper right corner.

4.4.3 Econometric effects: consumer preferences

There has been disconnecting between people's material desires and the physical world for quite some time. The widespread use of COVID-19 has compounded the

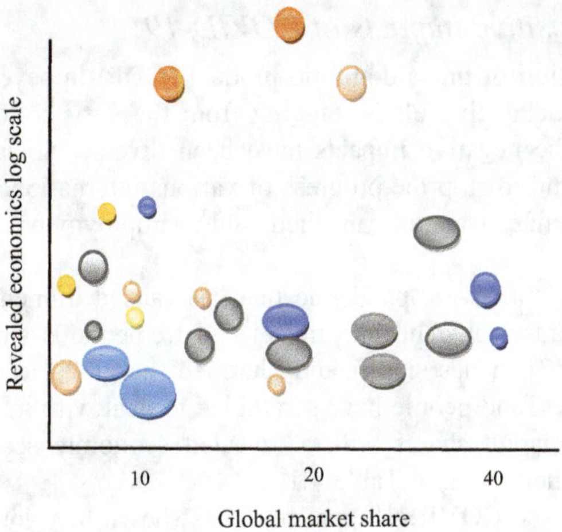

Figure 4.2 Global product export from China to other countries as [43]

increased focus on the societal consequences of individual behaviors. In many nations, the behavior of consumers was first panicky with significant purchases of food and sanitary supplies. Overall, consumer attitude is also shifting, both privately and in the marketplace. It has caused people to reevaluate their spending habits and requirements and prioritize the necessities more. Tech obsolescence is affecting both the linear economy model and the business-as-usual model. It predicts mobile phones with a normal lifespan of 2 years (1 year in the United States) depending on manufacturing and renovating facilities restrained by finance shutdowns.

Cottage industry production may solve crucial equipment costs, which are all too costly, rare, high-skilled, and material-intensive. In contrast, however, medical technology, which might greatly profit from gathering manufacturing and the customaries of high-tech tool, is saddled with the problem of patents. To assist cope with health issues like COVID-19, the problem of 3D printer in-frustration in Italy led to proposals for open pharmacy facilities.

In some countries, factories are running out of facemask inventory and have to ration their production and distribution. Interestingly, Livingston *et al.* [41] described that the handmade facemask business has sprung up to serve the more significant population. Still, it has also become important in ensuring the supply of resources and aiding an evacuation route if a lockdown is in place. The resurrection of traditional small house-built-up methods of manufacturing tools and simple but needed goods like facemasks might fundamentally alter the global manufacturing environment for decades to come, likely lowering levels of consumerism. Due to the high likelihood, a recession will result in short-term views, which will cause companies to cancel the long-term product. It is primarily for companies in the automotive and aerospace industries that previously endured recessions.

4.4.4 Nonpositive impacts of COVID-19

From a contraction of gross domestic product (GDP) in several nations to environmental and social difficulties, ranging from the very bottom of society to the upper classes, the negative impacts have been diverse. Socioeconomic activities effectively ground to stop the progress of various international event aspects. The entertainment venues were all cancelled, and unemployment claims went up in the millions.

COVID-19 is a severe pandemic that has caused immense human suffering, resulted in a catastrophic health, and placed tremendous strain on international economies [42,43]. It has significantly harmed the global economy, and governments, businesses, and people have scrambled to deal with it. Figure 4.2 identifies several global market shares with a revealed economic scale during pandemic COVID-19, as mentioned in Table 4.1.

As a result, the COVID-19 pandemic has shown the world's economic paradigm to be utterly vulnerable to unanticipated disruptions and catastrophes. It has highlighted the vulnerabilities of centralized global supply and production chains networks and instability in global economies. This has directly impacted employment, and as a result, has created an increased danger of food poverty for millions owing to the locking down of borders and the imposition of border restrictions. Some government interventions have brought to a leveling of the COVID-19 data (as mentioned in Table 4.2). As at the time of writing, new healthcare crises are continually occurring in various world regions.

Despite predicting a modest global economic growth rate of 3.3% in 2020, the IMF now says that the global economy would contract by 6.3% in the same period. The potential financial catastrophe this would cause is equivalent to a worldwide financial shock like the enormous despair and worse, which has already exceeded the severity of the international economic crisis of 2009 as in Tables 4.3 and 4.4. With caution, a detrimental impact is projected for emerging and developing economics, while recessions are seen to occur in China and India by the end of 2020.

Table 4.1 Different global products shared in a different country as Figure 4.2

S. no.	Global market share	Revealed economics scale	Colors
1	Fabricated metals	Kazakhstan ferroalloys	Blue
2	Machinery equipment	Bulgaria, Egypt, Hungary, Morocco, Romania	Gray
3	Textiles, footwear	Jordan sports clothing, Turkey	Green
4	Chemicals and pharmacy products	Morocco fertilizers	Light red
5	Motor vehicles and transport	Hungary, Poland, Romania	Yellow
6	Vegetable products	Uzbekistan frozen vegetables	Deep red
7	Other manufacturing	Lithuania, Poland, Romania	Light green

Table 4.2 Month-wise new COVID-19 cases in 10 most affected countries (as $k = 1{,}000$ values)

	Feb 2020	Mar 2020	Apr 2020	May 2020	Jun 2020	Jul 2020	Aug 2020
India	0	0.1	1	2	6	23	70
USA	0	0.1	30	31	20	60	70
Brazil	0	0.1	1	5	20	40	50
Mexico	0	0.1	1	5	8	5	4
Colombia	0	0.1	1	2	2	3	6
Argentina	0	0.1	1	2	2	3	3
Peru	0	0.1	1	2	4	3	3
South Africa	0	0.1	1	2	2	3	10
Iran	0	0.1	1	2	2	3	4
Russia	0	0.1	1	2	2	3	4

Table 4.3 Comparison finance effects between COVID-19 lockdown 2020 and global financial crisis 2009

Economics item	COVID-19 lockdown 2020	2009 global financial crisis
Global economic growth forecast	−3.0	−0.1
Advanced economics	−6.0	−3.2
Emerging market and developing economics	−1.0	2.8
Major economies in recession		
1. United States	−6.0	−2.5
2. Euro Area	−7.5	−4.8
3. Japan	−5.0	−5.4
4. China	0.1	9.2
5. India	2.0	8.2

Table 4.4 Economic loss over 2020 and 2021

	2018	2019	2020	2021
Expected GDP growth	97	100	104	107
Loss of GDP growth	97	100	97	102

The collective GDP loss due to COVID-19 might be over $9 trillion over the following year.

The current rise in worldwide poverty might be the first since 1998. Up to 49 million people might be forced into severe poverty because of the effect

COVID-19 is projected to have on sub-Saharan Africa. Using the most effective policy tools, the finance department predicts the growth rate of poverty, inequality, exclusion, and discrimination over the medium and long run. Global security structures used as a kind of automatic stabilizers can significantly lessen the occurrence of poverty and safeguard employees for several years to come.

In Table 4.2, all values are multiplied by 1,000 to make the number of people affected COVID-19.

4.4.5 Impact of international commercial trading

COVID-19 is expected to contribute to reducing the world economy. Fragmentation and geographic dispersion inherently plague supply systems. While it has made organizations more complex and interconnected, globalization has also made them more susceptible to upheavals. According to an examination conducted by the United States, most businesses have accounted for commotions in their trading. This has caused a supply-chain emergency that originated from the short-sightedness and inflexibility of various supply chains at different layers around the world and the limited supply diversity that companies use. These disruptions would affect the loss of production for enterprises in exporting nations and the unavailability of raw materials for enterprises in importing nations. In the end, this will result in a "momentary manufacturing desert" in which a nation, area, or city's production decreases considerably, resulting in a geographic restriction in which everything except basics, such as food items and prescription pharmaceuticals, may be obtained. Due to China's rise to prominence in global supply chains and the economy, this has resulted. Global commerce is expected to shrink by around 32% as a result of COVID-19.

A clear example of this is China's decreased exports, which have led to the worldwide decrease in economic activity. Trade has now contracted for the second time since the mid-1980s. Based on various pandemic waves and hazard levels, the picture illustrates how a pandemic affects global supply networks.

4.4.6 COVID-19's effect on the aviation industry

As a result of the massive movement and aircraft limitations in place, the transportation industry has borne the brunt of COVID-19.

Aviation, for example, has seen flight cancellations and prohibitions, resulting in fewer flights and significant revenue losses. The expenses of operating and maintaining an airport do not decrease as traffic demands fall, making it difficult for airports to lower expenses since running and maintaining an airport stays the same. The full-year 2020 maintains two scenarios for economic aspects: Scenario 1 (recovery in the latter part of May) and Scenario 2 (start again in the third quarter). It anticipated with Scenario 1 that the number of airline seats would be reduced between 39% and 56%, as well as the number of passengers between 872 and 1,303 million, failing disgusting functioning incomes of about \$153–\$231 billion. It is operating with Scenario 2 and predicts that there would be a loss of between 49% and 72% of airline seats: 1,124 to 1 with a

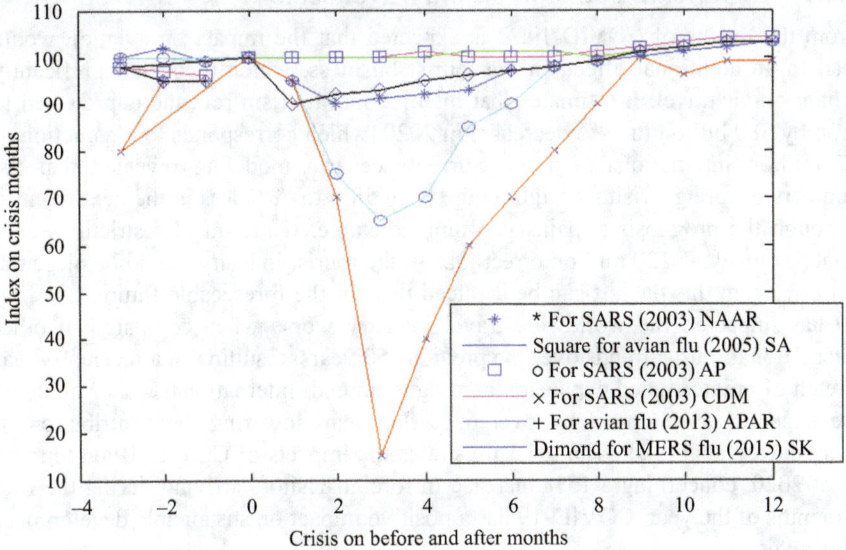

Figure 4.3 Effect of past disease outbreaks on aviation

corresponding loss in revenue of $198–$273 billion. They stated that the projected outcomes are dependent on the length and magnitude of the pandemic and on the number of funds put toward managing the crisis, the degree of consumer trust for air travel, the state of the global economy, and the speed of the country's economic recovery [44].

When losses occur in the aviation sector, it is essential to contextualize the situation, and various other comparisons have also been made about the airline business. Foreign passengers are expected to decrease from 44% to 80% between 2019 and 2020. Airports Council International predicted that air passenger traffic would decline by two-fifths and cost $76 billion in 2020 if airport revenues remain constant. IATA anticipated $113 billion in mislaid income and a 48% decrease in domestic and international flights. Predicting an epidemic scenario is mentioned in Figure 4.3. The history of prior illness outbreaks reveals the degree of their influence on aviation. The 8% drop in RPKs and $6 billion in incomes for Asia/Pacific airlines have all been down to COVID-19's influence. While the 6-month recovery road for SARS seems long, it offers an understanding of global markets.

However, the aviation industry also has an obligation for several economic aspects, such as fuel economy and waste utilization, and not just focus on income loss due to COVID-19. This is rather unfortunate news, as per economical air travel, since it will likely result in significant job losses. However, in the eyes of environmentalists, these projections are hopeful, and they should motivate the airline sector to examine greener, more sustainable methods.

4.4.7 Significant collision on the travel sector

From the results of COVID-19, it is expected that the impact on aviation would lead to an additional effect on the tourist business, which today is significantly reliant on air travel. It estimates that international tourism revenue is projected to drop by $80 billion (a 22% decrease) in 2020, which corresponds to a reduction of 67 million international visitors. Current scenario modeling revealed that the numbers of foreign visitors might range from 58% to 78% less in the next months, although the prognosis remains very unpredictable. If the travel restrictions continue, as many as 120 million direct jobs in the tourist industry would be placed at danger. From this data, it can be deduced that for the foreseeable future, COVID-19 has impacted the worldwide travel industry worse when compared to other international tourist trends over the previous 50 years, resulting in a recent 10-year stretch of uninterrupted expansion coming to an end. International visitor numbers are expected to plummet by over 60% this year, lowering the contribution of tourism to global GDP. Table 4.5 illustrates the impacts of COVID-19 on tourism in of 2020, concerning a 15% increase in foreign visitors arriving during the first 3 months of the year. COVID-19 has a positive impact on sustainable development objectives.

UN member states in 2015 agreed to set 17 Sustainable Development Goals (SDGs) to enhance the standard of living for people and the natural environment by 2030. The SDGs were constructed on two substantial assumptions: globalization and economic development. The fact that COVID-19 has already hindered this assumption has been covered in the preceding sections. Coverage provided by COVID-19 is drawing attention to the fact that the SDGs presently exist cannot cope with epidemics. Progress was at a standstill before COVID-19, since the SDGs had not been fully established.

Here we have covered some of the benefits of COVID-19. Despite the vast array of problems caused, COVID-19 has resulted in some good improvements in behavior and attitudes. The following topics are on the rise because of the flu, and they help illustrate the increasing pace incorporate functions that have decreased productive operations. This has caused considerable decreases in exhaust emissions from autos, other forms of fuel burning. Earth Observatory satellites demonstrate significant decreases in air pollution across China and important European towns as indicated in Figure 4.4. Air pollution in China was reduced by 20%–30%, with similar reductions in the United States and India, while in Rome, Milan, and Madrid the air pollution concentration fell by 45%–54%, while Paris had a

Table 4.5 The impact of COVID-19 on tourism in quarter 1 of 2020

	World	Europe	Asia and the Pacific	Americas	Africa	Middle East
January	2	6	−2	0	4	6
February	−9	6	−37	3	4	5
March	−57	−60	−64	−46	−44	−41

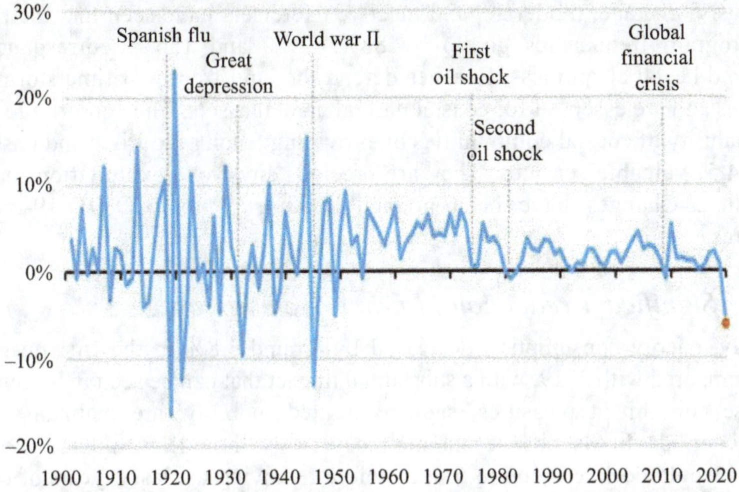

Figure 4.4 Yearly rate of change with effecting energy demand highlighted

tremendous drop of 54%. Air pollution caused by NO_2 dramatically decreased in significant cities in the United Kingdom. Note that in some regions of China, pollution mitigation measures are inadequate because of the harmful environmental impacts; the reduction in human activities cannot wholly compensate because of adverse alterations to the environment.

The preceding possibilities emphasize the dangers of our current lifestyles and strong dependence on fossil fuel-based transportation systems. This kind of pollution created a plethora of respiratory illnesses, including respiratory disease, coronary heart disease, lung cancer, and asthma, among others. Air pollution has shown to be a substantial environmental hazard to the general health and well-being of the population. According to research conducted in the United Kingdom, approximately between 28,000 and 36,000 fatalities per year is associated with enduring disclosure to air pollution. It has been stated that the decrease in air pollution during the lockdown time in conjunction with the subsequent developments in air excellence had saved more lives than would have been spared, otherwise due to COVID-19 in China.

Air pollution has decreased; however, the reduction in ambient noise has been minimal. A significant number of Europeans, about 20% of the population, suffer long-term exposure to harmful noise levels. About 48,000 new occurrences of ischemic heart disease each year and approximately 12,000 early deaths are due to environmental noise pollution. Over 22 million individuals are chronically irritated while around 6.5 million individuals are impacted by severe restlessness. About 12,500 pupils had noise-induced hearing loss as a result of the planes flying over them.

According to a recent survey, pandemic COVID-19 enhanced global levels of physical activity by less traffic congestion and lower noise and pollution. As seen previously, average, moderate, and inactive exercisers have seen that their exercise program frequencies go up by 88%, 38%, and 156%, correspondingly improved beach cleanliness. Beaches defend the land from maritime storms and cyclones and are essential for coastal natural capital assets. They contribute to the sustainability of coastal communities by providing (such as tourism and leisure as Table 4.5) valuable services. They are precious since overexploitation must be controlled. Changes have been noticed because of the COVID-19-induced measures.

4.4.8 Significant reduction in primary energy usage

Globally, energy consumption decreased by around 3.8% in the first quarter of 2020 compared with 2019, with a substantial impact that can be seen in March [45]. Suppose curtailment measures, such as limited mobility, are maintained over lengthy periods. In that case, economic recoveries will be delayed, and the energy demand would decline by up to 6%; therefore removing the last 5 years of energy required increases. In Figure 4.4, IEA predicts that global energy demand would plummet to levels not seen in the last 70 years if their predictions come to fruition. The impact will be 7.4 times greater than the 2008 financial catastrophe. Alternatively, if COVID-19 is discovered sooner than expected and the economy experiences a rapid recovery, the drop in energy might be limited to around 4% [45].

Although 8% less coal was produced in the first quarter of 2019 compared to the same period last year, overall demand was higher owing to China's heavy reliance on coal, cheaper gas, renewable energy growth, and warm weather conditions. Oil consumption fell by over 5% in the first quarter as a result of transportation and aviation-related constraints accounting for over 60% of global oil consumption [45]. Some road and air transportation industries activity was about 50% and 60% below the 2019 average. With complete lockdown limitations in place, global power consumption decreased by nearly 20%. This corresponded with a spillover impact on the energy mix. Similarly, renewable energy sources' proportion in the overall energy supply expanded due to increasing capacity and more priority dispatch, given that their outputs are generally unhampered by consumer demand [45].

4.4.9 Record decrease in CO_2 emissions

COVID-19's massive drop in energy consumption was the primary cause of the substantial decrease in worldwide greenhouse gas emissions. Although no such event has occurred, CO_2 emissions are forecast to continue falling at a pace never seen before. The 8% emissions reduction will likely lead to the most considerable emission decrease ever recorded (Figure 4.5). That rate of decline is also expected to be greater than the sum of the five deepest recessions that the United States has experienced since the 1950s [45]. Because of this, there will be an increase in emissions after the economic downturn has ended, unless interventions are based on greener and more robust energy infrastructure [45].

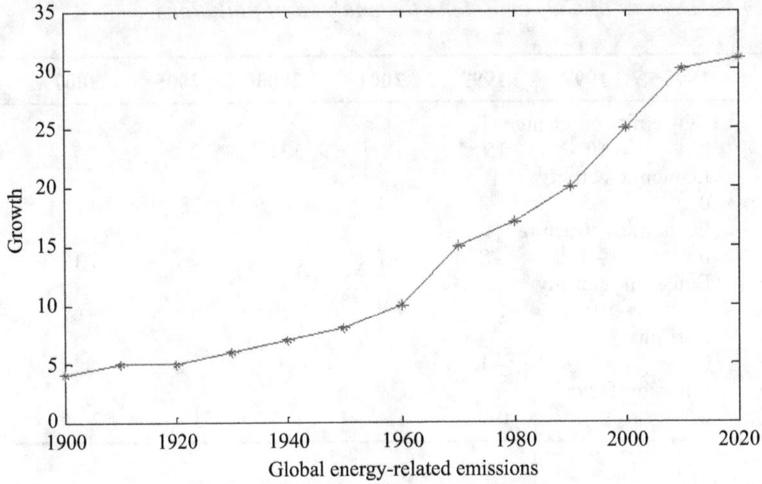

Figure 4.5 Global energy-related emissions provide a sense of scale [45]

4.4.10 Rise in digitalization

One aspect of the decline in air pollution after the COVID-19 introduction directly resulted from the reduction in economic activity caused by the lockdown. While this effect is temporary, though, there is a difference in the structure of the global economy, as demonstrated by the improvement in air quality after the introduction of COVID-19. The improvements are not the result of appropriate climate change policies enacted by governments, and as such, should not be seen to represent a victory in this area. More crucially, economies will need to recover, and emissions will rise. To emphasize our thesis, we carried out a decomposition study of four worldwide air pollution drivers (accelerators or retardants) with the findings presented in Tables 4.6 and 4.7.

For example, although global CO_2 emission increased by 32% from 1995 to 2009, economic activity and emission factor accelerated the increase as shown in Figure 4.5. Still, the economic structure, emission intensity, and fuel mix each had a role in slowing down the increase. Although economic activity with emission factor boosted emissions, the addition of driving variables, such as economic structure, emission intensity, and fuel mix, mitigated this upward impact. Reducing flying and driving in response to COVID-19 helped reduce emissions by around 8%. However, zero-emissions are unattainable due to these actions alone. It means emissions reduction is only possible when an ideal balance is found among the following four drivers: the economy, policy, technology, and innovation.

Typically, following a recession, such as the global economic crisis of 2008, the environment experiences an increase in pollution. However, the substantial and persistent reduction necessary to establish a low-carbon economy will not be caused by societal reactions. This is visible since we have interconnected supply networks, multidimensional manufacturing methods, and nonlinear consumer

Table 4.6 Drivers of CO_2 emissions for analysis of pollutions

S. no.	1995	1997	1999	2001	2003	2005	2007	2009
1	CO_2 emission change							
	0	10	15	18	13	2	−7	−10
2	Economic activity							
	0	−5	−2	−1	10	28	48	50
3	Economics structure							
	0	−5	−8	−7	−11	−7	−10	−10
4	Emission intensity							
	0	10	15	17	12	0	−6	−10
5	Fuel mix							
	0	0	−1	−1	−1	−2	−3	−4
6	Emission factor							
	0	0	0	1	1	1	2	2

Table 4.7 Drivers of NO_x emissions for analysis of pollutions

S. no.	1995	1997	1999	2001	2003	2005	2007	2009
1	NO_x emission change							
	0	−5	−12	−10	−5	−4	−20	−30
2	Economic activity							
	0	11	19	17	27	43	57	34
3	Economics structure							
	0	0	−5	−8	−2	0	−2	−5
4	Emission intensity							
	0	−10	−7	3	−8	−25	−32	−12
5	Fossil fuel dependency							
	0	0	−0.5	0	−0.1	−0.1	0	−0.2
6	Emission factor							
	0	−10	−18	−16	−20	−24	−40	−42

behaviors. While this might enhance the number of environment-friendly alternatives available to customers, it may also cause a rise in vehicle ownership and hence an increase in carbon emissions. Suppose sustainability principles inspired by the concepts of low-carbon CE are to be expanded. In that case, proper methods to maintain the right balance in the ecological life that the world can endure are imperative. Next, the possible use of the CE in combatting such pandemics as COVID-19 is addressed.

4.5 The role of circular economy

The conventional linear financial system has long been the foundation of the industrial economy. The unrestricted use of natural resources, regardless of their long-term sustainability, puts a strain on the planet's capacity to produce such resources. Let us take the manufacturing industry example; around 90% of raw materials are considered trash before leaving the production facility, yet in manufacturing, 80% of things made have been disposed of during the first 6 months of their existence. Similarly, Hoornweg and Bhada-Tata [46] have found that an annual quantity of 1.3 billion tonnes of solid waste with a total price tag of $205.4 billion. They estimate that the total quantity of this waste could grow to 2.2 billion tonnes by 2025, which would increase the total price tag to $375.5 billion. Thus, worldwide demand for resources is expected to increase by 2-fold by the year 2050. Under these circumstances, it maximizes the ability to decouple financial development from raw materials and reduce waste and building capital has intensified.

These three ideas are key in developing a comprehensive environmental system design: create goods and materials out of waste, utilize goods and materials, and regenerate natural systems. CE is focused on (i) I helping companies maximize the ecological benefits of their manufacturing and product recovery activities; (ii) bringing about a harmonious ecological partnership between corporations, consumers, and governments; and (iii) moving to a manufactured goods worth that takes into consideration the environmental impact from inception to end-of-life.

Now is the perfect opportunity to study how the CE principles may be used in the actual world when the global economy rebounds. The pandemic has made it abundantly clear financial system, which is falling short on solving environmental and social problems. Humans have only intensified their interconnections and interdependencies in the current global pandemic, with their natural environment, economy, and social systems. This chapter will briefly explore the several possible uses of CE as a tool in terms of mitigating climate change, helping construct well financial system, and fostering socially equitable and inclusive societies.

4.5.1 *The circular economy for slowing the onset of climate collapse*

The abnormal finding from the shutdown is that while the limitations to movement and other leisure activities were in place, emissions were at 92% of the starting figure. Worrying climate change mitigation measures have often been framed as "prohibiting the beautiful things of life," yet, as shown, merely cutting off 8% of these "good things" provides an actual decrease in greenhouse gas emissions. Thus, reducing emissions from power plants has a cost of around $3,200–$5,400 per tonne of carbon dioxide in the United States, for example, as reported by the Rhodium Group [47]. It states that, if an 8% CO_2 emission decrease occurs, it would release an equivalent of about 172 billion tonnes of CO_2 instead of 187 billion tonnes of CO_2. This implies that a completely new strategy is necessary in the effort to tackle the climate challenge.

Therefore, as a result, a more robust low-carbon CE model must be widely adopted in order to combat the findings of researchers who believe climate breakdown, rather than COVID-19, will be the largest danger to world health. A considerable reduction in greenhouse gas emissions cannot be achieved with renewable energy just but with CE methods. Reduce emissions while promoting climate change mitigation by putting pressure on product life cycle management, like (i) material recirculation (reducing the production of primary materials while increasing the use of recycled materials); (ii) with a link to using more recycled materials while decreasing primary material production; (iii) product material efficiency (optimizing production processes, utilizing recycled components, and designing products with fewer materials). Credible remedies to the bulk of the structural vulnerabilities highlighted by COVID-19 are offered by comprehensively adopting these principles. Green and CE investment and climate-resilient infrastructure go hand in hand, playing the twin function of providing new jobs while also boosting environmental and economic advantages. It is hoped that by adopting a CE, countries could create more robust economies.

It found that if we use short-term remedies to address subsequent shocks, it will be greater than the capacity supposed to address them. It means that we have to come up with long-term risk mitigation and budgetary strategies designed to replace short-term profit-oriented thinking. When it comes to food goods, locally sourced things have an advantage since they do not need the rest of the supply chain to operate. On the other hand, the whole supply chain may be a better alternative for other things. As COVID-19 continues to indicate, specific individual cycles have the inappropriate scale level, and this means that a reexamination of cycle capacity might be seen as an invitation to do so.

The world is seeing a growing realization of interconnectivity among ecological life due to the consequences of COVID-19. This supports the use of the ideas of resilience thinking in enhancing social innovation. It will aim to benefit the population's overall well-being rather than only increase the competition and the market size.

4.5.2 Social finance system

On the other hand, advanced economies have mainly concentrated on helping families keep their purchasing power. Many emerging nations have also used similar tactics by including significant increases in social welfare expenditures in their containment strategies. Nonetheless, such prevention measures also bring attention to how inequitable the global economy is, since their deployment in more developed nations would have a devastating effect on poorer nations and people. Second, in developing countries, working from home is limited due to poor infrastructure and healthcare access. Such a course of action, which governments have used over the short term, is thus inadequate at remedying long-term inequalities and social injustices.

This goal may be reached via CE strategies, which identify resources and resources/wastes as wastes and then turn them into something useful to decrease pollution and help meet social inclusion objectives. Several businesses are adopting this concept. To avoid potential looping and neediness, this closes all loops and returns sustenance to the hungry. The development of a country's digital and materials innovation can be expedited by increasing investment in the CE. Even more so, it believes that the CE can promote socially equitable and costs that will be involved in applying various end-of-life treatments and automation to these processes.

Furthermore, as CE offers workarounds for all these issues, it has the capacity to give rise to local employment and help "reindustrialize" an area by using labor instead of energy, materials instead of labor, and local businesses instead of centralized factories. However, some people would rather see more automation rather than less. However, this is a political and economic issue rather than a scientific or technical one in practice.

4.5.3 Hurdles to CE for context of COVID-19

CE's primary purpose is to generate three victories in three different categories: social, economic, and environmental. Constraints do, however, remain at every stage of the transition from the linear economy to the CE. Within these actors and interactions within the actors, the obstacles reside. Some of the nontrivial factors identified by Korhonen *et al.* [48] in their COVID-19 report include (i) limitations impressed by recycling or remanufacturing (as with combustion in material and energy); (ii) with material and energy footprints; (iii) with organizational culture and management methods, which may use recycled materials and energy; (iv) consumer and organizational inertia (as with business models that utilize recycled materials and energy, as well as management and culture); (v) fragile industrial ecosystems (as with cooperation between the organization, region, and subregions along with pubic authorities); and (vi) the need of standard agreement on what all the Rs. Manufacturing or supply chain challenges such as unclarity in product history through time, difficulties in data exchange between product endpoints, and high start-up costs have also been seen in other countries.

To ground the paradox of COVID-19, the researchers also had to design a system that would provide a one-time chance to reexamine some of these obstacles. Still, CE strategy proponents applauded some sharing economy models as outstanding examples. Ride-sharing modes might help to boost demand in transportation. Use as pay performance may have a reduction in total bookings by Airbnb of 416% occurs with every doubling of new COVID-19 instances.

As long as greenhouse gas emissions are reduced, this will need significant investment by developing and implementing new, low-carbon technologies and infrastructure. Now that COVID-19 has resulted in a worldwide economic crisis, it is expected that the chances for large low-carbon investments from the business sector would be less than prior to the slump. This perspective may be used to both the corporate and governmental sectors as shown by Naidoo and Fisher [5]. Also, as COVID-19 concludes, one way to accelerate progress in achieving CE is by providing local, regional, and national governments with decisive financial and legal as well as a positive environment. By implementing this, the community will have increased capacity to respond to future pandemics, and it also helps integrate with several current resource efficiency roadmaps. Several detection phases of COVID-19 are mentioned in [49]. The classification data and privacy of data can be used for COVID-19 record as [50,51].

4.6 Chances financial support after COVID-19

Local industry has been encouraged for job development, which has inspired a behavioral shift in customers and necessitated more variety and circular supply chains. There is no longer an issue of whether we should rebuild, but how. As a result, it is just as crucial for governments to decide whether or not they will form a new route toward socioeconomic progress as it is for local companies and their customers to collaborate to facilitate the transition to a CE. The pandemic effects of COVID-19 are already well documented. The various monetary policies used by various countries to mitigate these short-term implications are presented in previous parts of this study.

Nevertheless, it has the prospect of fostering a desirable technical and behavioral shift across many countries in the long run. To learn more about pandemics, reference COVID-19, which deals with pandemics, not all of them, and medical accessory production, when product development and manufacture occur in the same location.

For the enormous demand, panic purchasing and the purposeful stockpiling of crucial medical items for profit are all blamed on the COVID-19 incident. We will advocate for creative and environment-friendly alternatives to the shortages, such as reuse and recycling, since reputable entities like the United States centers for Disease Control and Prevention have already made these recommendations. However, medical accessories like PPE are created and manufactured using non-compliant procedures, which means that they are hard to repair and reuse without causing substantial deterioration in their performance. Design solutions to close resource loops, such as the McDonough and Braungart model, are helpful in accomplishing some of the required competencies.

One other rising piece of evidence favoring CE is being embraced without considering it in the current influenza outbreak: a few different companies could easily repurpose their manufacturing floors to produce new items to meet the medical accessory shortage. Notable examples include, but are not limited to, AMTICO (flooring manufacturing) reconfigured their production lines; BARBOUR (a clothing company) redeployed their manufacturing resources.

4.6.1 Several solutions to manage hospital medical and general waste

Because of its toxic, caustic, infectious, corrosive, potentially radioactive, and to character, it is common for HCI wastes to invoke fears about security. So, healthcare waste generated distant from traditional municipal garbage has to be managed according to severe regulatory models. On pre-COVID-19, it is stated that the startling amount of HCI waste reaches a large amount of annual waste product, and several studies have examined possible solutions for this problem at the national level. However, in this new era of the pandemic, the other one of the related problems is the worrying trend among consumers that places emphasis on personal cleanliness at the price of the environmental effect caused by the plastic packaging used in food delivery and grocery shopping. We have hardly given attention to the disposal of these nonbiodegradable plastics, yet most of these items are created from them. Reaction in the environmental community has arisen due to the treatment of these types of waste, resulting in reasonable apprehension in several sectors. Even frustratingly, there are not many things that can be done in the present. All that can be done is to devise appropriate waste management policies for these potentially dangerous materials. When confronted with the complexities of typical HCI waste management procedures, the effort is overwhelming. Another critical step in implementing waste reduction and recycling strategies is reducing the physicochemical complexity of HCI waste. These goals correlate with the CE mission, which stresses waste reduction above all else.

In a study conducted by Wong *et al.* [52], the researchers discovered that different materials were found in hospital wastes. Medical device manufacturers may take steps to address the COVID-19 threat by increasing the amount of bioproducts. In fact, even with use of bioplastics and recyclable materials, there will be medical devices and supplies that cannot be made from them. On the other hand, there is also a lot of resistance to CE in the healthcare business (HCI). However, environmental gains may be outweighed by health and safety risks and rules that need for strict compliance. On the other hand, though, CE is beginning to gain traction in HCI, helping hospital supply chains run more efficiently while reducing operational costs while at the same time doing good with good life.

For the most part, the use of finance system is related to the movement of materials and waste evaluation. Classifying 80% of hospital garbage as general garbage, along with the remaining 20% as infectious trash, has shown that in recent years, hospitals have almost doubled their general garbage generation since the 1990s. There are two kinds of HCI waste: incineration is a popular way to deal with both of them. Large quantities are not problematic for incineration since it creates such toxic products. Thus, lowering the amount of nonhazardous waste by using green buying practices or lowering waste input in the manufacturing and supply chain is molded by adopting such activities. While this might be of use in the short term, we must take a long-term approach in tackling this problem, adopting CE. This will enable an eventual shift to environment-friendly HCI, beginning with the life cycle evaluation of medical products and working our way up to the concept of reusable medical equipment. Voudrias [53] provides several CE solutions for hospital waste management, as outlined by Kane *et al.* [54]. The proportion of infectious trash increases because hospitals are doing everything they can to keep the epidemic under control. However, it is still possible to realize the potential of recycling large amounts of general trash using thermal, microwave, or biochemical sterilizing methods. It should go into all aspects of building and the built environment to embrace resource efficiency.

Based on the financial section, COVID-19 has called attention to the failings of present practices in ecology, especially regarding affordable housing and inflexible building stocks. In some instances, people who lived in inadequate housing and tiny dwellings with inefficient energy consumption become infected with the virus. The situation is most apparent in impoverished nations where people cannot access proper sanitary facilities, hindering them from adhering to safe practices that are essential to fighting the spread of disease. Despite these concerns, a rising worry over the industry's resource-wasting character, coupled with the increasingly prevalent belief that something must be done, make a compelling argument for reconsidering it. As a result, the CE will be positioned to propose viable solutions to these issues.

Occupancy requirements may provide behavioral issues, and CE may assist to balance them. Research has shown that humans spend around 90% of their time inside. It is also probable that office and commercial space renovations need adapting them to varying demands, such as change in occupant density, social distance, ventilation, and the like. When there is not enough air, healthcare staff and patients at temporary hospitals might get infected. The measure's influence on energy consumption must be assessed because of social distancing strategies, which might need lower population density but higher ventilation rates. Therefore, despite improved energy recovery being very relevant for the built environment, reducing mechanical ventilation needs for a lesser number of people places extra requirements on building energy consumption. Some academics have advocated that buildings should utilize 100% fresh outside air instead of recirculation (important for energy savings). It helps to circulate resources and better utilize resources, helping to reduce CO_2 emissions and provide employment opportunities. In the case of a warehouse, an ARUP study calculated that planning for steel reuse may lead to a 6%–27% and 9%–43% savings, resulting in material cost reductions of up to 25%. Policies that the EU is advocating would make recycled materials (a concept known as material looping) a mandatory component in certain building goods once safety and functionality have been checked. To help designers and researchers to make their objects suited for circulation, projects of this kind should encourage them to use material looping in their entire design approach, beginning at the product design stage and on through the whole value chain. It has been shown that by using this material winding process, costs for disposal are reduced and secondary materials may provide new sources of revenue. Reducing building waste will assist to cut solid waste by a third in India.

4.6.2 Facilities for CE in communication sector

The transport was one of the most severely affected industries as a result of COVID-19. A range of CE initiatives will likely be employed in the future in order to help maintain and strengthen the transport industry. It will assist to reorganize urban fabric and improve transportation infrastructures that have already been built. These kinds of cities have a higher amount of infrastructural sprawl, need greater overall mobility, and more operational vehicle usage, causing a rise in traffic congestion, resource depletion, and pollution. To a certain extent, "social separation" impacts many urban residents' perceptions; however, this shift may result in behavior change for individuals.

A transport sector plan based on urban freight strategies that also benefit environmental noise, air quality, and waste management is possible for providing

CE services. Transportation may be informed by using the availability of rich transport data and AI-enabled sophisticated data-processing technology. Routing traffic in real time and rules on traffic flow, route planning, dynamic pricing, and parking spot allocation may all be done in real time using real-time data. Because these innovations involve CE, it is not surprising that there is still a lack of coordination among them. Because governments usually deal with urban planning, the government must establish an integrated strategy for mobility to guarantee efficient resource flows. Innovation and improved utilize of advantages and big data solutions are possible through stakeholder involvement in the transport industry. Developments in air excellence must be sustained.

One of the beneficial developments owing to the COVID-19-imposed shutdown was improved air quality. A heightened focus on investment in cleaner modes of public transit, including sidewalks and bike routes for health benefits, as well as cities are redesigned to make it more difficult for polluted automobiles to enter inhabited areas. To improve this much, we must increase the adoption of electric cars via making more ambitious objectives for the use of electric cars and providing more charging stations for electric cars as well as actively advocating for the use of alternative fuels with lower emissions.

Batteries provide a big contribution to the drive to a renewable energy system and decarbonization of road transportation. It is critical to develop a circular, responsible, and fair battery value chain to actualize these transformations. This means determining which of the batteries is the one to be identified. Such batteries are inexpensive and sustainable and provide a framework that supports the implementation of renewable energy technologies powered by batteries, which results in more widespread taking of non-petrol vehicles for pollution free. We acknowledge that, in the case of an electric car ubiquity, the total number of vehicles will remain constant, as would the number of materials used in their production, which might lead to substantial social, environmental, and integrity threats to the whole supply chain. One way to do this is by the use of the levers as mentioned earlier, which may assist with overcoming these obstacles and with achieving a sustainable battery value chain. Removing greenhouse gas emissions during developed, addressing public abuses, providing security situations, and increasing manufacturing, recycling, and remanufacturing are all aspects of this project.

4.6.3 Use digitalization after COVID-19

Supply chain digitalization is enabled by using disruptive digital technologies (DDTs). Computing environments are all considered a key step in a company's efforts to plan for and deal with disruptive events like COVID-19, which is expected to emerge globally shortly. Ways to help a company generate value in a circular supply chain include prolonging the usable lifetime of an item and maximizing the use of all assets. Gathering information about the location, condition, and availability of assets is a source of intelligence. The many possibilities afforded by cutting these cogs might impact both the product and the business model, which may lead to innovation and value creation. One wonderful example of big data analytics in the workplace is the ability to speed up procurement decisions; it is now utilized to help organizations organize and manage their supply-chain interactions in the cloud. Predictive maintenance is enabled by digitalization, allowing the addition of manufactured goods and avoiding breakdowns. For that reason, it is a perfectly suitable delivery vehicle for circular supply chains, which allows the possibility of closing material loops and improving operations.

Movement toward 5G adoption causes setbacks such as delays in completion of use cases, a wait for the answers to security, competition, and other wireless communication regulatory challenges. The development of automation and robots to combat supply-chain disruptions will be much more important because of COVID-19. Many organizations are automating their manufacturing processes in order to save costs. COVID-19 is anticipated to have an effect on the speed with which regulators provide new rules for 5G. That, in turn, will expedite the adoption of IoT-enabled monitoring devices.

Despite the advantages of DDTs, a conflict remains between their abilities to produce quantifiable environmental advantages and the issues they involve, resulting in rebound effects. It utilizes digital services that must be analyzed for not aggravating the current problems caused by using and discarding so many resources. Contingencies arise across supply chains when products must be designed, procured, distributed, used, disposed of, and recycled in ways that may not account for contingencies. Incentives, regulations, and public policies to help producers shift from traditional CE.

Researchers identified seven primary forms of policy intervention to support, progress, and steer the movement toward a CE. They included both impediments and regulatory failures that try to fix the market and market action that encourages. The policies were recommended to include integrating systems such as life cycle engineering education, public communication and information campaigns, and educational curricula with associated research. It develops to establish platforms for collaboration and knowledge sharing; also, implementing a variety of initiatives, incubation of various types of sustainability initiatives, including financial/technical support, incentive programs. Regulatory models like product registration, and warranty extensions, are also implemented. At the sectoral level, resource productivity strategies and associated targets are put in place. Also, reductions in VAT or excise taxes are introduced for manufacturing natural elements.

4.7 Conclusions

The wastefulness of paradigm has been shown in COVID-19. While short-term plans for coping with the rapid spread of the pandemic are unlikely to be long-term solutions, the approach might work for a while until something better comes along. Their findings underscore crucial concerns, such as the vital relationship between pollution in the environment and the pollution generated by cars and industry. Unrestricted air travel is clearly implicated in the spread of many viral epidemics, with industries like tourism and aviation being seriously impacted owing to decreasing passenger numbers. The long-term consequences for the aviation industry have proven to hit financially, but resulting in positive environmental effects, will reshape the sector. Sharing economy or P2P models such as Uber, Airbnb, and many others have emerged and continue to expand with a new generation of service providers and workers, although these platforms are very unstable in the face of worldwide systemic shocks.

A simultaneous increase in demand and supply resulted in an overall decline in cargo transportation and an increase in airfreight, with transatlantic cost per kilogram tripling overnight. Additionally, there have been jobs lost, income inequality increased, mass increases in global poverty levels, and industry-wide and supply chain-wide economic shocks. The capability to work remotely has been explored and tested in several industries/professions and has shown to provide benefits for employees with regard to decreased commute. Remote healthcare and telemedicine are no longer considered impractical due to the success that has been shown in a 4-month worldwide lockdown. There was a commensurate drop in primary energy use. Machine learning, IoT, and robots have the ability to increase the efficiencies of production processes and speed up supplier selection procedures while also boosting supplier relationship management and logistics.

Hospital JIT procurement has failed to provide big quantities of necessary medical and emergency supplies at short notice owing to shortcomings in current healthcare delivery systems. Millions of patients and healthcare personnel died due to a failure to plan and prepare for PPE with clinical tools adequately. Preventive measures to manage the increase of the disease necessitated an increase in infectious hospital waste, but proper/advanced sterilization processes using radiation procedures assist in recycling discarded or retrieved items and PPE.

An ecosystem-based food system resiliency requires the following: (i) an end to the nutrient loop by using regenerative agriculture, anaerobic digestion facilities, and organic nutrients; (ii) increased value from and organic nutrients through the use of anaerobic digestion facilities. International collaboration and mutual interests would be harmed; long-term planning would be put at risk, and a balance would have to be struck between outsourcing/importing and local manufacturing/productivity. There is a likelihood of a realignment of value chains since resource-rich nations may capitalize on this global epidemic to drive sustainable prosperity, and a new world order will develop independent of the influence of major powers in technology.

While most buildings were occupied throughout the lockdown, business and commercial areas were underused, increasing the amount of ventilation needed in hospitals. For flexible usage, however, buildings may be redecorated to include flexible walls. Modular construction methods such as those used in China are anticipated to become more prevalent in the future. Refurbishment and renovation will highlight newfound energy with decreased carbon emissions and new employment being generated as old buildings are given a new lease of life.

In the future, it is recommended that those who use circular thinking put their knowledge and lessons learned into practice in the broader public's benefit, not only for the advancement of corporations with finances. Post-COVID-19 speculations are required to move the world toward extra flexibility.

References

[1] Sohrabi, C., Alsafi, Z., O'Neill, N., *et al.*, World Health Organization declares global emergency: a review of the 2019 novel coronavirus (COVID-19). *Int. J. Surg.* 2020, 76: 71–76.

[2] WHO, *Coronavirus Disease (COVID-19) Pandemic*. World Health Organization, 2020. https://www.who.int/emergencies/diseases/novel-coronavirus-2019.

[3] Gopinath, G., *Limiting the Economic Fallout of the Coronavirus With Large Targeted Policies*. IMF. March 10, 2020.

[4] JHU, MAPS & TRENDS: New Cases of COVID-19 In World Countries. Coronavirus Resource Center, Johns Hopkins University (JHU) 2020. https://coronavirus.jhu.edu/map.html.

[5] Naidoo, R. and Fisher, B., Reset sustainable development goals for a pandemic world. *Nature* 2020, 583(7815): 198–201.

[6] Sarkis, J., Cohen, M.J., Dewick, P. and Schröder, P., A brave new world: lessons from the COVID-19 pandemic for transitioning to sustainable supply and production. *Resour. Conserv. Recycl.* 2020, 159: 104894.

[7] Anderson, R.M., Heesterbeek, H., Klinkenberg, D. and Hollingsworth, T.D., How will country-based mitigation measures influence the course of the COVID-19 epidemic?. *Lancet* 2020, 395: 931–934.

[8] Piguillem, F. and Shi, L., The optimal COVID-19 quarantine and testing policies. *EIEF Working Papers Series* 2004, Einaudi Institute for Economics and Finance (EIEF), 2020.

[9] Ibn-Mohammed, T., Application of mixed-mode research paradigms to the building sector: a review and case study towards decarbonising the built and natural environment. *Sustain. Cities Soc.* 2017, 35: 692–714.

[10] Snyder, H., Literature review as a research methodology: an overview and guidelines. *J. Bus. Res.* 2019, 104: 333–339.

[11] Grant, M.J. and Booth, A., A typology of reviews: an analysis of 14 review types and associated methodologies. *Health Inf. Libr. J.* 2009, 26: 91–108.

[12] Bloom, D.E. and Cadarette, D., Infectious disease threats in the 21st century: strengthening the global response. *Front. Immunol.* 2019, 10: 549.

[13] Bloom, D.E. and Canning, D., Epidemics and economics. In *Interactions between Global Change and Human Health*, 2004, Scripta Varia 106. pp. 304–331. Vatican City: The Pontical Academy of Sciences.

[14] Hotez, P.J., Alvarado, M., Basáñez, M.-G., *et al.*, The global burden of disease study 2010: interpretation and implications for the neglected tropical diseases. *PLoS Negl. Trop. Dis.* 2014, 8: e2865.

[15] Saunders-Hastings, P.R. and Krewski, D., Reviewing the history of pandemic influenza: understanding patterns of emergence and transmission. *Pathogens* 2016, 5(4): 66.

[16] Horrox, R., *The Black Death*. Manchester University Press, 2013, pp. 1–364.

[17] Wagner, D.M., Klunk, J., Harbeck, M., *et al.*, *Yersinia pestis* and the Plague of Justinian 541–543 AD: a genomic analysis. *Lancet Infect. Dis.* 2014, 14: 319–326.

[18] Gibbs, M.J., Armstrong, J.S. and Gibbs, A.J., Recombination in the hemagglutinin gene of the 1918 "Spanish flu". *Science* 2001, 293: 1842–1845.

[19] De Cock, K.M., Jaffe, H.W. and Curran, J.W., The evolving epidemiology of HIV/AIDS. *AIDS* 2012, 26: 1205–1213.

[20] Lee, J.-W. and McKibbin, W.J., Estimating the global economic costs of SARS. *Learning from SARS: Preparing for the Next Disease Outbreak: Workshop Summary*. National Academies Press, Washington, DC, 2004, pp. 92.

[21] Baseler, L., Chertow, D.S., Johnson, K.M., Feldmann, H. and Morens, D.M., The pathogenesis of Ebola virus disease. *Annu. Rev. Pathol.* 2017, 12: 387–418.

[22] Murray, N.E.A., Quam, M.B. and Wilder-Smith, A., Epidemiology of dengue: past, present and future prospects. *Clin. Epidemiol.* 2013, 5: 299–309.

[23] Fernandes, N., Economic effects of coronavirus outbreak (COVID-19) on the world economy. 2020. Available at SSRN 3557504.

[24] McKee, M. and Stuckler, D., If the world fails to protect the economy, COVID-19 will damage health not just now but also in the future. *Nat. Med.* 2020, 26: 640–642.

[25] McKenzie, B., Beyond COVID-19: supply chain resilience holds key to recovery. *Oxford Econ.* 2020, 24: 20.

[26] Muhammad, L.J., Ebrahem, A.A., Sani, S.U., Abdulkadir, A., Chinmay, C. and Mohammed, I.A., Supervised machine learning models for prediction of COVID-19 infection using epidemiology dataset. *SN Comput. Sci.* 2021, 2(11): 1–13. https://doi.org/10.1007/s42979-020-00394-7.

[27] Gupta, A.K, Chinmay, C. and Gupta, B, Monitoring of epileptical patients using cloud-enabled health-IoT system. *Trait. Signal, IIETA* 2019, 36(5): 425–31. https://doi.org/10.18280/ts.360507.

[28] Sukanya, R. and Chinmay, C., Panic buying situation during COVID-19 global pandemic. *J. Inf. Technol. Manage.* 2021, 13(2): 231–44. DOI:10.22059/jitm.2021.80625.

[29] Chinmay, C. and Abougreen, A.N., Intelligent Internet of Things and advanced machine learning techniques for COVID-19. *EAI Endorsed Trans. Pervasive Health Technol.* 2021, 7: 1–14. http://dx.doi.org/10.4108/eai.28-1-2021.168505.

[30] Bhuyan, H.K., Kamila, N.K. and Jena, L.D., Pareto-based multi-objective optimization for classification in data mining. *Cluster Comput.* 2016, 19(4): 1723–1745.

[31] Bhuyan, H.K., Kamila, N.K. and Pani, S.K., Individual privacy in data mining using fuzzy optimization. *Engineering Optimization*, Taylor & Francis, May 2021. pp. 1–19.

[32] Baldwin, R. and Evenett, S., *Covid-19 and Trade Policy: Why Turning Inward Won't Work*. CEPR Press, London, 2020.

[33] Ranney, M.L., Griffeth, V. and Jha, A.K., Critical supply shortages—the need for ventilators and personal protective equipment during the Covid-19 pandemic. *N. Engl. J. Med.* 2020, 382(18): e41.
[34] Bhuyan, H.K. and Kamila, N.K., Privacy preserving sub-feature selection in distributed data mining. *Appl. Soft Compu.* Elsevier, November 2015, volume 36. pp. 552–569,
[35] Bhuyan, H.K. and Kamila, N.K., Privacy preserving Sub-feature Selection based on fuzzy probabilities. *Cluster Comput.* 2014, 17(4): 1383–1399.
[36] Bhuyan, H.K., Chakraborty, C., Pani, S.K. and Ravi, V.K., Feature and sub-feature selection for classification using correlation coefficient and fuzzy model. *IEEE Trans. Eng. Manage.* 2021. 10.1109/TEM.2021.3065699.
[37] Iyengar, K., Bahl, S., Vaishya, R. and Vaish, A., Challenges and solutions in meeting up the urgent requirement of ventilators for COVID-19 patients. *Diabetes Metab. Syndr.* 2020, 14(4): 499–501.
[38] Solomon, M.Z., Wynia, M. and Gostin, L.O., Scarcity in the Covid-19 pandemic. *Hastings Cent. Rep.* 2020, 50: 3.
[39] Bown, C.P., COVID-19: demand spikes, export restrictions, and quality concerns imperil poor country access to medical supplies. In *Trade Protection in the Age of COVID-19*. CEPR Press VoxEU.org eBook, 2020, volume 31, pp. 1–179.
[40] Browne, M., Sweet, M., Woodburn, A. and Allen, J., Urban freight consolidation centres final report 10 Transport Studies Group, University of Westminster, 2005.
[41] Livingston, E., Desai, A. and Berkwits, M., Sourcing personal protective equipment during the COVID-19 pandemic. *JAMA* 2020, 323(19): 1912–1914.
[42] WHO, Coronavirus disease (COVID-19): situation Report – 107, 2020, pp. 1–17.
[43] Javorcik, B., Global supply chains will not be the same in the post-COVID-19 world. COVID-19 and Trade Policy: Why Turning Inward Won't Work 111, 2020.
[44] Wang, P., Chen, K., Zhu, S., Wang, P. and Zhang, H., Severe air pollution events not avoided by reduced anthropogenic activities during COVID-19 outbreak. *Resour. Conserv. Recycl.* 2020, 158: 104814.
[45] IEA, Global Energy Review, The impacts of the COVID-19 crisis on global energy demand and CO_2 emissions. *International Energy Agency*. IEA Publications, 2020, pp. 1–56.
[46] Hoornweg, D. and Bhada-Tata, P., What a waste: a global review of solid waste management, 2012.
[47] Gates, B., COVID-19 is awful. Climate change could be worse. *Climate and the Coronavirus*, GatesNotes, 2020. https://www.gatesnotes.com/Energy/Climate-and-COVID-19.
[48] Korhonen, J., Honkasalo, A. and Seppälä, J., Circular economy: the concept and its limitations. *Ecol. Econ.* 2018, 143: 37–46.
[49] Bhuyan, H.K., Chakraborty, C., Shelke, Y and Pani, S.K., COVID-19 diagnosis system by deep learning approaches. *Expert Syst.* 2021: e12776. https://doi.org/10.1111/exsy.12776.

[50] Bhuyan, H.K. and Ravi, V., Analysis of sub-feature for classification in data mining. *IEEE Trans. Eng. Manage.* 2021: 1–15 (Early Published).
[51] Bhuyan, H.K., Dash, S.K., Roy, S. and Swain, D.K., Privacy preservation with penalty in decentralized network using multiparty computation. *Int. J. Adv. Comput. Technol.* 2012, 4(1): 297–303.
[52] Wong, K.-F.V., Narasimhan, R., Kashyap, R. and Fu, J., Medical waste characterization. *J. Environ. Health* 1994: 19–25.
[53] Voudrias, E.A., Healthcare waste management from the point of view of circular economy. *Waste Manage.* 2018, 75: 1–2.
[54] Kane, G.M., Bakker, C.A. and Balkenende, A.R., Towards design strategies for circular medical products. *Resour. Conserv. Recycl.* 2018, 135: 38–47.

Chapter 5

Early diagnosis and remote monitoring using cloud-based IoMT for COVID-19

Madhura S. Mulimani[1], *Shridhar Allagi*[1,2] *and Rashmi R. Rachh*[1]

Abstract

The entire globe has been battling with deadly coronavirus disease 2019 (COVID-19) pandemic from the time December 2019. Around 190 million people have been affected by the virus, and 4 million have lost their lives to it. It has adversely influenced the socio-economical lives of people in almost all countries across the world. Hence, it is essential to detect the disease at an early stage and ensure that the transmission of the virus is curbed, in turn, saving the lives of many other people. With the advancements and developments in the information technology field, it is possible to diagnose infectious diseases like the current COVID-19 pandemic at an early stage and give proper treatment to the infected. In addition to analyzing the disease early, many other approaches are employed to deal with this deadly disease. In this chapter, various Internets of Things that are being used to track the patients' health and provide them the necessary care and treatment even in remote locations have been discussed. Also, machine learning and deep learning for early diagnosis and remote monitoring have been discussed. An experimental case study using COVIDX dataset has been discussed along with the results. Comprehensive experiments have been carried out with varying computed tomography (CT) sizes of CT images and an average accuracy of above 80% has been achieved. In all, how the use of technology in the medical field proves beneficial and how it can be leveraged even further to control the spread of the diseases has been elucidated in this chapter.

Keywords: Internet of Medical Things (IoMT); COVID-19; Early detection; IoMT devices; Machine learning COVID detection

[1]Department of Computer Science, Visvesvaraya Technological University, Belagavi, India
[2]Department of Computer Science, KLE Institute of Technology, Hubballi, India

5.1 Introduction

An unusual coronavirus called the very severe acute respiratory syndrome coronavirus-2 (SARS-CoV-2), initially discovered in China's Hubei province, Wuhan, at the end of December 2019, has caused a calamitous event and impacted entire world economy to collapse adversely, further engendering the societal and political disruptions. As of July 16, 2021, more than 190 million people worldwide have been infected with coronavirus disease 2019 (COVID-19), and around four million have succumbed to it, as per the John Hopkins University and Medicine, Coronavirus Resource Center, United States [1,2].

Once an individual is exposed to the virus, it may usually take about 5–6 days to show signs. Individuals with slight symptoms may recoup independently, but others may suffer from severe symptoms, especially if they already suffer from other health ailments such as diabetes or heart problems. Animals, too, can get affected by this virus and can transmit the infection [3].

The pandemic has been rising mainly due to global travels and exploitation of the environment. Hence, it is crucial to recognize any emergent epidemics and formulate policies to restrain and thwart the spread of COVID-19 contamination and save the lives of individuals worldwide, which can be done by detecting the disease early and ensuring proper treatment for the patients diagnosed with COVID-19 as well as for the safety of public health [4].

Since there was no vaccine for COVID until recently, the only way to cure or prevent it was through its early diagnosis. This helps to avoid its further spread wherein the patients are advised to quarantine or isolate themselves. Most of the patients with COVID-19 stay asymptomatic. Others demonstrate mild-to-moderate symptoms with high fever, shortness in breathing, mild cough, and signs alike oxygen capacity dipping or sometime lung auscultation. These all signs and indications play a decisive role in ascertaining any infection and execution of further diagnostic tests [5].

Several preventive tools and measures that are being used to prevent the infection from spreading use personal protective equipment, properly used face-masks, face-shields, use of gloves, and ventilators [4], washing hands repeatedly with soap for 25–30 s, continuing social distance, masking mouth and nose with a disposable tissue paper while sneezing and so on [6]. In addition to all this, to curb the spread of the disease, there is a need for expeditious and precise testing of COVID-19 in people, considering the furious spread of the disease.

This major contribution of the chapter includes a comprehensive coverage of various Internet of Medical Things (IoMT) devices that are being used in the medical field for diagnosing and remote monitoring of patients with different diseases, procedures carried out during early diagnosis of COVID-19 and remote monitoring of home isolated or quarantined patients, an experimental case study that uses machine learning (ML) with deep learning (DL) techniques to distinguish between the computed tomography (CT) images of normal and COVID-19-infected patients mainly to identify and diagnose if the patient has been infected with COVID-19, and various measures that different countries are adopting to thwart the spread of the virus from affecting more people.

The organization of the chapter is as follows: Section 5.2 discusses about techniques used for COVID-19 detection. Section 5.3 presents an architecture of IoMT devices. In Section 5.4, we discuss about various medical devices with Internet connectivity that are used for identifying COVID-19 symptoms and remote monitoring. Section 5.5 presents the phases that occur during the identification and treatment of patients affected with COVID-19. In Section 5.6, we briefly discuss about how ML and DL techniques can be used or are being used for early detection of COVID-19. Section 5.7 lists the works of different authors who have used ML and DL techniques in COVID-19 prediction. In Section 5.8, we provide details about the experimental case study that was conducted using ML with DL techniques on COVIDX dataset containing numerous CT images of varying sizes. Section 5.9 lists various preventive measures adopted by different countries for controlling the spread of the virus. Section 5.10 lists the limitations encountered when using IoMT devices. Section 5.11 concludes the chapter and gives a brief idea about how the current work can be enhanced or improved in future scenarios using recent or emerging developments in the information technology field.

5.2 Detection techniques

People who are infected by the virus and exhibit symptoms such as fever, cough, body aches, running nose, headache, and sore throat undergo specific tests. The following two categories of tests are used for COVID-19 detection:

1. Diagnostic tests: Reverse-transcription–polymerase-chain-reaction (RT-PCR) is a diagnostic test used for detecting an active coronavirus infection. Reverse real-time PCR assay, a typical molecular-based assay, is a standard diagnostic testing method widely used to screen COVID-19. Generally, it provides results in 4–6 h. This test has several drawbacks: time-consuming, reliance on well-equipped laboratories and trained specialists, manual, expensive, ineffective, laborious, and complex. Additionally, the number of available test kits is limited in quantity, and to make things worse, domain experts cause further delay in the situation as the test is manual, laborious, complex, expensive, and ineffective.
2. Antibody tests: Here, tests look for antibodies formed in the body with response to the disease. The antibodies usually take several days or even few weeks to grow well and may remain in the blood for a long time even after recuperation. Hence, these tests cannot be used to detect COVID-19. With certain limitations in the current investigative techniques and a rapid increase in number of infected patients, it is a paramount prerequisite that the physicians use certain alternate automatic screening systems to quickly detect and isolate patients infected with COVID-19 [5].

The purposes of the two classes of tests overlap in the supervision of the COVID-19 pandemic. The first class of testing recognizes persons infected with SARS-CoV-2 during the critical phase of contamination. In contrast, the second class of testing recognizes individuals within whom antibodies to the virus have developed, and hence, could be prospective convalescing plasma donors. It can trace and observe the status of immunity of individuals and assemblages over a certain period. Hence, to manage COVID-19, it is essential to have an appropriate identification, active treatment, and future anticipation. This has led to a competition to establish economical and point-of-contact test kits and well-organized laboratory practices to confirm SARS-CoV-2 infection [7].

Thorax CT is more reliable, functional, and quicker than RT-PCR to classify and assess COVID-19 in an epidemic region. Nearly all hospitals carry out CT image screening. Hence, to detect COVID-19 patients early, thorax CT can be used. However, a radiology expert and ample time are required to classify COVID-19 on the basis of thorax CT. Since COVID-19 test results take a complete day to sense the virus in the human body, it is vital to identify the disease in the initial period and instantaneously quarantine the infected patients as there are no drugs that are explicitly existing for COVID-19. As per the government of China, RT-PCR can be used to diagnose the confirmation of COVID-19. However, the RT-PCR test does not yield satisfactory results due to its higher false-negative rates. Also, it is time-consuming because it takes around 4–8 h for the machine to process the samples of patients. Perhaps, in certain cases, the diseased may not be identified on time and, hence, may not obtain appropriate treatment. A diseased may be ascribed as COVID-19 negative due to the false-negative outcome. Hence, in such cases, it is necessary to analyze the thorax CT images in an automated manner, which can be time-saving for the specialist medical staff as well as avoid delays in starting the treatment [3].

Another drawback of RT-PCR is that it needs a laboratory kit that cannot be easily provided to several countries, especially during crises and epidemics. Another matter of concern is that this test is not error-free and is prejudiced. In this test, a skilled laboratory technician extracts the nasal and throat mucosa sample. Since this method is painful, many people refuse to undergo the test. Also, the RT-PCR test has a sensitivity of 35–65%, which indicates a diminution in the accuracy of COVID-19 diagnosis [2].

Since patients with COVID-19 generally remain asymptomatic, diagnosing COVID-19 early is challenging. It is hard to distinguish between patients having symptoms and those having various respiratory infections like pneumonia and severe flu. Since the wet-lab tests for diagnosing COVID-19 are highly priced and time-consuming, there needs to be some substitute that is noninvasive and fast as well as a discounted automatic screening system. As a substitute model to detect and determine COVID-19 infection, a chest CT (CCT) scan can be exploited.

Medical practitioners use imaging modalities such as X-ray and CT as diagnostic techniques that do not require any instruments to be introduced in the body to analyze and cure many diseases. They use these imaging modalities to even determine COVID-19. However, since the CCT scans are 3D images and contrast dyes, their performance in diagnosing COVID-19 is significantly improved compared to the simple 2D chest X-ray (CXR). Meanwhile, COVID-19-infected patients' CT scans show disparate features with subtle variations and make it quite challenging to interpret these scans manually. Additionally, the current immense increase of infected patients has made it more difficult for domain experts to complete the diagnosis on time. Hence, some computer-aided diagnostic systems that generally use CT scans are needed to manipulate better and understand the CCT images. ML approaches have been successfully applied to diagnose lung diseases. They have also been used to analyze COVID-19 using CCT images with unpredictable sources and amounts of data [5].

The sensitivity of CT scan images in diagnosing and detecting COVID-19 cases is higher. However, their low-specificity represents that CT scan is extra precise in COVID-19 cases but less in nonviral pneumonia instances [2]. CCT scans have been used to detect COVID-19-related lung damage effectively. However, this diagnostic has some limits.

The CT findings are conventional in a few patients at the beginning of the infection. Hence, using the CT alone causes it to have a negative prognostic value. Since the CT scans have a high false-positive rate, it could lead to difficulties in detecting non-COVID-19 cases. Moreover, if it necessitates for patients to have manifold CT scans in the course of the disease, the CT scanner rays can harm them and cause complications.

Hence, the American College of Radiology advises against CT scans as the first line of diagnosis. Since a CT scan is expensive and there is disease transmission risk while using the CT scan device, it leads to serious complexities for the patient and the healthcare systems. Hence, it is advisable to replace a CT scan with CXR radiography if medical imaging is needed.

Compared to CT scans, X-ray imaging is inexpensive and has widespread usage. Since the digital image need not be transferred from the contact point to the examination point, the diagnostic process is accomplished much more swiftly. Chest radiography is beneficial and quick for the medical triaging of patients. X-ray imaging expects less occasional and less affluent equipment [2].

5.3 Internet of Medical Things

Internet of Thing (IoT) is an emerging technology in which devices that collect and share real-time data without human intervention are interconnected and build a system. Such a system can control various healthcare systems, logistics, traffic congestion, retails, emergency service, smart cities, etc. The Internet provides an infrastructure with many benefits such as state-of-the-art connectivity, services, and systems and, thus, drives past machine-to-machine evolution and is interconnected with other services. Therefore, it is feasible to introduce automation practically in almost all fields, and as a result, IoT offers an extensive variety of applications and solutions [8].

Smart devices, smart sensors, and progressive lightweight communication protocols have made it conceivable to interconnect medical things and monitor biomedical signals, which can further be used to analyze patients' diseases without any human involvement. Such medical things combined with intellectual devices are together labeled as the IoMT. They can transfer data over a system without insisting on the interaction between humans or between humans and computers [9]. They find healthcare and medical care applications and are based on communication between machines through wireless connectivity to transfer data. IoMT finds usage potentiality in various applications such as health monitoring, home medication, fitness projects, chronic ailments, elderly care, and compliance with treatment. Hence, smart devices include multiple sensors and medical devices, imaging devices, and diagnostics, and they form a primary part of the IoMT, the major benefits of which include an increase in the standard of living, reduced cost, and increased user's knowledge in healthcare systems [8]. Hence, an IoMT platform can be defined as an intelligent system comprising various elements such as sensors and electronic circuits, a processing unit, a network device, a storage component, and a visualization platform. Sensors and the electronic circuits procure biomedical indicators from a patient that are operated on by the processing unit. A network unit transmits the biomedical information over a network and stores it in a storage unit that may either be temporary or permanent. A visualization framework with artificial intelligence (AI) schemes decides as per the convenience of the physician. The IoMT architecture is presented in Figure 5.1.

IoMT systems are used in varied areas and are very ubiquitous. They play a crucial role in the healthcare sector and provide real-time surveillance using wireless body area networks, AI and the cloud-based remote health testing, remote-healthcare-monitoring (RHM), and wearable health-monitoring devices. They also

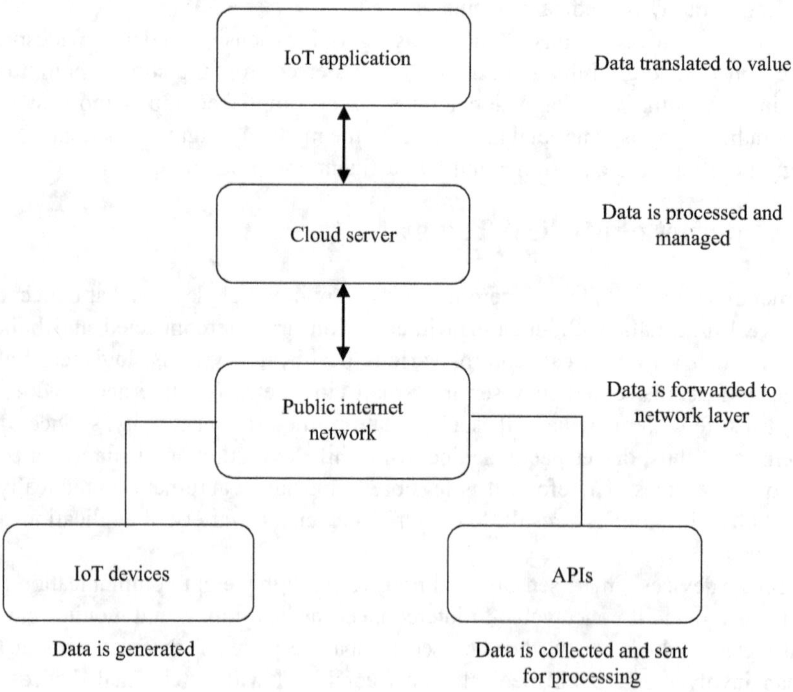

Figure 5.1 Architecture of IoMT

provide real-time, continuous, and remote monitoring of patients. They can make healthcare more convenient and efficient, especially regarding accuracy, visibility, accessibility, reliability, continuity, and real-time tracking. For example, hospitalized patients suffer massive money on the patients, healthcare centers, and insurance companies. In addition, it is extremely difficult for all those patients who live in remote locations and cannot easily access either the hospitals or caregiver centers. In such cases, they may need to travel lengthy distances to pursue healthcare. However, with the advancement in IoT, they are being used for RHM due to their characteristic features such as interoperability, communication, and information exchange. This, in turn, has enabled RHM to provide an enhanced and continuous monitoring for chronic diseases. Hence, they qualify to be excellent candidates that can predict, prevent, and monitor any emerging transmissible diseases such as COVID-19. In the IoMT system, end-user devices such as health monitors, tags, or cell phones use wearable sensors/devices to gather the remote data for patients. They then store the collected data in the cloud databases and send the data to the cloud platform for real-time analysis and application, i.e., for caregivers' decision-making and analytics. Hence, the IoMT devices can be leveraged as an early indication system to control infectious diseases [10].

5.4 IoMT devices for the identification of COVID-19 symptoms and remote monitoring

Millions of people worldwide are using smartwatches and other wearable devices that detect and gage many physiological parameters like sleep, skin temperature, and heart rate. Consumer wearable devices continuously measure vital signs, which can monitor the onset of infectious diseases. For example, consumer smartwatches are being used to detect coronavirus disease pre-symptomatically. These devices determine individual baseline parameters of health and detect any substantial aberrations from the reference physiology readings at the start of infection. Hence, they are a widely deployed technology. These parameters can be used in a retrospective manner to detect COVID-19 early and for real-time health monitoring and surveillance. For example, fitness trackers acquire the heart rate signals that can be used well in advance of symptom onset to detect COVID-19 infection.

Wearable devices have sufficient potential to diminish the ill effects of COVID-19. Since the commencement of the pandemic, millions of people have been infected, and millions of people have succumbed to this deadly disease. Hence, it is vital to have an improved infection-tracking system. It can be done using population-scale technology solutions to identify the infected cases in real-time and track them. Currently, PCR assays are used to identify active infections, and after illness, they require 3–4 days for a dependable positive signal. In addition, since PCR tests are rarely used and most infections become obvious just upon the onset of symptoms, the existing testing procedures may not detect pre-asymptomatic carriers. Hence, it is incredibly challenging to implement intrusions at an early stage to reduce transmission. Supposedly, almost 60% of persons with COVID-19 are asymptomatic and, thus, enable more viral spread. Nevertheless, to detect COVID-19 early on in real-time, there is a contingency for accessible and inexpensive methods [11].

5.4.1 Wearables

The fight against the COVID-19 pandemic may be easier when apposite wearable devices are used. The usage of wearable devices has proved to be an efficient and effective way to diagnose the disease early during the pandemic as they can detect the COVID-19 symptoms of the patients. For instance, a wearable IoT device can be used to determine whether the respiratory symptoms of a patient are normal or not, which, in turn, can help the patient to witness changes, if any, in their health state and accordingly choose to have a medical appointment prior to the appearance of any other symptoms.

These technologies are defined as a blend of electronics and anything that can be worn. They may be described as app-enabled computing technologies that use built-in Bluetooth wireless technology to receive and process input when worn on the body or stuck. These intelligent wearables include bands, glasses, and watches and are designed for various purposes to be used in diverse domains like healthcare, fitness, and lifestyle. IoT-wearable devices include smart wearable tools such as smart helmet, smart thermometers, IoT-Q-band, smart glasses, proximity trace, and EasyBand [12].

5.4.1.1 Smart thermometers

These devices are used to record constant measurements of body temperatures and are accurate, affordable, and user-friendly and can either be worn or stick to the skin below the apparel. Touch, patch, and radiometric are various forms in which they are available. These smart thermometers are highly recommended for capturing the body temperature against the infrared thermometers that may probably spread the virus more as the patients and healthcare providers are quite close to each other when checking the temperature. Some smart thermometers can post the body temperature on a smartphone at any time, including Ran's Night, iFever, Tempdrop, and iSense. By means of these devices, the likelihood of detecting novel patients at an initial phase of the infection can drastically improve in our daily existences.

5.4.1.2 Smart helmet

These wearable devices have a thermal camera and lower human interactions and are safer to use than the infrared thermometer gun. For example, KC N901, a smart helmet manufactured by China, detects high body temperature with an accuracy of 96%. The thermal camera on the intelligent helmet detects a high temperature, and an optical camera within the helmet sends the locale and picture of the person's face together with an alarm to the assigned mobile device, which is usually to the diseased person's health officer who can take appropriate action. Figure 5.2 illustrates the process. To obtain all the places that a suspected person has visited, the smart helmet can be incorporated with Google Location History.

5.4.1.3 Smart glasses

This is another type of wearable device. These devices have lesser human interactions when compared to thermometer guns. Smart glasses use optical and thermal

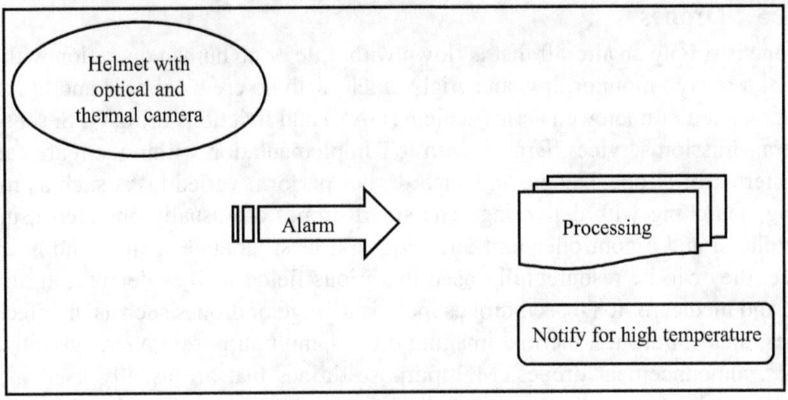

Figure 5.2 Smart helmet

cameras, and the built-in face detection technology makes it easy to monitor crowds, and the tracking procedure once suspicious cases are detected. Moreover, since Google Location History can capture the places visited by the suspicious subject, it can effectively empower further actions with more excellent reliability. An example of such a smart glass is the Rokid that uses infrared sensors and monitors up to 200 people. Once these devices detect people with elevated temperatures, they make the recorded information available to medical centers or authorities.

5.4.1.4 Robots

A robot is often "a machine bearing resemblance to a living being in its capability to move independently." The evolution in the robotic field has led to the development of networked robots within the cloud, and such robots are called the Internet of Robot Things. These robots can perform various repetitive tasks, make life easy and simple. Considering the current COVID-19 pandemic situation, different robots such as telerobots, autonomous robots, social robots, and collaborative robots are being used.

IoT-linked robots can be used in the initial diagnosis of the infection. These robots remarkably process a patient's treatments and lower work stress levels for the healthcare workers. These autonomous robots can help in combating all phases of COVID-19. For example, autonomous swab test robot can collect throat swabs samples from patients and help in the process of diagnosis, and as a result, it can prevent the medical team from getting infected. Vayyar Imaging and Meditemi are the two companies that have jointly developed a robot to carry out this process, called the Intelligent Care Robot. It uses a quick scanning of a person within a span of 1-m without touching any control or interface and captures the breathing signs and thermal reading to detect the COVID-19 symptoms in just 10 s. Xenex disinfection robot is used to sterilize virus and bacteria-contaminated areas like hospitals and helps in reducing the possibility of infection for the healthcare staff.

5.4.1.5 Drones

A drone is simply an aircraft that is flown with little or no human operation with the help of a remote monitor. It is an aerial vehicle with no crew onboard and is called the unmanned or uncrewed aerial vehicle (UAV) and functions using GPS, sensors, and transmission services. Drones with IoT implementation within them are called the Internet of Drone Things, and such drones perform varied tasks such as monitoring, searching with delivering. The smart drones are usually operated using a smartphone and a controller unit and require a least amount of time and energy. Hence, they can be resourcefully used in various fields such as defense, agribusiness, and medicare. IoT-based drones include a range of drones such as disinfectant drones, medical drones, thermal imaging drones, multipurpose drones, surveillance drones, announcement drones. Multipurpose drones that are usually used in the healthcare domain are now primarily being used to combat the COVID-19 pandemic.

In the initial diagnosis phase of COVID-19, it is imperative to find the infected people in the crowd. To hasten the process of finding the infected people and areas, the most common way is to use the UAV, and more specifically, the IoT-based drones during the pandemic. Since drone technology reduces human communications and reaches difficult-to-access locations, it is much more useful, especially during the COVID-19. Combining such drones with virtual reality (VR) as a vesture gadget can help detect individuals with elevated thermal readings. A Canadian company has developed the Pandemic Drone application that remotely monitors and detects any cases of infection. It captures the biological parameters such as temperature, any sneezing or coughing, and respiratory signs such as heart rate [12].

5.4.1.6 IoT buttons

These are small, programmable, electronic buttons that are usually connected to the cloud via wireless communication. Each IoT button has an associated code written on the cloud to perform different repetitive tasks. Hence, pressing a button enables the code to be executed, and as a result, the intended task is completed. For instance, Visionstate has produced an IoT button called Wanda QuickTouch. This IoT button, installed as a cleaning alert system in hospitals, alerts the authorities regarding the necessary sanitation or public safety concerns [13]. Another IoT button may enable the patient to indicate a drop in his oxygen level when undergoing a COVID-19 treatment just by pressing a button. Sefucy IoT button, initially designed to track missing children, is now being used during quarantine for emergency notifications as a rejoinder to COVID-19 pandemic. If the patient's condition, secluded at home gets worse, he can press the IoT button, which will immediately alert the healthcare provider or the family members [12].

5.4.1.7 WHOOP strap

It is a wearable strap with a photoplethysmography sensor and is worn on the wrist. The device contains a thermometer, photoplethysmogram, capacitive touch sensor, gyroscope, and accelerometer. This small strap, which is waterproof and rechargeable, can be comfortably worn 24 h per day, with each charge lasting up to 5 days. It collects the metrics such as resting heart rate (RHR), respiratory rate, and heart rate variability (HRV) and transfers data via wireless communication to the mobile devices on which the connected WHOOP app runs. From that point onward, data is conveyed to a WHOOP system that consists of protected cloud-based data storage and processing server. The system provides physiological data as follows:

- Respiratory rate: The average number of respirations per minute represents the respiratory rate. The photoplethysmogram present in the strap uses photoplethysmography to derive this value every single night for the key sleep period duration.
- Resting heart rate (RHR): It represents the average values of beats per minute (bpm) inspected in the previous 5-min duration of the past occurrence of slow-wave sleep each night.
- Heart rate variability (HRV): It uses the root mean square of successive RR interval difference method to investigate the slow wave sleep sample during the last 5–10 min of the previous incident each night. It is expressed in units of milliseconds.

WHOOP system is usually used to track physiological data automatically. With additional functionality, it has been able to track COVID-19 symptoms as well as test outcomes during the ongoing COVID-19 pandemic. Since the primary stages of the infection may have measurable signs, recognizing SARS-CoV-2 condition before and during the first days of symptoms could help recognize all those entities who need to self-isolate or quarantine and seek testing [14].

5.4.2 Smartphone applications

They are application-software intended to perform restricted tasks inside a mobile gadget such as a smartphone. Since there are more than 3 million operational smartphones in 2021, IoT-based smartphone applications are being efficiently used in numerous domains like retail, healthcare, and agriculture. Among them, smartphone applications such as Stop Corona, nCapp, DetectaChem, Aarogya Setu, SelfieApp, StayHomeSafe, TraceTogether, HaMagen, Coalition, BeAware Bahrain, Social Monitoring, and Civitas have been advanced especially for the healthcare purview and used exclusively in response to COVID-19 [12].

5.5 Early diagnosis of COVID-19 and remote monitoring procedures

Early detection of COVID-19 among infected individuals and their remote monitoring during home isolation or quarantine treatment can be divided into different phases as early diagnosis, quarantine time, and post recovery. The procedures carried out during each stage have been explained in the following:

1. **Phase 1: Early diagnosis**
   The essential step that can be taken to battle the COVID-19 pandemic and prevent the dispersion of the virus is to diagnose it early. This can be a

considerable help to the healthcare providers as it will enable them to plan better treatment and arrangements, rescue more lives, and reduce uncleanliness and infections. As an initial step toward early diagnosis, understanding the symptoms is most crucial as COVID-19 has wide-ranging symptoms, along with fever, cough, chills, tiredness, muscle or body aches, headache, etc. Among all these symptoms, fever or elevated body temperature is one of the most prevalent COVID-19 signs, and when gauged, it surpasses 38°C or 100.4°F. The detection process can be faster and more efficient when IoT devices are used as they use sensors within them to capture data that is analyzed for healthcare providers, patients, and authorities, who will further detect, control, and eventually end the transmission of the deadly virus that has caused the pandemic and affected so many lives [12].

The first and foremost task is the collection of real-time symptom data using a set of vesture sensors on the user body. To detect these symptoms, several biosensors are available. For instance, various sensors can be used to detect different symptoms like temperature-based sensors to detect fever, auditory sensors with acoustic and aerodynamic prototypes to detect cough along with its classification, locomotion-based and heart rate sensors to sense weariness, image-based classification to detect sore throat, and lastly, oxygen-based sensors to detect difficulty in breathing. Mobile applications may be used to gather the travel and contact history in the past 3–4 weeks duration on an ad hoc basis as such data is also relevant for early diagnosis [15].

Many patients at their homes or hospitals can be monitored with support from IoT devices. They can collect various vital signs such as blood pressure, heartbeat and transmit them to the cloud so that the healthcare workers can analyze the data. This avoids exposing the healthcare workers to the infection. In one study, it has been demonstrated how IoT was used to detect a fever and how it automatically uploaded the readings to an Android-based smartphone and then to a worldwide network via wireless Bluetooth communication. Consequently, the results were quickly available anywhere, at any time immediately. Such an IoT system is vital in tackling infectious diseases, especially for medical practitioners [16].

2. **Phase II: Quarantine time**

Once an infected person is detected, it is mandatory to isolate them and then monitor the patient at home or in a hospital. This quarantine is applicable to the confirmed patients, doubted patients, and diverse areas, cities, or nations. This is mainly carried out to impede the likely spread from suspected cases or zones to others. Employing the IoT devices during this period can help alleviate critical tasks like spread of virus. Hence, patients are monitored skillfully, and their respiratory signs, heart rate, blood pressure, etc. are controlled [12]. Hence, data is collected from quarantined or isolated users who are in a healthcare center during the quarantine time. The data consists of both technical and nontechnical information. While the technical data includes the time-series data of various symptoms, the nontechnical data includes information about the travel and contact history in the former 3–4 weeks duration, age, long-standing diseases, gender, and any other pertinent information like a family record of ailment [15].

During the COVID-19 pandemic, most IoMT systems have been used as digital surveillance systems to track and locate the infected individuals. IoMT has also been used to detect, monitor, and test, to curtail the possibility of infection or to accelerate the assessment procedures [17]. Though it has steered to some privacy issues, many citizens have accepted it as they understand that it is much needed to end the pandemic.

3. **Phase III: Post recovery**

To restrict the spread of the COVID-19 pandemic, many restrictions like lockdowns, social distancing had/have been imposed, resulting in an adverse consequence on many businesses, markets, and the economy.

After many months, the restrictions are being lifted, and countries are slowly and prudently opening again. During this phase, all and sundry must stay with extra cautiousness following societal distancing and restrictions on physical amenities to ensure that the virus will not spread again [12].

Wearable devices such as smartwatches produce much larger datasets that are almost impossible for humans to analyze. Data mining and computational approaches based on ML come to the rescue and have been in continuous demand in such cases. These approaches help analyze the complex relationships between sensor data and the patients' physiological status, thus leading to more accurate predictions that were previously unknown. Wearable electronic devices in healthcare have a great potential to monitor physical as well as biochemical markers continuously. COVID-19 pandemic has emphasized such capability in the current wearable devices, and through their continual innovation and development, they could play a significant part in fighting any future pandemic.

Though it may be easy to collect the physiological data of individuals, making accurate predictions about the infected individuals using population-based data and modeling may be inadequate. To decide regarding an individual's health, collecting and processing large volumes of data from every individual are essential. The cost of low-power silicon electronics is reducing continuously, and computational power is increasing. This makes it possible to process the data locally and, thus, decentralize and accelerate the decision-making process [17].

5.6 Machine learning and deep learning in COVID-19 diagnosis

Clinical testing and image testing, which do not have many transformations, differ mainly in their procedures. In clinical testing forms, filing procedures take a long time and are annoying, especially in urgent situations. In contrast to this, image testing does not have long processes to be followed. In clinical testing, doctors themselves analyze the reports. This testing is slightly more accurate than image testing. One needs to rely on the computer, which will intelligently perform tasks until precise instructions are given. These two types of tests differ mainly in terms of cost. Image testing is more economical than clinical testing. CT scans can also be evaluated for other viruses to distinguish them from the coronavirus using different DL-based techniques [3].

ML and DL approaches have established themselves as valuable approaches that can assess gigantic high-dimensional features of medical images. CT or X-ray discoveries of COVID-19 sufferers and that of other uncommon diseases like pneumonia are quite alike. ML and DL approaches can be used to discern between COVID-19 and other pneumonia conditions robotically. COVID-19 can also be discerned from other diseases using drug-induced viruses or immune-pneumonitis. Various DL approaches such as VGG-16, Ensemble, InceptionNetV3, MobileNet v2, ResNet, Xception, CNN, *K*NN, and Truncated Inception Net have been used to evaluate chest images of COVID-19 patients, and their solicitation has produced hopeful results. This is significant as X-rays are easily acquirable and cost little. The significant advantage of these methods are that in addition to diagnosing COVID-19 patients, they can even forecast the austerity of COVID-19 pneumonia and the threat of fleeting mortality. The number of studies conducted to measure each of the X-ray and CT images is almost the same, even though the X-rays are less expensive when compared to the CT images. Some other research studies have applied procedures on both kinds of images. Several independent studies have shown that convolution neural networks (CNN)-based methods have classified COVID-19 patients from further causes of pneumonia or even related ailments with an accuracy of 99.99%. This means that these approaches can be used as screening procedures for the primary assessment of COVID-19 cases.

Though both ML and DL approaches can be used for the stated objective, they vary in some regards. For example, ML can use a minor amount of data from the users, while DL requires a massive volume of labeled training data for a succinct denouement. ML methods require the users to accurately define the features. However, DL methods require high-performance hardware. DL generates features on its own and, hence, consumes more time to train when compared to ML. ML divides the tasks into smaller ones and later combines the obtained results into one conclusion. On the contrary, DL uses end-to-end principles to resolve the problems.

DL is a rapid and efficient method used for the identification and forecast of various ailments mainly due to its good accuracy rate. Hence, it can be used in medical science as the most efficient technique. Models are explicitly trained to categorize the inputs into various classes as per the programmers' preference. Such models are used in the medical field for multiple tasks such as detecting heart problems, diagnosing cancer and tumors using image analysis, and several additional applications. They are also exploited to discriminate between CT scan images of the patients diseased with COVID-19 as positive or negative. In the medical field, DL method such as CNN efficiently processes CT scan images to the particular model. Since a CT scan image gives a detailed image of a specific area, it helps to detect internal defects, tumors, measurements of the parts, injuries, etc., and thus, a CT scan proves to be more reliable than RT-PCR method in the case of

COVID-19 and efficiently classifies the images of COVID-19 patients with great accuracy at a faster rate.

Additionally, during the COVID-19 pandemic, they were able to detect the reticular pattern, ground-glass-opacities, alliance, and crazy tiling pattern, which are the hallmarks of COVID-19 infection. However, CT scans have side effects, such as patient exposure to radiation when numerous CT scans are conducted. Diagnosing the disease early largely increases the chances of treating the disease or the virus in a better way. Sometimes a few minor symptoms can steer in diagnosing a major illness like cancer or a minor disease like a simple viral, which can be wrongly predicted [3].

5.7 Related works

Muhammad *et al.* [18] have developed various supervised learning models using epidemiology labeled dataset to predict COVID-19 infection and evaluated their performances. Their results show decision tree, support vector machine, and naïve Bayes to be the best among all others in terms of accuracy, sensitivity, and specificity, respectively. Dash *et al.* [19] have developed a model that predicts the outbreak of COVID-19 and is used to predict the daily-confirmed cases for 90 days future values, thus, helping to plan and manage the healthcare systems and infrastructure. Chakraborty and Abougreen [20] have presented a review of the AI and ML contributions to confront the pandemic disease. Dhawan *et al.* [21] have proposed a secure technique that uses IoT protocol and steganography to transfer the stego images to their destination using the secure transmission of hidden images. Kumar *et al.* [22] have proposed to classify and audit the coughing sound investigation, AI models, and information assortment strategies through IoT to group the pulmonary sicknesses. They have tested the feasibility of the model by comparing it with other models that have used data from a pediatric office and wearable sensors. Shelke and Chakraborty [23] have presented a review to evaluate the relevance of augmented reality and virtual reality in spinal navigation.

5.8 Experimental case study

In this section, a case study has been discussed and experimental results are provided.

5.8.1 Dataset description

COVIDX dataset that is publicly available on GitHub has been used. Our experiment used only a subset of the COVIDX CT dataset due to the limited computation facility. For the analysis, we have used 100,500 CT slices that span across 4,000 patients. All the CT images are labeled manually with the assistance of medical professionals, and some are labeled using automatic labeling models. Table 5.1 gives the instances of labeled images used in experimentation.

The dataset is categorized into two variants: A and B. Variant A consists of COVID confirmed cases certified by medical professionals. The second variant, B,

Table 5.1 Instances of labeled images

Patient id	Source	Country	Finding	Verified finding	Slice selection	View	Modality
CP_0	CNCB	China	Pneumonia	Yes	Expert	Axial	CT
CP_10	CNCB	China	Pneumonia	Yes	Automatic	Axial	CT
CP_1068	CNCB	China	Pneumonia	Yes	Automatic	Axial	CT
CP_1070	CNCB	China	Pneumonia	Yes	Expert	Axial	CT
CP_1071	CNCB	China	Pneumonia	Yes	Expert	Axial	CT
CP_1072	CNCB	China	Pneumonia	Yes	Expert	Axial	CT
CP_1073	CNCB	China	Pneumonia	Yes	Expert	Axial	CT
CP_1075	CNCB	China	Pneumonia	Yes	Expert	Axial	CT
CP_1076	CNCB	China	Pneumonia	Yes	Expert	Axial	CT
CP_1077	CNCB	China	Pneumonia	Yes	Expert	Axial	CT
CP_1081	CNCB	China	Pneumonia	Yes	Automatic	Axial	CT
CP_1082	CNCB	China	Pneumonia	Yes	Expert	Axial	CT
CP_1083	CNCB	China	Pneumonia	Yes	Automatic	Axial	CT
CP_1087	CNCB	China	Pneumonia	Yes	Automatic	Axial	CT
CP_1088	CNCB	China	Pneumonia	Yes	Expert	Axial	CT
CP_1091	CNCB	China	Pneumonia	Yes	Expert	Axial	CT
CP_1092	CNCB	China	Pneumonia	Yes	Expert	Axial	CT
CP_1093	CNCB	China	Pneumonia	Yes	Expert	Axial	CT
CP_1094	CNCB	China	Pneumonia	Yes	Expert	Axial	CT
CP_1095	CNCB	China	Pneumonia	Yes	Expert	Axial	CT
CP_1097	CNCB	China	Pneumonia	Yes	Automatic	Axial	CT
....							
...							
study_0621	MosMedData	Russia	COVID-19	No	Automatic	Axial	CT
study_0622	MosMedData	Russia	COVID-19	No	Automatic	Axial	CT
study_0623	MosMedData	Russia	COVID-19	No	Automatic	Axial	CT

has all image sets of A with additional images confirmed to be diagnosed as COVID but no validation. These other images are used as a part of the testing dataset. Figure 5.3(a) and (b) provides the data distribution across normal, pneumonia, and COVID.

5.8.2 Methodology

In this segment, we discuss the proposed model for screening patients' CT scan images using DL models such as CNN. The model is iteratively trained with normal and COVID-infected CT images. The images in the dataset are preprocessed to fit in the considered model. The proposed model consists of the following stages: (1) Preprocessing and (2) EfficientNet-B0 architecture.

The flow diagram for the proposed model is given in Figure 5.4.

1. Preprocessing:
   The image dataset has been captured in real time. The intensity of pixels across an image varies. For any CNN, it is essential to normalize the pixels across the

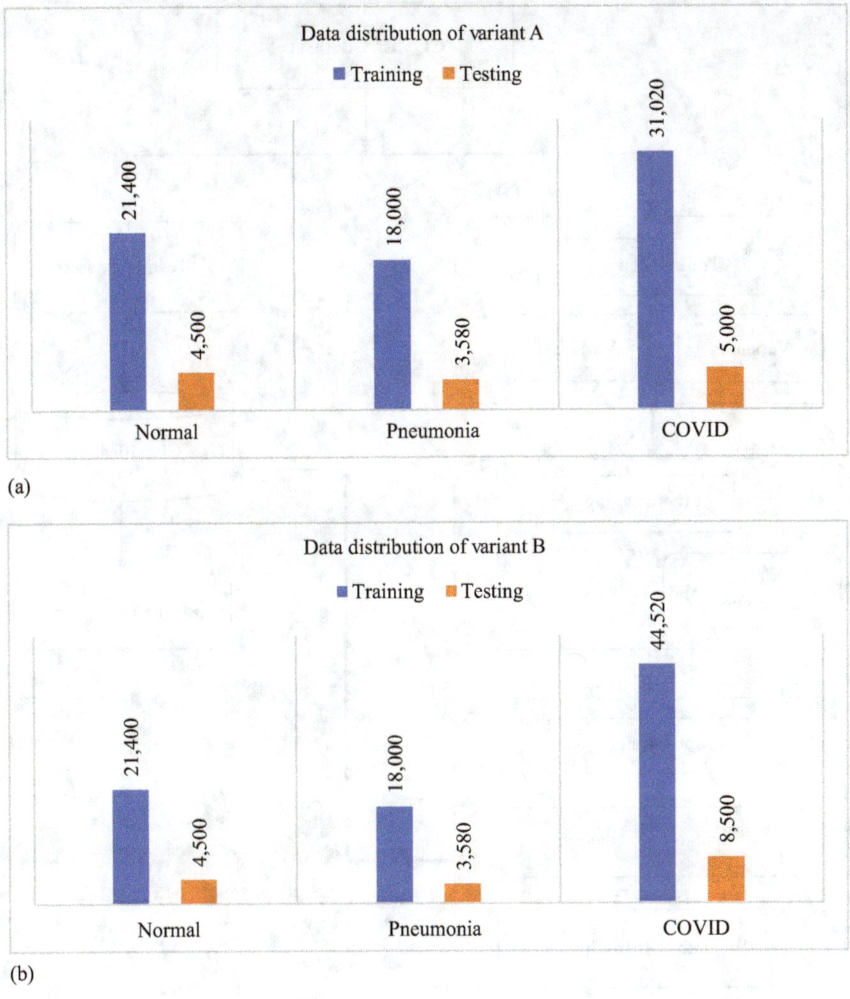

Figure 5.3 (a) Data distribution of variant A and (b) data distribution of variant B

image. For this purpose, we have used pixel intensity normalization of all pixels in the range [0, 1]. This process also helps in the training stage of model convergence.

For any of the CNNs, images are to be reduced to standard size. Once the images are reduced, there is a scope of loss of data. Since the cost involved in EfficientNet is low in terms of memory and latency, we do not have to reduce the size of the image. Thus, the information in image can be retained. Figure 5.5(a) and (b) shows the sample images of COVID CT scan and Normal CT scan, respectively.

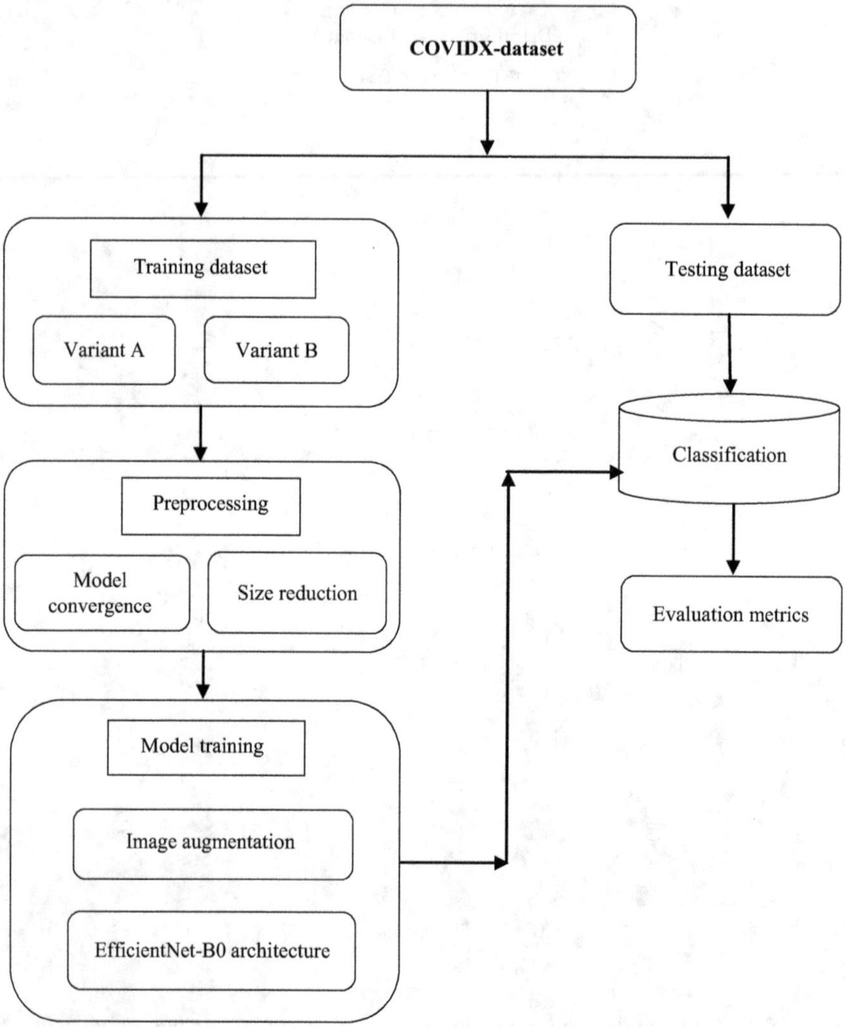

Figure 5.4 Flow diagram for proposed model

2. EfficientNet-B0 architecture:
   The EfficientNet-B0 baseline architecture belongs to the family of multi-objective neural networks. It is further developed for B1–B7 to achieve a higher accuracy rate. Table 5.2 describes the architecture.

The three parameters, width, depth, and resolution are scaled using compound coefficient parameters ∅ for the proposed model. The alpha, beta, and gamma scaling multipliers are used as per (5.1)–(5.3) to compute the depth, width, and resolution.

$$Depth\ D = \alpha^{\varnothing} \tag{5.1}$$

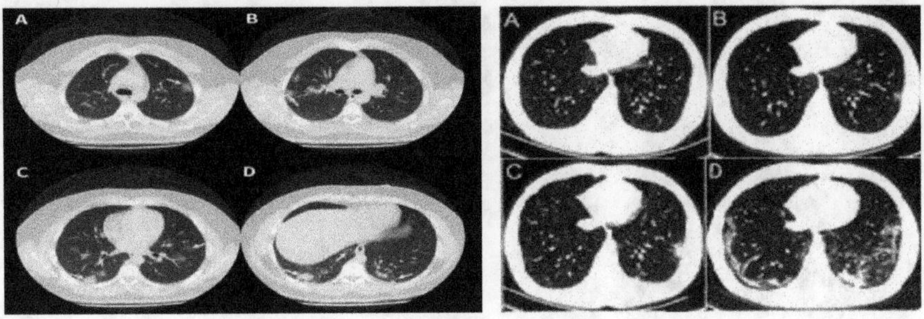

(a) (b)

Figure 5.5 (a) COVID-19 CT scan and (b) non-COVID-19 CT scan

Table 5.2 Efficient Net baseline network-B0 architecture

Stage-X*i*	**Operator *F^i***	**Resolution *H^iXW^i***	**Channels C*i***	**Layers L^*i***
1	Conv 3 × 3	224 × 224	32	1
2	MBConv1, k3 × 3	112 × 112	16	1
3	MBConv6, k3 × 3	112 × 112	24	2
4	MBConv6, k5 × 5	56 × 56	40	2
5	MBConv6, k3 × 3	28 × 28	80	3
6	MBConv6, k5 × 5	14 × 14	112	3
7	MBConv6, k5 × 5	14 × 14	192	4
8	MBConv6, k3 × 3	7 × 7	320	1
9	Conv1 × 1/Pooling/FC	7 × 7	1,280	1

$$Width\ W = \beta^{\varnothing} \tag{5.2}$$

$$Resolution\ R = \gamma^{\varnothing} \tag{5.3}$$

$$w.r.t.\alpha * \beta^2 * \gamma^2 \approx 2, \alpha \geq 1, \beta \geq 1 \text{ and } \gamma \geq 1$$

The proposed model uses various residual blocks with different configurations with swish activation functions and inverted residual blocks. Using swish activation is to minimize the error and increase the accuracy as ReLu produces unexpected changes. The Swish activation function can be represented as (5.4). Here, it does not nullify the negative values as ReLu:

$$S_x = X * Sigmod(X) \tag{5.4}$$

5.8.3 Training

In DL models, large datasets need to be used in the training model because of the complexity in computations involved. But, in real time, availability of a large dataset is challenging, and hence, to address this issue, we employ the technique of data augmentation. We increased the sample size by transformation operations over

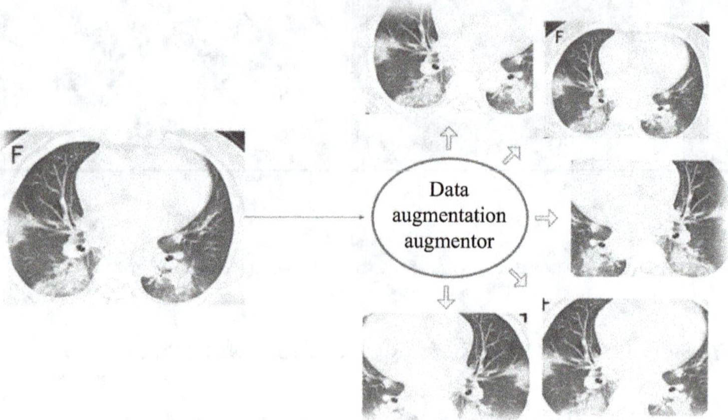

Figure 5.6 Image augmentation operation

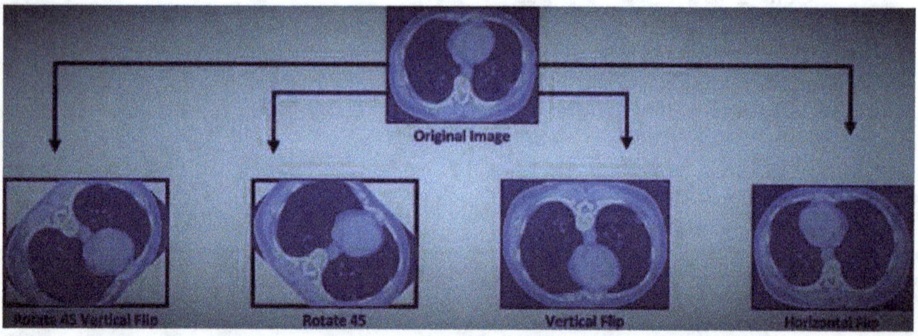

Figure 5.7 Augmented image in dataset

images such as rotation, scaling, and flip. Figure 5.6 gives the sample instance of data augmentation operation.

The image augmentations are performed using the python augmenter package. The transformation parameter applied for rotation is 0–20° anticlockwise. For scaling, it is up to 30% zoom. The operations are involved in different probability orders on samples. Figure 5.7 shows an augmented image in the dataset.

5.8.4 Experimental setup and results

Experiments have been accompanied on an Intel® Core™ i7-5820K CPU with 3.30 GHz, Titan X Pascal with 12 GB, 64 GB Ram, and the TensorFlow with Keras framework for Python. The training model initiates with a limit learning rate of 0.001 with the Adam-Optimizer for 15 epochs using categorical cross-entropy loss.

The experiment for the proposed model is carried out with varying input image sizes, and various performance metrics are computed and shown in Table 5.3. Figure 5.8 gives the ROC curve for the proposed approach.

Table 5.3 Performance metrics for various input image sizes

Input size	Accuracy	Sensitivity	Prediction	*F*1-score
250 × 250	69.41	60.41	74.15	76.70
300 × 300	72.81	69.39	78.00	74.12
350 × 350	75.49	72.59	80.41	78.00
400 × 400	81.25	85.61	94.01	92.49
450 × 450	88.55	89.63	93.43	92.17
500 × 500 (original)	94.74	94.67	98.93	93.55

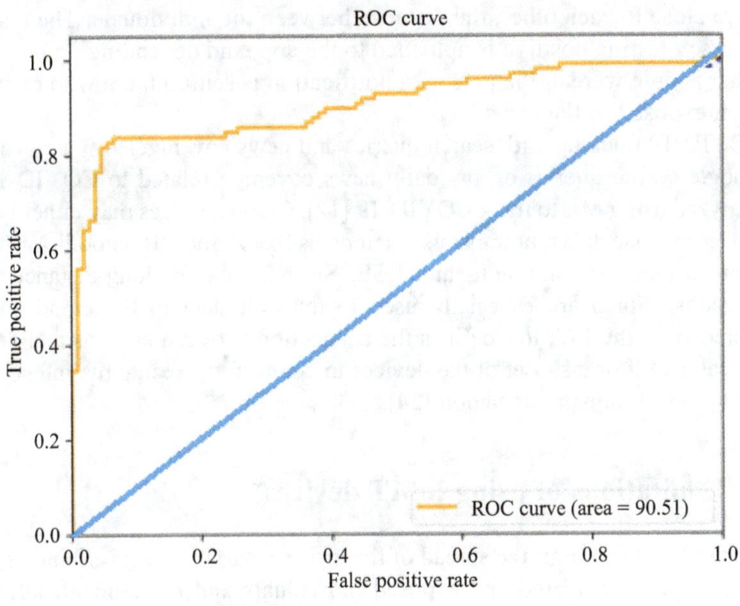

Figure 5.8 ROC curve

5.9 Measures for monitoring and tracking COVID-19

To prevent the transmission of the virus and affecting more people, various digital monitoring tools are used, such as

1. Social contact tracing: To inhibit the transmission of the virus, many countries have imposed lockdown rules. However, the lockdown has many downsides too, such as it interrupts productivity, affects people's living conditions, and brings down the economy for the nations. The contact tracing method has been imposed in a lot of places to control the spread of the virus while simultaneously permitting people to live a new normal. This approach is used to identify potentially infected people based on the study of people's social

interactions. Thus, the information obtained from the approach can be used to notify the healthcare workers and people of their risk of infection [4].

2. COVID-19 monitoring using smartphones: Around the world, several smartphone applications have been developed and deployed. Official governments in China, India, and Singapore support some of them. Different countries have used different approaches to monitor the spread of COVID-19. Some countries have made it mandatory for citizens to enter their data. Other countries are automatically tracking the movement of citizens with the help of authorities who monitor law enforcement. These tracing applications locate phones using Bluetooth in the vicinity that uses the identical application. The Bluetooth signals contain data such as how often individuals were close to each other, the distance between the individuals. The result of a person testing positive is uploaded to the app, and depending on how close other people were to the person, a notification is sent to them who may have been exposed to the virus.
3. COVID-19 tracking with search queries and news coverage: Any keywords in Google search queries or any daily news coverage related to COVID-19 are analyzed using ML to track COVID-19 [12]. Cloud services may either be paid or free and use different transmission models like Zigbee, Bluetooth, Wi-Fi, for short-distance transmissions and LTE, Sigfox, etc., for long-distance transmissions, which are especially used to transmit data to the cloud and are included on the IoT. IoT defines the connection between humans and devices that allow all or a subset of the devices to connect to execute the intended job exclusive of human interaction [24].

5.10 Limitations of using IoMT devices

One method that can limit the spread of the disease is to use a surveillance system that can track the infected and exposed individuals and the clinical outcomes. However, since these surveillance systems have limitations regarding factors such as spatial resolution, timeliness, and scalability, reporting in these systems has the tendency to be specific to a nation or a region. They may not have adequate evidence about maladies at the community or city level. This affects the social distancing and quarantine measures, and as a result, the disease cannot be contained [16].

IoT and innovative medical devices can monitor and screen patients' health conditions anywhere, anytime. As a result, the healthcare systems have improved tremendously and can provide timely services in various locations. However, due to the novel COVID-19 pandemic, there has been an unexpected and massive increase in patients. Hence, it is imperative to constantly monitor the patient's health conditions to avoid any serious disorder or infection. The IoT and smart medical devices produce gigantic volumes of sensitive information about patients. However, the patients do not want their personal and sensitive information to be disclosed. This raises serious security concerns concerning IoT data [25].

5.11 Conclusion and future scope

COVID-19 has afflicted the lives of many people across the globe. Almost all countries are taking various measures to control the virus from spreading and to save peoples' lives. In this chapter, the advancements in information technology being leveraged in various ways to diagnose the diseases and monitor the patients even if they are in remote locations have been described. Wearable devices are being used to collect the patients' data that is analyzed using ML and DL techniques to make predictions about the diseases. As a result, it helps to adopt measures to curb the infection from spreading even further. Additionally, a case study along with experimental results has also been discussed.

In the current work, ML and DL techniques have been used with available dataset. However, in real time, since a large amount of data is being continuously generated on a number of devices, the current work can be extended to deploy continual machine learning (CML) models in the production environment where the data is generated, i.e., on the edge devices. CML can retrain the ML model periodically with new data and trends to build a more accurate model with improved performance, thereby saving the retraining time. In other words, CML can be combined with edge computing to provide autoadaptive models on the edge devices with some processing occurring at them rather than sending all the data to the cloud and as a result, data can remain secure as it is processed on the edge devices.

References

[1] Seshadri DR, Davies EV, Harlow ER, *et al.*, Wearable Sensors for COVID-19: A Call to Action to Harness Our Digital Infrastructure for Remote Patient Monitoring and Virtual Assessments. *Frontiers in Digital Health*. 2020; 2: 8.

[2] Ghaderzadeh M and Asadi F, Deep Learning in the Detection and Diagnosis of COVID-19 Using Radiology Modalities: A Systematic Review. *Journal of Healthcare Engineering*. 2021: 1–10.

[3] Shah V, Keniya R, Shridharani A, Punjabi M, Shah J and Mehendale N, Diagnosis of COVID-19 Using CT Scan Images and Deep Learning Techniques. *Emergency Radiology*. 2021; 28: 497–505.

[4] Allam M, Cai S, Ganesh S, *et al.*, COVID-19 Diagnostics, Tools, and Prevention. *Diagnostics*. 2020; 10(409): 1–33.

[5] Abbasi WA, Abbas SA, Andleeb S, *et al.*, COVID: An Expert System to Diagnose COVID-19 and Predict Its Severity Using Chest CT Scans: Application in Radiology. *Informatics in Medicine Unlocked* [Internet]. 2021; 23(100540):1–8. Available from: https://doi.org/10.1016/j.imu.2021.100540.

[6] Khanday AMUD, Rabani ST, Khan QR, Rouf N and Mohi Ud Din M, Machine Learning based Approaches for Detecting COVID-19 Using Clinical Text Data. *International Journal of Information Technology* (Singapore). 2020; 12: 731–9.

[7] Carter LJ, Garner LV, Smoot JW, *et al.*, Assay Techniques and Test Development for COVID-19 Diagnosis. *ACS Central Science* IN FOCUS [Internet]. 2020; 6: 591–605. Available from: https://pubs.acs.org/doi/10.1021/acscentsci.0c00501.

[8] Bharati S, Podder P, Mondal MRH and Paul PK, Applications and Challenges of Cloud Integrated IoMT. In: *Studies in Systems, Decision and Control* [Internet]. Springer International Publishing; 2021. p. 67–85. Available from: http://dx.doi.org/10.1007/978-3-030-55833-8_4.

[9] Vishnu S, Jino Ramson SR and Jegan R, Internet of Medical Things (IoMT) – An Overview. In: *ICDCS 2020–2020 5th International Conference on Devices, Circuits and Systems*. 2020. p. 101–4.

[10] Aman AHM, Hassan WH, Sameen SAL, Attarbashi ZS and Alizadeh M, IoMT amid COVID-19 Pandemic: Application, Architecture, Technology, and Security. *Journal of Network and Computer Applications*. 2021; 174: 1–20.

[11] Mishra T, Wang M, Metwally AA, *et al.*, Pre-Symptomatic Detection of COVID-19 from Smartwatch Data. *Nature Biomedical Engineering* [Internet]. 2020; 4: 1208–20. Available from: https://www.nature.com/articles/s41551-020-00640-6.

[12] Nasajpour M, Pouriyeh S, Parizi RM, Dorodchi M, Valero M and Arabnia HR, Internet of Things for Current COVID-19 and Future Pandemics: an Exploratory Study. *Journal of Healthcare Informatics Research*. 2020; 4(4): 325–64.

[13] Chai PR, Zhang H, Jambaulikar GD, *et al.*, An Internet of Things Buttons to Measure and Respond to Restroom Cleanliness in a Hospital Setting: Descriptive Study. *Journal of Medical Internet Research*. 2019; 21(6): 1–10.

[14] Miller DJ, Capodilupo JV, Lastella M, *et al.*, Analyzing Changes in Respiratory Rate to Predict the Risk of COVID-19 Infection. *PLoS One* [Internet]. 2020; 15(12): 1–10. Available from: http://dx.doi.org/10.1371/journal.pone.0243693.

[15] Otoom M, Otoum N, Alzubaidi MA and Etoom Y, An IoT-based Framework for Early Identification and Monitoring of COVID-19 Cases. *Biomedical Signal Processing and Control*. 2020; 62(102149): 1–16.

[16] Gong M, Liu L, Sun X, Yang Y, Wang S and Zhu H, Cloud-based System for Effective Surveillance and Control of COVID-19: Useful Experiences from Hubei, China. *Journal of Medical Internet Research*. 2020; 22(4): 1–9.

[17] Ates HC, Yetisen AK, Güder F and Dincer C, Wearable Devices for the Detection of COVID-19. *Nature Electronics*. 2021; 4(1): 13–4.

[18] Muhammad LJ, Algehyne EA, Usman SS, Ahmad A, Chakraborty C and Mohammed IA, Supervised Machine Learning Models for Prediction of COVID-19 Infection using Epidemiology Dataset. *SN Computer Science* [Internet]. 2021; 2(1): 11. Available from: http://link.springer.com/10.1007/s42979-020-00394-7.

[19] Dash S, Chakraborty C, Giri SK, Pani SK and Frnda J, BIFM: Big-Data Driven Intelligent Forecasting Model for COVID-19. *IEEE Access*

[Internet]. 2021; 9: 97505–17. Available from: https://ieeexplore.ieee.org/document/9474452/.

[20] Chakraborty C and Abougreen A, Intelligent Internet of Things and Advanced Machine Learning Techniques for COVID-19. *EAI Endorsed Transactions on Pervasive Health and Technology* [Internet]. 2021; 21(26): e1. Available from: http://eudl.eu/doi/10.4108/eai.28-1-2021.168505.

[21] Dhawan S, Chakraborty C, Frnda J, Gupta R, Rana AK and Pani SK, SSII: Secured and High-Quality Steganography Using Intelligent Hybrid Optimization Algorithms for IoT. *IEEE Access*. 2021; 9: 87563–78.

[22] Kumar A, Abhishek K, Chakraborty C and Kryvinska N, Deep Learning and Internet of Things based Lung Ailment Recognition through Coughing Spectrograms. *IEEE Access*. 2016; 4: 1–12.

[23] Shelke Y and Chakraborty C, Augmented Reality and Virtual Reality Transforming Spinal Imaging Landscape: A Feasibility Study. *IEEE Computer Graphics and Applications* [Internet]. 2021; 41(3): 124–38. Available from: https://ieeexplore.ieee.org/document/9112351/.

[24] Hasan MW, Covid-19 Fever Symptom Detection based on IoT Cloud. *International Journal of Electrical and Computer Engineering*. 2021; 11(2): 1823–9.

[25] Akhbarifar S, Javadi HHS, Rahmani AM and Hosseinzadeh M, A Secure Remote Health Monitoring Model for Early Disease Diagnosis in Cloud-based IoT Environment. *Personal and Ubiquitous Computing*. 2020.

Chapter 6

Blockchain technology for secure COVID-19 pandemic data handling

Agbotiname Lucky Imoize[1,2], *Daisy Osarugue Irabor*[3], *Peter Anuoluwapo Gbadega*[4] *and Chinmay Chakraborty*[5]

Abstract

In recent times, COVID-19 pandemic data collected via the Internet of Medical Things–enabled channels can be transmitted seamlessly and processed remotely by medical practitioners globally. However, the confidentiality and integrity of these channels pose serious security concerns. The transmission of medical information, which comprises highly sensitive personal data, must meet stringent security requirements. In order to achieve this, blockchain has been deployed to enhance the security, confidentially, trust, and integrity of sensitive data being transmitted over insecure channels as a result of its cryptographic characteristics. Blockchain is regarded as a protected and distributed structure of data, which enhances security, simplifies the tracking, and analyses the stored medical information independently. Additionally, blockchain allows the transmission and exchange of messages between two parties in a network configuration, independent of sole trusted authority. Blockchain technology is verifiably safe against an attacker who mismanages the scheme and compromises the central controller. Furthermore, blockchain technology has been deployed to handle distributed medical data in standard medical laboratories. The decentralized and immutability features of blockchain have facilitated the rapid development of the beyond 5G wireless services for health-related data sharing and processing. However, the adoption of blockchain technology in medical data handling is still in its infancy, and the need for a

[1]Department of Electrical and Electronics Engineering, Faculty of Engineering, University of Lagos, Lagos, Nigeria

[2]Department of Electrical Engineering and Information Technology, Institute of Digital Communication, Ruhr University Bochum, Bochum, Germany

[3]Department of Electrical and Computer Engineering, Tandon School of Engineering, New York University, New York, USA

[4]Discipline of Electrical, Electronic & Computer Engineering, School of Engineering, Howard College Campus, University of KwaZulu-Natal, Durban, South Africa

[5]Department of Electronics and Communication Engineering, Birla Institute of Technology, Mesra, Ranchi, India

rigorous study in this domain cannot be overemphasized. Toward this end, this chapter first highlights how blockchain technology has developed in recent times and how it is applied in the medical data-handling space. Further to this, the chapter examines the potential benefits, key challenges, and prospects in blockchain technology. Additionally, the chapter highlights research efforts in blockchain in healthcare, especially as it relates to the dreaded COVID-19 pandemic. The chapter also discusses the application of blockchain technology in healthcare data-handling practices that can build trust with automated tracking of integrity and responsible credential verification. Finally, practical COVID-19 pandemic data were analyzed and presented to motivate the chapter further.

Keywords: Blockchain technology; Security; COVID-19 pandemic; Medical information; Distributed data handling

6.1 Introduction

The present inconsistencies of channels through which COVID-19 pandemic data are transmitted and collected have given rise to the increasing need for better secured, yet more reliable, data accessible to health professionals and policy makers [1]. Globally, these data help manage the spread of COVID-19. Through the Internet of Medical Things (IoMT), they can be received and processed for health and environmental benefits. The sensitivity of these data demands the highest level of channel confidentiality and integrity, which are currently inadequate. In addition, the health data transmission and processing systems designed to improve treatment outcomes may suffer centralization and licensure that invariably leads to failure at one or more points in the transmission or collection process [2]. In response, blockchain technology addresses this by improving the reliability of health logistics, supporting early detection of an outbreak, and protecting users' privacy during the pandemic [3].

Blockchain is a system of distributed databases that work using stable decentralized servers and a computer network [4]. Blockchain technology manages a record of chronological data transactions that are distributed among available nodes in a verifiable, node-synchronized, decentralized, cost-effective, and timely manner [5–7]. As the pandemic prevails even with control measures being developed, the global healthcare system is consistently strained, and characteristic data have become a precious resource to curb the spread of the virus. We also live in a technology-driven world that is transforming rapidly. It is valuable to collect and record digital activities like sensitive data through smart devices and digital monitoring tools. Individuals give these devices access to manage their personal and business data directly or indirectly, and even though the devices appear reliable, data may not be handled appropriately. This gives rise to the misuse of sensitive data that other digital or examining systems collect the data of users and their network. In most cases, they use these data dishonorably [8]. Although this may be a common occurrence within social Internet channels, several sensitive data have still been lost, broken, or diverted within healthcare transmission or processing systems due to mishandling data.

Blockchain technology consolidates data security such as locations visited by people who have been infected; medications and test kits from manufacturer to users; records of remote patient–doctor consultation; credential verification of healthcare specialists; and the source of malfunctioned test kits [9]. Unarguably, this technology handles data with a high level of confidentiality, transparency, and improved system integrity. We shall soon see that these may be optimized for even more efficiency and better security that may accommodate more data and challenging situations. With this, blockchain technology may streamline the operations of handling medical information [10]. Blockchain can be private, public, or consortium [11]. In a private blockchain that may be preferred for handling sensitive data due to its high throughput and low-energy consumption, the network is controlled by a specific provider who is trustworthy and manages preselected participants connected to the Internet. While the public blockchain operates in contrast, the consortium combines both operations over a network. While healthcare systems may choose any of these blockchain types, there are specific requirements and cases, like handling the COVID-19 pandemic data that may demand the operation of a particular blockchain, according to the size of participants, the strength of the network, and available resources. A summary of the key benefits of the three categories of blockchain technology in relation to medical information management is presented in Figure 6.1.

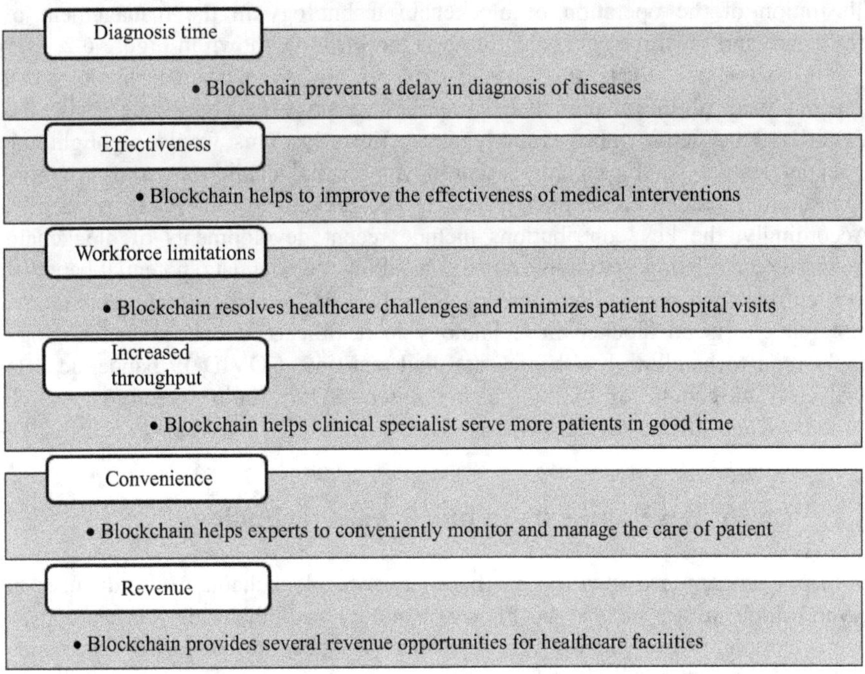

Figure 6.1 Key benefits of blockchain in the management of medical information

After Bitcoin and Ethereum, the applications developed as the third blockchain technology have been instrumental to healthcare, supply chain, and Internet of Things (IoT) [8]. In Section 6.6, an explanation will be provided on how blockchain can be used to handle healthcare data across the network to build trust. For many years, the IoT has been revolutionizing the healthcare industry to improve medical information records, collect data for prescribed drugs, and provide insurance information [12,13]. For handling COVID-19 data, the IoMT collects important data of patients, provides disease symptoms and trends, automates process logistics, facilitates remote caring, and gives patients access to control their healthcare [14–16]. Hence with one or more of these devices, it is possible to monitor patients in real time, enable treatments, conduct check-ups, and even follow up on the progress of improvement. In turn, this helps to deliver faster healthcare while reducing hospital costs. With sensors in medical devices, data can be collected and securely sent over a wireless network to a health specialist who would then analyze the data for possible anomalies. Essentially, this has a higher potential to manage the COVID-19 pandemic and reduce the spread of the virus more securely and reliably than conventional strategies employed to address the widespread epidemic experienced in the past. This is evident in the operation that expands technology capabilities while minimizing the risk of exposing patients, medical practitioners, and health specialists to COVID-19 since contact is only established on a critical need basis. Patients can also improve their self-care and easily access support using digital and communication tools developed using blockchain technology [17]. An illustration of the operation of blockchain technology in the management of healthcare and sensitive data using through the IoMT is shown in Figure 6.2.

In content and focus, this chapter explores how blockchain technology can transmit medical information that comprises sensitive data associated with the COVID-19 pandemic more securely and efficiently. This would highlight the essential features of blockchain technology, potential challenges, and emerging opportunities related to healthcare data of the prevailing COVID-19 pandemic. Accordingly, the key contributions include recent developments of blockchain technology in relation to its application to handling medical data, potential benefits, key current and impending challenges, prospects of blockchain technology, research efforts on blockchain technology in healthcare, blockchain technology application to handling healthcare data, and real-time COVID-19 pandemic data analysis. The conclusion of this chapter reiterates key findings, future research directions, and further reading.

6.2 Recent developments in blockchain technology

In recent times, more attention has been given to blockchain. As it advances in several applications such as healthcare, banking, manufacturing, computer networks, communication, and governance, there has been an increasing acceptance globally [18]. The popularity of blockchain technology rose from its capability to improve service security, efficiency, and scalability in applications. This has made

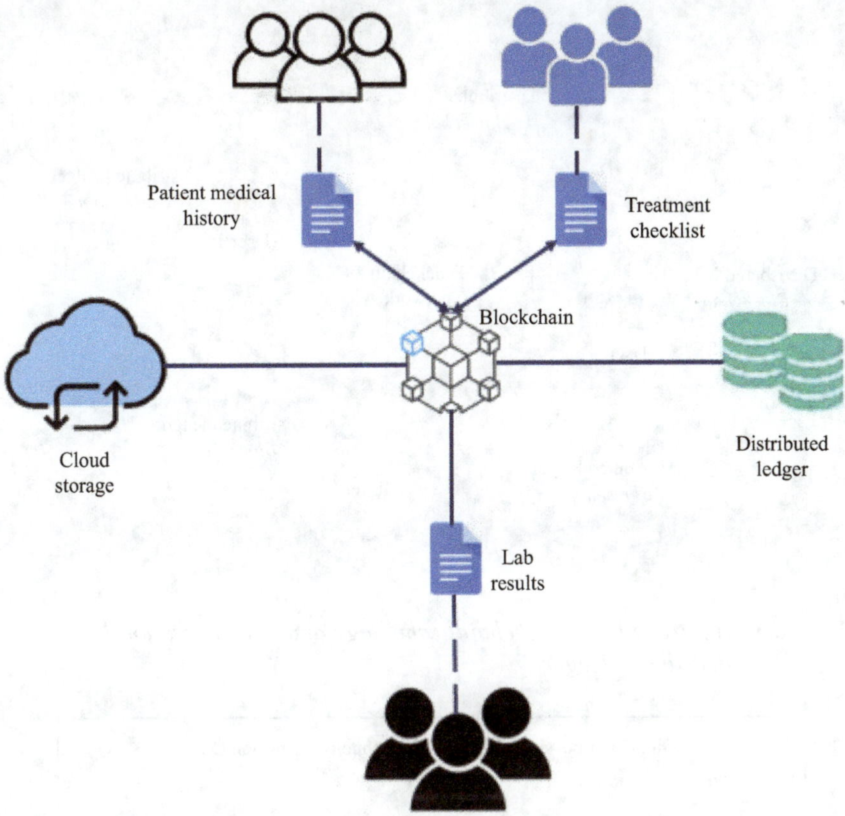

Figure 6.2 An illustration of the management of healthcare data using blockchain technology

it a top choice for incorporating decentralized ideas and procedures in various domains. Since 2019, blockchain technology has developed into a strategic industry that can be integrated into cross-chain, open sources, and various industrial applications [19]. In these applications, blockchain provides distributed data handling of protected and time-marked records of information, which could be sensitive like patients' personal information in healthcare. A typical example of this is shown in Figure 6.3, where the data of users are stored on a distributed ledger in each blockchain, which is all directly connected to a common network, without an intermediary.

In this case, blockchain combines separated health records on the network to track the personal health progress of an individual. Although the first blockchain technology named Bitcoin was introduced in 2009 [19], several unexpected events have occurred over the years that have given blockchain technology an upward trend. This intensified with the emergence of the COVID-19 pandemic, with high expectations of the blockchain domain beyond 2021, as statistics reveal an

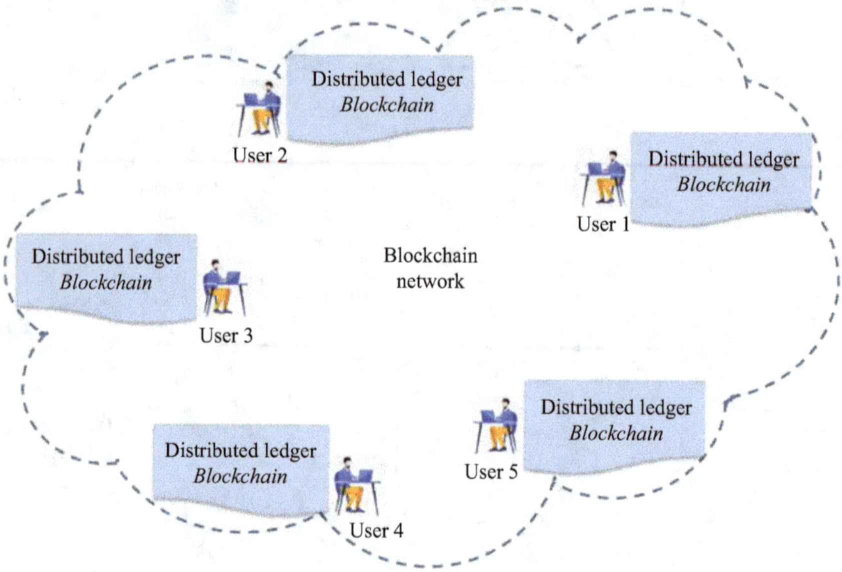

Figure 6.3 An example of blockchain technology and data stored on the distributed ledger

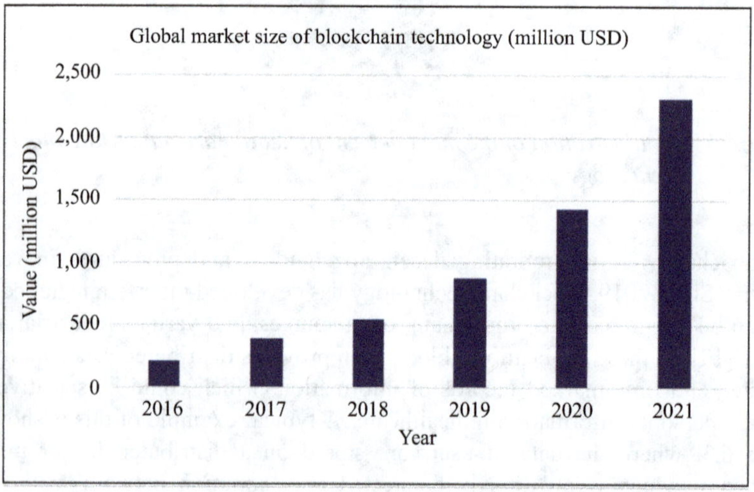

Figure 6.4 Global market size of blockchain technology (2016–2021)

estimated 1 000% increase in the size of blockchain technology from the year 2016 to the year 2021 worldwide [20], as shown in Figure 6.4.

The application of blockchain technology in the handling of medical data is constantly transforming healthcare. As new measures are developed to manage the spread of COVID-19, this has been an invaluable tool to medical experts, healthcare specialists, policy makers, and patients. In these times, digital transformation is more than just a choice for any business. It has become essential for survival in a rapidly changing environment with limited resources, as the COVID-19 pandemic increasingly puts a strain on everyday companies. In healthcare, blockchain technology is making remarkable changes in managing health issues and the provision of care. In effect, the sector is looking to become more digital with blockchain help in data exchange, supply-chain management, and contracts [21].

The autoregression integrated moving average (ARIMA) model with machine learning is another recent development that can be integrated into blockchain technology. Using the available sensitive data, this model contributes to COVID-19 data handling by forecasting its outbreak or predicting the reported cases of COVID-19 in a certain region [22]. It does this through phases of transformation, model identification, estimation of the best suited ARIMA, and diagnostics.

6.2.1 Healthcare data systems

The control and management of the COVID-19 pandemic have seen a consistent development of healthcare data systems. They combine the generation, access, and storage of an individual's medical information digitally. They are designed to operate in real time as a patient-centered record that authorized users can access instantly [23,24]. This has helped to manage the spread of the pandemic better since it includes a broader view of the healthcare condition and exposure of each COVID-19 patient. These systems are developed by blockchain technology that further helps authorized clinical specialists remotely create, manage, and share medical information across multiple health institutions. Another form of these systems developed recently is an optimized version of Personal Health Records, where patients can control who has access to their medical information and remotely manage and track their healthcare, regardless of the healthcare institution providing their care. The recently developed healthcare data systems combine both functions, which can address a health situation at a given time, where more sensitive sensors are used on healthcare devices or in health institutions, and patient-centered healthcare is provided [25,26]. For COVID-19, this may involve infected and noninfected individuals.

An individual's healthcare data can be generated from medical devices at a different location or while that individual receives the provision of healthcare services in a medical institution. However, the dire need to implement optimized blockchain technology in the handling of medical information systems during the COVID-19 pandemic arose because most of the systems before the advent of the pandemic were not interconnected, leaving critical players in healthcare provision with restricted, fragmented, or compromised information, despite having their private database [27]. In response, new health blockchain architectures have been developed, with others underway. A general scenario of these architectures in relation to securely handling data is shown in Figure 6.5.

In this architecture, the blockchain stores medical information in a digital electronic format. The health elements stored have network applications and

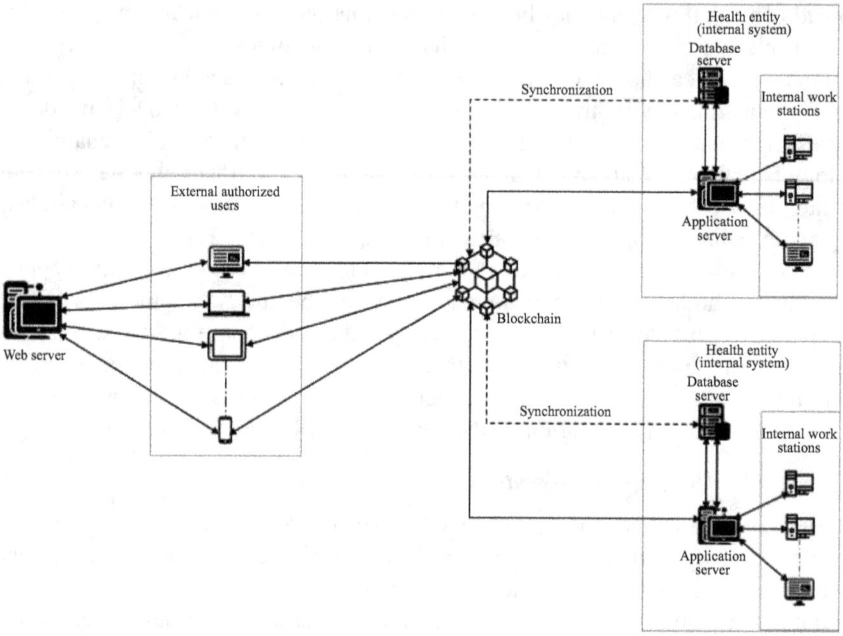

Figure 6.5 Blockchain architecture in healthcare

database servers connected to the blockchain to store and process this medical information. Through another application server within, authorized clinical personnel can communicate with the data system. At the same time, the medical information from the databases of medical devices in their institutions is combined with that of the blockchain, using a synchronizing component. This setup guarantees a high level of security and data integrity in the event of breakage or connectivity loss in the chain [27].

Systems for ensuring that previous analyses are not used for new diagnostic processes have also been developed to support data handling. While these systems have been developed over the last decade, it has also been accompanied by challenges such as incapacity for early detection of disease, poor data quality, high cost, patient privacy, lack of interoperability, and inefficient patient data management [28,29]. The blockchain-developed eHealth system of today improves the system's intervention by supporting electronic medical information solutions that overcome the limitations of power while synchronizing clinical research and information technology. In effect, more privacy, better scalability of data, and less fragmentation are experienced. Blockchain technology maintains integrity by securely storing data that otherwise may be inappropriately accessed due to the instability of communication networks or intermittent connection failures [27]. Other healthcare data systems developed using blockchain technology are being applied to medical records of several individuals at the risk of exposure to COVID-19 for swift intervention and addressing connectivity and data transmission issues.

6.2.2 Healthcare data exchanges

As the number of patients infected with COVID-19 increases, the provision of adequate medical care becomes a challenge in the area of diagnosis, monitoring, treatments, and cost [30]. This is particularly because healthcare services cannot securely send and receive sensitive data across trustworthy channels to improve their services in the overwhelming times imposed by the pandemic. However, recent reports show that healthcare providers have adopted blockchain technology to enable network access among medical practitioners, patients, and healthcare specialists while maintaining the security of data and the integrity of the system. This comes in designed products that give access rights and manages permissions of medical information exchanges. In contrast, others manage the information of the medical provider in terms of storage and transmission [31]. In order to reduce the load of reported cases, a few health groups are also coming together to ensure an up-to-date directory where essential information is shared among themselves and accessible from a database. Additionally, blockchain technology is used to develop a credential verification system that allows medical practitioners at the forefront of COVID-19 pandemic cases to prove their license for the operation [32].

Although in the past few years, the quality of healthcare has improved with wearable devices, implantable devices, and the IoMT [33], blockchain technology helps to authenticate and secure healthcare data that may be otherwise accessed inappropriately [30]. This is highly instrumental, as securing patients' personal information requires healthcare systems to meet the unique requirements of data transfer and interoperability, which the concept of decentralization achieves excellently.

6.2.3 Healthcare administration

Following data-handling standards, including privacy, security, transmission, exchange, content, and terminology, blockchain technology is employed to speed up some healthcare processes and reduce transaction costs [34]. The rise in the spread of COVID-19 accompanied an urgent need to exchange data through healthcare systems efficiently. To combat the pandemic, healthcare providers, health policy makers, health insurance companies, and healthcare institutions collectively understand the complete picture of the pandemic through the exchange of essential data. These are only achieved by implementing standards that guide the capture and transfer of medical information, where blockchain technology significantly impacts today. Typically, patients' medical information is grouped to form a dataset to evaluate the quality of care provided, measure healthcare outcomes, and report on the safety or progress of health [35]. Prior to the active integration of blockchain technology in healthcare and the inception of the COVID-19 pandemic, healthcare support was more complex, costly, and slow, which invariably generated a lower quality of healthcare provided and an incapacity to manage the ranging spread on COVID-19 when it was first discovered.

Although these healthcare standards and their administration in the provision of healthcare have been in place before the pandemic, the need and challenges have only intensified with the COVID-19 pandemic. Following the required procedure and consent, several representatives work to enforce the standardization of sensitive data transactions, which, for the most part, requires access to complex data through a high level of transparency, confidentiality, and integrity. Intelligent Healthcare Networks are being developed to track data gathered, transmitted, received, revenue, and permission status using blockchain technology. As expected, this comes with an improved scalability and speed of health administrative process that can also be employed in a larger situation like the fight against the spread of COVID-19.

6.2.4 Pharmaceuticals

Pharmaceuticals and drug production play a significant role in managing the COVID-19 pandemic, and the industry is fast moving toward blockchain technology. Given that large data are a big part of pharmaceuticals, the management of data is essential. Aspects of the industry that may generate a large amount of data include pharmaceutical research for the production of vaccines and suppressants; clinical testing; development of applications for healthcare like the IoT; and the expansion of new regulations for drugs and supply chain. As large as these data may be in many cases, it must also be maintained and organized. Blockchain technology is currently improving this and providing smart security of data and transparency in data handling and logistic activities [36]. In effect, safer drugs production can now be enforced with minimum errors that can be detected and traced, if any. This is important to deliver quality healthcare and minimize unsafe drugs, especially in curbing the spread of COVID-19. Accordingly, several initiates are currently being developed to support this. Some of these projects track and verify pharmaceutical returns using blockchain technology that detects when a drug is touched and the person who did. This is expanding to other applications as in the year 2020, blockchain technology helped to combat the production of counterfeit COVID-19 drugs, while sophisticated tools like machine learning are employed to optimize this function in this present time [37,38]. This would require training deep learning models using the interpreted COVID-19 dataset within the network for data-transfer learning and data augmentation [39].

With the increase in the number of individuals vaccinated against COVID-19, blockchain technology is implemented to accurately manage medical information on the storage and transportation of several batches of vaccines. This is done using the IoT through sensors affixed to the storage containers and transport vessels of the vaccines. While helpful data are collected, transmitted, and stored on the blockchain, healthcare institutions, regulators, and distributors can instantly view this information to affirm the safety and effectiveness of how the vaccines were stored and transported. This has dramatically minimized the spread of COVID-19 and maximized clinical research and trials. These require the careful handling of a large amount of sensitive data from various sources. Blockchain functions to connect these disparate data from different clinical research facilities and then create a traceable record with an in-built safety mechanism and an audit framework

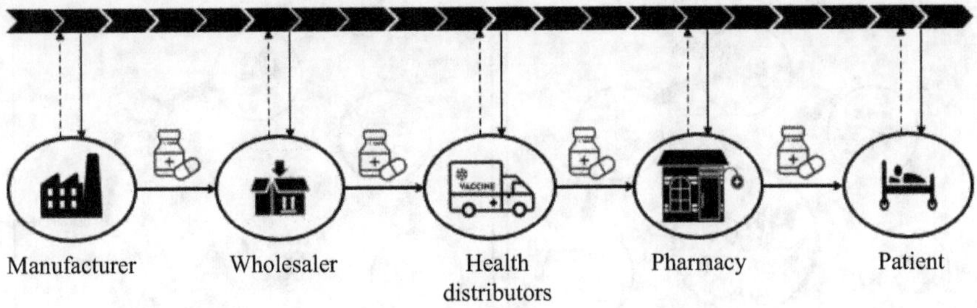

Figure 6.6 Blockchain technology healthcare supply-chain management system

accessible to regulatory bodies and healthcare services. The basic structure of how blockchain technology securely handles data through a supply-chain system is shown in Figure 6.6.

In order to carry out this function for data security, blockchain technology is developed to instantly alert authorized individuals when any attempt to alter data at any point of the chain is detected. In compliance with regulatory requirements, this has improved the authenticity, confidentiality, and trust in the data from healthcare systems currently managing the COVID-19 pandemic.

6.3 Potential benefits of blockchain technology in data handling

Blockchain technology provides healthcare data systems with adequate access control, data security, data integrity, auditing access, and data sharing [40,41]. It includes the security of sensitive data in a supply chain by leaving all added data to the blockchain unchanged once they are added. This has the potential to automate data exchange log instances and policies on data access for subjects and professionals in healthcare to access and verify at any time. Given that the COVID-19 pandemic has strained healthcare systems globally, and healthcare professionals are pressured to control the spread of the pandemic, relevant data access must be adaptable to changing healthcare conditions. In handling these data securely, blockchain technology may help integrate COVID-19 pandemic data generated from different health service providers and several healthcare intermediaries [42]. Such systems may also store patients' health histories, which can be useful to health service providers, pharmaceutical companies, and medical product consumers. In this case, blockchain technology may offer the advantage of establishing interoperability. The potential benefits of blockchain technology in healthcare can be summarized in Figure 6.7.

Healthcare systems use different approaches to prepare for unforeseen occurrences like the COVID-19 pandemic and medical emergencies in mitigation, recovery, and response. In critical situations, blockchain technology tools provide the benefits of cooperation and sound communication between critical elements of

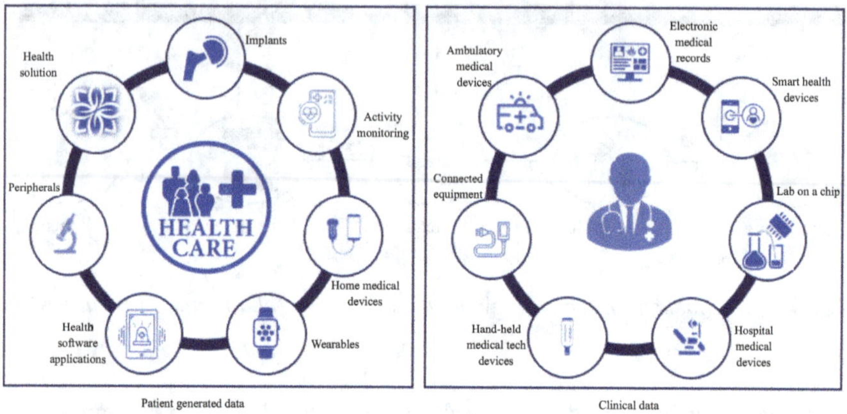

Figure 6.7 Potential benefits of blockchain technology in healthcare

healthcare provision like finance, logistics, health workers, back-end data input, and management for decision-making [43]. Generally, this improves data integrity, reduces medical costs, and decentralizes operations. Blockchain also can deliver precision that is essential to improve the care of patients and management of critical health situations. At the same time, records of medical information are connected across networks. Using the IoMT to track the different data nodes and update patient data, these benefits consolidate real-time monitoring of health and the measures adopted to inhibit the pandemic. Globally, blockchain technology adds benefits of high data accuracy and reliable data security when health systems are developed based on seamless data sharing [44,45]. Hence, blockchain technology can be used in any data-driven areas of healthcare, including health claims, supply chain, healthcare records, and supply chain. Top-rated potential benefits of blockchain technology in securely handling COVID-19 data may be seen in the following.

6.3.1 Better exchange of healthcare data records

In the exchange of health records, blockchain technology can potentially address interoperability challenges by securely distributing healthcare data [31]. A big challenge of achieving healthcare data interoperability is the inadequate capacity for healthcare data systems to share their healthcare data, especially during a pandemic like COVID-19. While this may vary from one health facility to another, clinical specialists or specific doctors at the forefront of combating COVID-19 need sensitive data that must be recent in most cases. However, health services often experience redundancy that delays the care delivery process. Nevertheless, blockchain technology helps to easily manage this easily by creating a seamless and secure access to healthcare data and treatment records [46].

6.3.2 Validating trust in medical research and supplies

Health facilities that have handled COVID-19 cases experience challenges in shifting health results and accessing reliable data. This makes it difficult for them to maintain and expand their capacity to provide adequate care for patients and control a critical situation like the COVID-19 pandemic. Blockchain technology has the potential to enable the secure transfer of valuable records of research outcomes and clinical trials, which minimizes the possibility of errors or interference in healthcare data records. This is possible because of the encryption associated with blockchain. In effect, previous clinical trial logs can be tracked by blockchain while avoiding redundant clinical trial outcomes or data that have been altered [31]. Given that this area of healthcare management is guided by manufacturing, distribution, and administration regulations, the government may provide the needed assistance for health facilities to meet the challenges of the COVID-19 pandemic.

The fight against COVID-19 has led to several clinical trials to develop a partial remedy for the virus. This is known to yield so much data that those may be challenging to track. These data may also be hidden, corrupted, forged, or erased by external influences and some researchers. In the consideration of this in handling COVID-19 pandemic data, blockchain technology has the potential to confirm any document transmitted through the network authentically. Blockchain may first maintain an inalterable record of data that can all be verified for approval [47]. In turn, the transparency and accuracy of these data build confidence in researchers, policy makers, and medical supply firms.

6.3.3 Validating correct billing management

Blockchain technology offers a high-integrity option for the tracking and refreshing of data at a given time. The correctness of billing can be validated by improving the auditability and security of billing while supporting seamless billing processes and efficiency and avoiding theft. An integration of blockchain technology to handle this kind of healthcare data has the potential of adequately detecting fraud and related activities [48]. It simplifies billing tasks and engages with sound network access to adapt to healthcare demands that are constantly changing, particularly in the COVID-19 pandemic. Apart from fraudulent activities, the complex yet a large amount of data from the pandemic and healthcare field, in general, may also generate financial mishaps. However, recent blockchain technology developed can improve billing using automated paying processing based on the data received.

6.3.4 Internet of Things (IoT) in healthcare

The use of blockchain technology in handling COVID-19 data provides the potential benefits of tracking emergency room occupancy, inventory, patients, availability of medical devices, and health progress. This is improved with the IoT that are the key elements that capture and transmit data to an authorized clinical destination. The pandemic has driven more visits to health institutions more than ever before, with more in-hospital stays and beds occupied. Hence, responding to health issues and tracking patients may be difficult for doctors around the world. IoT in blockchain technology can make these responsibilities easier by providing access to secure and relevant data when needed [49]. These benefits can also be extended to temperature control in the rooms occupied by patients and medical supply availability. Predictably, several technology firms are developing IoT-based blockchain technology systems that would support adequate healthcare in the present uncertain times of the COVID-19 pandemic.

As an advantage, these systems work in a distributed and decentralized way, maintaining data that cannot be altered and, therefore, not misleading. With a good setup of the IoMT, fraudulent activities could also be detected easily because blockchain allows one to efficiently track the source and prescription of drugs at any time within the network. Optimizing blockchain IoT technology with machine learning could enhance these benefits and make medical operations of controlling COVID-19 more efficient.

6.3.5 Optimized privacy and data security

For the effective management of COVID-19, collaboration and coordination must be established between health facilities, health specialists, and authorities in different regions [50]. This would be impossible with data security and integrity issues, which has been the case before now. Although sufficient data are constantly exchanged in managing a global pandemic, those are often not trusted due to the data system inconsistencies, giving rise to experiences of delayed interventions, inaccurate diagnosis, and healthcare errors. However, through private and public chains, blockchain technology presents the potential benefit of an authorized data access control and the control of cyberattack threats that limit data distribution while maintaining interoperability standards. For a strong security of data and improved privacy, the private blockchain encrypts sensitive medical information that is only accessible by authorized users.

Data privacy and security are also demanded in the flow of healthcare services overwhelmed with insurance, medical claims, and finances issues, which can expand to lose and fraud running into outrageous sums of money. This can be experienced because of the poor transparency of data that are incomplete or inadequately stored. Blockchain technology may recover lost funds, monitor care received by patients within and outside a health facility. With blockchain technology, medical events and clinical operations can be evaluated from the data of care that are provided from the blockchain across the network. Accordingly, systems that enhance data transparency are being developed to control the spread of the COVID-19 virus better.

6.4 Key challenges of blockchain technology in data handling

Implementing blockchain technology in healthcare applications like secure handling of the COVID-19 pandemic data comes with some limitations that prevent meeting the goals of managing the spread of COVID-19 in part or totally. Key challenges identified include security, speed, interoperability, stringent data protection regulations, scalability, and privacy [51].

6.4.1 *Security*

While blockchain technology provides data encryption, there are possibilities of revealing the identity of individuals or other sensitive data, mainly when separate medical information of an individual is linked within a network, and a public blockchain is adopted for healthcare data [52]. Some health facilities have also experienced attacks on their healthcare blockchain from fraudulent organizations, and this breaches the security of sensitive data leading to a compromise of privacy. This may also be due to a compromised data decryption and encryption function in the blockchain, which these organizations leverage by gaining unauthorized access to sensitive healthcare data stored. In most cases, this may not be detected early on if the blockchain is not maintained for optimized functions. This is a significant challenge as several reports of cyberattacks on blockchain networks control the data functions of cryptocurrencies [53].

6.4.2 *Speed*

In many cases, the performance of the blockchain technology system is compromised with a low processing speed. Although the blockchain may have great potential benefits for combating COVID-19, inadequate data-processing speed is considered a major challenge [54]. For health cases like the COVID-19 pandemic, more data should be processed at high streaming speeds in data collection and transmission to the appropriate destinations. This is because processing in blockchain technology may introduce some latency, particularly in cases where all network nodes participate in a data validation process during and after blockchain setup [53]. In addition to the data load, this results in a significant processing delay. The tradeoff in improving the speed may consider a few nodes in the data validation or consensus processes, which may not be sufficient to deliver an optimized data function of the size of data generated from the COVID-19 pandemic. While the public blockchain may require any node to participate in these data processes, the security and content of data transmitted may be inadequate to meet the need of managing the pandemic.

6.4.3 *Interoperability*

In order to manage the COVID-19 pandemic, it can be challenging to implement blockchain technology where there is no existing standard for developing secure handling of data. This makes interoperability a major challenge for developed applications that securely handle a large amount of data. There is a lack of interoperability between two blockchain systems, so the exchange of relevant data becomes difficult [54]. In most cases, it is impossible for one platform to synchronize with another. This results in loss of data, inaccurate data, or delay in obtaining data. In turn, this generates an inconsistent provision of healthcare and control of the pandemic, which is both critical end-products of handling the pandemic data securely.

6.4.4 *Stringent data protection regulation*

The General Data Protection Regulation (GDPR) supports the right of users to request a total erase of their data. This is against the operations of blockchain that leaves data unaltered once it has been saved. As a result, implementing blockchain technology to handle data securely can be challenging given the sensitivity of the COVID-19 data pandemic. Although, in some cases, this regulation may not be considered when other people have to make data privacy decisions for patients who are unable to do so, historic data for medical record purposes may be altered when data protection regulations are effected. Nevertheless, this would be counter-productive when erasing a medical history is desired by patients or their representatives. In turn, it would be difficult to control the spread of COVID-19 and develop future preventive measures with accurate data.

6.4.5 Scalability

This is another major challenge when implementing blockchain technology in secure data handling. The scalability of blockchain technology data systems is the capacity to handle the changing demands of handling data resources. While scalability requires specialized techniques to deliver as it should, it is a significant challenge in healthcare solutions because of the high volume of data handled in the COVID-19 pandemic. Generally, the blockchain was built with the capacity to store a too high volume of medical data than it can take, leading to severe performance degradation [6]. Given the conditions of the COVID-19 pandemic, the traffic on the blockchain would become bulky with an increasing number of transactions daily. As each node stores all validated data transactions, a restriction would be experienced on the size of the block and the time taken to create a block [54]. In turn, there would be a delay in validation and data processing since the management of the pandemic is accompanied by a high data load [55]. Hence, the challenge of scalability also affects the speed of transactions on the network.

6.4.6 Privacy

As key data balances and details are validated by authorized network users, blockchain technology may have privacy leakages. Although blockchain technology has the potentials to offer patients and clinical specialists better control over the healthcare data of individuals, which translates to better management of the COVID-19 pandemic, it is not originally designed for this function, so at an initial stage, sensitive data can be stored on a distributed log that is accessible to any user on the network. This limits the privacy function of blockchain technology, especially with a weak network. Hence, the privacy function of blockchain technology can be supported when the blockchain network is developed to have nodes that process data without revealing any of it. This may be a good measure to handle this challenge, but more resources would be demanded optimum function. Nevertheless, systems that provide this optimization service to blockchain technology have been developed with newer systems underway. However, they offer no guarantee of perfection with the optimized networks.

While implementing blockchain technology in healthcare applications persist, some solutions have been developed to manage them. In order to prevent fraud or unauthorized access to data in the blockchain, a mixing solution system is proposed. It transfers a given fund to an output address from multiple input addresses to maintain data anonymity in the network. To improve scalability, encrypted healthcare data can be stored outside the blockchain, where condensed medical information from the dataset and an access guide are both stored on a blockchain at a given time [56,57]. This also provides a solution to the stringent data protection regulations as the stored data can be deleted while leaving data pointers on the blockchain. The tradeoff in this is the partially lost redundancy that may enhance data availability in the blockchain. From a legal perspective on data handling, the concerns that arise in the COVID-19 pandemic are storing, sharing, and accessing data from the distributed database of a blockchain network [54]. This is owing to the data laws and policies that invariably limit the function of blockchain technology. The solution to this would be to revise these policies by international health organizations, policy makers, and country leaders, which may have to introduce new health policy regulations on digital health, digital connectivity, data sharing, and the digital divide.

The security of healthcare data and privacy protection issues can be resolved using a permission consortium blockchain for digital healthcare applications like the secure handling of COVID-19 data. Most of the threats to security may also be contained by applying known security measures to develop software and codes to optimize blockchain technology functions. This also helps to reverse traces of fraudulent transactions. Smart contracts of the blockchain technology can also help to define and program rules that may help to control the behavior of the blockchain in the data handling of COVID-19 patients.

6.5 Prospects of blockchain technology

Blockchain technology can assist in modifying the current healthcare data–handling systems to combat the COVID-19 pandemic in more productive ways. The current systems have adopted efficient measures to manage the global condition, which is evident in the rollout of vaccines that would help to manage the effects of the virus in infected individuals [58]. However, these potential improvements of blockchain technology are expected to yield better results that would be evident in a progressive decrease to the number of COVID-19 cases, which would also inhibit the spread of the virus to a minimum than ever before. The major areas of improvement are summarized in Table 6.1.

These prospective areas of improvements by blockchain technology are already being explored, and several ideas have been developed to support the efficient control of the COVID-19 pandemic. Noteworthy is the role of elements in a blockchain-based medical information management system, which are important to convey certain functions in implementing blockchain technology. These blockchain elements include storage memory, cloud storage, distribution ledger, and hardware. All these have their functions in the overall impact of blockchain technology in healthcare. A displacement of any element in the data-handling frame can potentially compromise the blockchain technology operation. A summary of how

Table 6.1 Prospects of blockchain technology in data handling

S. no.	Blockchain technology prospects	Improvements to the healthcare data handling system
1.	Protection of digital healthcare data systems	Digital healthcare systems are susceptive to cyberattacks globally, leading to a compromise of sensitive medical information [59]. This mostly occurs in a compromised network connection. When concerns on security and privacy are addressed, digital healthcare data systems will improve. Blockchain technology can help provide the highest standards of privacy protection, trust, security, and optimization in these systems, leading to better protection and privacy of data. Further to this, an exchange of data can be optimally established without an intermediary, enabling the storage of all patients' healthcare history and treatment records securely accessible, decentralized, and traceable. However, where there are limited resources, the cost of implementation may be increased
2.	Healthcare invoicing	Fraudulent activities are common in the healthcare billing system [60]. More so, the financial transaction processes are time-consuming and require more resources. While measures like complex codes programming help structure healthcare billing systems, they may also come with delayed inaccurate, duplicate, or unintentional billings [10]. Integrating program codes in blockchain technology systems can optimize healthcare billing. It could help make the billing and payment process more secure and easier than the conventional billing systems in most healthcare facilities. For example, a delay in paying the bills of insurance claims is often experienced. An implementation of an automated blockchain technology system can speed up invoicing and payment processes of insurance claims by storing data in a manner that cannot be altered. This decreases the excess resources, saves time, and helps insurance providers make payments faster
3.	Drug traceability	There have been cases of detected counterfeit drugs entering the market in the supply-chain cycle for the distribution of drugs for healthcare purposes [61]. From the manufacturing to the distribution phase, the supply of fake drugs has become a business for many years and is estimated at several billions of dollars globally [62]. As a result of this, it can be deduced that the pharmaceutical industry is weakly protected. Blockchain technology can help track the manufacturing of these drug chains since blockchain stored data transactions cannot be altered. According to business needs, blockchain technology offers pharmaceutical companies the option of employing private

(Continues)

Table 6.1 (*Continued*)

S. no.	Blockchain technology prospects	Improvements to the healthcare data handling system
		or public blockchain systems that can help them obtain a complete clinical trial of a drug. When the drug is touched or moved, this information is stored as unalterable data on the blockchain database. These can significantly improve drug traceability and minimize the risk of supplying and distributing fake drugs
4.	Healthcare data management	COVID-19 healthcare and the management of the pandemic require access to a patient's full medical records to provide patient-centered care that would be different from another patient. Handling these data can be challenging because healthcare data systems are not equipped with the needed privacy, security, and trust that the sensitivity of the data demands [63]. In most cases, this data may also be altered or deleted, thereby incurring an extra cost when patients need to move from one health facility to another since there may be no records of tests and medications from past healthcare provided. Blockchain technology has the potential to overcome this challenge, owing to its decentralized peer-to-peer network structure, which can only be accessed using smart platforms [64]. In addition, the record of healthcare provided is stored on several blockchain nodes within the network. This way, data transfer can be done from one health facility to another securely and transparently. Blockchain technology can also help to reduce cost since patients would not have to repeat some clinical tests or diagnostics that have been done earlier
5.	Precision medicine	Precision in medicine and the outcome of clinical trials is an essential part of healthcare monitoring and provision. The process of clinical research and trials can be optimized with blockchain technology by potentially addressing incorrect clinical trial data and supporting data integrity [65]. Often, inaccurate clinical trial outcomes lead to inefficient interventions, and for a case like the COVID-19 pandemic, this should be encountered. With a programmed blockchain technology system, more transparency can be provided to improve analytic data accuracy. Other areas of precision medicine that can be potentially improved with blockchain technology are clinical supply audit, reducing clinical trial time, recruiting patients, and tracking prescriptions. It may also be used to control genomic sequences [66], which may be used to treat different genetic disorder-induced illnesses and infections. Blockchain technology can capture the genetic data of an individual that would help generate more

(Continues)

Table 6.1 (Continued)

S. no.	Blockchain technology prospects	Improvements to the healthcare data handling system
		accurate results. More so, the interoperability function in most blockchain technology systems ensures that individuals can control their own data while it is being shared between health organizations. With this, there would be no need for a central database managed by an intermediary but susceptible to cyberattack
6.	Data access permission	Permission to access the medical data of a patient may be required in emergencies. When this is inconsistent, human life may be in danger due to the limited access to relevant medical information that can assist medical professionals in providing the needed healthcare. For secure and seamless data access permission, blockchain technology has the potential to create a contract consisting of set rules that grant access to data through smart platforms. These contracts could be designed to include an automated schedule of different workflows and conditions for specific cases, like when two medical specialists need access to private data at the same time for the provision of specialized healthcare. Access control can be managed by the patients themselves using cryptographic master keys, which are entered to unlock healthcare data within a preferred length of time [10]. With this, a patient can share any data with healthcare facilities or clinical specialists as needed. In emergency cases where a patient is indisposed to grant access, blockchain technology systems can be programmed as robots for certain functions, which may assist in saving the life of a patient. Thus, access privileges of reading and writing can be added to the blockchain. All these prospects can help minimize human-imposed errors and save time needed to collect patient data

blockchain is used to access and transfer data stored and processed by blockchain elements in a typical healthcare scenario is shown in Figure 6.8.

6.6 Research on blockchain technology in COVID-19 healthcare

The ongoing research on blockchain technology in COVID-19 healthcare has revealed innovations that support a better quality of healthcare and inhibit the spread of the pandemic. Identified areas of these researches include pharmaceuticals, healthcare data processing, billing, cyber security, and healthcare data system optimization. Some of these studies have already tested and implemented outcomes in

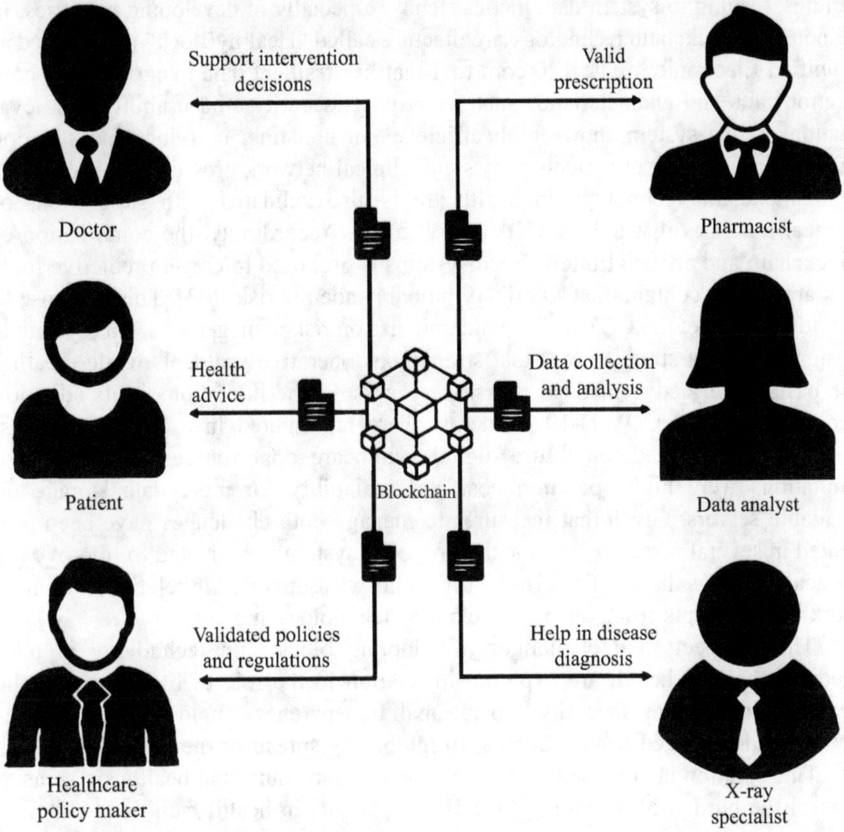

Figure 6.8 Blockchain technology-enabled healthcare data management

real-time health applications, while others may be undergoing revision. In relation to the prevalent COVID-19 pandemic, health research outputs help provide evidence-based healthcare, treatment plan, and health prevention options [67]. They also guide doctors and other clinical specialists on the best treatment options for their patients. New healthcare tools, the development of medicine, the adoption of new care procedures, effective interventions, and preventive disease strategies are all possible due to constant clinical research outputs [68]. In turn, healthcare becomes more efficient, personalized, and convenient. A few recent research works on blockchain technology in healthcare applications is highlighted as follows:

The blockchain-network Electronic Medical Record system is created as a proposed solution for the security, privacy, and fragmentation of medical information from different databases, limiting effective treatment and disease prevention that arise from issues like data leaks, data loss, or misinformation [27]. This system was developed to prevent the direct risk that these issues pose on individuals and to reduce public health costs. The proposed system may be vulnerable to connectivity failures, leading to system data inconsistency, especially in developing countries. In response, a blockchain technology architecture called "HealthyBlock" is presented as a unified Electronic Medical Record tool that has resilient data integrity when connection fails and characteristics such as privacy, security, and usability. The evaluation of this system shows high efficiency in updating, unifying, and securing medical information of patients across any clinical network provided connected.

Blockchain technology in healthcare is also validated with suggestions of clinical practices that uphold COVID-19 safety. Accordingly, the combination of blockchain and artificial intelligence systems is proposed to create predictive tools that are able to contain the COVID-19 global pandemic risks [43]. This response to the adverse effect the COVID-19 pandemic has on risk management. This system is designed to be a strategic tool that strengthens operative protocols while creating the basis for effective medical decision processes. The limitations in its adoption for managing the COVID-19 pandemic were highlighted in a SWOT analysis, which also presented top future digital healthcare opportunities. Two of these limitations were high operation cost and scalability for more data storage on available servers. Given that measures to manage both challenges have been presented in several research outputs, the proposed system is evaluated to improve the clinical practices that are COVID-19 safe. This was supported in relation to clinical workflow concepts from various blockchain technology models.

The prospects and challenges of adopting blockchain technology in telemedicine and telehealth are explored in relation to the role of blockchain in the provision of privacy, security, operational transparency, fraud detecting traceability, and unaltered health records, to inhibit the spread of the COVID-19 virus [9]. This solution is proposed to manage the scarce resources in healthcare so as to control the burden of managing COVID-19 patients in health facilities. Although there are concerns about issues related to patients' insurance claims and the verification of credentials, the evaluations of the proposed solution reveal that integrating blockchain technology improves telehealth care services by providing remote, decentralized, reliable, and trustful health services. The further assessment shows good security and accuracy in detecting faults in medical test kits for diagnosis outside health facilities. As a future development area, the global adoption of blockchain technology in healthcare was encouraged if the challenges identified in the implementation process are resolved.

Another solution is modeled for sharing, analyzing, and organizing COVID-19 data with interoperability and privacy-preserving methods. This is aimed at improving the time, cost-effectiveness, and outreach for treatment and disease-control interventions. Accordingly, a blockchain system is proposed as a promising technology to drive effective disease control and monitoring [4]. For a disease like the COVID-19 virus, a health surveillance system is required for regular diagnosis, control, and treatment interventions. This solution was presented because of the blockchain features such as data immutability, decentralization, cryptography, and data provenance. In effect, a literature bibliometric analysis of integrating blockchain technology in the data management system of a disease like the COVID-19 virus was performed. The suitability of many existing blockchain platforms was also evaluated in relation to disease data storage, processing, and sharing. Also addressed were optimization models on the blockchain application, like the design of machine learning models that preserve data privacy better, which can also support collaborative learning. Overall, a disease data-handling system that integrates machine learning models on blockchain was recommended [4].

Other studies identified new characteristics of blockchain that are of great benefit to healthcare systems, including healthcare industry collaboration, health business models, optimized auditability, disintermediation, and continuity [18]. Results from statistical models identify blockchain technology as a platform also created to provide reliable recording, where initially fragmented medical information records would be combined to easily track the health records of an individual [69,70]. The difficulty of building a tracking capable foundation of high integrity has led to an inconsistency in accessing healthcare records. Further to this, history-based diagnoses are costly because of the complexity of medical information records, privacy issues of the network, and fragmentation. Blockchain technology offers a system to address all these through the continuous track of services, which it provides [18]. The combination of blockchain and artificial intelligence can also offer a solution for these healthcare data problems while also supporting the seamless access and storage of data on the blockage. However, these ideas can be implemented when regulatory barriers from data privacy policies are addressed or revised to deliver healthcare or mitigate COVID-19 spread.

While many more research outputs have been presented, it is worthy of considering collaboration in healthcare to drive the development of brilliant ideas and effect the needed change. In managing the COVID-19 pandemic by exploring secure data handling, this is highly critical considering that a large amount of medical data are shared among healthcare facilities and clinical experts expeditiously across several miles globally.

6.7 Real-time analysis of COVID-19 pandemic data

The global situation of COVID-19 pandemic cases is explored in statistical terms to give a broader perspective of integrating blockchain technology to the secure handling of data. Across the globe, there have been a rise and fall in the number of infected individuals recorded. Therefore, a regular analysis of COVID-19 patient data is critical for understanding clinical progress, measuring how effective the strategies for mitigating the spread are, potential effects of treatments, and expected outcomes [71]. Accordingly, adequate statistical models are necessary to affirm data in health facilities at a given time. In-line with this, real-time clinical examples are used to evaluate standard statistical models and their mathematical framework regarding real-time COVID-19 pandemic data.

6.7.1 The susceptible recovered infectious (SIR) model

This is a simple model used for the analysis of COVID-19 pandemic data, where the population is divided into three parts: the susceptible but not infected, the infected, and the recovered (or deceased) [72]. Several research outputs have been generated by modeling the outbreak using the basic susceptible recovery infectious (SIR) model. Examples include the estimation and simulations of all the symptomatic cases of the COVID-19 virus in Wuhan [73]; the identification of contagion, death rates, and recovery of COVID-19-infected individuals in Italy [74]; the combination of a basic SIR model with probabilistic methods for the estimation of the number of infected people in France [75]; and the use of the SIR model with a parameter to maintain social distancing measures, in order to forecast the outbreak stages of COVID-19 in Brazil [76]. The SIR model is more appropriate for a localized epidemic outbreak because mostly it only examines temporal dynamics. Hence, it can be most effective for analysis at a country, city, or state level.

Noteworthy is that the SIR model simplifies COVID-19 data analysis. Inferentially, the model also assumes that recovered individuals who were infected can be immune to COVID-19. While unconfirmed reports support this, the model can capture relevant data that can be viewed to make healthcare decisions in the control of the COVID-19 pandemic.

6.7.2 Standard logistic regression model

This tool examines the available healthcare data of COVID-19 patients. It aligns risk factors with certain events like the point of entry, exposure to another infected person, and the presence of an underlying health condition. The major limitation of the model is the unavailability of sufficient data or data exclusions that are unaccounted for [71]. As a result of the high likelihood of selection bias created by these limitations, COVID-19 risk estimates may be inaccurate. Hence, the standard logistic regression model may not be suitable for examining the connection between the medical predictors of a patient and COVID-19-related health events concerning that patient. If logistic regression must be used in this case, some patients or some of their healthcare data may be excluded. This may omit the effects of certain predictors, which would not present a holistic picture of the situation of the COVID-19 virus in a certain place.

However, the standard logistic regression model is most suitable in predictive situations to determine one outcome or another [77]. This implies that there can often always be two possible outcomes. In managing the COVID-19 pandemic, this may still be useful for clinical trials that generate the presence of the disease or not.

6.7.3 Time-to-event analytics model

This is an alternative to the standard logistic regression model, where the outcome includes the time of the event occurrence along with details on whether an event occurred or not. In addition, the time-to-event analysis considers censoring data that is captured when a patient does not experience effects of the virus at follow-up times. This analytics model was designed to address time of origin, advance technique assumptions, and healthcare predictors. Accordingly, estimation techniques for time-to-event data are developed to use the available medical information on censored patient data for unbiased survival estimates. From multiple points across the COVID-19 healthcare for a patient, the techniques can incorporate data to estimate time ratios, infection rates, and hazard ratios [78].

The models discussed earlier have been used to analyze several COVID-19 data for targeted interventions to mitigate the spread globally. Recent real-time COVID-19 data from a few European countries are presented and analyzed as a sample to make health-related and COVID-19 safety decisions.

6.7.4 Results of major real-time analysis

Figure 6.9 is the generated chart from Table 6.2, which highlights the data of recorded COVID-19 cases in several European countries since its global inception in March 2021. Figure 6.9 is highly instrumental to clinical experts and policy makers as the number of cases indicates the rate of spread, what regions or areas are most vulnerable, and how effective curbing strategies are. These all influence their decisions about where to invest more resources and what change needs to be made toward the management of COVID-19. In Table 6.2, the most valuable data are the absolute change that guides interventions at a given time while considering details such as the identification of the virus, the number of an infected individual that has recovered, and the death figures [74]. Hence, the SIR model can be used for its analysis. First, experts divide the population of a certain area of the region into groups of those susceptible to getting infected, those already infected, and those who have recovered or are deceased. Thereafter, data are drawn at each month and analyzed in relation to data from the previous month. This identifies what is working, what is not working, and issues that need to be addressed to curb the spread of the virus. Given the sensitivity of these data, blockchain technology may be implemented to extract, store, securely transmit and access them [55].

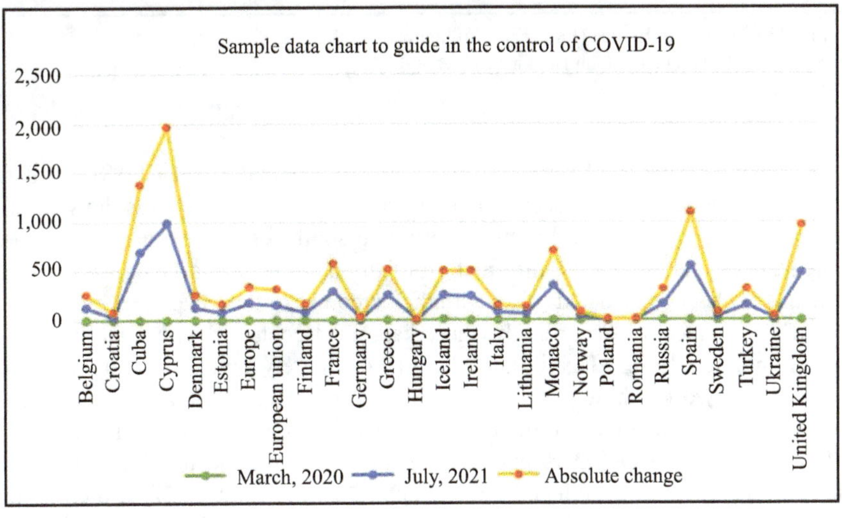

Figure 6.9 COVID-19 pandemic data (March 2020 to July 2021)

Table 6.2 Data on COVID-19 cases in European countries from March 2020 to July 2021

Country	March 2020	July 2021	Absolute change	Relative change (%)
Belgium	0.01	127.64	127.63	1 063 558
Croatia	0.24	37.65	37.41	15 331
Cuba	0.06	688.72	688.66	10 931 105
Cyprus	4.18	983.42	979.24	23 410
Denmark	0.15	126.62	126.48	85 456
Estonia	0.21	81.2	80.98	37 667
Europe	0.39	172.46	172.07	44 120
European Union	0.62	156.32	155.7	25 195
Finland	0.13	76.36	79.23	61 420
France	0.25	288.81	288.56	115 887
Germany	0.19	19.87	19.68	10 144
Greece	0.1	225.92	255.82	266 479
Hungary	0.13	5.9	5.77	4 336
Iceland	10.88	249.5	238.62	2 192
Ireland	0.17	251.56	251.38	144 474
Italy	3.64	75.52	71.89	1 977
Lithuania	0.05	71.89	71.84	138 156
Monaco	3.64	353.1	349.46	9 601
Norway	0.66	41.9	41.24	6 258
Poland	0.06	2.77	2.71	4 512
Romania	0.02	5.78	5.75	26 159
Russia	0	159.03	159.03	–
Spain	0.25	547.89	547.64	218 185
Sweden	0.18	40.67	40.48	22 002
Turkey	0.03	155.85	1 555.82	519 413
Ukraine	<0.01	25.78	25.77	859 100
United Kingdom	0.04	482.1	481.96	346 737

New confirmed cases in Europe (for every 1 million people).
Source: CCSE COVID data, John Hopkins University.

Figures 6.10 and 6.11 represent the results of the analysis of COVID-19 data recorded in Table 6.3. This accumulated data from 2020 to 2021 was drawn from the central, eastern, northern, northwestern, and southwestern regions of Virginia, United States and covers the information of the number of individuals who have been and not been vaccinated along with the outcomes of their experiences with the COVID-19 pandemic. Accordingly, these data must contain the personal information of individuals in Virginia and should be securely and effectively handled across the network. These data are valuable to pharmaceuticals and useful in the several clinical trials involved in developing vaccines that are in global circulation to fight against the COVID-19 pandemic. Although when infected, living with the COVID-19 virus and experiencing its symptoms is unavoidable since there is no proven cure [79], the measure of vaccine effectiveness is evident in the reduced number of COVID-19 cases, hospitalization, and death rates altogether. Hence, the

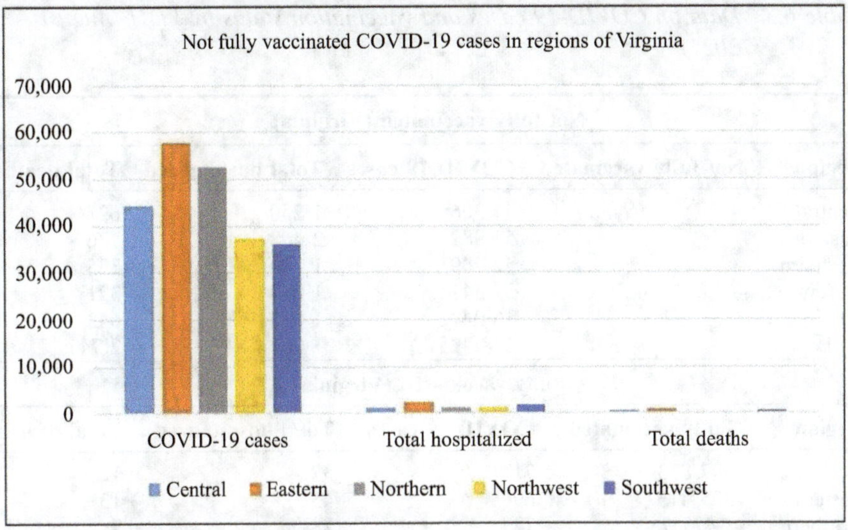

Figure 6.10 *COVID-19 cases and vaccination status in Virginia—not fully vaccinated*

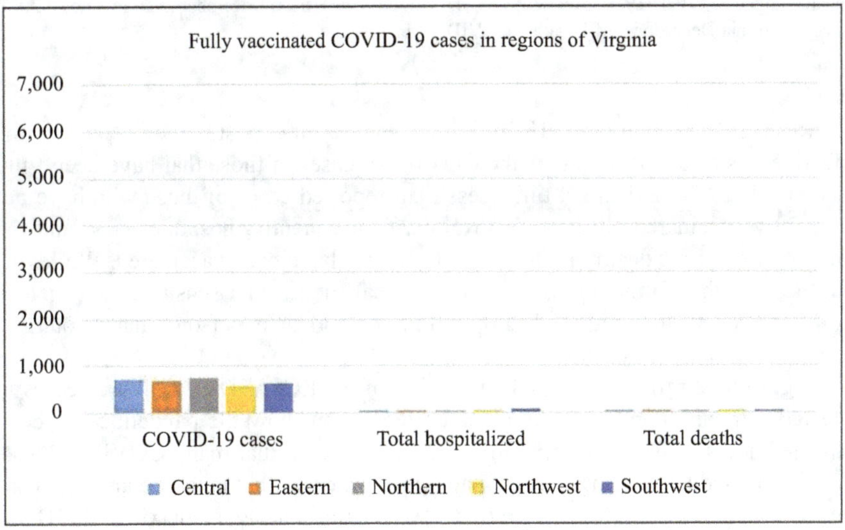

Figure 6.11 *COVID-19 cases and vaccination status in Virginia—fully vaccinated*

data in Table 6.3 can be analyzed using the time-to-event analysis, which captures the effects of the virus experienced by individuals while using estimation techniques to incorporate data time ratio, spread rates, and hazard ratios [78]. With this model, clinicians and healthcare researchers can interpret outcomes appropriately to influence the management of the pandemic.

Table 6.3 Data on COVID-19 cases and vaccination status by VDH (August 2021)

Not fully vaccinated (Virginia)				
Region	**Not fully vaccinated**	**COVID-19 cases**	**Total hospitalized**	**Total deaths**
Central	–	44 306	1 250	622
Eastern	–	57 982	2 468	776
Northern	–	52 749	1 280	335
Northwest	–	37 341	1 088	371
Southwest	–	36 047	1 865	643
ALL	–	228 425	7 951	2 747
Fully vaccinated (Virginia)				
Region	**Fully vaccinated**	**COVID-19 cases**	**Total hospitalized**	**Total deaths**
Central	697 833	713	37	12
Eastern	805 413	699	45	13
Northern	1 427 757	747	28	7
Northwest	632 690	571	33	4
Southwest	543 183	629	75	14
ALL	4 642 482	3 359	218	50

Updated data on COVID-19 cases in Virginia, the United States, from December 2020 to August 2021.
Source: Virginia Department of Health—COVID-19 in Virginia.

Results from Figures 6.10 and 6.11 show some positive evidence in the effectiveness of the vaccines, as the COVID-19 cases of those that have been fully vaccinated are more than six times less than reported cases of those who have not been fully vaccinated all through Virginia. Consequently, hospitalization and the amount of recorded deaths are lower in those who have been vaccinated. While this may be enough information to influence clinical trials, other sensitive data such as the history of an individual's health conditions and their personal data would be needed for other control modalities.

Figure 6.12 reflects the updated records of total COVID-19 tests and cases in selected African countries. This gives an idea about how the pandemic has been managed across Africa. From Figure 6.12, it is evident that many COVID-19 tests have been conducted across Africa, and while the cases that emerged are a lot less, the test numbers are a good move toward the management of COVID-19. Figure 6.13 also reflects data of the number of individuals who have recovered and died of the disease. Results generated from Table 6.4 show that the critical cases from COVID-19 complication may lead to death. While extensive research on the different variants of COVID-19 is ongoing [80], these data may help clinical experts consider preventive measures or adopt interventions to manage the disease better for the purpose of reducing the number of reported COVID-19 cases. Hence, risk factors and underlying health conditions that increase the susceptibility of an individual getting infected are important medical information. To analyze these

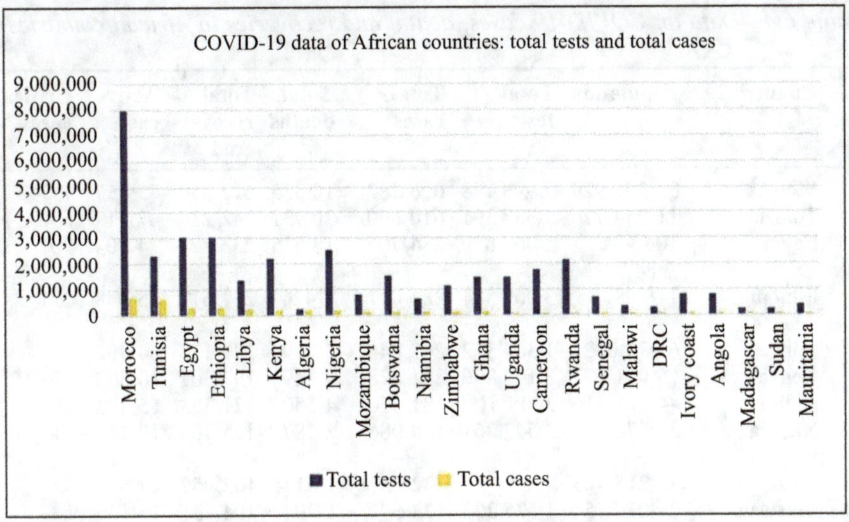

Figure 6.12 COVID-19 data of African countries showing total tests and cases

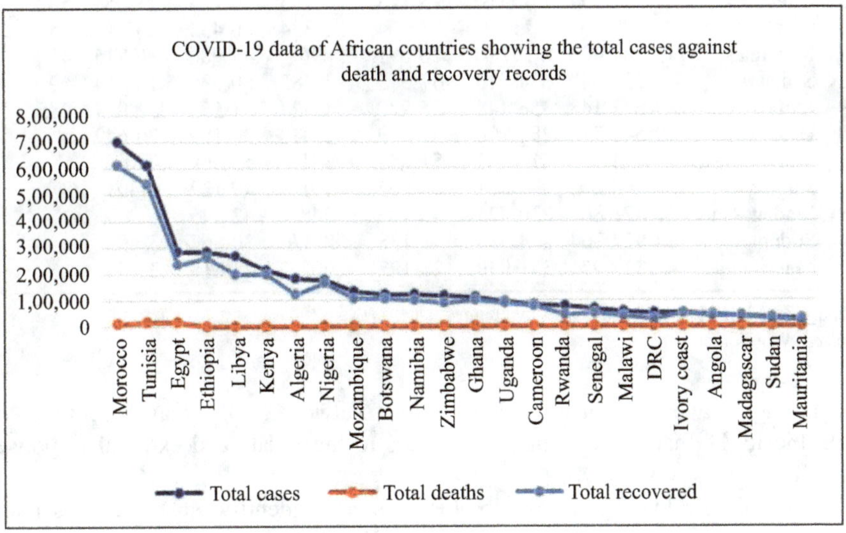

Figure 6.13 COVID-19 cases and effects in African countries showing the total cases vs. death and recovery records (August 2021)

data from Table 6.4, the standard logistic regression model is most suitable, given that predictive analysis for possible future outcomes is often implemented on these data. Given that this medical information is shared among health experts managing a COVID-19 patient, it should be handled securely. Blockchain technology provides a distributed data handling that addresses this. For a robust blockchain

Table 6.4 Data on COVID-19 cases, death, and recoveries in African countries

S. no.	Country	Population	Total tests	Total cases	Total deaths	Total recov-ered	Active cases	Critical cases
1	Morocco	37 391 929	7 998 148	696 282	10 335	612 390	73 557	1 042
2	Tunisia	11 954 726	2 337 391	610 660	20 931	542 210	47 519	630
3	Egypt	104 454 842	3 068 679	284 706	16 575	233 227	34 904	90
4	Ethiopia	118 087 799	3 069 384	284 091	4 426	264 617	15 048	291
5	Libya	6 974 062	1 364 372	267 846	3 719	199 135	64 992	–
6	Kenya	55 071 577	2 190 806	211 828	4 149	197 307	10 372	133
8	Algeria	44 721 116	230 861	181 376	4 550	121 353	55 473	48
9	Nigeria	211 744 938	2 542 261	178 086	2 187	165 763	10 136	11
10	Mozambique	32 215 423	776 609	132 452	1 613	102 957	27 882	32
11	Botswana	2 403 775	1 525 222	122 574	1 704	104 731	16 139	1
12	Namibia	2 591 466	625 854	121 043	3 191	99 191	18 661	76
13	Zimbabwe	15 100 848	1 149 029	116 327	1 900	88 829	23 598	12
14	Ghana	31 785 183	1 459 845	108 226	874	100 383	6 969	36
15	Uganda	47 323 337	1 499 619	95 723	2 793	90 225	2 705	542
16	Cameroon	27 270 802	1 751 774	82 064	1 334	80 433	297	152
17	Rwanda	13 304 466	2 157 915	76 091	890	44 986	30 215	41
18	Senegal	17 227 840	674 910	67 579	1 482	50 533	15 564	69
19	Malawi	19 672 148	356 144	55 920	1 828	41 155	12 937	285
20	DRC	92 544 772	282 990	51 889	1 048	30 189	20 652	–
21	Ivory Coast	27 094 912	813 541	51 380	341	50 069	970	–
22	Angola	33 986 273	821 071	43 662	1 049	40 122	2 491	8
23	Madagascar	28 471 860	230 721	42 776	948	42 445	–	27
24	Sudan	44 972 864	234 414	37 138	2 776	30 867	3 495	–
25	Mauritania	4 783 697	391 940	28 197	605	23 818	3 774	16

Reported COVID-19 cases and deaths by country.
Source: Worldometer.

technology network, a software development network (SDN) may be combined with the IoMT that reduces unsecure access to these data and external response time [81].

The SDN technology also helps health experts identify what countries may require the investment of more resources, as Figure 6.13 highlights the most vulnerable countries. These are countries with the highest number of reported COVID-19 cases and have recorded the highest number of COVID-related deaths.

6.8 Recommendations and future directions

A discussion of how blockchain technology can be applied to real-time healthcare data-handling practices is presented as a recommendation and direction for future practice, to manage COVID-19 and inhibit the spread. These are drawn from the analysis of COVID-19 data illustrated in the previous section and the limitations of blockchain technology to be addressed.

First, blockchain technology protects the privacy of patients and authorized users while preserving data consent and automated provenance in areas such as healthcare, wherewith strong security, medical information can be shared between doctors and health facilities; IoMT, where privacy is maintained for the preference of any IoMT device; and data storage, where there are data protection and data access control across the network. In-line with this, more blockchain technology application systems should be built and optimized for better healthcare support that reduces COVID-19 cases to the lowest minimum and improves other sectors. It has been established that the potential benefits of blockchain transcend the healthcare sector to practically all sectors that operate with data and things across a network. Therefore beyond the COVID-19 pandemic, blockchain technology should be adopted for better cyber security, data privacy, and communication.

However, limitations such as data policy and regulations, interoperability, scalability, and response time are acknowledged as the major challenges to be addressed. For stringent data policies and regulations, extensive research and healthcare influence may introduce operational standards of blockchain technology for handling sensitive data like that of the COVID-19 pandemic. Perhaps, only permissioned blockchain should be adopted for the handling of COVID-19 pandemic data to avoid cyberattacks and unauthorized data sharing. Alternatively, the medical information of patients can be protected by blockchain encryption that should be updated or maintained regularly. The interoperability still experienced in some blockchain systems prevents optimal operational communication between two frameworks, while the synchronization of blockchain with healthcare facilities persists, particularly in developing countries. This can be addressed with the introduction of a few subchains that would reduce the pressure on the blockchain network and allows smaller and quicker transactions on the blockchain. The processing speed and efficiency of the system can also be improved with interoperability when fewer nodes are involved in the validation process. However, other optimization tools should be in place to control the tradeoff.

Scalability also limits the operation of blockchain on the network as it affects the processing speed and the validation of transactions. It has been established that larger networks are more costly to run nodes and take more response time. To address this, using smaller blocks can help to provide a better scale without compromising the response time or increasing the processing cost. Smaller blocks are also compatible with cloud solutions, thereby also providing better interoperability. Future research direction may be in the design of blocks that provide optimal scale and interaction within the network.

Existing healthcare applications also experience some security concerns following the detection of several data leaks and attacks on blockchain applications across networks. This is critical because valuable data runs blockchain technology systems. So compromised data defeat one of the main purposes of adopting blockchain technology to handle data as sensitive as that of the COVID-19 pandemic. The integration of machine learning and other system security optimization programs in the blocks are likely to better secure data on the network.

Given that blockchain technology systems can solve most real-world problems, future research areas may focus on optimization strategies in areas of privacy, security, data access, and block size. Furthermore, extensive research on blockchain technology implementation to improve data handling may be considered since there are currently only a few ongoing developments of working prototypes that go through a series of clinical trials and system testing to manage blockchain limitations. The integration of blockchain technology in big data–processing functions is also yet to be explored. Therefore, working models for the best data management implementation practices are needed. This can play a vital role in future healthcare, communication, IoMT, and identity management systems. However, the acceptance of these new models would need new data regulations that support blockchain technologies operations. Nevertheless, blockchain technology systems must comply with the GDPR in their existing and impending solutions.

6.9 Conclusion and future scopes

Blockchain technology is evolving to revolutionize data handling within and outside of healthcare. As seen, it can be directly applied in several applications where an unalterable record of data is useful. To evaluate blockchain application in COVID-19 data handling, recent developments, potential benefits, key challenges, prospects, and the data-handling application of blockchain have been highlighted in this chapter. Practical solutions for the limitations of implementing blockchain and productive research focus were also identified. Overall, integrating optimization programs in the blockchain to help expand its privacy, security, authenticating, interoperability and scalability functions were recommended. For implementations in other sectors where seamless data management is vital, operational standards for handling data effectively may be introduced for blockchain implementation. Although some working prototypes to improve, the functions of blockchain technology have been developed, while others like permissible blockchain, off-chain storage, and smart contracts have been tested in many real-world applications. Nevertheless, more research is needed for optimization and evaluation of blockchain implementation and supporting ongoing efforts. This is aimed at addressing issues with blockchain technology use such as interoperability, response delay, security, scalability, and privacy.

For healthcare data handling, as in the case of the COVID-19 global pandemic, blockchain technology is increasingly implemented to create a reasonable basis for an effective evidence-based treatment or intervention process. Existing research has shown that a blockchain is an effective tool for safe data storage and sharing between authorized users. It can also be used to improve the protocols of risk management. It can then be concluded that blockchain technology is highly instrumental in the clinical practice of controlling COVID-19. However, a few issues that have been experienced in the pandemic are data manipulation, miscommunication, delayed response time, and failure at single points. This study has also shown that blockchain can be used for other healthcare functions like pharmaceutical supply-chain management, counterfeit drug detection, remote health monitoring, and biomedical research. Therefore, it is important to regularly update or maintain these systems for optimal functions in controlling the COVID-19 and tracking other infectious diseases. As evidence, key elements of the blockchain, like already existing smart contracts, may be expanded to enable easy interaction between users and the blockchain, while blockchain applications may be extended to accommodate a larger amount of data.

Acknowledgments

The work of Agbotiname Lucky Imoize is supported by the Nigerian Petroleum Technology Development Fund (PTDF) and the German Academic Exchange Service (DAAD) through the Nigerian-German Post-graduate Program under grant 57473408.

References

[1] A. Azim, M. N. Islam, and P. E. Spranger, "Blockchain and novel coronavirus: Towards preventing COVID-19 and future pandemics," *Iberoam. J. Med.*, vol. 03, pp. 215–218, 2020, [Online]. Available: http://creativecommons.org/licenses/by/4.0/.

[2] N. T. Lee, J. Karsten, and J. Roberts, "Removing regulatory barriers to telehealth before and after COVID-19," *Brookings Inst.*, pp. 1–24, 2020, [Online]. Available: https://www.brookings.edu/wp-content/uploads/2020/05/Removing-barriers-to-telehealth-before-and-after-COVID-19_PDF.pdf.

[3] D. C. Nguyen, M. Ding, P. N. Pathirana, and A. Seneviratne, "Blockchain and AI-based solutions to combat Coronavirus (COVID-19)-like epidemics: A survey," *IEEE Access*, vol. 9, pp. 95730–95753, 2021.

[4] M. Hiwale, S. Phanasalkar, and K. Kotecha, "Using blockchain and distributed machine learning to manage decentralized but trustworthy disease data," *Sci. Technol. Libr.*, vol. 40, no. 2, pp. 190–213, 2021, doi: 10.1080/0194262X.2020.1859046.

[5] A. Hasselgren, K. Kralevska, D. Gligoroski, S. A. Pedersen, and A. Faxvaag, "Blockchain in healthcare and health sciences—A scoping review," *Int. J. Med. Inform.*, vol. 134, p. 104040, 2020, doi: 10.1016/j.ijmedinf.2019.104040.

[6] C. Agbo, Q. Mahmoud, and J. Eklund, "Blockchain technology in healthcare: A systematic review," *Healthcare*, vol. 7, no. 2, p. 56, 2019, doi: 10.3390/healthcare7020056.

[7] A. F. da Conceição, F. S. C. da Silva, V. Rocha, A. Locoro, and J. M. Barguil, "Electronic health records using blockchain technology," 2018, [Online]. Available: http://arxiv.org/abs/1804.10078.

[8] P. V. Kakarlapudi and Q. H. Mahmoud, "A systematic review of blockchain for consent management," *Healthcare*, vol. 9, no. 2, 2021, doi: 10.3390/healthcare9020137.

[9] R. Wasim, K. Salah, R. Jayaraman, I. Yaqoob, S. Ellahham, and M. Omar, "Since January 2020 Elsevier has created a COVID-19 resource centre with free information in English and Mandarin on the novel coronavirus COVID-19. The COVID-19 resource centre is hosted on Elsevier Connect, the company's public news and information," January 2020.

[10] I. Yaqoob, K. Salah, R. Jayaraman, and Y. Al-Hammadi, "Blockchain for healthcare data management: Opportunities, challenges, and future recommendations," *Neural Comput. Appl.*, 2021, doi: 10.1007/s00521-020-05519-w.

[11] M. S. Ali, M. Vecchio, M. Pincheira, K. Dolui, F. Antonelli, and M. H. Rehmani, "Applications of blockchains in the Internet of Things: A comprehensive survey," *IEEE Commun. Surv. Tutorials*, vol. 21, no. 2, pp. 1676–1717, 2019, doi: 10.1109/COMST.2018.2886932.

[12] P. P. Ray, Di. Dash, K. Salah, and N. Kumar, "Blockchain for IoT-based healthcare: Background, consensus, platforms, and use cases," *IEEE Syst. J.*, vol. 15, no. 1, pp. 85–94, 2021, doi: 10.1109/JSYST.2020.2963840.

[13] M. G. R. Alam, S. F. Abedin, S. I. Moon, A. Talukder, and C. S. Hong, "Healthcare IoT-Based Affective State Mining Using a Deep Convolutional Neural Network," *IEEE Access*, vol. 7, pp. 75189–75202, 2019.

[14] F. Ali, S. El-Sappagh, S. M. Riazul Islam, *et al.*, "A smart healthcare monitoring system for heart disease prediction based on ensemble deep learning and feature fusion," *Inf. Fusion*, vol. 63, pp. 208–222, 2020, doi: 10.1016/j.inffus.2020.06.008.

[15] H. Tao, M. Z. A. Bhuiyan, A. N. Abdalla, M. M. Hassan, J. M. Zain, and T. Hayajneh, "Secured data collection with hardware-based ciphers for IoT-based healthcare," *IEEE Internet Things J.*, vol. 6, no. 1, pp. 410–420, 2019, doi: 10.1109/JIOT.2018.2854714.

[16] C. Chakraborty and M. Rathi, "Smart healthcare systems using big data," In *Demystifying Big Data, Machine Learning, and Deep Learning for Healthcare Analytics*, (pp. 17–32). London: Academic Press; 2021.

[17] V. Chamola, V. Hassija, V. Gupta, and M. Guizani, "A comprehensive review of the COVID-19 pandemic and the role of IoT, drones, AI, blockchain, and 5G in managing its impact," *IEEE Access*, vol. 8, pp. 90225–90265, 2020, doi: 10.1109/ACCESS.2020.2992341.

[18] W. Chen, Z. Xu, S. Shi, Y. Zhao, and J. Zhao, "A survey of blockchain applications in different domains," *ACM Int. Conf. Proceeding Ser.*, pp. 17–21, 2018, doi: 10.1145/3301403.3301407.

[19] D. B. Rawat, V. Chaudhary, and R. Doku, "Blockchain technology: Emerging applications and use cases for secure and trustworthy smart systems," *J. Cybersecur. Priv.*, vol. 1, no. 1, pp. 4–18, 2020, doi: 10.3390/jcp1010002.

[20] M. C. Suciu, C. Năsulea, and D. Năsulea, "Is blockchain a new creative industry?," *Collab. Res. Excell. Econ. Soc. Sci.*, pp. 154–163, 2021, doi: 10.2478/9788366675322-019.

[21] M. Gaynor, J. Tuttle-Newhall, J. Parker, A. Patel, and C. Tang, "Adoption of blockchain in health care," *J. Med. Internet Res.*, vol. 22, no. 9, pp. 1–10, 2020, doi: 10.2196/17423.

[22] S. Dash, C. Chakraborty, S. K. Giri, S. K. Pani, and J. Frnda, "BIFM: Big-data driven intelligent forecasting model for COVID-19," *IEEE Access*, vol. 9, pp. 97505–97517, 2021, doi: 10.1109/ACCESS.2021.3094658.

[23] Q. Li, H. Lin, X. Wei, *et al.* "MaraVis: Representation and coordinated intervention of medical encounters in urban marathon," In *Proceedings of the 2020 CHI Conference on Human Factors in Computing Systems*, (pp. 1–12). New York, NY: ACM; 2020.

[24] X. Yue, H. Wang, D. Jin, M. Li, and W. Jiang, "Healthcare data gateways: Found healthcare intelligence on blockchain with novel privacy risk control," *J. Med. Syst.*, vol. 40, no. 10, 2016, doi: 10.1007/s10916-016-0574-6.

[25] A. H. Mayer, C. A. da Costa, and R. da Rosa Righi, "Electronic health records in a Blockchain: A systematic review," *Health Informatics J.*, vol. 26, no. 2, pp. 1273–1288, 2020, doi: 10.1177/1460458219866350.

[26] S. Dash, C. Chakraborty, S. K. Giri, and S. K. Pani, "Intelligent computing on time-series data analysis and prediction of COVID-19 pandemics", *Pattern Recognit. Lett.*, vol. 151, pp. 69–75, 2021, https://doi.org/10.1016/j.patrec.2021.07.027.

[27] O. Gutiérrez, G. Romero, L. Pérez, A. Salazar, P. Wightman, and M. Charris, "HealthyBlock: Blockchain-based it architecture for electronic medical records resilient to connectivity failures," *Int. J. Environ. Res. Public Health*, vol. 17, no. 19, pp. 1–38, 2020, doi: 10.3390/ijerph17197132.

[28] M. M. Qureshi, A. Farooq, and M. Mazhar, "Current eHealth challenges and recent trends in eHealth applications," February 2021.

[29] B. J. Nievas Soriano, S. Garcia Duarte, A. M. Fernandez Alonso, A. Bonillo Perales, and T. Parron Carreno, "eHealth: Advantages, disadvantages and guiding principles for the future," *J. Med. Internet Res.*, pp. 1–23, 2019, doi: 10.2196/preprints.15366.

[30] P. Ratta, A. Kaur, S. Sharma, M. Shabaz, and G. Dhiman, "Application of blockchain and Internet of Things in healthcare and medical sector: Applications, challenges, and future perspectives," *J. Food Qual.*, vol. 2021, 2021, doi: 10.1155/2021/7608296.

[31] S. Shi, D. He, L. Li, N. Kumar, and M. Khurram, "Since January 2020 Elsevier has created a COVID-19 resource centre with free information in English and Mandarin on the novel coronavirus COVID-19. The COVID-19 resource centre is hosted on Elsevier Connect, the company's public news and information," January 2020.

[32] A. Grech, I. Sood, and L. Ariño, "Blockchain, self-sovereign identity and digital credentials: Promise versus praxis in education," *Front. Blockchain*, vol. 4, pp. 1–12, 2021, doi: 10.3389/fbloc.2021.616779.

[33] S. Parvathavarthini, N. Karthikeyani Visalakshi, S. Shanthi, and J. Madhan Mohan, "An improved crow search based intuitionistic fuzzy clustering algorithm for healthcare applications," *Intell. Autom. Soft Comput.*, vol. 26, no. 2, pp. 253–260, 2020, doi: 10.31209/2019.100000155.

[34] W. Bible, J. Raphael, M. Riviello, P. Taylor, and I. O. Valiente, "Blockchain technology and its potential impact on the audit and assurance profession," *CPA Canada, AICPA*, pp. 1–28, 2017, [Online]. Available: https://www.aicpa.org/content/dam/aicpa/interestareas/frc/assuranceadvisoryservices/downloadabledocuments/blockchain-technology-and-its-potential-impact-on-the-audit-and-assurance-profession.pdf.

[35] Institute of Medicine. *Patient Safety: Achieving a New Standard for Care.* Washington, DC: National Academies Press; 2004. https://doi.org/10.17226/10863.

[36] M. L. Jochumsen and A. Chaudhuri, "Blockchain's impact on supply chain of a pharmaceutical company," *EUROMA Conf. 2018*, pp. 1–8, June 2018.

[37] M. Sahoo, S. S. Singhar, and S. S. Sahoo, "A blockchain based model to eliminate drug counterfeiting," *Adv. Intell. Syst. Comput.*, vol. 1101, pp. 213–222, 2020, doi: 10.1007/978-981-15-1884-3_20.

[38] A. Sanghi, Aayush, A. Katakwar, A. Arora, and A. Kaushik, "Detecting fake drugs using blockchain," *Int. J. Recent Technol. Eng.*, vol. 10, no. 1, pp. 100–109, 2021, doi: 10.35940/ijrte.a5744.0510121.

[39] H. K. Bhuyan, C. Chakraborty, Y. Shelke, and S. K. Pani, "COVID-19 diagnosis system by deep learning approaches," *Expert Syst.*, pp. 1–18, 2021, doi: 10.1111/exsy.12776.

[40] S. G. Alonso, J. Arambarri, M. López-Coronado, and I. de la Torre Díez, "Proposing New Blockchain Challenges in eHealth," *J. Med. Syst.*, vol. 43, no. 3, 2019, doi: 10.1007/s10916-019-1195-7.

[41] A. A. Vazirani, O. O'Donoghue, D. Brindley, and E. Meinert, "Implementing blockchains for efficient health care: Systematic review," *J. Med. Internet Res.*, vol. 21, no. 2, pp. 1–12, 2019, doi: 10.2196/12439.

[42] P. E. Velmovitsky, F. M. Bublitz, L. X. Fadrique, and P. P. Morita, "Blockchain applications in health care and public health: Increased transparency," *JMIR Med. Inform.*, vol. 9, no. 6, 2021, doi: 10.2196/20713.

[43] A. Fusco, G. Dicuonzo, V. Dell'atti, and M. Tatullo, "Blockchain in healthcare: Insights on COVID-19," *Int. J. Environ. Res. Public Health*, vol. 17, no. 19, pp. 1–12, 2020, doi: 10.3390/ijerph17197167.

[44] R. S. Evans, "Electronic health records: Then, now, and in the future," *Yearb. Med. Inform.*, pp. S48–S61, 2016, doi: 10.15265/IYS-2016-s006.

[45] A. Sheikh, M. Anderson, S. Albala, *et al.*, "Health information technology and digital innovation for national learning health and care systems," *The Lancet Digital Health*, vol. 3, no. 6, pp. e383–e396, 2021, doi: 10.1016/S2589-7500(21)00005-4.

[46] D. Tith, J.-S. Lee, H. Suzuki, *et al.*, "Application of blockchain to maintaining patient records in electronic health record for enhanced privacy, scalability, and availability," *Healthc. Inform. Res.*, vol. 26, no. 1, pp. 3–12, 2020, doi: 10.4258/hir.2020.26.1.3.

[47] J. Taskinsoy, "Blockchain: A misunderstood digital revolution. Things you need to know about blockchain," *SSRN Electron. J.*, 2019, doi: 10.2139/ssrn.3466480.

[48] S. Halilbegovic and A. O. Arapovic, "Impact of blockchain technology on the payment management systems – What future holds?," *Eur. J. Econ. Stud.*, vol. 8, no. 1, 2019, doi: 10.13187/es.2019.1.43.

[49] H. F. Atlam, M. A. Azad, A. G. Alzahrani, and G. Wills, "A review of blockchain in Internet of Things and AI," *Big Data Cogn. Comput.*, vol. 4, no. 4, pp. 1–27, 2020, doi: 10.3390/bdcc4040028.

[50] M. Nicola, C. Sohrabi, G. Mathew *et al.*, "Health policy and leadership models during the COVID-19 pandemic: A review," *Int. J. Surg.*, vol. 81, pp. 122–129, 2020, [Online]. Available: /pmc/articles/PMC7366988/%0A/pmc/articles/PMC7366988/?report=abstract%0Ahttps://www.ncbi.nlm.nih.gov/pmc/articles/PMC7366988/.

[51] M. N. Kamel Boulos, J. T. Wilson, and K. A. Clauson, "Geospatial blockchain: Promises, challenges, and scenarios in health and healthcare," *Int. J. Health Geogr.*, vol. 17, no. 1, pp. 1–10, 2018, doi: 10.1186/s12942-018-0144-x.

[52] I. Radanović and R. Likić, "Opportunities for use of blockchain technology in medicine," *Appl. Health Econ. Health Policy*, vol. 16, no. 5, pp. 583–590, 2018, doi: 10.1007/s40258-018-0412-8.

[53] J. Yli-Huumo, D. Ko, S. Choi, S. Park, and K. Smolander, "Where is current research on Blockchain technology? – A systematic review," *PLoS One*, vol. 11, no. 10, pp. 1–27, 2016, doi: 10.1371/journal.pone.0163477.

[54] D. Marbouh, T. Abbasi, F. Maasmi, *et al.*, "Blockchain for COVID-19: Review, opportunities, and a trusted tracking system," *Arab. J. Sci. Eng.*, vol. 45, pp. 9895–9911, 2020, doi: 10.1007/s13369-020-04950-4.

[55] Z. Zheng, S. Xie, H. Dai, X. Chen, and H. Wang, "An overview of blockchain technology: Architecture, consensus, and future trends," *Proc. – 2017 IEEE 6th Int. Congr. Big Data, BigData Congr. 2017*, pp. 557–564, July 2017, doi: 10.1109/BigDataCongress.2017.85.

[56] Q. Xia, E. B. Sifah, A. Smahi, S. Amofa, and X. Zhang, "BBDS: Blockchain-based data sharing for electronic medical records in cloud environments," *Information*, vol. 8, no. 2, 2017, doi: 10.3390/info8020044.

[57] W. J. Gordon and C. Catalini, "Blockchain technology for healthcare: Facilitating the transition to patient-driven interoperability," *Comput. Struct. Biotechnol. J.*, vol. 16, pp. 224–230, 2018, doi: 10.1016/j.csbj.2018.06.003.

[58] E. Pritchard, P. C. Matthews, N. Stoesser, *et al.*, "Impact of vaccination on new SARS-CoV-2 infections in the United Kingdom," *Nat. Med.*, vol. 27, pp. 1370–1378, 2021, doi: 10.1038/s41591-021-01410-w.

[59] S. T. Argaw, J. R. Troncoso-Pastoriza, D. Lacey, *et al.*, "Cybersecurity of hospitals: Discussing the challenges and working towards mitigating the risks," *BMC Med. Inform. Decis. Mak.*, vol. 20, no. 1, pp. 1–10, 2020, doi: 10.1186/s12911-020-01161-7.

[60] T. K. Mackey, K. Miyachi, D. Fung, S. Qian, and J. Short, "Combating health care fraud and abuse: Conceptualization and prototyping study of a blockchain antifraud framework," *J. Med. Internet Res.*, vol. 22, no. 9, pp. 1–24, 2020, doi: 10.2196/18623.

[61] P. Pandey and R. Litoriya, "Securing E-health networks from counterfeit medicine penetration using blockchain," *Wirel. Pers. Commun.*, vol. 117, no. 1, pp. 7–25, 2021, doi: 10.1007/s11277-020-07041-7.

[62] H. I. Miller and W. Winegarden, "Fraud in your pill bottle the unacceptable cost of counterfeit medicines," October 2020, [Online]. Available: https://www.pacificresearch.org/wp-content/uploads/2020/10/CounterfeitMed_F.pdf.

[63] S. Tanwar, K. Parekh, and R. Evans, "Blockchain-based electronic health-care record system for healthcare 4.0 applications," *J. Inf. Secur. Appl.*, vol. 50, 2020, doi: 10.1016/j.jisa.2019.102407.

[64] P. Pandey and R. Litoriya, "Implementing healthcare services on a large scale: Challenges and remedies based on blockchain technology," *Heal. Policy Technol.*, vol. 9, no. 1, pp. 69–78, 2020, doi: 10.1016/j.hlpt.2020.01.004.

[65] I. A. Omar, R. Jayaraman, K. Salah, and M. C. E. Simsekler, "Exploiting Ethereum smart contracts for clinical trial management," *Proc. IEEE/ACS Int. Conf. Comput. Syst. Appl. AICCSA*, vol. 2019, August 2019, doi: 10.1109/AICCSA47632.2019.9035341.

[66] F. Carlini, R. Carlini, S. Dalla Palma, R. Pareschi, and F. Zappone, "The Genesy model for a blockchain-based fair ecosystem of genomic data," *Front. Blockchain*, vol. 3, pp. 1–13, 2020, doi: 10.3389/fbloc.2020.483227.

[67] H. Szajewska, "Evidence-based medicine and clinical research: Both are needed, neither is perfect," *Ann. Nutr. Metab.*, vol. 72, no. Suppl. 3, pp. 13–23, 2018, doi: 10.1159/000487375.

[68] S. Tian, W. Yang, J. M. Le Grange, P. Wang, W. Huang, and Z. Ye, "Smart healthcare: Making medical care more intelligent," *J. Global Health*, vol. 3, no. 3, pp. 62–65, 2019, doi: 10.1016/j.glohj.2019.07.001.

[69] N. G. Badr, "Blockchain or distributed ledger technology what is in it for the healthcare industry?," *IC3K 2019 – Proc. 11th Int. Jt. Conf. Knowl. Discov. Knowl. Eng. Knowl. Manag.*, vol. 3, pp. 277–284, 2019, doi: 10.5220/0008348902770284.

[70] Deloitte, "Blockchain—A New Model for Health Information Exchanges," pp. 1–12, 2016. Available from: https://www.healthit.gov/sites/default/files/4-37-hhs_blockchain_challenge_deloitte_consulting_llp.pdf.

[71] M. Wolkewitz, J. Lambert, M. von Cube, *et al.*, "Statistical analysis of clinical covid-19 data: A concise overview of lessons learned, common

errors and how to avoid them," *Clin. Epidemiol.*, vol. 12, pp. 925–928, 2020, doi: 10.2147/CLEP.S256735.

[72] J. Chu, "A statistical analysis of the novel coronavirus (COVID-19) in Italy and Spain," *PLoS One*, vol. 16, no. 3, p. e0249037, 2021.

[73] J. T. Wu, K. Leung, M. Bushman, *et al.*, "Estimating clinical severity of COVID-19 from the transmission dynamics in Wuhan, China," *Nat. Med.*, vol. 26, no. 4, pp. 506–510, 2020, doi: 10.1038/s41591-020-0822-7.

[74] G. C. Calafiore, C. Novara, and C. Possieri, "A Modified SIR Model for the COVID-19 Contagion in Italy," *Proc. IEEE Conf. Decis. Control*, vol. 2020-Decem, pp. 3889–3894, 2020, doi: 10.1109/CDC42340.2020.9304142.

[75] L. Roques, E. K. Klein, J. Papaïx, A. Sar, and S. Soubeyrand, "Using early data to estimate the actual infection fatality ratio from covid-19 in France," *Biology (Basel)*, vol. 9, no. 5, pp. 1–11, 2020, doi: 10.3390/biology9050097.

[76] S. B. Bastos and D. O. Cajueiro, "Modeling and forecasting the early evolution of the Covid-19 pandemic in Brazil," *Sci. Rep.*, vol. 10, no. 1, pp. 1–15, 2020, doi: 10.1038/s41598-020-76257-1.

[77] M. E. Shipe, S. A. Deppen, F. Farjah, and E. L. Grogan, "Developing prediction models for clinical use using logistic regression: An overview," *J. Thorac. Dis.*, vol. 11, no. Suppl. 4, pp. S574–S584, 2019, doi: 10.21037/jtd.2019.01.25.

[78] J. Le-Rademacher and X. Wang, "A Time-to-event data: An overview and analysis considerations," *J. Thorac. Oncol.*, vol. 16, no. 7, pp. 1067–1074, 2021. doi: 10.1016/j.jtho.2021.04.004.

[79] L. J. Muhammad, E. A. Algehyne, S. S. Usman, A. Ahmad, C. Chakraborty, and I. A. Mohammed, "Supervised machine learning models for prediction of COVID-19 infection using epidemiology dataset," *SN Comput. Sci.*, vol. 2, no. 1, 2021, doi: 10.1007/s42979-020-00394-7.

[80] A. S. Lauring and E. B. Hodcroft, "Genetic variants of SARS-CoV-2 – What do they mean?," *JAMA – J. Am. Med. Assoc.*, vol. 325, no. 6, pp. 529–531, 2021, doi: 10.1001/jama.2020.27124.

[81] A. Rahman, C. Chakraborty, A. Anwar, *et al.*, "SDN–IoT empowered intelligent framework for industry 4.0 applications during COVID-19 pandemic," *Cluster Comput.*, pp. 1–18, 2021, doi: 10.1007/s10586-021-03367-4.

Chapter 7

Social distancing technologies for COVID-19

Aumnat Tongkaw[1]

Abstract

Because of the COVID-19 scenario, the viral infection rate in Thailand has sky-rocketed as people commute to work and go about their everyday lives. Social divides have a role in illness prevention. As a result, Thailand is focusing on adopting different technologies to assist us in managing the gap and support everyone's ability to work. Adopting this technology has resulted in it being the New Normal in use as a substitute for older systems. It also plays a role in instilling everyone a sense of social responsibility and caution to avoid near individuals from becoming infected; it has become an accepted part of daily life. This chapter offers a template analysis of stakeholder interviews conducted with the aid of technology to accomplish social distancing, which is divided into three categories: educational, public health, and social distancing, as well as manufacturing employees. A software usage pattern has been developed due to data analysis utilizing the content analysis to help create social distancing for job planning and everyday use. It can also be used to plan future smart cities.

Keywords: COVID-19; Social distancing; Healthcare; Education; Manufacturing

7.1 Introduction

Since the spread of the COVID-19 pandemic, the government in several nations has adopted the phrase "social distancing." Social distancing is a physical distancing technique that involves establishing a distance between two individuals or among people to limit their interaction with one another. This scenario has a considerable influence on how the population work and interact with one another. The acceptability of the distance is no more than 6 ft apart. In public health, social distancing is frequently referred to as physical distancing. In a collection of non-pharmaceutical measures aimed at preventing the transmission of a contagious illness by keeping a physical barrier between individuals, minimizing the number

[1]Faculty of Science and Technology, Songkhla Rajabhat University, Songkhla, Thailand

of times people came into contact with one another, and limiting huge crowd gatherings. Scientists and engineers are using all available technologies to combat the virus's spread; ICT can provide valuable tools for ensuring social distancing. To be a generation in which technology has improved hardware and software, including mobile applications and many Internet of Things (IoT) sensor actuators in devices. Artificial intelligence (AI) techniques such as machine learning, data mining, deep learning, and other AI approaches are also included in some technologies. For 2019-nCoV pandemic patients, these options would make diagnosis and prognosis easier. In one study, for example, supervised machine learning models for COVID-19 infection were developed [1]. People are using social media more than ever before during COVID-19. Technological developments and social media platforms give opportunities to keep people safe, informed, and connected. Working from home has become possible because to access to social media during COVID-19. Furthermore, technology enables people to interact online or work from home in order to preserve social distance. Every firm in Thailand, both government and commercial, has embraced social media and technology to improve work efficiency even further.

7.2 Methodology

The content of this chapter came from the 30 participants in three sectors: education, industry, and healthcare. The literature draws the theme of interview questions and analysis by using template analysis that is a part of thematic analysis [2,3]. Template emphasizes hierarchical coding while balancing a high level of organization in the process of analyzing textual data with the flexibility to adjust it to the needs of a specific study [3]. Researchers questioned 30 persons involved in utilizing technology to assist in times of need social distance, interpreting the details from the interview, recording it, and documenting it. Subsequently, preliminary coding was performed for important information the interviewees had discussed the same issue or are essential or a focus, which may lead to the main point of using those technologies. The researchers recorded the respondents' remarks regarding problems of interest and impediments to leadership. Following that, the researcher gathered several issues—both primary and sub-issues—which were discussed, and the intricacies of each issue were discovered in depth. The researchers then published this article based on the resultant template to demonstrate to readers the uniformity of technology implementations utilized in three areas: education, public health, and manufacturing.

7.3 Social distancing technologies for education

During the COVID-19 epidemic, many institutes must teach entirely online at all educational levels, from preschool to university. As a result, the ministry of education employs social distancing to employ social distancing between individuals, which significantly influences learning activities at higher institutions. Colleges replace in-person meetings with online networking and homework obligations. This study attempts to characterize the various models and platforms utilized in online learning for future instructors during the social distance phase [4]. Many online teaching and learning tools are proliferating. Some university courses that need practice laboratories must consider how to isolate classes of students and how to alert when students are close to one other in the lab. As a result of the COVID-19 epidemic, many nations have had to adjust to new conditions in various fields, including education. The Indonesian government has decided to shift education away from face-to-face meetings and video conferencing using various learning management systems (LMSs) such as Moodle and Google Classroom.

7.3.1 Learning management system

During COVID-19, LMSs made a significant contribution. Furthermore, keeping all of the course information, videos, and activities in one location might help manage the course and stick to the lesson schedule. Students may access them anytime, from anywhere in the globe, with security remaining the primary concern. Students can access the Internet using suitable devices such as computers, tablets, or even mobile phones. Students can utilize LMS to learn while schools are closed due to social distancing. Furthermore, school teachers can reduce the administrative burdens involved with keeping instructional resources in their classrooms, saving educational institution's costs. The benefits of the LMS system include the ability for schools to administer the system themselves, alter the system to suit the learners and the environment of each school without too much effort, and the fact that it does not require as many computer specialists as other systems. The LMS is designed to enable integrated teaching techniques, which combine self-paced eLearning with instructor-led online instruction. Teachers may utilize the integrated authoring tool to import current courses or build completely new ones from the start and then establish adjustable student paths that determine when and how learners can take them. Discussion forums and private chats increase class participation, and teachers may plan live webinars to teach students real time. Automated grading streamlines homework assignment evaluations, while detailed data and student analytics aid professors in evaluating which students need more help and which courses may be improved. Many countries must adjust to changing conditions in a variety of sectors, including education. As a consequence of the COVID-19 epidemic, LMS is being utilized in Thailand education for teaching and learning, contributing to teacher self-improvement. The LMS system can also plan education until the conclusion of the semester online. As a result, research has proven that a completely online education system is feasible [5]. Indonesia's government has held online meetings and has made all schooling available online. They make use of platforms like massive open online course (MOOC) Moodle and Google Classroom [6].

7.3.1.1 Massive open online course

MOOCs have emerged as one of Thailand's most effective online learning techniques following COVID-19. The Thai MOOC platform includes a large and approved library of educational content that may be accessed in various ways [7].

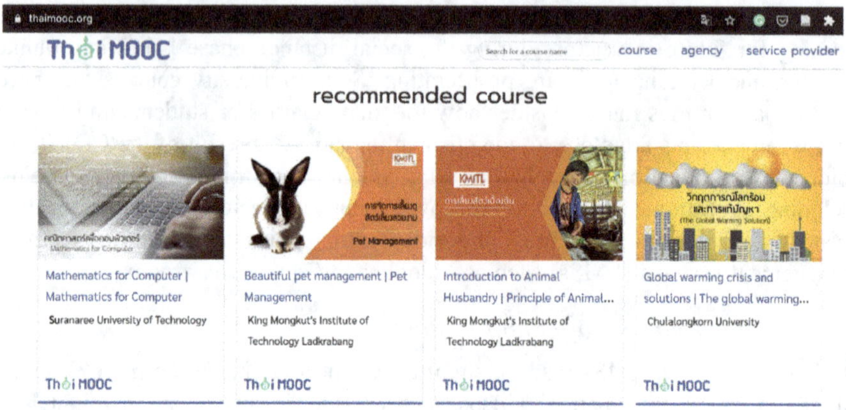

Figure 7.1 Thai MOOC platform

Following COVID-19, MOOCs emerged as one of Thailand's most effective online learning platforms. The Thai MOOC platform provides a vast and approved library of educational resources that may be accessed in various ways. See Figure 7.1 that shows Thai MOOC platform. The effectiveness of the MOOC on the learners depends on the learn–certify–deploy ideology. The quick process helps people integrate their knowledge gained from the class to help them do their job better or follow their interests. Interestingly, Thais people who take MOOC courses tend to follow their interests rather than other goals. Fast implementation is an important factor contributing to MOOCs' success during the pandemic. Most people stepped out of their normal lives before and exerted their willingness to learn something new [8].

Lessons obtained through designing instructional technology and guiding articles, on the other hand, may be implemented in a variety of situations in primary care education. It is discovered that MOOCs provided the freedom to adjust the content, modify the instructional phases, and adjust the components based on the pandemic's progress as well as learners' requirements and suggestions. Furthermore, MOOCs are ideal for rapid information distribution. Learner participation in virtual group discussions was advantageous and was widely recognized by users as an effective tool to share insights globally [9].

7.3.1.2 Google Classroom

Google Classroom is a free online service for schools, nonprofits, and anyone with a Google account. Google Classroom makes it easy for students and teachers to stay connected, both inside and outside the classroom. It is a hybrid learning platform originating from Google that promises to facilitate the creation, distribution, and assignment of assignments in a paperless way. Using this teachers can create virtual classes, invite students to join classes, and provide information about the teaching and learning process. It can also provide teaching materials that students can learn in the form of material presentation files and learning videos, give assignments to

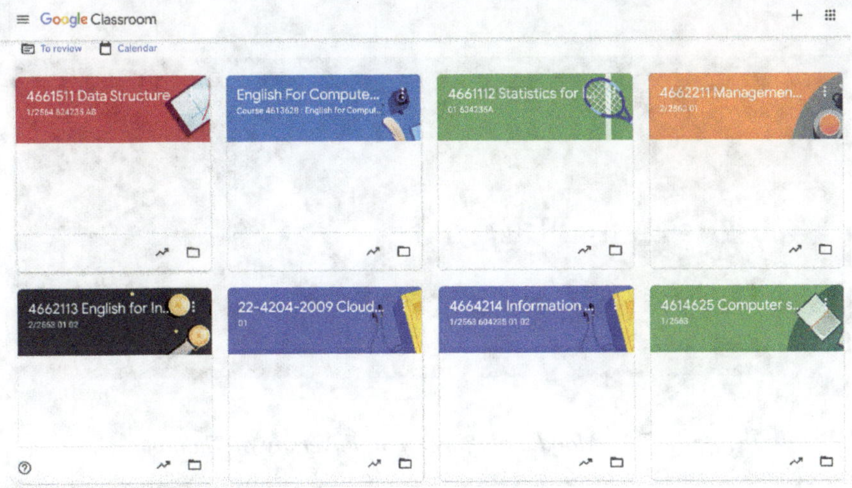

Figure 7.2 Google Classroom

students, and make a schedule for collecting assignments and others. Being a relatively new platform for learning, the need for Google Classroom in online Indonesian learning is worth investigating from various perspectives, both from the side of students, teachers, and supporting facilities. For example, from the student aspect, active student involvement, accuracy in doing assignments, student enthusiasm, and student learning outcomes. From the teacher's perspective, for example, the teacher's mastery of information technology, the teacher's skills in preparing lesson plans, implementing learning, and providing evaluations. Meanwhile, in terms of infrastructure, the examples are the availability of a strong network, Internet connection, and the financial readiness of parents and perhaps teachers to purchase data packages. This Best Practice will not reveal all aspects related to the implementation of online learning using Google Classroom during the COVID-19 pandemic but is only limited to increasing student activity and learning outcomes through online learning using Google Classroom [10]. Google Classroom is a free application that allows teachers to create courses, give and mark homework, and offer feedback to students. Instructors may set permissions for students, parents, and co-teachers, share their display, connect a student's screen and lockdown for a pop quiz. Teachers can also employ digital learning to augment classroom education. Figure 7.2 shows many classes in a Google Classroom in a university of Thailand.

7.3.1.3 Moodle

Moodle is a program that manages the LMS, or for short, the LMS. That is the LMS Martin Dougiamas created for use in online teaching and learning. The system management structure is a Web-Based Instruction that has a vital component in the writing language, which includes PHP and MySQL database, which provides

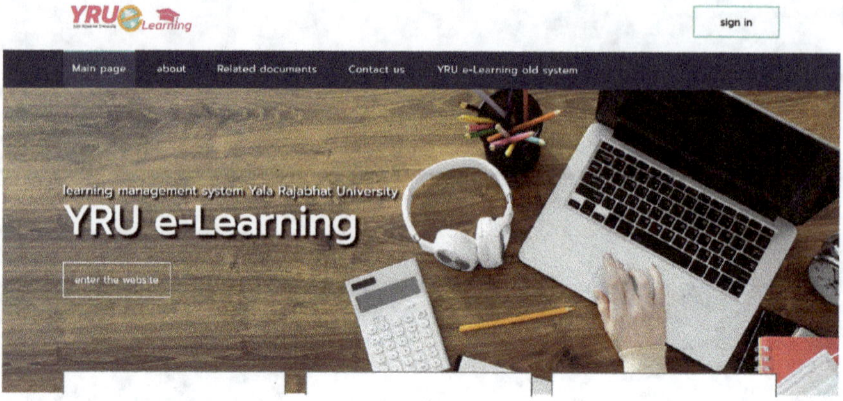

Figure 7.3 Moodle platform in a university of Thailand

administrators, instructors, and students, the three user groups. Interaction is prioritized in network-based teaching and learning. Moodle is open-source software, which indicates that it is free to use. The license is a GPL (General Public License) that users can download. The program is free to use and can develop additional programs according to users.

Moodle-based LMS is effective for improving students' argumentation skills. It is supported by the statement of many researches which state that learning using LMS can be used to train students' thinking skills in various courses. Furthermore, based on the results of [11], it demonstrates that the usage of Moodle in blended learning has an average degree of effectiveness in terms of student motivation, with a mean of 3.216, a mean of 3.164 in terms of student success, and a mean of 3.199 in terms of student interaction and coordination. Several theoretical reasons can be used to justify that the student's argumentation ability has moderate improvement criteria. Moodle and its procedures are associated with the application of learning through the use of a Moodle-based LMS. A well-designed Moodle-based LMS will facilitate learning by leveraging self-service and self-guided services, quickly collecting and distributing learning information, and facilitating knowledge reuse. This idea allows teachers to manage classwork and communicate with students in a flexible and timely manner. Figure 7.3 shows an own Moodle-based in a university in Thailand.

7.3.2 Social networking and conference software for education

In the Thai education system, there are two levels of LMS: school and undergraduate and above. In Thailand, Google Classroom is largely utilized. However, there is a difficulty in that most instructors cannot use Google Classroom since pupils do not have personal computers. Then, the usage of LMS is restricted, as it does not cover all courses. During the lockdown, Thai schools allow pupils to study online using various technologies. According to the interview data, the most commonly utilized system is a social media platform that parents or kids use on a daily basis to contact friends or teachers at school, such as LINE or Facebook. Students utilize social media to connect with one another and form groups for teaching and learning. Students also utilize conference software for communicating and teaching, such as Google Meet, Zoom, Webex, Team, or LINE Group call.

7.4 Social distancing technology in healthcare

Many patients require hospitalization, particularly in underdeveloped countries. The following examples demonstrate how technology may help with social distancing policies by lowering the number of people queuing at the hospital, waiting for prescriptions, or completing payments.

7.4.1 Wearable technology

Wearable technology is becoming more prevalent in our daily life as well as the healthcare profession. These regions can benefit from on-time remote access, symptom prognosis, and interaction tracking enabled by technology. The IoT plays an important part in tracking a person's health and diagnosing COVID-19. ML is a sophisticated AI technique that can be used to detect and diagnose COVID-19 from X-ray and CT pictures reliably, and it could be a possible diagnostic method in the radiology department [12]. Moreover, to assist coronavirus-infected patients, different wearable monitoring devices such as medical devices respiration rate, heart rate, temperature, and oxygen saturation, and respiratory assistive technologies (ventilators, CPAP machines, and oxygen treatment) are routinely employed [13]. A patient can be fully monitored by a doctor using wearable technology during the quarantine or self-treatment time. Wearable technology is the least expensive and most often used option for social distancing. Any device issued by the company could legally be tracked within the premises of the workspace, which could be integrated with a site-wide notification system of potential health risks or any alerts that adhere to the social distancing guidelines. A smart system could also be used in conjunction with the wearable device to enable real-time and analytical solutions to social distancing guidelines. A similar approach has already been implemented in healthcare for the elderly, preventing potential hazards within the residences, such as stairs, railings, and power cords. This technological answer has helped the elderly in their daily lives; such devices monitor the person's activity if they are stationary or moving. If the surrounding area is mapped, then these activities could be discretely identified as sitting or running. These aspects of wearable gear in healthcare might serve as a model for developing social distancing technologies, which enforce workplace standards and comprehend employee behavior, resulting in the best outcome for everyone. However, the question of privacy still lingers when presenting a perfectly manageable engineered solution, which is a bigger concern when monitoring larger crowds in a bigger facility compared to a single resident [14]. The concept is applied in research by integrating low-cost and ever higher quality based metadata for patient monitoring. Future patient monitoring and health information delivery systems will be dramatically impacted by advances in communications combined with IoT and embedded system technologies [15]. This can provide services through a smartphone theory of growth for chronic wound image processing at the patient's side, as well as providing better integration between doctor and patient remotely, end-to-end daily schedule-based diagnostic, and sustaining patient history [16].

7.4.2 Screening system

Most hospital screening methods before the COVID-19 circumstance allow for patients to inadvertently come into contact with one another. Pressure measurement and preliminary history recording may require being in close proximity to the ill individual for less than 1 m, a distance that has the potential to be infected after the occurrence. Because the number of medical workers is limited and cannot provide comprehensive services, the world has focused on limiting exposure as a result of the pandemic. Various sensor technologies have been used to assess patients before they begin treatments.

Many Thai hospitals include patient screening systems that are linked to the central hospital database, such as a service queue booking system that allows patients to get a queue before visiting the hospital, as detailed in the following section. Patients can make an appointment to visit the hospital or simply stroll in. Then they must pass via the hospital's screening procedure. The hospital uses smart video analytics to monitor temperature and can inform the nurse if the patient has a high temperature. If the patient does not have a fever, the patient can proceed with the screening procedure by using the following steps: a sensor or actuator for weight and blood pressure measurement.

7.4.3 Queue systems

While the government is dealing with the COVID-19 crisis, several hospitals have implemented screening systems using sensor devices. As the hospital has a limited number of medical professionals, the hospital uses technology to assist with the process, which queuing systems are increasingly being utilized in Thai hospitals. The system connects with the hospital's HIS system, which includes a registration system. When arriving at the hospital, the queuing system software integrates with a mobile application and a kiosk register, which uses an ID card in front of the kiosk. Using the kiosk reduces social interaction and maintains the social distancing procedure without the need to see a nurse. The system also includes a web-based system accessible via a web browser. A queue system through a mobile app is a method in which patients may use their phones to make appointments with doctors in various departments, which can now be used to develop models for predicting clinic selection. In terms of patient guidance, if the patient is still unable to select which clinic to visit, the system may recommend a clinic and time for the appointment. Furthermore, the system will communicate the patient's information to the examination room. The system will also transmit a LINE to alert patients when it is nearing the end of the wait. As a result, the patient does not need to sit

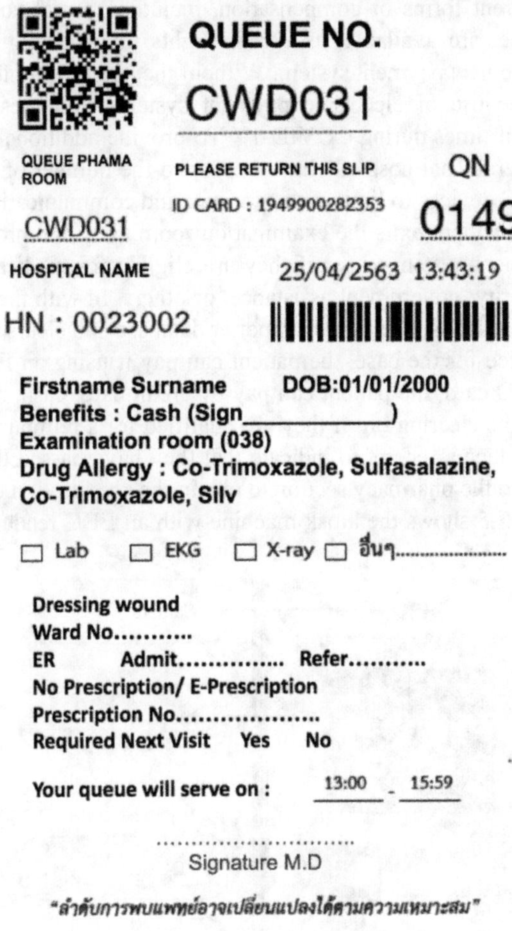

QUEUE NO.
CWD031

QUEUE PHAMA ROOM
CWD031

PLEASE RETURN THIS SLIP
ID CARD : 1949900282353

QN
0149

HOSPITAL NAME
25/04/2563 13:43:19

HN : 0023002

Firstname Surname DOB:01/01/2000
Benefits : Cash (Sign________)
Examination room (038)
Drug Allergy : Co-Trimoxazole, Sulfasalazine, Co-Trimoxazole, Silv

☐ Lab ☐ EKG ☐ X-ray ☐ อื่นๆ......................

Dressing wound
Ward No...........
ER Admit.............. Refer...........
No Prescription/ E-Prescription
Prescription No...................
Required Next Visit Yes No

Your queue will serve on : 13:00 - 15:59

....
Signature M.D

"ลำดับการพบแพทย์อาจเปลี่ยนแปลงได้ตามความเหมาะสม"

Figure 7.4 Slip queue

and wait at the hospital for an extended period of time and may conduct errands elsewhere first As a result, this method provides social distance control to minimize the transmission of COVID-19. Figure 7.4 shows the slip queue that notified the patient when the patient queue was nearly called.

7.4.4 Payment system

The payment system described earlier aids in cashless transactions, or if the organization wishes to decrease paper usage to save the environment. These computerized payment methods can also assist in driving social distance. Because patients may engage with the kiosk or electronic data capture (EDC) machine rather than the cashier, the payment method has the potential to minimize the number of infections during the COVID-19. Electronic payment methods are increasingly being employed in some hospitals. The system will be linked to the hospital's central database.

Furthermore, different forms of compensation, including social compensation and government service, are available, as certain rights may be eligible for medical assistance under the new payment system. Without the need to pay for medical costs or medications, the use of electronic payment systems promotes efficiency and reduces patient wait times during COVID-19. To provide additional electronic payment services, several Thai hospitals have expanded the number of payment kiosks equipped with EDC devices to limit cash exposure and communication with hospital cashiers. When the patient exits the examination room, they can proceed straight to an electronic payment system to see if they are eligible for medical compensation such as social security, government assistance, or others. In with the patient's rights and supports, the kiosk connects to the supporter database and clears the cost. If there is an additional price for the case, the patient can pay it using an EDC machine or cash. Using their ID card, the patient can pay by credit card, cash, or bank transfer. They will receive the clearing bill if they are qualified for a reimbursement scheme. The kiosk will produce a receipt to indicate that they have passed this process, and the patient can go to the pharmacy section to obtain the prescription or other medical necessities. Figure 7.5 shows the kiosk machine with an EDC reader.

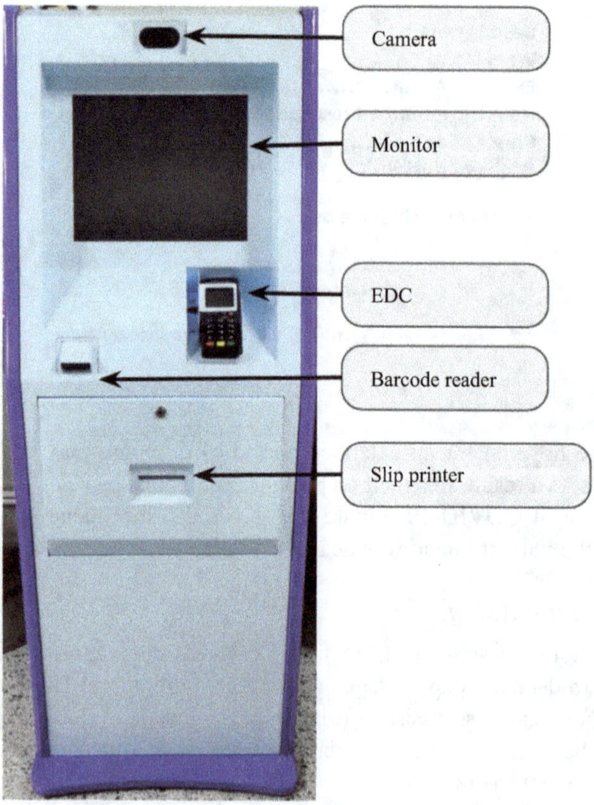

Figure 7.5 Kiosk of EDC

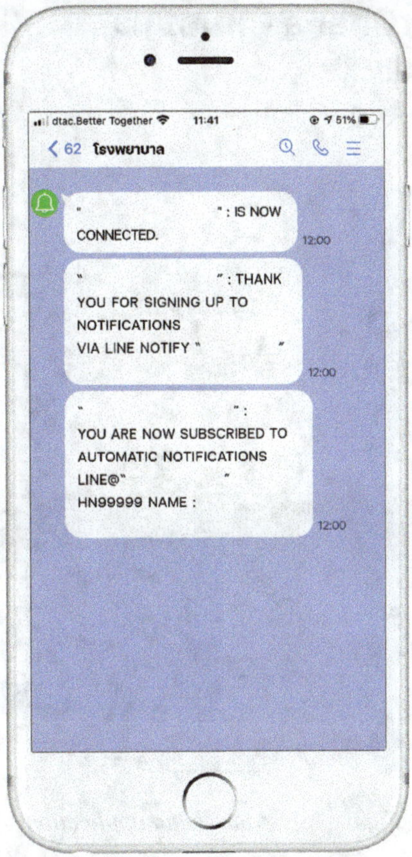

Figure 7.6 LINE notifier

Patients will be assigned a number once they have made a payment in the financial system. The LINE notification system will remind the patient within a few minutes to pick up the medication. See Figure 7.6. Moreover, the patient can also use delivery to deliver medicines at home.

7.4.5 Social distancing notified people in public

Thailand adopted the MorChana program as a tool to assist medical personnel, government agency operators, and, most importantly, individuals in caring for and protecting themselves from the COVID-19 pandemic. See Figure 7.7.

By tracking infection information, the program collects, utilizes, and disseminates just the information required to avoid or suppress threats to each individual's health, as well as the others around them and the general public. The system assesses chances or risks of infection and monitors the situation of the COVID-19 outbreak by providing the information to the user. The program also

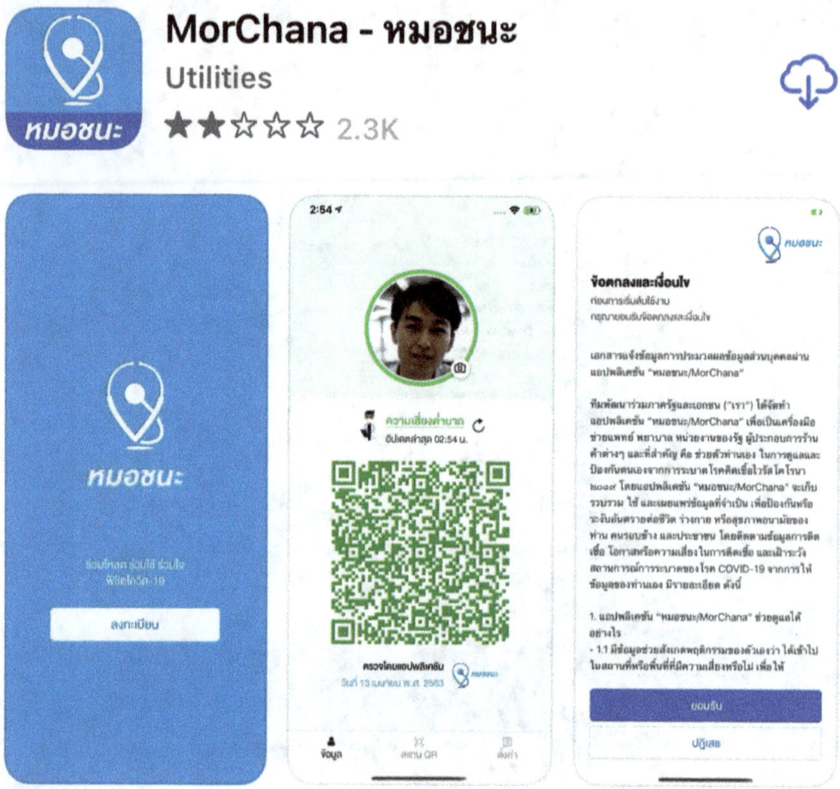

Figure 7.7 MorChana application

includes a QR code scanner for checking in and out of places such as shopping centers or supermarkets, which would update the user's timeline. If there were an infected individual in the area, the application would send the information to the Ministry of Public Health Database and notify the citizens of the immediate area to evacuate the area. The update notification relies on mobile functions such as GPS and Bluetooth to relay updates to users quickly. The infectious rate of the virus decreased significantly with the use of the ThaiChana application. In the future, this application may monitor the COVID-19 vaccine and others at risk of becoming infected. Those who contact the disease avoid crowded locations, where patients would be restricted to a particular area of mobility such as the hospital or at home. The New Normal has proved to be a time of new technological advancement with the advent of COVID-19, making technology a part of everyday life. Not only can the latest mobile apps make life easy, but they also aim to keep people safe and healthy. This issue government introduces an application worth downloading and installing to help people deal efficiently with present and potential developments.

7.5 Social distancing technology in manufacturing

Remote work is virtually never a possibility for production line employees, which is not ideal for the COVID-19 situation. Manufacturing employees are still adjusting to their jobs, with a particular emphasis on social distance as a result of working in industrial factories. To prevent viruses from spreading on the manufacturing line, only a few personnel must be stationed on duty. A research study opted to monitor worker behavior and detect breaches of social distancing guidelines on CCTV feeds using computer vision, resulting in real-time voice notifications on the manufacturing line. It is critical to keep personnel safe while still keeping the business running. The research that follows is an efficient and cost-effective approach to using AI to create a safe environment in an industrial setting. It demonstrates how to develop a strong social distance evaluation technique by combining contemporary deep learning and traditional projective geometry methodologies [17]. The four technologies listed later have changed manufacturing workforce management while keeping everyone safe in the process.

7.5.1 Checking the distance using wearable device

Wearable devices, as discussed before, are one of the common approaches when implementing social distancing guidelines. Due to its lower cost, lower maintenance, and efficiency in tracking, it is deemed the most appropriate solution within workspaces. Before COVID-19, wearable devices are used in healthcare for monitoring patients, including symptoms and patient movements. Since these features are nothing new and are used to assess health risk, it is easy to deploy in any facility. Nowadays, digital tools and technical solutions play an important part in detecting distance between various components of society, such as vehicle firms employing sensors to avoid collisions. The audio tether can also be used to notify employees if their personal gadgets are in close proximity to one another. Another option is to attach a sounding device to helmets equipped with distance-sensing devices, and light may be emitted as well. Another attribute that could be used to monitor health risks is temperature. Products such as TempTraq or Oura ring are wearable devices to measure skin temperature, which are used within the Cleveland Medical Center for medical professionals who are working on the frontline. The temperature sensors nowadays operate on low power, small in size, and they are reliable and incorporated with existing wearable devices. The smart features, the devices would be much helpful to detect abnormal body temperature changes. In this case, it would be much easier to detect and isolate individuals before an outbreak began [18]. However, some plants in Thailand adapt existed technologies to make social distancing between the workers. During the COVID-19, most of the plants remained open, according to one interviewer. Employees must record their travel or reveal the timeframe of 14 days before visiting the factory as a precautionary step against infection. When workers request access to the facility, a reasonable practice would be to provide a 14-day timeframe, maybe using an application designed particularly for the company and for this purpose. Each zone in the facility should be distinguished by partitioning or zone management, which may decrease the risk of worker infection and product contamination.

7.5.2 Distance monitoring using Wi-Fi

Since Wi-Fi operates using radio signals, it is possible to locate heavy usage based on the radius of the Wi-Fi. Some companies use existing Wi-Fi communication systems to check Wi-Fi distances between people. It can view the location of devices such as tablets, laptops, or smartphones and shows where each user is frequented. Zigbee, for example, utilizes signal propagation to detect the location of the users [19]. This approach allows employers to monitor employee positions. The number of workers congregating in some areas employee movement and the elapsed time in a particular location when one or more limits have been violated. The system will display a notification. The advantage is that employers can identify points of interest in their factories where large numbers of people gather and provide them with vital information to manage the distribution of workers in the factory, also saving costs. Because it uses the existing Wi-Fi communication system and no upfront investments or employees wear sensors, no personal information is collected [20]. Therefore, the privacy of the user is preserved.

7.5.3 Distance monitoring using video analytics

Some areas can use video analysis or high-resolution cameras instead of wearable devices or Wi-Fi-connected apps; companies may choose to use video analytics. Using AI to monitor video and analyze the distance between people, the system can alert supervisors when social distancing limits are violated. Research on a real-time social-distance and pedestrian density detection system was presented. Using modern video surveillance cameras and a deep learning-based computer vision model can evaluate the pedestrian density and social-distance patterns. Models such as YOLO v3 and DeepSort are deployed to separate people from the surroundings and then identify them by individuals with their bounding boxes. These boxes are then used to calculate the distances between each person in real time, then the results are evaluated [21]. The proposed technique for measuring social distancing patterns is based on the assumption that by combining a pretrained object detection model, precise range approximation, and post-processing filtering, one may get pedestrian densities and range between each pedestrian pair [22]. The benefit is that video analytics allow people to use their existing office camera system. It does not require a smartphone or wearable app, while it requires investment, inspection, and maintenance. The system can now identify social distance and deliver real-time warnings. It can also predict the distance to the safe zone using data integration and machine learning. Management may utilize this information to plan task management in the company. However, because video analytics implementation is pricey, some Thai businesses are unable to pay, and management refuses to proceed in this fashion because it is unnecessary.

7.5.4 Social distancing by replacing some work with a robot

According to research, labor is one of the most important elements in manufacturing costs. If the firm wishes to expand its product line, it must hire more workers throughout the manufacturing process. Investment in purchasing robots to replace human labor has grown, but not to the extent that it should have. There may be a large investment, but when the virus COVID-19 arises, individuals face a high risk that impacts productivity and cannot address the problem even if those individuals are vaccinated; nevertheless, another new virus strain may emerge in the future. Both the client and the manufacturer are interested in intelligent automation. People, particularly customers, seek alternatives where human interaction is as minimized as possible. Furthermore, there are increasing automation products and solutions, which people of all levels have to access. Some examples include self-checkout at grocery stores or online business systems, which are more used apparently. Robots are also being used in airport hospitals using robots for temperature screeners and food delivery bots to reduce manual labor and induce social distancing. However, big-scale operations are also slowly being replaced by robots and automation systems. Considerable cooperation such as Amazon or Walmart has already started using robots to operate most of their warehouses for shipping products. Sadly, most of those jobs replaced with automation, especially after the recession, are fully depleted for good. Therefore, the decision to use robots to replace workers in some industrial plants tends to rise significantly [23]. Even though the rise of automation is prevalent, the reliability is not fully appreciated due to many factors such as the limitation to the tasks that the robots are assigned or extensive data availability and proper usage. Indeed, implementing robotics and automation has many benefits to many agencies during COVID-19, but entirely relying on the nature of automation might not be a worthwhile investment.

7.6 Social-distancing technologies for supporting everyday life

The Johns Hopkins University and the Centers for Disease Control and Prevention describe Social Distancing as a public health practice that isolates infectious patients from healthy individuals in order to reduce the danger of the virus spreading. Group activities should be canceled or done in enclosed areas, and crowded venues should be avoided, in addition to being at least 2 m apart from other individuals. The goal of social distance is to reduce COVID-19 transmission. Suppose it is done correctly to reduce the risk of infection among high-risk groups and healthcare professionals. In that case, the infection rate will be lower, resulting in fewer individuals being admitted to the hospital.

Government policy in every country tries to introduce everybody to have social distancing to decrease spread infections that are as follows.

7.6.1 Technologies support working at home

7.6.1.1 Remote working

The spreading and deadly coronavirus, also known as COVID-19, has profoundly impacted the global economy. All countries are trying to find alternatives to deal with this challenging situation. There is an urgent need to protect employees in offices. In Thailand, both the public and private sectors have adopted Internet-based front-end technology as an integral part of their services for employees and public users. COVID-19 compelled every country to enter the New Normal phase, which may not be optimal for countries where technology is scarce. As a result, digitizing all aspects of the organization is difficult. Working from home still has network security concerns while transitioning to the New Normal because developing countries' network structure and design are inadequate. As a result, network security problems have become increasingly frequent since beginning work from home; most work from home is not linked through virtual private network (VPN) and still uses the Internet. As working from home becomes more critical and security features are introduced, a VPN is built on a packet-based network and consists of some selected packet-based network resources. VPN is the most simple and efficient tool for people to safeguard their Internet data and conceal their identity online. When a device connects to a secure VPN server, the user's Internet data is routed through encrypted tunnels that no one can see, including hackers, governments, and ISPs. However, VPN technology and support systems are not without security dangers and risks. People and business persons who are working from home use computer networks and virtual environments that hackers or cybercriminals have abused. One of the biggest challenges facing any organization in adopting VPN technology is VPN gateway location and access control. It is a policy challenge directly related to the nature of the network security infrastructure that organizations deploy to secure knowledge, applications, and networks. The remote access technology and security checklist consist of 13 main security feature categories the organizations provide to their staff, administrator, and authorized users. Details of each category within the checklist are displayed in Tables 7.1 and 7.2.

7.6.2 Applications support work from home (WFH) service

7.6.2.1 Call center

Call center personnel are now regarded as the organization's beating heart. Call centers keep businesses running, with no set work hours and few holidays to guarantee that customers are satisfied. However, suppose call center employees are required to remain up late at night. In that case, there will be issues with the safety of returning home, and the majority of them work in congested areas that are vulnerable to COVID-19 spread. The call center turnover rate is quite high; the firm requires technology that allows employees to work from home in order to maintain social distance. Voice over IP (VoIP), often known as Voice over Internet Protocol, is a means of communicating over the Internet using voice. It is a novel method of making calls via the Internet network, with the first evident advantages. Because utilizing the Internet to make a phone call eliminates the need to travel via a

Table 7.1 Remote access security feature categories

Number	Category name	Description
1	General organization remote access instruction available to their remote access users	• Staff remote access • Administrator remote access • Authorized users remote access
2	Organization provides remote access hardware to its authorized users	• Staff remote access • Administrator remote access • Authorized users remote access
3	The organization has a different group's level of remote access users	• Administrator • Staff • Other authorized users
4	Remote access technology	• Customer managed solution • Virtual private network (VPN) and encryption methods • Cloud-based technology
5	Central remote access architecture, mechanism, and integration system	• Remote access gateway architecture • Gateway DNS name • Remote access mechanism • Remote access system integration
6	End device software and system requirements	• Operating System (OS) support • User remote access software application
7	End device security control	• Operating System (OS) security • Use well-known strong personal firewall/antivirus/malware • Web browser security (clientless mode) • Vendor or built-in remote access client software (IPSec/SSL)
8	Central site authentication technology	• Employed encryption and digital certificate technologies
9	User site authentication technology	• Logon to remote access server requirement • Using two-factor (2FA) authentication as second security logon layer • Logon failure limitation • Logon user input type • Password restriction/requirement • Single sign on (SSO)
10	Central site network access and system security	• Pre-logon • Host Information Profile (HIP) control • Internal firewall in-place • filtering • Block malicious domains (DNS filtering)

Table 7.2 Remote access security feature categories (Cont.)

Number	Category name	Description
11	Central site application security	• Client image application (i.e., Citrix, VM) • Automatic timeout feature for inactivity Web browser/Client Software/Idle timeout • Session timeout • Multiple concurrent sessions • Bandwidth rate limiting to priority remote access users • Password policy management • Logging information and alert • Vulnerability protection • File blocking • Deep content inspection
12	IT assistance, monitoring, and support	• Hotline/helpdesk service availability for personal help
13	Remote access IT policy and procedure	• Use of remote access and Internet usage policy • Use of information security policy (remote access related) to the university's staff and lecturers • Use of information security policy—technical to the university's IT staff • Regular update or review the remote access related policy • Advise general remote access and • Internet usages, including security awareness to new remote access user • Frequent advice to staff, lecturers, and students for IT security information including remote access, Internet related

telephone network, it can help reduce the cost of calling, whether it is an international or domestic call. IP network communication requires the employment of a router (Router) with a specific purpose to ensure the quality of the IP channel in order for the information to be sent or returned correctly. Furthermore, there may be privileges before other IP packets (quality of service: QoS) to provide high-quality services, which will be seen in the development of current network equipment switches, which have included Port QoS. Employees at businesses utilized VoIP phones; when working from home, they may continue to use the phone as if they were at work. A program named SIP Client must be installed on the mobile system. To communicate with the device, the user may also utilize the SIP Client program if they wish to use it from their computer.

7.6.2.2 E-Documents

During the COVID-19 epidemic, medium-sized and big companies prioritized IT systems, working on papers online. Electronic Document Management System

(EDMS) improves the organization's working system by making it more convenient, faster, and efficient. It reduces the time spent searching for documents, which reduces the number of staff in operations and the cost of purchasing document management resources. It also reduces the amount of paper used. The benefits of adopting an EDMS include the ability to effectively add, remove, modify, and search documents saved in the database. It is simple and quick to use the software installed on the computer or operate through the browser at the organization. As a result, there is no issue with the original document being destroyed or damaged as a result of poor storage, poor quality, or loss without anybody being able to discover it. System security regulates system usage by granting rights to different groups of users, such as admin groups, data collector groups, and general user groups. EDMS also backs up the work, and the database may be utilized in the event of a system crash or damage as well.

7.6.2.3 Cloud service

The term "public cloud" refers to a cloud service that is available to anybody. Dropbox, Amazon, OneDrive, and Google Drive are all examples of completely public cloud services. Everyone who uses the public cloud is renting a shared server space. As a result, the public cloud may be thought of as a shared environment, similar to information stored in the main office. Private clouds vary from public clouds in that all virtual machines and cloud infrastructures are exclusively available to the customer. Everyone has access to anything on the Internet, but the server hosting only corrects the customer data. Because the server holding your data is not shared among numerous customers, some people may want to utilize a private cloud for added security, whilst others may require a personal cloud for increased productivity. The private implementation may need a significant expenditure, such as a data center, server, and IT administrator. In addition, unlike the public cloud, the private cloud provides clients control over how their servers are managed, kept secure, or entirely backed up. Most people use public clouds; however, private clouds are ideal for individuals that manage large amounts of data on a large scale. Using cloud services is a technology that may embrace social distance by allowing employees to work in multiple locations without limits while also decreasing congestion among employees who must work in the same location. As a result, the proliferation of COVID-19 is reduced.

7.6.2.4 Management information system

A management information system (MIS) is a system that gives executives the information they need to work effectively with both internal and external data. The data is about the firm, both in the past and in the present, as well as what is expected in the future. Furthermore, the MIS system must provide data at key times so that administration may make sound decisions about guaranteeing the security and functioning of the company. Although the highest MIS system will benefit middle management the most, the MIS system will be a system that can assist information executives at all three levels: top-level executives, middle management, and senior management. The MIS system will create a report that is a summary of data gathered from all corporate databases. The objective of the report is to provide executives with an evaluation of current developments, an overview of the company, and drive management and audit operations. On the other hand, the report's breadth is defined by the nature of the data and its intended purpose. Reports may be issued on a regular basis (e.g., an income statement or a balance sheet), on-demand, or in response to specific situations or occurrences. An MIS can be designed to allow the user to access anywhere by accessing through a web browser and the MIS client system installed on the computer. To safeguard access to information, the user may need to utilize a VPN. MIS is a technology that allows people in many departments to work from home as if they were in an office.

7.6.3 Conferencing application

Due to the extreme COVID-19 virus outbreak, several firms are requiring their workers to work from home. Although online meetings are popular, they are not as productive as face-to-face meetings. Furthermore, many organizations' policies are to begin work from home procedures, participate in conferences, and hold meetings, whether in or out of the office. Video conferencing has become the standard, and with it, online meetings and seminars will become part of the New Normal workplace culture. This does not just apply to working in a corporation but also to study at a university or a high school. Many people, even those with impairments who need to be with their families, may benefit from this technology. This is not just an in-company only, but studying in the university or school as well. This tool may benefit many people, such as people with disabilities and who need to be with their families. Today, practical meeting tools for social distance are widely used, as described in the following subsections.

7.6.3.1 LINE

Thailand already had a high number of LINE users prior to the COVID-19. However, it is not yet obvious for academic purposes. After the lockdown, LINE has played a larger part in education, and teachers must develop ways to communicate with pupils about homework and assignments. All the school directors, instructors, and educational staff interviewed stated that by using the group LINE to establish a group with students, LINE returned to play a role in teaching and learning. A new LINE feature is the ability to use group calls that appear like teleconferencing. LINE groups make it easy to arrange online courses. Online tutoring through LINE's group sessions, on the other hand, is exclusively offered to primary school pupils. Teachers will seldom utilize LINE with kindergarten children. Teachers may only meet with pupils for 10–20 min so that kids may go to activities or worksheets, and parents can send worksheets to the teachers via LINE. In addition, LINE also plays a role in many other meetings because it can be used for unlimited meetings. Furthermore, a small group can meet together without many of the advanced features, allowing for communication individually. Parents could conveniently send files and images for meetings. Both large and small entrepreneurs use LINE as their main communication service since the lockdown.

7.6.3.2 Zoom

In Thailand, many universities consider using Zoom applications. The user who has created the room is considered an administrator or host of the room. When a person enters a Zoom conference room, they are considered an attendance hosted by another user. The meeting organizer or substitute host (if the original host is unable to attend) will have host controls, such as the capability to silence audio, utilize video, share your screen, and more. The attendance microphone can be muted and unmuted by the host. The host can also control the room's sound by clicking on the arrow next to the mute button, and the host will get further audio settings options. The host, for example, can change the attendance microphone, switch off the computer's audio, or access the audio settings. Attendees can switch on or off the camera by pressing the Start/Stop Video button. By pressing the arrow adjacent to the start/stop video button, attendees can swap showing cameras, adjust Zoom video options, or change a virtual background. The attendance can see who is presently in the meeting by clicking on participants and raising their hand or changing the name on the participant's list. Moreover, the attendance can share their screen in the meeting if the host allows it. The attendance screen share will be able to be stopped by the host. Other features of Zoom include a breakout room assignment. Zoom allows the host to assign participants into groups which encourages a smaller and active learning environment. The host or the instructor could quickly assess each student of their understanding, which is proven to be a convenient online alternative learning experience for college taught subjects that require active participation and higher level understanding, such as medicinal chemistry [24].

7.6.3.3 Google Meet

During the COVID-19 epidemic, the Google Meet application provides secure video conferencing for teams and companies while remaining simple for students to utilize. Organizations may use enterprise-grade video conferencing based on Google's secure global infrastructure to keep employees securely connected and on the go. It is backed up with safe design architecture.

Many Thai institutions have Google Education licenses, which are part of the Google Meet platform. Google Meet uses self-security and a well-known worldwide network to secure data and privacy to the greatest extent feasible. During transmission, Google Meet uses an encrypted video session, and various anti-abuse measures are activated by default. Google Meet is offered at no cost to educational institutions. However, in order to host a virtual meeting for up to 250 participants, the institution must register as an enterprise. Google Enterprise also includes features such as internal live broadcasting and the ability to save call recordings to Google Drive and the ability for room creators to invite up to 100 people to each Google Meet session without requiring them to install the Google Meet app on individual devices. Users can join the conference using only a web browser; moreover, room creators in Google Meet Enterprise can add group members for up to 24 h of video chatting. Meeting room organizers may now view all of the day's scheduled meetings in one place and join with a single tap from the dedicated Gmail mobile app or Meet app. Google Workspace also assigns a phone number to each meeting, ensuring that all attendees have a positive experience. Meetings may be joined immediately via calendar events, email invitations, or Gmail, which is also linked to Google's infrastructure. Those in attendance can join the meeting from any computer, phone, or conference room. All event details will be consistent. With live captioning, low-light mode, and noise suppression are employed, meetings become more productive.

7.6.3.4 Webex

Customers may need to hold an online conference when they begin to work from home. The school should invest more in online instruction and has begun to employ video conferencing software for distant sessions. During this time, one of the most popular programs is "Webex," which can hold continuous meetings for 50 min and handle 100 devices. Webex may be accessible via a variety of channels, including installing an app on a Tablet or Smartphone for both iOS and Android or using a web browser on a PC, Windows, or MAC OS, and there is software available to download into the device for convenience.

7.7 Social distancing and smart city

7.7.1 AI and big data

Various sensors and IoT devices are instruments that might be quite useful during the COVID-19 epidemic. Whether via shortwave radio networks such as Wi-Fi, NB-IoT, or cellular, these devices serve to notify the distance between individuals; if these devices join with the Internet system across the city, data from these devices may be gathered for processing. Furthermore, the data collected may be utilized with machine learning to develop a model to anticipate various clusters and infections and utilize GPS to notify individuals in close vicinity by putting them on a map or even creating a model for vaccine planning. The information might be used to create a quarantine plan for affected people or even to allocate hospital beds to deal with future epidemics. Thailand, for example, has a MorChana application that can monitor the course of infection from one person to another and is used for vaccine registration, which may be assigned to multiple medical facilities. Big data refers to information gathered through data gathering across the country and is used to plan vaccine allocation. The data can also be used to forecast the number of epidemic infections in the future by developing a machine learning model, such as linear regression or artificial neural network, with the input layer consisting of the number of infected people at the time, the number of classes, the infection rate, the vaccination rate, the death rate, the number of hospital visits, and the number of people who have been screened.

7.7.2 Implementation and usability

The COVID-19 problem in Thailand prompted application developers to construct an application (MorChana) for the government in a short period, despite the public's lack of knowledge of the usage. User-friendliness and UX/UI compatibility are critical for the major aspects of the application, which allow users to encounter minimal issues in order to receive correct and timely information. Furthermore, the adoption of this technology across the country causes frequent network failures and the delivery of erroneous SMS messages, resulting in the message not being verified. There was an issue with data handling, and the service had to be terminated. These applications rely on Google Maps for network services in order to use the maps. Furthermore, alerts from LINE apps and Facebook improve efficiency.

7.7.3 Privacy and security

When a huge volume of data is gathered, it is possible that it will contain illegal personal information. It is an issue in terms of violating personal rights, regardless of its stated goal of giving useful information for tracking the spread of COVID-19. As a result, privacy checks and the partial deactivation of personally identifiable information are necessary. Another consideration is the exchange of information across organizations. The link between government agencies such as hospitals, schools, subdistrict administrative organizations, and volunteers, the information transmitted may contain personal information that will impact that individual in the future.

7.7.4 Policy and legislation

Thailand passed the Personal Data Protection Act in 2019 to protect the personal information stored by government agencies. Citizens will be allowed to defend their privacy under the new law. The law, however, has been delayed for another year and will go into effect in 2022. Opening personal data regarding travel routes, work, and places is a breach of personal data, even if the individual did not intend to expose the information. As a result, after COVID-19, the government must account for data utilized for future epidemic prevention. During the COVID-19 period, people experience a variety of emotional reactions, including fear and anxiety. Because of the cognitive effect, COVID-19 has an impact on purchase decisions during lockdowns. One study examined the content of online newspapers and concluded that it is an important emotional component in individual purchase decisions. Incorrect belief rumors/false news, various types of viral social media news, and survival psychology are all key cognitive variables [25]. Furthermore, resolving the COVID-19 infection must not infringe on individual rights and must be supported by legislation in each nation. Major firms agreed that partial information must be disclosed in the form of an aggregate that does not identify a person. This information must be used to observe the distribution of COVID-19 clusters or other information that is used ethically.

7.8 Conclusion and future works

Amidst the unexpected crisis that arises from COVID-19, humanity looks for technology to solve problems, especially in their daily lives. Education is the first aspect where technology could be used to mitigate the health risks of crowded classrooms and auditoriums, but it also presents alternate solutions for those who seek further knowledge and fill educational gaps. LMSs are used widely by educational institutions to ease the access of course materials and to provide a simple tool for instructors to use; examples mentioned include Google Classroom and Moodle. MOOC is another alternative to regular classroom settings, allowing students to be able to access university-level course content onlinc for free, which promotes self-learning during the closure of schools and university campuses due to COVID-19. Along with the education sector, healthcare is in need of technological solutions to manage social-distancing guidelines in facilities and the management of patients. Wearable technology becomes a commodity for both patients and healthcare workers, which allows the administration to track movements and location and notify if a health policy has been a breach or if there is a potential health risk. In large healthcare facilities, a system is put in place to guide patients through the medical process easily. This includes a screening system to scan patients upon arriving at the facility, a queue system to manage the order of patients receiving medical care, and a payment system to ensure a safe and efficient checkout. However, protecting the public interest in health and safety from COVID-19 extends beyond the hospital walls. Some applications manage the general population's well-being by notifying them of potential health risks and organizing other health services in one system, such as vaccination registration. Another sector that employs the use of technology is manufacturing. Some technological solutions include using big data and AI such as video analytic and Wi-Fi monitoring to mitigate infection rates within manufacturing facilities. Some manufacturing firms also require employees to have a wearable device to monitor their conditions and their location for the best of the employee's interest and safety in the workspace. While health safety is important for the human workforce, intelligence systems are being used in all systems where human labor is redundant. These systems not only reduce the risk of mass infection within factories but also save cost and time. Nevertheless, many firms allow employees to work from home, which will help reduce employee interaction. To ensure protection from a data breach or other technological threats while working from home, VPN access and entitlements are given to each employee. Access to sensitive information is very limited. Different applications that would support remote work are also mentioned. These include VoIP, e-documents apps, cloud service, MIS, and conferencing apps, such as Zoom, Google Meet, and Webex. VoIP is very beneficial for call center applications, where existing Internet service and all voice calls are processed through the same channel. E-documents applications enable online collaborative documents to work to be done remotely, which could be a part of cloud services where file-sharing is made easier through the cloud. Meetings and conferences could also be held online due to in-person limitations by apps such as Webex, Zoom, and Google Meet. Achieving a fully hi-tech "New Normal" society requires a smart city framework. Agencies on many levels tend to lean in on AI and big data solutions. Still, intelligence systems tend to have limitations, and understanding the usage would be key to solve necessary tasks. The understanding of technology should also be given to the general public if technology is being implemented for their purpose. Other factors that should be considered are the privacy and security of the users, which are required by laws and policies.

References

[1] Muhammad L., Algehyne E.A., Usman S.S., *et al.* Supervised Machine Learning Models for Prediction of COVID-19 Infection Using Epidemiology Dataset. *SN Computer Science*. 2021; 2(1): 1–13.

[2] King N. *Template Analysis*. Sage Publications Ltd; 1998.

[3] Brooks J., McCluskey S., Turley E., *et al.* The Utility of Template Analysis in Qualitative Psychology Research. *Qualitative Research in Psychology*. 2015; 12(2): 202–222.

[4] Gunawan G., Suranti N.M.Y. and Fathoroni F. Variations of Models and Learning Platforms for Prospective Teachers During the COVID-19 Pandemic Period. *Indonesian Journal of Teacher Education*. 2020; 1(2): 61–70. Available from: https://journal.publication-center.com/index.php/ijte/article/view/95.

[5] Raza S.A., Qazi W., Khan K.A., *et al.* Social Isolation and Acceptance of the Learning Management System (LMS) in the Time of COVID-19 Pandemic: An Expansion of the UTAUT Model. *Journal of Educational Computing Research*. 2020; 59(2): 183–208. Available from: https://doi.org/10.1177/0735633120960421.

[6] Octaberlina L.R. and Muslimin A.I. EFL Students Perspective towards Online Learning Barriers and Alternatives Using Moodle/Google Classroom during COVID-19 Pandemic. *International Journal of Higher Education*. 2020; 9(6): 1–9. Available from: http://www.sciedu.ca/journal/index.php/ijhe/article/view/18485.

[7] Hermanto F. and Putri N.A. Learning Ability and Supporting Capacity of Online Learning In Students during Covid-19 Pandemic. *3rd International Conference on Environmental Geography and Geography Education IOP Conf. Series: Earth and Environmental Science*. 2021; 747(1): 012080. Available from: https://doi.org/10.1088/1755-1315/747/1/012080.

[8] John C., Staubitz T. and Meinel C. Took a MOOC. Got a Certificate. What Now?. In: *2019 IEEE Frontiers in Education Conference (FIE)*; 2019. p. 1–9. ISSN: 2377-634X.

[9] Razai M.S., Kankam H.K.N., Hourston G.J.M., *et al.* Lessons Learned From Producing Guidance Articles and Rapid Massive Open Online Courses During the Covid-19 Pandemic in Primary Care. *Journal of Primary Care & Community Health*. 2020; 11: 2150132720963624. Available from: https://doi.org/10.1177/2150132720963624.

[10] Sutrisno S. Increased Learning Activities and Outcomes Through Online Learning with Google Classroom in The Covid-19 Pandemic Period. *Ideguru: Jurnal Karya Ilmiah Guru*. 2020; 5(1): 95–106. Available from: https://jurnal-dikpora.jogjaprov.go.id/index.php/jurnalideguru/article/view/151.

[11] Filippidi A., Tselios N. and Komis V. Impact of Moodle Usage Practices on Students' Performance in the Context of a Blended Learning Environment. Proceedings of Social Applications for Life Long Learning; p. 2–7.

[12] Chakraborty C. and Abougreen A.N. Intelligent Internet of Things and Advanced Machine Learning Techniques for COVID-19. *EAI Endorsed Transactions on Pervasive Health and Technology*. 2021; 7(26).

[13] Islam M.M., Rahaman A. and Islam M.R. Development of Smart Healthcare Monitoring System in IoT Environment. *SN Computer Science*. 2020; 1(3): 185. Available from: https://doi.org/10.1007/s42979-020-00195-y.

[14] Alarifi A. and Alwadain A. Killer Heuristic Optimized Convolution Neural Network-Based Fall Detection with Wearable IoT Sensor Devices. *Measurement*. 2021; 167: 108258.

[15] Chakraborty C., Gupta B. and Ghosh S.K. A Review on Telemedicine-Based WBAN Framework for Patient Monitoring. *Telemedicine and e-Health*. 2013; 19(8): 619–626. PMID: 23841489. Available from: https://doi.org/10.1089/tmj.2012.0215.

[16] Chakraborty C., Gupta B. and Ghosh S.K. Mobile Metadata Assisted Community Database of Chronic Wound Images. *Wound Medicine*. 2014; 6: 34–42. Available from: https://www.sciencedirect.com/science/article/pii/S2213909514000445.

[17] Khandelwal P., Khandelwal A., Agarwal S., *et al.* Using Computer Vision to enhance Safety of Workforce in Manufacturing in a Post COVID World; arXiv:2005.05287. https://arxiv.org/abs/2005.05287.

[18] Seshadri D.R., Davies E.V., Harlow E.R., *et al.* Wearable Sensors for COVID-19: A Call to Action to Harness Our Digital Infrastructure for Remote Patient Monitoring and Virtual Assessments. *Front Digit Health*. 2020; 2: 8.

[19] Nguyen C.T., Saputra Y.M., Van Huynh N., *et al.* Enabling and Emerging Technologies for Social Distancing: A Comprehensive Survey and Open Problems. *IEEE Access*. 2020; 8: 153479–153507. Comment: 43 pages, 21 figures, journal.

[20] Venkatnarayan R.H. and Shahzad M. Demo: Measuring Distance Traveled by an Object Using WiFi-CSI and IMU Fusion. In: *2019 IEEE 27th International Conference on Network Protocols (ICNP)*; 2019. p. 1–2.

[21] Punn N.S., Sonbhadra S.K., Agarwal S., *et al.* Monitoring COVID-19 Social Distancing with Person Detection and Tracking via Fine-Tuned YOLO v3 and Deepsort Techniques. *arXiv*:200501385 [cs]. 2021.

[22] Zuo F., Gao J., Kurkcu A., *et al.* Reference-Free Video-to-Real Distance Approximation-Based Urban Social Distancing Analytics amid COVID-19 Pandemic. *Journal of Transport & Health*. 2021; 21: 101032. Available from: https://www.sciencedirect.com/science/article/pii/S2214140521000268.

[23] Coombs C. Will COVID-19 Be the Tipping Point for the Intelligent Automation of Work? A Review of the Debate and Implications for Research. *International Journal of Information Management*. 2020; 55: 102182.

[24] Singhal M.K. Facilitating Virtual Medicinal Chemistry Active Learning Assignments Using Advanced Zoom Features during COVID-19 Campus Closure. *Journal of Chemical Education*. 2020; 97(9): 2711–2714.
[25] Roy S. and Chakraborty C. Panic Buying Situation During COVID-19 Global Pandemic. *Journal of Information Technology Management*. 2021; 13(2): 231–244. Available from: https://jitm.ut.ac.ir/article_80625.html.

Chapter 8

Social health protection in touristic destinations during COVID-19

Zaklina Spalevic[1], Aleksandra Stojnev Ilic[2] and Milos Ilic[3]

Abstract

COVID-19 pandemic has caused huge economic losses in almost all industries. Thus, the economic crisis caused by this pandemic has modeled huge challenges for leisure industry. Travel bans, closed borders, mandatory quarantine after border crossing, reduced contacts are just some of the problems that citizens around the world have encountered. Observed from the point of view of tourism, a special problem was curfew and quarantine closure of cities and areas. All these significantly disrupted global tourism, which have been in full upswing in the years before pandemic. The research described in this chapter aims to give a description of the proposed software solution intended for better control and records of infected persons. The straightforward use of the proposed software solution aims to reduce the potential for the virus to spread among tourists. In order to reduce the potential for the spread of the virus, the proposed software solution needs to enable a better control of the movement of infected persons. Proper control of the movement of infected persons reduces the pressure on the tourism sector and opens the possibility of reoperation of tourist facilities for persons who are not infected. The proposed system is based on mutual cooperation of several actors. Thus, at the local and state level, the healthcare system can be singled out. Actors acting only at the local level are tourism organizations and local governments, while the actor acting only at the state level is border control. When it comes to the process of collecting personal data of patients, the bearer of this task within the system is the local health organization, which is certainly the first in contact with infected patients. In this way, the role of the healthcare organization is the proper registration of infected patients, and their entry into the proposed system. This part of the system also provides data on vaccinated and revaccinated patients. In order not to further burden the healthcare system, proposed software solution will use existing data and

[1]Faculty of Tourism and Hospitality Management, Singidunum University, Belgrade, Serbia
[2]Department of Computer Science and Informatics, Faculty of Electronic Engineering Niš, University of Niš, Niš, Serbia
[3]Department of Computer Science and Informatics, Faculty of Technical Sciences, University of Pristina, Kosovska Mitrovica, Serbia

will not require additional tests. Based on provided data from all actors, the integrated management system will create a database with vaccinated or tested positive persons. This database will be obtained by merging several databases into one so-called centralized register. However, each of the actors in the system has the right to use only that part of the data that is essential for their work. In this way, the system is able to protect personal patient data from unauthorized access. The system will allow one to check vaccination or home isolation status of an individual and, based on the results, approve or deny reservations. The edge/cloud architecture at the same time will provide data availability, and data access control.

Keywords: e-Health; COVID-19; Cloud; GDPR; Software application

8.1 Introduction

When this software solution is proposed (May 2021), 168 million people were infected by COVID-19 virus. In the same time this virus caused the deaths of around 3 million people worldwide. From the start of the 2020 year, more precisely after the onset of the COVID-19 virus, a mass pandemic people's daily activities were disordered with different constrains and rules. People's daily activities like interacting with each other, traveling, having fun have taken on a whole new form or have been banned. COVID-19 also affects different fields of world economy. From the aspect of human health, the COVID-19 virus has endangered both the physical and mental health of the world's population. In addition to physical and mental health, the fight against the pandemic also affected personal data privacy. Personal data were found in one chain cycle, where on the one hand it is necessary to preserve those, while, on the other hand, it is necessary to enable their processing in order to reduce pandemic [1].

One of the ways to fight the pandemic proposed by the World Health Organization is to close the borders of many countries around the world. Their borders remained closed for a long period of time for both visitors and tourists. This move has caused great economic losses, especially for those countries that base most of their budgets on tourism. Furthermore, the pandemic affected the tourism sections of these countries significantly, making it harder for economy. For the first time ever all global tourist destinations have introduced some form of restriction [2]. Restrictions in terms of movement, gatherings, travel did not bypass domestic tourism either. Revenues from domestic tourism have decreased significantly. The easing of measures enabled the reopening of tourist destinations. Of course, the emphasis on reopening was placed on respecting the prescribed measures and respecting the imposed restrictions. The overall situation with the pandemic has led to the fact that there are a large number of individuals who, despite the easing of measures and the opening of borders, do not dare to go on international trips. There is also a group of people who cannot afford international travel given that they have lost their jobs or their incomes have been significantly reduced. Prior to the pandemic, tourism was considered the sector with the highest economic growth. In support of this are the data that in 2018 alone, 1,407 million international departures were made. For the sake of comparison, some of the most popular countries in terms of the number of tourists such as France, China, Spain, during 2020 faced a large number of infected patients and the closure of borders, which led to a huge drop in visits compared to 2019. The extent to which the pandemic caused economic losses to the tourism sector is also shown by the fact that a loss of $297 billion was recorded in the United States alone, as a result of the suspension of tourism in the first quarter of the year [3]. Furthermore, for a very large number of countries, tourism represents the main income for their citizens, and in the same time basic government revenue, based on the fact that tourism is one of the industries that employ a significant number of workers. Without such a key type of earnings, many countries experienced significant losses in gross domestic product.* One of the partial solutions for economic and psychological crisis is to gather necessary information about tourists and use them to allow or deny different activities. By providing a solution for simplification and organization of patient data, categorization of individuals tested positive or negative, without compromising privacy rights. All these will be achieved within the proposed software solution by introducing different privacy policies. This will provide greater travel opportunities for individuals tested negative for COVID-19 or vaccinated ones. Viewed from the point of view of patients whose results have shown to be positive for the virus, the proposed software solution enables a better control of the movement of such patients, as well as a better control of compliance with measures to prevent the spread of the virus.

The proposed software solution described in this chapter is based on the use of data obtained from different sources. The data obtained from the health system database represent the backbone of the entire system. In practice, these data are crucial in separating people positive and negative for the COVID-19 virus. The data obtained from the health system within the proposed software solution are combined with the points obtained by the local administration, tourist organizations, as well as border control. In this way, the possibility of monitoring the movements of infected persons is realized. The contribution of the proposed system is primarily reflected in providing better data protection for persons registered as COVID-19 positive. In addition to data protection, the proposed software solution should reduce the spread of the virus by ensuring a better monitoring of infected persons and preventing their reckless behavior. Finally, for all those who are not infected, as well as for tourism in general, the contribution of the software solution is to ensure the reopening of tourist destinations and the free movement of all persons who are negative for the COVID-19 virus or vaccinated against it.

The chapter is organized as follows: the second section of the chapter provides an overview of the literature as well as relevant papers related to the research presented in this chapter. The third section describes the architecture of the proposed software solution intended for use in order to reduce the spread of viruses

*OECD Better Policies for Better Lives, Retrieved 15.10.2020, from http://www.oecd.org/.

and increase opportunities for tourism recovery. An overview of legal norms, laws, and bylaws related to the protection of personal data during the pandemic of the COVID-19 virus is given in the fourth section. The fifth section of the chapter summarizes key benefits of proposed system, key conclusions, and plans for future research.

8.2 Related work

The traditional approach to monitoring the health status of patients, as well as their treatment, has changed a lot during the last 2 years. A large number of medical institutions have switched from the traditional to the remote approach to treating patients, in all those cases where this was possible. A significant number of studies conducted on this topic have contributed to this treatment system. One of the researches on this topic described in [4] presents system for home healthcare. Practically, this is a system with remote access whose task is to provide assistance in the healthcare home. Within this chapter, the authors proposed a software system whose task from the patient's point of view is to obtain a prescription for medications without going to the doctor. System enables monitoring of the patient's health status in order to determine the right therapy. The software solution is based on the Android mobile application. This application connects to a web-based application. In this way, mutual communication between the doctor and the patient is possible. The collection of data relevant to the determination of therapy is done automatically using sensors. These sensors record the psychophysical parameters of the patient. In order to provide accurately read data of psychophysical parameters, the authors performed the installation of a HAC monitoring framework. With the implementation of this framework, the performance of the system itself has been improved. The proposed software solution aims to monitor patients remotely, without any contact with them. The proposed mobile platform enables the sending of daily values of parameters, as well as communication between the doctor and the patient, during the period of time that the patient spends in isolation.

The use of telemedicine to improve health services in rural and highly occupied areas of India was one of the topics of research presented in [5]. Within this chapter, the authors emphasized the possibilities of using new technological solutions in order to improve the healthcare system of India. The authors also emphasized that the use of technological solutions is especially visible during epidemics and pandemics. Epidemics and pandemics pose a kind of challenge for both the healthcare system and healthcare workers. The conclusion of the author is that the need for new information and communication solutions leads to quality changes in the management of the healthcare system. The research highlighted potential challenges, as well as the opportunities offered by the use of telemedicine in order to improve the healthcare system during a pandemic.

In the study conducted by the group of authors, a system aimed to detect COVID-19 virus based on thermal image processing is shown. Reduction of interference among people is provided by the use of a smart helmet [6]. The technologies on which the proposed solution is based included a thermal camera built into the smart slam and IoT technology. The task of IoT technology is reflected in monitoring the scanning process itself, as well as collecting data in real time. Also, the use of the mentioned technologies enabled another functionality that is reflected in the impregnation of faces. Practically, by impregnating the face, it is possible to obtain personal information of the person who is being scanned, and whose temperature is being measured. Such a system can be especially important when it comes to scanning the temperature of passengers at border crossings, as well as at airports of known tourist destinations.

Author in [7] presented the implemented information and communication technology system for remote monitoring of intensive care unit. The operation of the proposed system is based on the use of specially designed cameras and smartphones. The use of closed-circuit television cameras is suggested. Such high-resolution cameras are installed throughout intensive care. More precisely, a camera that monitors the operation of mechanical ventilation is placed above each bed in the intensive care unit intended for patients. The monitoring itself is organized cyclically.

In another study, the authors used cameras as a form of audiovisual communication with patients. Their goal was also to increase the level of protection of medical staff, as well as to monitor the condition of patients from a remote location [8]. In addition to the cameras, the use of the system itself required the installation of a server, which was used to store the values of the measured parameters. The group of vital patients parameters that were monitored by the proposed system included the patient's temperature, ECG, SpO_2, blood pressure, CO_2 and respiratory rate. The values of all parameters can be checked by the medical staff on a mobile phone. In this way, the mobile phone is a special tool used to monitor the patient's condition, as well as to alert medical staff if the patient's condition has deteriorated. The key thing in the whole system is the fact that for their own safety, the fashion staff dreams of contact with patients using such a system [9].

Authors in the one of the researches proposed a smart medical system for monitoring both the patient's condition and the condition of the room in which the patients are. The system is based on the use of the IoT platform and a set of selected sensors. The system was intended to monitor the condition of patients in hospital [10–12]. The given system also monitored the situation in their rooms. A total of five sensors were used to measure: heart beats, body temperature, room temperature, the amount of CO in the room, the amount of CO_2 in the room [13]. The use of such a system made it possible to monitor the condition of patients using a web portal. In this way, the medical staff was able to analyze the patient's condition at any time, which increased the effectiveness of treatment. The error rate within the system was below 5%.

In one of the researches, the authors created a mathematical model intended for the analysis of future growth of epidemic. In the same time, this model needs to predict how fast epidemic will grow. This model based on machine learning was applied during 2020. The main task of the created prediction model was to assess the speed of spread and danger of this virus in countries around the world [14]. The entire process of creating, training and using the prediction model was performed on the cloud platform in order to obtain more accurate results in real time. This approach to data storage and processing is beneficial to both government and citizens. Cloud computing within this model offers access capabilities regardless of user location.

The research presented in [15] was conducted in two major directions. The first direction was the challenges that the hospitality and tourism industry have due to the new situation with the COVID-19 virus pandemic. The second line of research concerned the vital industry. The research was based on interviews in which 15 participants participated. Participants were people in senior positions in hospitality and tourism. By analyzing the results obtained after all the interviews, 27 subtopics were created, which were later grouped into four larger groups. Out of the total number of 27 subtopics, some dominant subtopics singled it out. The main goal of the research was to determine the basic topics for combating a further decline in the tourism and hospitality rate caused by the COVID-19 virus pandemic.

Author in [16] presents latency minimization in e-healthcare through fog computing. More precisely, the authors presented a new scheme that uses machine learning, more precisely the *k*-fold random forest algorithm, to segregate multimedia data. The authors also presented models for calculating the total latency. By the simulation procedure, they repented that it is possible to create a model that will have a classification accuracy of 92%. The model also created showed a reduction in latency of approximately 95% compared to previously existing models. In this way, the quality of services belonging to e-health has been increased.

Authors in research presented in [17] show their model that should allow for anonymity. This model is based on the use of IoT technologies. The authors presented the RFID concept by which it is possible to track nonhuman virus carriers. Practically in this way, it will be possible to follow both animals and objects that move like cars. By applying the model, animals and moving objects will be able to send or receive notifications if they approach the marked area. The simulation results showed very high efficiency.

Panic shopping at the beginning of each of the pandemics can cause great logistics and supply to stores. The authors in one of the researches dealt with the analysis of panic purchases during the corona virus pandemic [18].

The contribution of machine learning applied to data obtained during a pandemic can facilitate decisions about its further course. The aim of one of the papers was to review the contribution of machine learning and IoT in the fight against the COVID-19 epidemic [19].

8.3 Proposal of software solution for health protection

The main global focus of actions for almost all countries in the world in the last 2 years was how to prevent the spread of a pandemic, and how to minimize its effect to different sectors such as economy, tourism, healthcare, and education. One of the greatest challenges almost all countries faced was how to protect the economy, when almost all industry stops working. As tourism, given the specificity that characterizes it (travel, gatherings of people, social events, etc.), is largely affected by the pandemic, it can be said that it has suffered the greatest losses compared to other industries. The collapse of the economy coming from tourism has directly affected a large number of families [20]. As the economies of almost all counties worldwide rely directly on the revenues that are generated from the tourism sector, it is necessary to find the best possible solution to relax the measures introduced in response to the corona virus pandemic. Given the seriousness of this pandemic, the opening of tourist destinations for tourists as well as the relaxation of the introduced measures must be carried out in a way that will not endanger the health of both natives and tourists.

Observed from the stakeholders' point of view and principally having in mind the current knowledge about the way the coronavirus spreads, as well as the ways to fight against it, some of the key factors can be singled out. In the first place, special attention should certainly be paid to tourists as potential carriers of the corona virus. Viewed from the point of view of tourists as carriers, tourists can bring the virus with them to the tourist destination where they are staying. Also, if, during their stay at a specific tourist destination, they come into contact with the virus and become infected, they can bring it home when they return and thus continue to spread it. In this regard, a very important aspect in the protection of the health of the population is certainly the precise testing and records of health institutions in terms of tested and positive people for COVID-19.

Immunization of the population as one of the key measures in the fight against the coronavirus opens up opportunities for easing measures, and restarting tourism, as well as for facilitated travel and movement of tourists. This practically means that it is necessary to establish a system that will provide facilities both in terms of performing daily activities and in terms of enabling travel to the immunized part of the population. Based on the regulations in force at the time of writing, persons who have a certificate are not COVID-19 positive, as well as persons who have been vaccinated, do not need to be in self-isolation. Each of the actors in the system has a clearly defined role. Also, each of the actors in the proposed software system has a predefined set of data with which it operates and for which it is responsible. The system itself is organized as a series of services, grouped by levels. Mutual interconnection of all actors could be seen from Figure 8.1.

8.3.1 System architecture

The entire system is organized as a collection of different services, each one of them providing different functionality. The architecture of this system is designed to control access to sensitive data to various actors and provide valuable information for each of them. Systemenables data travel toward the central storage system and back to the actors. This component is organized as a set of services available to other actors. The functionality of this component is based on four levels. These four levels are named: core, support, analysis and application.

Core level may contain certain services like core data, commands, and metadata. Services on core level provide intermediary communications between the actors of the system. The core data service family provides a centralized persistence

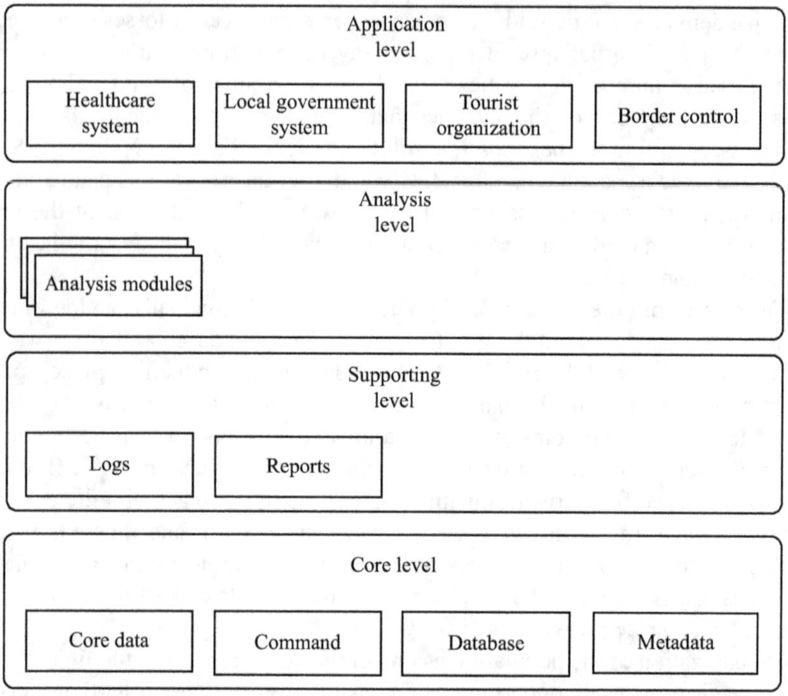

Figure 8.1 Architecture of the proposed software solution

facility for data readings and also implements different protocols for data protections. If the data need to be preprocessed for clarification, or if there are invalid instances that must be processed, this is where such a service will be logically located. Command represents a service family that facilitates and controls action requests from one side of the system to another. It should expose the commands in a common, normalized way to simplify communications between the actors. Metadata represent a repository and associated management service of metadata about the actors that are connected to platform. Metadata provide the possibility to create new sources, and store and manage information about the services that serve as platform interfaces to the actual actors. Database services are other services that communicate directly with the actors and normalize information and communications.

The service layer provides support for the operation of software applications such as logging, data cleaning, data scheduling. In our cases, supporting service cannot be considered optional, as it is necessary to provide legal traces for data sharing. These services can be fundamental because they could provide valuable evidences in case of data leak or breach. Furthermore, this type of application features can be very important for maintenance, bug tracing and further development of the system. Service architecture can allow each of the actors to have their own settings for logging and log file storage.

Since we created a system that has access to global data, it will be useful to perform different analytics tasks on the collected and shared data. In this way, we can get useful insights from the data that are relevant not only to public health, but also for the entire human existence and well-being. Services in this level can use data for which they have access permissions, making this entire system more resilient for data breaches. Although this level is rather optional, we expect it to become main focus of development in the future. With the increased data, the demand for analysis will be brought to the fronts, because the knowledge extracted from confirmed accurate data can be valuable for the entire population.

The role of application level is to extract, process/transform and send data from platform to an actor. Services on the application level should be adjusted to meet different requirements from different users. Furthermore, special attention must be given to data privacy and data access control services. Each actor of the system will be represented as a service on this level. This is the most efficient way to control shared data and data access among the participants. Furthermore, services on this level can use results and models created in analysis level to create different actions or to generate comprehensive reports that can provide useful knowledge.

This way of organizing the management system was chosen to support expansions while taking data privacy in mind. Each of the individual actors of the system is enabled to operate on data on different devices. More about the individual functionalities of each part of the system from the point of view of individual actors will be given in the following sections. Each component on the application level will be explained. Components on the other levels in this system are very general and not specific to this particular implementation and usage and thus are not explained in detail in this chapter.

8.3.2 Healthcare service

The proposed system identifies the healthcare system of each of the countries as a stakeholder. As we mentioned earlier, the role of the healthcare system is to create a register of infected people and enter the personal data of each of the patients who are positive for the COVID-19 virus. These data are crucial in the fight against this virus [21]. The healthcare service would have access only to the data for individuals who were tested positive to the virus. In this way, unnecessary sharing of patients' personal data will be reduced. Other actors need data on persons currently positive for the COVID-19 virus as a starting point for future use. Each of the actors in the system uses the obtained data in order to control and reduce the possibility of irresponsible movement and spread of COVID-19 virus by infected persons. Such tourists, depending on the competent authorities who discover their movements in the period in which they should be in isolation, will be processed in an adequate manner.

Another part of the healthcare service is a communicator for the IoT system intended for monitoring the health condition of patients who are being treated within a tourist destination. Practically, if tourists are hospitalized during their stay, the system enables the collection of parameters such as body temperature, CO_2

emissions and storage of all measured values on the cloud via a central software platform. In this way, after they recover and return home, the local health institution has data on the patient's condition and all the treatments he has undergone. Data of this type can be entered within the system either by healthcare professionals, if their additional processing is required before the entry or automatically using a data logger after each reading from the installed sensors. The role of the data adapter as well as the filters shown in Figure 8.1, which belong to the healthcare system, is reflected in the processing of data about each patient. In this way, the recorded data on each individual patient required for the treatment of the patient are processed so that only those data that are relevant will be forwarded to the central system. The use of the mentioned adapter and filter prevents the exchange of irrelevant data on patients of a specific healthcare institution. For example, data on patients not recorded as COVID-19 positive would be considered irrelevant data. Also if a person is recorded as COVID-19 positive, data on his or her previous medical history will not be relevant within the proposed system and should therefore certainly not be taken from the system of the healthcare institution. Operating exclusively on approved data, as well as their targeted use by specific system actors, reduces the possibility of their misuse.

Regarding the processing of data on the immunized part of the population, depending on the immunization policy and recognition of vaccines of individual manufacturers, each of the holdings within the system will define the rules according to which other system actors will be guided when checking a particular tourist. The task of the healthcare system within the immunization process is to accurately record data on each person who received both the first and second doses of the vaccine. Observed from the angle of the proposed software system, the healthcare institution records data on each individual patient after vaccination. After receiving the second dose, the healthcare institution should, in accordance with the regulations issued by the state authorities of the country to which it belongs, issue a certificate of vaccination to the patient. It should also add the electronic data from the certificate to the central software platform of the proposed software system. Electronic data on each vaccinated citizen in this way would become available to all other actors in the system, which would enable easier control of potential tourists, as well as tourists whose period of stay has already begun.

8.3.3 Tourist service

Travel agencies as one actor of the proposed system have the task of entering data on each individual reservation in the central register. In this way, anyone who makes a reservation for accommodation or tourist tours can be checked through the system by looking for matching personal data on the cloud. The task is to find potential matches. Match detection refers to the search of data on the traveler who wants to book accommodation, travel tickets, tourist tour and the like within the proposed system. The first check that is made is whether there is a person within the system who registers it as COVID-19 positive. If the person is COVID-19 positive or if he has been in contact with positive people, the reservation will not be approved. Exceptions are cases when a COVID-19 positive person creates a reservation for the period of stay that will be realized after the anticipated period of isolation. Potential tourists who submit a negative PCR test or vaccination certificate are checked within the proposed system. Practically in this way, the authenticity of the attached document is checked. If a person is indeed negative for COVID-19 or has been immunized with one of the vaccines, it must be added to the system by a healthcare institution that has performed either testing or immunization. The employee within the travel agency forwards the data for verification within the proposed system and receives a confirmation of the authenticity of the documents. Vaccinated tourists must submit the green certificate or QR code in order to prove that they received both doses of the vaccine. The speed of checking the data of each of the tourists largely depends on the uniformity of the document on the performed vaccination, which is issued by the authorized health institution. This is especially reflected in cases when it comes to checking data for tourists who are residents of another country or have not been vaccinated in their own country.

The application of such a system reduces the pressure on hoteliers, tourist organizations as well as staff employed within tourist destinations. If each individual tourist who paid for the stay through the agency has previously checked the task of local tourist organizations, the hotel staff is reflected only in checking tourists who have organized specific activities within the tourist destination (accommodation, tourist tours, transportation, etc.) using various applications or in person at the tourist place.

8.3.4 Local government service

As tourists can independently organize their stay in a tourist destination, the task of local self-government is reflected in the entry and verification of data for each tourist when registered by hoteliers. Practically, these are tourists who did not book their stay through a travel agency, so they found accommodation upon arrival in the desired tourist place. In order to take advantage of the services of a specific accommodation, they must submit either a certificate of negative PCR test results or a vaccination certificate. On the other hand, every registered hotelier must register his guests in the branch office of the local tourist organization that operates within the local government of the municipality in which they are located. The tourist organization in cooperation with the local government institutions can check the fulfillment of the conditions of stay of each individual guest. When registering its guests and based on checking, the match of personal data of the guest with the data available in the database of the proposed software system, the local tourist organization using the software system received information whether a particular person registered as COVID-19 is positive. In order to successfully perform the test, they must have appropriate access to the system. By entering the data belonging to a specific guest, as well as scanning with the reader both personal documents and QR code on the certificate of negative PCR test, or certificate of vaccination, the process of checking all documents begins. Also, the appropriate institutions of local self-government are informed if the check shows that the vaccination certificate has been falsified. Such an organized check once again shows that uniformity is needed when it comes to documents confirming the performed vaccination or negative results of the PCR test.

8.3.5 Border control

Border control between countries where there are border crossings can be said to be the first barrier on which the separation of positive from nonpositive passengers can be made. The primary goal of such screening is to keep positive individuals within their country and prevent the spread of coronavirus. By doing this, it is possible to contain the virus on geographic basis and to track its spread across the countries.

Border control needs to enter the data into the proposed system of all their citizens who enter or left the country. The task of border control is reflected in the fact that when checking the identity of a person entering or leaving the country, he also checks whether a specific person is in the database of the proposed system, and whether that person is registered as COVID-19 positive. Verification is used by accessing the proposed software platform of the proposed system. If the passenger is not in the system as a person whose test results have shown that he is positive for COVID-19, the authenticity of the vaccination document is checked if the person has been vaccinated and if he has the given document. Also, if the person is not registered as COVID-19 positive, it is checked whether he has a certificate of negative PCR test, the authenticity of which should be confirmed. In case when passenger met all the conditions for entering in the country, the same will be approved. Another functionality of the proposed system by the border control is the entry of data on persons who were randomly tested when crossing the border. If such persons are found to have tested positive at the border to be COVID-19, they will notify the local self-government to which the place where the specific tourists stayed is in order to locate them and quarantine them. Applying this principle reduces the possibility of crossing borders for those people who are positive and thus reduces the potential for the spread of the virus.

8.4 Data protection

The COVID-19 virus pandemic has undoubtedly affected daily activities in people's lives and work. Normal activities quite normal for the human race have become something that must be avoided. On the other hand, something that is personal and that should not be important to others has become a topic of the majority. Among other things, the pandemic did not bypass human rights and personal data protection. Many individuals and various organizations, under the pretext of preventing the spread of the pandemic and its consequences, have given themselves the right to access and publicly disclose the personal data of persons infected or who have died from the COVID-19 virus. Precisely for this reason, the question has been asked about the data that relate to others, which can be used in cases of epidemics and the protection of humanity, and for what purpose they can be used. On the other hand, it is necessary to clearly emphasize what are the personal data that, regardless of the situation, no one would have the right to use without the prior consent of the person to whom they relate [22]. From the point of view of the healthcare system, it can be said that in the event of a pandemic, the health system is the one that has the most sensitive data of people infected with the virus. A number of studies have shown that data on infected people are crucial in order to create opportunities for their publication to process them and draw conclusions that can reduce the pandemic and thus reduce the number of infected people. Also, monitoring the condition of patients using digital devices that log each read parameter is of undoubted importance to the scientific community in the process of creating predictive models that would much more accurately predict the future condition of patients. Observed from the point of view of patients, and based on published experiences, it is concluded that in the case of the COVID-19 virus pandemic, the publication of data on infected people led to alienation and distance between people, which greatly affected the psyche of patients and their environment.

This way of collecting and processing data obtained in digital form by the health system can lead to the fact that a large amount of both personal and non-personal data from the group of sensitive data can be found in the data. If such data are not used exclusively for the purpose of suppressing the spread of the pandemic, but are misused, then such a processing procedure can lead to a serious violation of human rights.

A potential problem that may arise in the process of collecting, publishing and processing personal data of patients as well as data on their health status is the use of these data even after the end of the epidemic. More precisely, the problem that may arise is the public availability of data, which can enable individuals or organizations to use them even after the approval issued during the epidemic, has formally ceased to be valid. Precisely for these reasons, it is necessary to unequivocally adopt laws and bylaws that would regulate this area, as well as that would regulate cases in which it is possible to make exceptions. It is of utmost importance to control the access to these data, if possible only to machines, which will generate summarized and anonymized results when possible. Regarding the healthcare system, it is advisable to apply the principle of patient data confidentiality.

In response to the problems of digital personal data protection during the COVID-19 pandemic, a European Union directive on the privacy of electronic communications was adopted. Within the framework of this directive, it is explicitly defined that data obtained from any source for processing for the purpose of combating the COVID-19 pandemic may be used only if they are anonymous. More precisely, if any information that may indicate which person is in question has been removed from the data itself. If it is not possible to make the data anonymous by removing information about the person in question, each of the member states should prescribe special regulations that will regulate how to act in such situations. Transferred to medical data, by removing the personal data of the patient or his ID, it is possible to use all other information related to the example for diagnosis, measured values of various parameters and so on.

After the adoption of the directive, many countries of the European Union and beyond began to apply it, especially in the field of collecting the location of people of interest. For example, in Italy, mobile operators have made data on the locations of their users available to government services. This was of particular importance to the Ministry of Health as it made it possible to point out citizens who had disobeyed a restraining order or home isolation. Similar to the Italian model, the Polish authorities created a software solution that used mobile operators to wash citizens who should be in quarantine. The application is created so that from time to time, without the exact time interval, it requires citizens to take selfies with geolocation to determine whether the quarantine measure is adhered to or not. The authorities in China have gone even further, so that every citizen, when returning from abroad, receives an electronic bracelet that sends geolocation, as well as a warning to the authorities if there is a violation of the self-isolation measure. Singapore, on the other hand, has made all data on patients and citizens tested positive. This procedure is designed so that all citizens who are in the database can be followed and in order to discover which part of the country can be a potential hotbed.

Articles 6 and 9 of the GDPR define legal norms related to employers and healthcare organizations, which regulate the handling of personal data in the epidemic. However, the exchange of information in such cases must be proportional to the risk and the actual need for exchange, meaning that organizations must check regularly and carefully if the data access is absolutely necessary. It is up to employers to adopt the measurements that must be taken to protect their employees [23].

The protection of personal data was certainly one of the aspects when developing the proposed software solution. The use of data obtained from the healthcare system within the proposed system is done with special attention aimed at their protection [24].

8.5 Conclusion and future works

The corona virus pandemic has visibly disrupted people's daily routine, their habits and life plans. In order to prevent the further spread of the corona virus, measures have been introduced that restrict movement, travel, gatherings and everything that makes human beings the way we are. The tourism sector has suffered heavy economic losses by closing borders and banning the operation of accommodation facilities within tourist destinations. The proposed software solution aims to provide tools to system users to work together to reduce the impact of the pandemic on the work of the tourism sector and restart tourism. The main task is certainly to provide a mechanism to protect the health of the population, in order to prevent the re-expansion of the pandemic.

The proposed software solution is architecturally based on a service architecture to allow decoupling and expansion of the system. The service architecture of the proposed system is designed in a way that is suitable for adaptation and expansion. That is a very important property of a system that should be used for public data, because once integrated, it would not be easily replaceable or architecturally modified. The main task of this platform is to provide a mechanism of communication among several actors of the system taking into account the privacy of the data. As it works with data that belong to the group of personal data, mechanisms for the protection of this data must be provided, and the system must be developed with privacy in mind. By decoupling the entire system to different services with strict data access rights, actors in the system access only the set of data that is important to them. Also, if it is necessary to access a broader set of data, each access is recorded and searches over the data are performed independently of the system actors, while it presents the required results. Furthermore, it is possible to run an extensive analysis on the data that can be configured to only show results relevant to broad population and anonymize the data to hide personal information.

The use of such a system, both locally and globally, by as many countries in the world as possible will enable the relaxation of measures to combat the coronavirus, which further leads to greater travel opportunities and economic strengthening of tourist destinations. The basic precondition for the successful implementation of such a system, which would offer the possibility of relaxing measures and strengthening the collapsed tourism sector and the global economy of many countries, is the continuous and joint work of state and world institutions.

The problems caused by the COVID-19 virus pandemic are far from being solved. As the pandemic affected almost all branches of the economy, the economic consequences are still expected. In order to mitigate the economic consequences in the tourism sector, it is almost immediately necessary to act and enable unhindered travel and work of tourist destinations. On the other hand, given the fact that the spread of the virus has not stopped and that new strains of the virus are emerging, everything needs to be approached in the right way. The proposed solution requires mutual coordination and work of both the tourism sector and government institutions at the local and state levels. Further research will be focused on the full implementation of the proposed system and its application in real conditions. It is expected that the system can greatly contribute to preventing the spread of the virus by reckless behavior of individuals. The advantages of using such a system will enable its use in cases of other viruses, not only COVID-19.

Further continuation of the described research will include the implementation of the test model of the proposed system. The implementation of the test model of this system should show through a series of simulations and practical use what is the success rate of the application of such a system. A high success rate is expected, which would indicate the fact that the implementation of such a system in practice is justified.

References

[1] Ventrella E. 'Privacy in emergency circumstances: data protection and the Covid-19 pandemic'. *ERA Forum*. 2020; 21, pp. 379–393.

[2] Gössling S., Scott D. and Hall C. M. 'Pandemics, tourism and global change: a rapid assessment of Covid-19'. *Journal of Sustainable Tourism*. 2020; 29 (1), pp. 1–20. https://doi.org/10.1080/09669582.2020.1758708.

[3] Farzanegan M. R., Gholipour H. F., Feizi M., Nunko R. and Andargoli A. E. 'International tourism and outbreak of coronavirus (Covid-19): a cross-country analysis'. *Journal of Travel Research*. 2021; 60. https://doi.org/10.1177/0047287520931593.

[4] Olutosin T. and Absalom E. E. 'Smart healthcare support for remote patient monitoring during covid-19 quarantine'. *Informatics in Medicine Unlocked*. 2020; 20, pp. 1–11.

[5] Geetanjali S., Munish S. and Ajita K. 'Evolution of smart healthcare: telemedicine during COVID-19 pandemic'. *Journal of the Institution of Engineers (India): Series B*. 2021, pp. 1–6.

[6] Mohammed N. A., Halimatuz Z., Sairah A. K., Rusyaizila R. and Eddy Y. 'Novel covid-19 detection and diagnosis system using IoT based smart helmet'. *International Journal of Psychosocial Rehabilitation*. 2020; 24(7), pp. 2296–2303.

[7] Naveen N. R. G., Ajay S., Shiv L. S. and Puri G. D. 'Real-time smart patient monitoring and assessment amid COVID-19 pandemic – an alternative approach to remote monitoring'. *Journal of Medical Systems*. 2020; 44(131), pp. 130–131.

[8] Singh A., Naik B. N., Soni S. L. and Puri G. D. 'Real-time remote surveillance of doffing during COVID-19 pandemic: enhancing safety of health care workers'. *Anesthesia & Analgesia*. 2020; 131, pp. e112–e113.

[9] Zhang Y., Liu H., Su X., Jiang P. and Wei D. 'Remote mobile health monitoring system based on smart phone and browser/server structure'. *Journal of Healthcare Engineering*. 2015; 6(4), pp. 717–737.

[10] Rahman A., Chakraborty C., Anwar A., *et al.* 'SDN-IoT empowered intelligent framework for Industry 4.0 applications during COVID-19 pandemic'. *Cluster Computing*. 2021, pp. 1–18. 10.1007/s10586-021-03367-4.

[11] Dash S., Chakraborty C., Giri S. K., Pani S. K. and Frnda J. 'BIFM: big-data driven intelligent forecasting model for COVID-19'. *IEEE Access*. 2021; 9, pp. 97505–97517. 10.1109/ACCESS.2021.3094658.

[12] Aslam B., Javed A. R., Chakraborty C., Nebhen J., Raqib S. and Rizwan M. 'Blockchain and ANFIS empowered IoMT application for privacy preserved contact tracing in COVID-19 pandemic'. *Personal and Ubiquitous Computing*. 2021, pp. 1–17. 10.1007/s00779-021-01596-3.

[13] Islam Md. M., Rahaman A. and Islam Md. R. 'Development of smart healthcare monitoring system in IoT environment'. *SN Computer Science*. 2020; 1(185).

[14] Tuli S., Tuli S., Tuli R. and Gill S. S. 'Predicting the growth and trend of COVID-19 pandemic using machine learning and cloud computing'. *Internet of Things*. 2020; 11.

[15] Kaushal V. and Srivastava S. 'Hospitality and tourism industry amid COVID-19 pandemic: perspectives on challenges and learnings from India'. *International Journal of Hospitality Management*. 2021; 92, pp. 1–19.

[16] Kishor A., Chakraborty C. and Jeberson W. 'A novel fog computing approach for minimization of latency in healthcare using machine learning'.

International Journal of Interactive Multimedia and Artificial Intelligence. 2020, pp. 1–11. dx.doi.org/10.9781/ijimai.2020.12.004.

[17] Garg L., Chukwu E., Nasser N., Chakraborty C. and Garg G. 'Anonymity preserving IoT-based COVID-19 and other infectious disease contact tracing model'. *IEEE Access*. 2020; 8, pp. 159402–159414.

[18] Roy S. and Chakraborty C. 'Panic buying situation during COVID-19 global pandemic'. *Journal of Information Technology Management*. 2021; 13(2), pp. 231–44.

[19] Chakraborty C. and Naser Abougreen A. 'Intelligent Internet of Things and advanced machine learning techniques for COVID-19'. *EAI Endorsed Transactions on Pervasive Health and Technology*. 2021; 7, pp. 1–14.

[20] Gretzel U., Fuchs M., Baggio R., *et al.* 'e-Tourism beyond COVID-19: a call for transformative research'. *Information Technology & Tourism*. 2020; 22, pp. 187–203.

[21] Zwitter A. and Gstrein O. 'Big data, privacy and COVID-19 – learning from humanitarian expertise in data protection'. *Journal of International Humanitarian Action*. 2020; 5(4), pp. 1–7.

[22] Brouder P. 'Reset redux: possible evolutionary pathways towards the transformation of tourism in a Covid-19 world'. *Tourism Geographies an International Journal of Tourism Space, Place and Environment*. 2020; pp. 1–7.

[23] Fahey R. A. and Hino A. 'Covid-19, digital privacy, and the social limits on data-focused public health responses'. *International Journal of Information Management*. 2020; 55, pp. 1–5.

[24] Spalević Ž. and Ilić M. 'Management of tourist personal data protection in COVID 19 – it perspectives, legal and economic aspects'. *5th International Thematic Monograph – Modern Management Tools and Economy of Tourism Sector in Present Era*. 2020. pp. 409–424.

Chapter 9

Analysis of Artificial Intelligence and Internet of Things in biomedical imaging and sequential data for COVID-19

Sinthia Roy Banerjee[1], Saurav Mallik[2], Tapas Si[3], Arijit Banerjee[4], Shan Jiang[5] and Sudip Podder[6]

Abstract

Biomedical data analysis is an exceedingly broad field. It includes array data analysis, biomedical image analysis, integrated or hybrid data analysis, and patient data analysis using machine learning (ML) and artificial intelligence (AI). Array data analysis can be further classified into RNA-sequence, single-cell RNA-sequence, microarray, and ChiP-seq data analysis. Biomedical imaging encompasses different parameters like gathering of biomedical signal, formation of an image, processing of an image, display of image, and the medical diagnosis that are built on the features obtained from various images. AI was mainly used to break down healthcare data and used to track and screen patients while Internet of Things was used mainly for monitoring a patient remotely. There are different radiological imaging processes that include the radiography, ultrasound, thermography, magnetic resonance imaging, nuclear medicine and computed tomography. We, in this book chapter, provide a comprehensive survey (road map) on various array-based sequence data analyses and biomedical imaging along with their integrated studies for different tissue-specific dreadful diseases (such as cancer). We included the integrated studies of biomedical imaging and array-based data analysis for the same set of patients (samples) that covered the problem of combinatorial gene signature detection as well as disease subtype image classifications while specific multi-modal data from well-known data repository (e.g., TCGA, ICGC) had been

[1]Department of Computer Science and Engineering, University of Calcutta, Kolkata, India
[2]Center for Precision Health, School of Biomedical Informatics, University of Texas Health Science Center at Houston, Houston, USA
[3]Department of Computer Science and Engineering, Bankura Unnayani Institute of Engineering, Bankura, India
[4]Siemens Healthineers Pvt. Ltd., Bangalore, India
[5]Pamela Sklar Division of Psychiatric Genomics, Icahn School of Medicine at Mount Sinai, New York, USA
[6]Institute for Integrated Circuits, Johannes Kepler University Linz, Linz, Austria

provided. Finally, our book chapter covers the maximum area of biomedical imaging as well as array-based sequence data analysis along with the contribution of AI and ML in order to build a smart healthcare system, and provide a new dimension to the interested biomedical researchers.

Keywords: Biomedical imaging; Microarray; RNA-sequence (RNA-scq); Single-cell RNA-sequence (scRNA-seq); De novo mutation (DNM); Chromatin Immunoprecipitation Sequence (CHiP-Seq); Computed tomography (CT); Magnetic resonance imaging (MRI); Nuclear medicine imaging (NMI)

9.1 Introduction

The anthology of biomedical information is a major important element of research in the domain of both biological and social science. Both the collections and usage of biomedical information in social research have been growing rapidly. This increase reflects both the growing recognition of the importance of understanding the relationships between biomedical measures of health and individual outcomes and the growth of multidisciplinary research frameworks that blend social and medical paradigms of knowledge. The recent outbreak of COVID-19 pandemic has turned the world upside down. Biomedical data analysis helps in understanding the risks and signs with different consequences detected in patients with COVID-19. Image analysis, array analysis, and hybrid analysis play an equally important role in identifying the deadly COVID-19. Array data analysis is the procedure of exposing a DNA, RNA, or any peptide sequence to abroad range of analytical processes so that it can understand its features, its functionality, its structure, and its evolution. We have even observed that array is immediately competent to differentiate clean from recuperative COVID-19 subjects. Various methodologies used here include sequence alignment, search against different biological databases. Array data analysis can further be classified as RNA-seq, single-cell RNA-sequence (scRNA-seq), microarray, and ChiP-seq data analysis. Moreover, biomedical imaging as stated by Jiang [1] has been also undergoing a rapid technical advancement over the last couple of decades. It has been observed the development of various new applications to biomedical imaging. Different procedures such as functional imaging, imaging related to spectroscopy, optical imaging, and the various image-guided interventional techniques related to treatment or therapy have been attaining the recognition in different domains extending from fundamental research to clinical applications, and also from the cellular to the tissue and even to the organ level. Biomedical imaging is a multidisciplinary field that requires the efficient collaboration among researchers of different fields, including biologists, medical physicists, chemists, pharmacists, computer scientists, statistician, biomedical engineers, and other clinicians of different specialties. Efficacy, skill, and instruments provided by the different radiologists are an integral part of various clinical research programs [2]. Application of biomedical imaging is rising day by day and it is becoming an emerging research topic as an essential fundamental clinical investigational pro forma. Interestingly, biomedical imaging has a key role in cancer research. Array-based next generations sequencing data analysis is another hot biomedical research topic in this current era [3,4]. DNA microarray [5] is a structured and efficient technology that can simultaneously identify all levels of hundreds and thousands of transcripts (viz., miRNAs [6], genes, lncRNAs) across various sample groups or tissue samples [3,4,6,7]. Besides biomedical data analysis, artificial intelligence (AI) in healthcare primarily implies to physicians and medical service providers retrieving enormous datasets of hypothetically life-saving data. This involves medication techniques and their results, endurance levels, and pace of treatment collected around many patients, topographical sites, and numerous and at times interrelated well-being situations. Innovative processing capability can identify and evaluate huge and minor developments from the records and yet produce projections via machine learning (ML) that is intended to recognize prospective well-being results. Internet of Things (IoT)-supported machines have made remote monitoring in the healthcare sector possible, making it able to maintain patients secure and healthy, and enabling doctors to provide excellent treatment. It has also improved patient commitment and contentment as collaborations with doctors have turned out to be simpler and more effective. Moreover, remote monitoring of patient's well-being supports in decreasing the duration of hospital stay and avoids readmissions. IoT also has a key effect on lowering healthcare expenses substantially and thereby enhancing medication results.

A lot of works have been performed on all of these, but we think lots are yet to be done. Thereafter, there is a huge challenge for new researchers to grab these domains together, along with their integrated study to have a smooth progress in their research. Hence, in our book chapter, we portray a thorough survey or (road map) on various biomedical imaging and array-based sequence data analyses along with their integrated studies for different tissue-specific dreadful diseases (such as cancer) and usage of smart technologies. In this regard, initially, we provided different algorithms on biomedical imaging [8] that included multilevel thresholding [9,10], Markov random field (MRF) model [11], and clustering algorithms [12]. The advantages, shortcomings, and usages of different algorithms of biomedical imaging are demonstrated here. Second, we yielded a different array-based sequence data analysis algorithm that is very much useful for biomedical research. These array-based data might be divided into different categories, viz., single-cell sequencing data, RNA-seq data [6], microarray data. Various algorithms applied to each category of the sequence data have been notified here. This includes various computational problems such as gene signature discovering, biomarker discovery, disease classification or disease subtype classification, differential expression or differential methylation analysis, prognosis study, gene module detection [13,14], multi-modal data integration, etc. For each problem, specific algorithms (or, tools) have been mentioned here for the benevolent of the new researchers in this domain. The advantages, limitations, and overall usages of each category of the algorithms along with the corresponding comparative study of the different categories of algorithms are also described here. Furthermore, we

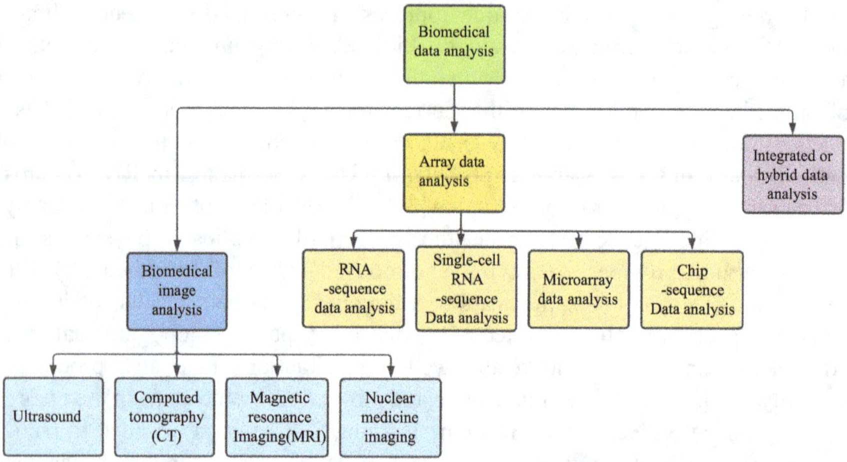

Figure 9.1 Classification of biomedical data analysis

included the integrated study of biomedical imaging [15,16] and array-based data analysis for the same set of patients (samples) that covered the problem of combinatorial gene signature detection as well as disease subtype image classifications while specific multimodal data from well-known data repository (e.g., TCGA, ICGC) had been provided. Finally, our book chapter covers the maximum area of biomedical imaging as well as array-based sequence data analysis along with the contribution of AI and ML in order to build a smart healthcare system and provide a new dimension [17] to the interested biomedical researchers. The chapter aims to provide researchers a review on various topics of biomedical data and the advancement of new technologies that can be used to assist in battling COVID-19 disease.

The major contributions of the book chapter include the following: the first section demonstrates the definition of various biomedical data and a comparative study on different computational algorithms (AI- and IoT-based techniques) applied to the biomedical data, while the second section of this book chapter covers the advent of smart technologies during COVID-19 [18,19]. The last chapter describes the conclusion regarding the empowerment of the new researchers to further work on evolving additional solutions to combat COVID-19 and its future applications in other biomedical applications (Figure 9.1).

9.2 Definition of biomedical keywords

9.2.1 Microarray and RNA-seq data

Microarray is a useful tool applied to determine the expression levels of thousands of transcriptomes (genes) in the same time. DNA microarrays are termed microscope slides that are used to print with thousands of tiny spots in specific predefined positions, while each spot consisting of a defined DNA sequence (gene). The microarrays are easier to use and cost-effective. They do not require huge scale of DNA sequencing.

RNA sequencing (RNA-seq) is a process that is used to study the magnitude and structures of RNA in a sample employing the next generation sequencing technique. We can get RNA-seq data from various sources like ICGC, TCGA, NCBI Gene Omnibus as stated by Geng *et al.* [2]. scRNA-seq is a demanding topic used since the last decade. The scRNA-seq data are a prevalent and robust technology that permits researchers to describe the entire transcriptome of a huge quantity of specific cells. scRNA-seq data are a popular dataset nowadays, but analyzing scRNA-seq data is difficult due to technical variability, high noise levels, and its massive sample sizes. scRNA-seq data have more dropouts and most often generate sparse matrix that makes it a challenging process to identify original zeros and dropouts.

9.2.2 De novo mutation

De novo mutation, as stated by Jiang *et al.* [1], refers to non-inherited mutation or most specifically a mutation that is not present in every cell of parents. So, it implies that the mutation happened in the sperm or the egg that generates the offspring. Basically, the genetic modification that occurred initially in one of the family members as an outcome of a metamorphosis in a germ cell, i.e., either egg or sperm of one of the parents, or any variation that develops in the fertilized egg by own through premature embryogenesis is termed de novo mutation. This is further detailed in Table 9.5.

9.2.3 ChiP-seq data

ChiP-seq stands for immunoprecipitation mixed with high-throughput sequencing. It detects the locations of genome attached by chromatin binding. ChiP-seq is a prevailing process to find the genome-wide DNA-binding sites for transcription factors (TFs) and many other proteins by combining chromatin immunoprecipitation (ChiP) with sequencing.

9.2.4 Biomedical imaging

Medical imaging is a procedure of generating visual interpretations of our interior body that is used for clinical diagnosis and medical research as well as the visual illustration of the function of few tissues or organs physiologically. Medical imaging tries to expose the internal structures that are hidden by our skin and bones as well as to detect and heal different diseases. Moreover, it also creates a database comprising normal anatomy and physiology to detect deformities. The localized measurement of a contrast generating biophysical effect in body or organ of living system is termed bioimaging. Now this contrast is basically the ability to distinguish tissue features against noise. Various modalities of medical imaging include X-rays, computed tomography (CT) imaging, ultrasound (US), magnetic resonance imaging (MRI), and nuclear medicine imaging.

9.3 Categories of computational algorithms in biomedical data

There are three kinds of data analysis available, viz., (i) algorithms for biomedical imaging data analysis, (ii) algorithms for array-based data analysis, and (iii) algorithms for hybrid data analysis containing same set of patients.

9.3.1 Biomedical data analysis

The biomedical data analysis plays an indispensable role in improving medical treatment, by data mining and integrating health records to reveal patterns that can be used to craft informed policy. Thereby learning the skills to help turns data into knowledge that can revolutionize the delivery of healthcare is of great importance. Biomedical analysis has multiple facets that help us in diagnosing ailing organs of human body. Hereby, we would like to throw some light on the way biomedical data analysis helps in detecting malignancy specifically in brain and breasts. The most widespread and important reasons for the rise in the death among adults and children around the whole world is brain tumor. Brain tumor is basically a cluster of unusual cells that expand inside the brain or around the brain. Few brain tumors are noncancerous (benign), whereas few are cancerous (malignant). Now computer-aided detection or diagnosis, i.e., CADe or CADx, systems can strengthen the diagnostic potentiality of doctors and minimize the time period necessary for the correct diagnosis. In the year 2014, Dahshan *et al.* [7] proposed a technique called the hybrid intelligent ML for CADe system meant for automatic recognition of brain tumor using MRI. The aforesaid method is basically based on the following computational procedures like the feedback pulse-coupled neural network used for image segmentation, then the discrete wavelet transform used for features extraction, then the principal component analysis used for reducing the dimensionality of the wavelet coefficients, and lastly the feed-forward back-propagation neural network to categorize the inputs into normal or abnormal category. Another most popular category of cancer found in women all around the globe is the deadly breast cancer. An initial discovery as well as the analysis of breast malignancy may lower the death ratio to a significant degree. Now to detect breast malignancy, various kinds of imaging modalities are being employed like CT, MRI, mammography, US, and biopsy. However, the different histopathological images are attained since the biopsy could impact the process cancer that is detected and the phase it is currently in. The computer-assisted diagnosis technique facilitates the diagnosticians in the early identification of the breast malignancy. The survey as stated by Kaushal *et al.* [3], in recent times, described various methods of the breast cancer analysis employing various histopathological images. Breast MRI possesses maximum sensitivity for breast cancer recognition among recent medical imaging modalities and is very crucial for the breast imaging practices. The foundation of breast MRI mainly consists of T1-weighted contrast-enhanced imaging, T2-weighted, ultrafast, and diffusion-weighted imaging out of which last one, i.e., diffusion-weighted imaging may be utilized to develop lesion categorization, as stated by Mann *et al.* [4].

9.3.2 Array-based data analysis

Array-based data analyses are used in deciphering the data generated from researches on DNA, on RNA, and on protein microarrays, which allows researchers to investigate the expression, basically the status of a larger gene sets—in most cases, or any organism's entire genome in one single experiment. There are three types of array data analysis, namely, microarray data analysis, the RNA-seq data analysis, and the scRNA-seq data analysis.

9.3.2.1 Microarray data analysis

There are lots of algorithms that have been developed by researchers in the last few years to identify the different gene modules. A new algorithm called WeCoMXP has been developed to assess assimilating co-methylation, co-expression, and protein-to-protein communications to identify modules of gene for multiomics dataset. The algorithm computes the respective divergent values from the intended indistinguishable values and detects the remarkable gene-modules from the network that regulates the gene using average linkage clustering. Subsequently, it looks out for literature and KEGG pathway. Gene-ontology evaluates to authenticate the genes depicting the modules. Moreover, it decides the TFs that control these gene-modules, and the miRNAs that aims for these genes-modules. But the major drawback is that connectivity measure for signed network is not taken into consideration at all. Then this chapter by Chandrashekar *et al.* [5] throws a light on guaranteeing precise results with minimal gene subsets allowing the doctors to identify the kind of datasets in cancer disease. It signifies the same classifier utilized for the selection and classification of gene, thereby improving the depth of the model portrayed by the results. Among various algorithms and tools that are used in recent times, Moonlight stated by Colaprico *et al.* [13] is a remarkable tool that uses multiomics data to recognize genes driving critical cancer. Moonlight analyzes more than 8,000 tumors from 18 kinds of cancer, thereby finding 3,310 oncogenic mediators and 151 possessing 2-fold roles. Moonlight basically targets to detect biological methods enhanced by a set of differentially expressed genes between couple of situations by means of functional enrichment analysis to detect the uphill regulators of the biological techniques that are significantly enhanced in contrast by means of upstream regulator analysis, and to detect "driver genes" having a double role that works as TSG or OCG in multiple stages or kinds of cancer. All the descriptions of the algorithms for microarray data along with their advantages and limitations are highlighted in Table 9.3.

9.3.2.2 RNA-seq data analysis

In the year 2015, Maulik *et al.* [14] came up with their method named as the statistical biclustering-based rule mining (StatBicRM) for detecting significant expressions of gene and the reports of methylation data. The main advantage of this method is the effectiveness of time consumption when dealing with bigger datasets. Then Mallik and Zhao [15] came up with an innovative idea for identifying methylation signs in various neurodegenerative diseases by using different systems that happen to use density-based clustering and reducing noise from the method. Their analysis discovered a methylation signature that comprises 21 genes for Alzheimer's disease commonly known as AD and a methylation sign containing 89 genes of down syndrome. Their assessment addressed the mentioned signs that can cause massive categorization correctness numbers (92% and 70%) for the abovementioned disorders. Precisely, this system will be beneficial as it improves detection outlier-free genetic as well as the epigenetic signs in many complicated disorders and with its respective progressive phases. Then in the year 2018, Bandyopadhyay and Mallik came up with Combinatorial Marker Discovery to research on tumorigenesis [9]. They proposed a unique computational framework, mainly used for detecting significant combinatorial markers commonly termed SCMs by utilizing the methylation data and the gene expression together. Both methylation data as well as gene expression remain combined in sole contiguous data and (after being approximated) propositional data founded on its respective inherent (i.e., reverse) affiliation. Thereafter, a collective count of expression and methylation figures (viz., CoMEx) have been created and calculated based upon continuous collaborative information for detecting an early set of necessary genes. This particular technique generates a lesser number of important nonredundant gene sets than produced by any different methods and it is comparatively quicker. However, the anticorrelation factor is not considered by them. Elaborate discussion on RNA-seq data is given in Table 9.2.

9.3.2.3 scRNA-seq data analysis

In this current era, scRNA-seq has turned out to be widely used for transcriptome analysis in numerous fields of biology. In the year 2017, Matsumoto *et al.* came up with an effective regulatory network inference algorithm from the scRNA-seq during their differentiation, i.e., SCODE as stated by Hirotaka *et al.* [10], which they applied to three scRNA-seq datasets and computed SCODE value by evaluating its implied associations using a DNA seq-footprint based network. SCODE performed well almost for couple of datasets and average for the rest of the datasets. This algorithm efficiently concludes regulatory network that is based on ordinary differential equation. This method fosters the growth of the single-cell differentiation analyses and bioinformatics method. Since each scRNA-seq profile represents a limited specimen of mRNA molecules from a distinctive cell that in no way can be retested and needs a strong assessment; thereby, it must split the sampling effect from the biological variance. Therefore, in 2019, Baran *et al.* [16] illustrate an approach for dividing the scRNA-seq datasets into separate as well as identical clusters of metacells that can be retested from the similar cell. This algorithm, on the contrary to clustering analysis, also focuses on achieving micro groups rather than the macro clusters. Here it portrays a way to utilize meta cells as building blocks for any complicated mathematical transcriptional plans by averting flattening of data. Now in the year 2021, Bhej *et al.* [8] establish an ML-based oversampling technique that utilizes a resultant expression of genes from previously discovered unusual cells as an input in order to produce the artificial cells to detect related unusual cells in other freely obtainable researches. They make the use of single-cell synthetic oversampling that is again created from the Localized Random Affine Shadowsampling algorithm. This algorithm rectifies the whole inequality ratio of the smaller and the bulk category. It also demonstrates the efficacy of the technique meant for a couple of individual use cases, every single comprising a couple of available set of data. For point-wise discussion on scRNA-seq data, see Table 9.1.

9.3.3 Hybrid data analysis

Hybrid data analyses have both imaging and array-based data for the same set of patients. The present technological advance is taking place in developing brain imaging data, across multiple modalities, as well as genomic data having high throughput. The study of brain tomography is an evolving and promptly expanding research area. It makes consolidative research that evaluates genetic differences like the single nucleotide polymorphisms or SNPs, epigenetic and copy number variations known as CNVs, the molecular features taken by the different omics data and the quantitative traits (QTs) of brain imaging, combined with more biomarkers, medical as well as ecological data. The main objective of genomics imaging is to obtain different perceptions from the phenotypic traits and the genomic and molecular structures of human brain, along with its effect on regular and disorderly brain functions as well as its behaviors. Taking into consideration the most exceptional magnitude and intricacy of the datasets having brain imaging genomics, most crucial computational and statistical trials have to be satisfied in order to achieve the complete ability of these useful data. Now surmounting these issues has turn out to be a foremost and demanding topic of study in the field of statistics and ML, where efficient and cost-effective data analytic techniques are used to disclose the genetic and the molecular underpinnings of neurobiological procedures, which may influence the advancement of the investigative, therapeutic, and the precautionary approaches for complicated brain syndromes. Shen and Thompson [6] have evaluated three main classifications of learning different problems in the genomics of brain imaging. First, it concentrated on understanding the problem of heritability approximation of the brain imaging QTs. The heritability of characteristic is mainly defended by the genetic factor. Second, it stresses on the issue of discovering the imaging genomics associations, an important topic explored in the brain imaging genomics to obtain innovative perceptions into the genomic and the molecular systems of the brain formation along with its purpose. Third, it concentrated on the knowledge problem of image integration and genomics for the outcome projection. This is a very vital issue studied related to brain imaging to attain significant perceptions onto the consequence-related neurobiological systems at the genetic, the molecular, and the macroscale brain structure degrees. Elaborate discussion on hybrid biomedical data analysis having biomedical data and array data together are given in Table 9.6.

9.4 Different techniques for diagnosis using biomedical imaging

9.4.1 Brain

Brain tumor is the extremely suffered disease that requires early and accurate detection techniques. Now most of the detection and diagnosis methodologies depend on the decision of neurospecialists as well as radiologists for the image assessment that leads to human inaccuracies and is also very time taking. Now CADx is basically ML and other computer algorithms that guide doctors to figure out what is going wrong in particular radiology images and other related areas. The CAD system improves investigative competencies of doctors and minimizes the span needed to analysis appropriately. The research paper as stated by Dahshan *et al.* [7] reveals the current available segmentation, categorization methods, and their advanced progression for human brain. The paper discusses the current segmentation as well as categorization methods and their existing advanced MRI images of human brain. On this context, this recommends a hybrid intelligent ML method based on CAD system used for detecting brain tumor automatically using MRI. The different computational techniques that have been proposed in this method for the image segmentation for reducing the dimensionality of the wavelet coefficients, for features extraction, are the feedback pulse-coupled neural network, the discrete wavelet transformation, and the principal component analysis, respectively, in order to classify inputs into normal or abnormal.

9.4.2 Breast

The usual type of cancer in the females across the globe is the deadly breast cancer. But the early discovery and identification of the breast cancer can minimize the mortality rate significantly. The various categories of imaging modalities that have been employed in order to detect and accumulate samples are mammography, US, CT, MRI, and many others. The CADx generally facilitates the doctors and pathologists in the detection of breast cancer. Kaushal *et al.* [3] report various methodologies for diagnosing breast cancer using various histopathological images. The important steps included in CAD analysis are preprocessing, segmentation, feature extraction, and classification. The digital image preprocessing is performed soon after the image is acquired. This plays the most essential part in detecting the organic tissues depicted in the image by enhancing its quality without obliterating the vital aspects. The second most essential stage is to detect the cells and the nuclei of various histopathological images that form the basis for the classification are called the segmentation stage. The third step, i.e., feature extraction phase, generally indicates the idea of getting prominent features that are immutable to the inappropriate changes of the input. Following the image segmentation stage, mostly the mining of features is done at the tissue level or could as well be done at the cellular level in order to quantify the changes. Finally, classification is used to classify which new instance belongs to which set of categories based on the existing dataset. For detecting abnormality in the images, different classifiers are used to classify tissues in various groups on the basis of the various kinds or grades of the breast malignancy.

9.4.3 Kidney

Another most common form of cancer is renal cancer as reported by the National Cancer Registry Program and Surveillance Epidemiology, and this renal cancer accounts for almost 3–4 percent of the entire fresh cancer incidents in Indian subcontinent and in the Western part of the world. We know that CADx systems can help enhance the abilities of physicians and also reduce the total span needed to conduct the exact analysis. Only way to survive for patients suffering from kidney cancer is premature discovery and therapy employing various imaging modalities that are noninvasive. Currently, renal cancer tomography mainly depends on CT. It basically is believed as the benchmark for identifying and categorization of kidney nodules. Kaur *et al.* [11] throw light on the massive role played by CADx for kidney nodules. It starts with an acquisition of image, preprocessing, segmentation, extraction of feature, selection, and categorization. Chaudhuri *et al.* [12] suggested another deep learning model known as U-Net for semantic segmentation of kidney. The main reason for selecting U-Net is that it is suitable for a smaller set of data, and it was initially devised for the process of biomedical image segmentation.

9.4.4 Ovary

Ovarian cancer is another most suffered disease. It can sneak up on us like a beast at night veiled as ordinary problems such prolonged bloating, then fatigue and the constant need to pee. The extremely common form of ovarian cancer initiates in aphelion cells, a particular type of cell that basically creates the tissue covering up the ovarian surface. To treat the ovarian cancers in the best possible way, doctors first confirm the identification and then discover the stage or the extent of the cancer that requires a technique called the surgical staging during which the doctor investigates the pelvic and the abdominal areas. The stage of the ovarian cancer is determined by the position of the cancer cells prevalent in our body. In the first stage, it is generally found on the upper surface of one or both ovaries or in the fallopian tube or in the abdominal fluid. In the second stage, the cancer gets propagated from the initial site to other nearby areas such as the ovaries, the fallopian tube, or even the uterus. In the third stage, cancer gets spread outside the pelvis like the lymph nodes or also on the surface of liver or spleen as stated by Togashi [17]. All modalities like CT, US, and MR imaging have almost equal precision rate when it comes to identifying stage of ovarian cancer.

9.4.5 Skin cancer

Skin cancer is any type of malignant growth that happens in skin. It can be broadly divided into two main categories that are melanoma and nonmelanoma skin cancer. Nonmelanoma skin cancer can further be categorized to basal cell cancer and squamous cell cancer. Most often basal cell cancer is diagnosed in any organ worldwide. Therefore, it is more common than the breast cancer, lung cancer, or even colon cancer. The second most common cancer diagnosed worldwide is squamous cell cancer. Mostly, patients will have either the basal cell cancer or the squamous cell cancer. Till date, biopsy technique is deemed as the benchmark used for detecting skin cancer in medical field. Although there are various anatomical imaging techniques available to assess the diverse kinds of skin cancer nodules, which include laser scanning, confocal microscopy, optical coherence tomography, high-frequency US, terahertz-pulsed imaging, MRI, and many more advanced procedures like the photoacoustic microscopy as stated by Hong and Cai [20], but the anatomical tomography may be inadequate in managing skin cancer detection as well as treatment. So, a variety of molecular imaging methods (like single-photon emission CT and the PET) are used to scrutinize the skin cancer imaging.

9.4.6 Soft tissue sarcoma

Soft tissue sarcoma is a sporadic type of malignant tumor of soft tissues at either of the extremities like arms or legs or in the central part of the body as well. They usually appear in the areas such as our muscle or in fat though they can occur in any other soft tissues also. Among the different types of sarcoma, probably liposarcoma is most frequently found. Mostly all soft tissue sarcoma is treated with surgeries where the doctors take out the tumor with a narrow zone of tissues around it to ensure the entire tumor and all of its cells are removed. Depending on multiple clinical factors like patients age or aggressiveness of the tumor addition of radiation or chemotherapy can also be followed. As stated by Afonso and Mascarenhas, Reference [21] throws a light toward the rational diagnostic tomography technique to patients having soft tissue tumors, underlining the basic principle that is an integral part of the soft tissue tumor imaging and diagnosis. In patients suspected with soft tissue lumps, US is well suited as the preliminary triage of the imaging modality, as the alleged tumor is available by using sonography though deeply seated tumors create apparent problems. Moreover, it is also a first-line analysis for children. MRI method provides finest contrast of soft tissue, has multiplanar capability, but is deficient in ionizing radiation and hence has become the most chosen modality to assess soft tissue masses. The CAD technology is another advanced digitized histopathology. Elaborate discussion on different modalities for biomedical imaging of various organs is given in Table 9.4.

9.5 Comparative review of computational algorithms

The different categories of computational algorithms have been reviewed and a comparative study is presented, as shown in Tables 9.1–9.6.

9.6 Role of CT in COVID-19 pandemic

We all know that in the month of December 2019, a tremendous epidemic of a novel infection was reported in China at the city of Wuhan, known as coronavirus or severe acute respiratory syndrome coronavirus 2 (SARS-CoV-2) as its origin. The international public health institution, World Health Organization (WHO), had thereafter identified the infection triggered by the novel coronavirus as coronavirus disease 2019 (COVID-19). Thereafter on March 11, 2020, WHO announced COVID-19 a pandemic, with approximately more than 10 lakhs confirmed cases and almost 5 lakhs deaths globally, within June 2020. Now, reverse-transcription–

Table 9.1 Different algorithms for single-cell RNA-sequencing (scRNA-seq) data

S. no.	Name of the method	Category	Description	Advantages	Limitations
1	Cell clustering [22]	Clustering of single cells	A fuzzy clustering technique based on multi-objective optimization (MOO) was built to identify the cell clusters in scRNA-seq data	Used to group the cells	Other biological challenges are not considered here
2.	Comparative study on dimension reduction and clustering techniques [23]	Dimension reduction and clustering strategies	Various methods like PCA are commonly used for unsupervised dimensionality reduction method	Data points are well distant when the dissimilar data points have been concentrated in the low-down dimensional area	More aspects need to be evaluated
3.	Meta as stated by Barang cell [63]	Graph partitioning using *K*NN graph	To partition multimodal scRNA-seq data profiles into several disjoint clusters of data profiles	• Used to partition the graph • Building blocks for complicated quantitative transcriptional maps	
4.	Clustering and classification algorithms scRNA-seq data as stated by Ren *et al.* [24]	Clustering scRNA-seq data	Discussed ML tactics for grouping and categorization of scRNA-seq and stresses on DR	Reviews nonsegregated methods and tools	Provides expression profile information of single-cell data
5.	SCODE as stated by Hirotaka et al. [10]	Regulatory network interference algorithm	Suggests an algorithm for scRNA-seq data, carried out on differentiating cells to revamp expression dynamics and concludes regulatory networks	Efficiently concludes regulatory network based on ordinary differential equations	
6.	Automated annotation as stated by Bej *et al.* [8]	ML-based oversampling method	Mentioned technique considers already identified rare cells and their gene expression count as input to produce synthetic cells, therefore identifying similar rare cells	• Rectifies the entire imbalance ratio • Recognizes unusual cell population with minimal false positive detection	• Time-consuming • Requires domain expertise knowledge

(Continues)

Table 9.1 (Continued)

S. no.	Name of the method	Category	Description	Advantages	Limitations
7.	Computational data analysis as stated by Geng *et al.* [2]	Data analysis of scRNA-seq data	Provides an outline of scRNA technologies, demonstrating the procedures for varied data of scRNA-seq analysis	• Ruling out cells that are inferior in quality	• Available scRNA-seq methods dropout, inadequate gene expression ignored
8.	Relevant datasets and analytical tools as stated by Peng *et al.* [25]	Clustering of scRNA-seq data	scRNA-seq clustering models comprising seven grouping methodologies are assessed on five public datasets	Improves the interpretation of treatment effectiveness	Lacking the gold standard benchmark datasets
9.	scRNA-seq analytical pipelines and computational methods as stated by Hie *et al.* [26]	Clustering and computational methods	Recommends the combined advancement of strong analytic pipelines, deals the challenges offered by investigative techniques, appropriate for genomic queries	• The computational technique findings are bench marked and potential prospects identified	
10.	Pathway analysis as stated by Zhang et al. [27]	Benchmarking algorithm for the pathway activity transformation of the scRNA-seq data	Broad framework to evaluate correctness, stability, and the scalability of the several pathway activity transformation algorithm	Selects appropriate methodologies that efficiently and accurately analyze scRNA-seq data	

Table 9.2 Different algorithms for RNA-seq data

S. no.	Name of the method	Category	Description	Advantages	Limitations
1	StatBicRM as stated by Maulik et al. [14]	Clustering of genes and samples	Computational framework for rule mining StatBicRM (i.e., statistical biclustering-based rule mining) utilizing cohesive methods of statistical as well as binary biclustering methods from the biological datasets	Execution time is saved and works on large datasets	
2.	Density-based spatial clustering of applications with noise (DBSCAN) as stated by Mallik and Zhao [15]	Hierarchical clustering	DBSCAN algorithm is applied to get rid of outliers; Limma statistical method is used to establish differentially methylated genes, and hierarchical clustering method was applied to identify gene modules	It is useful to detect outlier-free genetic and epigenetic signatures in several complicated disorders and respective evolving phases	Gene expression, copy number variation, chromatin remodeling, etc. are not part of the study
3.	H19-mediated multimolecular network analysis in pan cancer Li *et al.* [28]	miRNA-mediated lncRNA, TF, gene coregulation is complex but crucial in cancer	It established a unique analytic method by combining the synergistic rule amongst transcription factors (TFs), lncRNAs (e.g., H19), microRNAs (miRNAs), and target genes and then used it across datasets having cancer expression using linear regression from the Cancer Genome Atlas	• The effect of coregulation of multi-molecules can be determined • Effect of H19 on the biomolecules can be derived	

(Continues)

Table 9.2 (Continued)

S. no.	Name of the method	Category	Description	Advantages	Limitations
4.	Pareto-optimal cluster [29]	Cluster algorithm	It introduced a fresh structure for detecting signatures of gene employing Pareto-optimal cluster volume detection for RNA-seq data	It is valuable to discover signature for any microarray or RNA-seq data	
5.	Hypograph mining for obtaining the multiview cosimilarity gene modules as stated by Bhadra et al. [30]	Hypograph mining	It statistically identifies significant genes from each of the data profile and thereby calculates the set of union consisting of all the statistically meaningful genes	• Finds out the strength of co-similarity in multiview gene modules • Proposed a theoretic information naming MiNoMi	Gene expression, methylation, copynumber, etc. which are used to evaluate the inherent biological relations among profiles are not included in this chapter
6.	mRNA to miRNA regulatory network analysis as stated by Kandimallaand et al. [31]	Identification of miRNA panel	It explored a panel of miRNAs and meager molecular subtypes in PDAC	Used for the detection of risky patients and probable disorder monitoring in the patients with PDAC	Here subtype-specific miRNAs and their predictive implications remain unknown
7.	Combinatorial Marker discovery [9]	Gene expression and methylation data	Combines the score of gene expression and methylation data to compute the combined continuous data for discovering essential bunch of genes	• Method generates a smaller number of non-redundant gene sets • Faster	Strength of anticorrelation is not undertaken in this chapter

8.	Combined framework for accurate biological interpretation of DNA methylation, as stated by Mallik et al. [29]	DNA methylation and gene expression	Determines predicted gene expression number from the already filtered methylation information during linear regression by empirical Bayes test using Limma	Helps in better interpretation of DNA methylation study and gene expression in any disorder survey	The approach is performed on only a small dataset
9.	Seminoma and non-seminoma in testicular germ cell tumors as stated by Qin *et al.* [32]	Subtype classification	Extensively investigates the pair of TF and miRNA regulation, their FFLs, and TF-miRNA-mediated regulatory networks in two kinds of testicular germ cell tumors (TGCT): seminoma (SE) and non-seminoma (NSE)	Identifies the different regulatory particles, its interaction modules, along with few other characteristics of TGCT subtypes	Here dataset does not include matched control samples
10.	Identification of co-methylated and co-express genes as stated by Mallik et al. [29]	DNA methylation	It is a novel consolidative study of a framework to detect the co-methylated as well as the coexpress genes like mRNAs and microRNAs (miRNAs) modules in the TGCT subtypes, for example, non-seminoma and seminoma	Method is highly useful to obtain potential gene/miRNA modules as well as hubs for any kind of diseases	

Table 9.3 Different algorithms for microarray data

S. no.	Name of the method	Category	Description	Advantages	Limitations
1	Comparative study among different DMR finding algorithms, as stated by Mallik et al. [33]	Supervised and unsupervised consecutive clustering algorithm	Supervised DMR findings under 60 different parameter settings are used, which computes the strength and accuracy region. Compares results of many more features of analysis that includes the volume of the DMRs overlapping the approaches and the performance time	• Figure out the DMR finding tool, will be useful for finding which condition • Find optimal parameter setting of each DMR finding tool	It covers only four supervised DMR finding tool, rather than describing any other unsupervised tool
2.	Comprehensive survey on different parametric and nonparametric testing methodologies as stated by Bandyopadhyay et al. [34]	Microarray data	A thorough survey of several parametric and nonparametric approaches for finding differentially expressed transcripts	Useful for data with very few samples	Variability is ignored
3.	Differential methylated regions as stated by Gomezand et al. [35]	DMR analysis of array-based DNA methylation data	coMethDMR is a flexible and powerful tool for identifying DMRs. coMethDMR selects co-methylated subregions and tests association between methylation levels within the subregion and	The subregion identification phase in coMethDMR enhances power significantly	

			the phenotype		
4.	Regulatory analytical approach to detect the preserved regulatory networks in the human beings and the mice, as stated by Aimin et al. [36]	Gene regulatory mechanism	Here the regulatory mechanism is investigated with an analytic methodology to recognize the preserved supervisory links in human beings and rats to detect critical miRNAs, target genes and the regulatory motifs (miRNA-TF-gene)	Efficient	Time-consuming
5.	Moonlight as stated by Colapricoand et al. [13]	Detection of cancer driver genes	Analyzes more than 8 000 samples of tumors from 18 kinds of cancer, uncovering approximately 3 310 oncogenic negotiators, having 151 2-fold roles. Confirms various genes driving critical cancers by studying the cell-line datasets	It explains tumor heterogeneity and helps in therapeutic decisions	
6.	WeCoMXP as stated by Mallik and Bandyopadhyay [37]	Gene module detection	Develops a new weighted connectivity measure incorporating the comethylation, co-expression and the protein–protein interactions (called WeCoMXP) to identify the gene-modules for the multiomics dataset	It has got higher performance in terms of numerous clustering validity indices	WeCoMXP operates for only unsigned/undirected graph where the anticorrelation for the co-expression verses comethylation is not contemplated
7.	Distributed parallel algorithm as stated by Cao *et al.* [38]	A multi-objective feature selection model	Proposes a multi-objective feature selection model that concurrently considers the classification error, the feature number, and the feature redundancy	Highly effective and efficient	

(Continues)

Table 9.3 (Continued)

S. no.	Name of the method	Category	Description	Advantages	Limitations
8.	Distributed correlation based gene selection as suggested by Shukla and Tripathi [39]	Biomarkers detection from microarray	Newfound technique based on filter for selection of gene is presented. This picks appropriate genes to separate the tissues from the dataset having gene expression. This calculates the relation between the gene–gene and the gene–class to identify subset of essential genes	• High classification accuracy • High performance • Lower execution time	
9.	Disease prediction using deep learning technique, as stated by Chandrasekhar *et al.* [5]	Microarray classification	Evaluates the assessment period, the categorization, correctness and also the potentiality to detect the sickness to find out the stringency positions of illness and the empirical outputs, which signifies the deep neural network categorization execution	Accuracy rate is very high by using classification and feature selection	
10.	Heuristic algorithm as stated by Jia *et al.* [40]	Microarray data classification	Here a multi-objective heuristic algorithm named MOEDA is proposed according to analytic hierarchy process (AHP)	Various subsets of genes get high classification accuracies	High computational cost

Table 9.4 Different modalities for biomedical imaging of various organs

S. no.	Name of various organs	Modality used	Advantages	Disadvantages
1.	Brain [7]	• CT • MRI	CT acquires detailed images of bone, soft tissue, blood vessels, and various kinds of tissuesMRI offers better soft tissues comparatively and differentiate better between the fat, water, and other soft tissues	• CT involves radiation exposure • Artifact from metal implants will conceal the view in CT images • MRI scanners may cause a safety issue due to its strong magnets
2.	Breast as stated by Mann *et al.* [4]	• Mammography • US • MRI	• Lessens the probability of undergoing chemotherapy • US gives a clear picture of soft tissues and helps detecting lesions in women having dense breast • MRI delineates the true size of a cancer that often happens to be underestimated on mammography and US	• Mammograms expose the breasts to radiation over time • US cannot screen breast cancer as it misses early symptoms because it can only detect whether cyst is filled with fluid or a solid tumor • MRI cannot distinguish between cancerous abnormalities that lead to unnecessary biopsies known as false-positive results
3.	Kidney as stated by Nikken and Krestin [41]	• US • CT • MRI	• US modality helps in finding a kidney mass and shows whether it is a solid or a mass filled with a fluid • CT helps us to identify if the kidney has tumor or lesions or it has been through disruptive conditions like small stones, genetic variances, polycystic ailments, accumulation of water near kidney, or around abscesses MRI detects better contrast of soft tissue, thus identifying and categorizing renal lesions	• US overestimates kidney stone sizes • CT characterizes hypo-attenuation in masses generally smaller than 8–10 mm • In MRI, kidney seems as fuzzy signal voids, hence, gets overlooked with any other structures or artifacts

(Continues)

Table 9.4 (Continued)

S. no.	Name of various organs	Modality used	Advantages	Disadvantages
4.	Ovary as stated by Togashi [17]	• TVS • CT • MRI	• TVS acquires effective images that help differentiating simple cysts from complicated cysts • CECT studies can compare to lower dose of non-enhanced CT scans • MRI has higher sensitivity toward discovering blood-related products	• TVS is unreliable in differentiating benign from malignant ovarian tumors • CT scans do not show small ovarian tumors significantly • MRI detecting ovarian cancer includes higher cost, long acquisition time, and resultant motion artifact
5.	Skin cancer as stated by Hong *et al.* [20]	MRI	MRI offers extra ordinary soft tissue contrast with good spatial resolution (<100 m). Hence it discloses structural abnormality of skin tumors	Lower sensitivity that usually requires long scanning period even with exogenic contrasting agents

Table 9.5 Mutation table

S. no.	Name of the method	Category	Description	Advantages
1.	Whole genome sequencing as stated by Jiang *et al.* [1]	De novo mutation	Whole-genome sequencing was conducted for as good as 23 families belonging to two cohorts having siblings and parents with no impact. SCZ patients were found to have couple of nonsense de novo mutations (DNMs) in GJC1 and HIST1H2AD	The method suggests that GJC1 a DNM-implicated gene could possibly be a probability gene for Schizophrenia and its respective responsibility could indulge in fetal and premature neuro-development, an endangered time span for advancing diseases such as Schizophrenia
2.	Differential expression of triggering receptor on TREM2 cells in irregular-AD cases versus ADTREM2 carriers as stated by Aguil *et al.* [42]	Mutation in TRE-M2	It inspected the RNA-seq data in the parietal lobe tissue of the brain from AD patient having TREM2 variants from three different datasets expending Kallisto as well as R package import to establish the count of every transcript as well as quantify abundant transcript in terms of transcripts per million	The method explains the expression belonging to the three transcripts TREM2 in the post-mortem of human brain and also includes the resolvable Transcript, which does not incorporate a trans membrane domain It also observed the AD-risk types inclined to the expression of explicit transcripts

polymerase chain-reaction (RT-PCR) is the universal technique that is applied to create a complete detection of SARS-CoV-2 disease. But regrettably, RT-PCR results could be altered by inaccurate sampling and minimal virus burden. Therefore, radiological investigations, particularly chest computed tomography (also known as CT) scans, play an essential part in diagnosing the initial stage of lung disease, assessing the infection advancement, and directing medical conclusion for COVID-19 patients. Now owing to the minimal divergence of the disease areas in the CT images and significant alterations in both forms and locations of nodules in various patients, the demarcation of infected areas in CT scans of the chest is extremely tricky. Li *et al.* had described primary encounters of tools that are based on AI to detect COVID-19 pneumonia on radiological illustrations. There are many ongoing research works and out of those we would like to put forward few researches. Zhang *et al.* [27] discovered a uAI Intelligent Assistant Analysis

Table 9.6 Algorithms for hybrid biomedical data having biomedical data and array data together

S. no.	Name of the method	Category	Description	Advantages	Limitations
1.	A gradual analysis involving brain transcriptome and neuroimaging as stated by Aurina [43]	Review paper	Compares how different processing choices influence the resulting data of brain wide transcriptomic and neuroimaging data	The main advantage is that Allen Human Brain Atlas (AHBA) works toward a unified data processing pipeline to assure consistent and reproducible results	Detailed work is missing in the development of the techniques meant for the spatial correlations of data as well as a standardized workflow is very much needed to guarantee reproducibility
2.	Statistical and machine learning methodologies for the brain imaging genomics as stated by Shen and Thompson [6]	Review paper	It performs integrative examinations that evaluate genetic changes, molecular features seized by the several omics data and brain imaging quantitative traits (QTs) that are paired with other biomarker like clinical and environmental data	The main aim of the imaging genomics is to obtain an additional perception into the phenotypic traits as well as the genetic and molecular mechanisms of our brain and their effect on the normal and on disordered brain function and behavior	Though deep learning models are phenomenally effective in stating data-driven problems in medicine, but they were not broadly utilized in the brain imaging genomics because of the restricted sample range and elevated dimensionality of the prevailing imaging and the genomics datasets
3.	An evaluation of radiogenomics in oncology [44]	Review paper	Provides thorough picture of the tumor through radiomics and radiogenomics. It offers precise imaging associated with	Radiogenomics provides accurate imaging biomarkers, substituting for genetic testing, also predicts risks	Gene expression and signaling pathways are extremely complex

Table 9.6 (*Continued*)

S. no.	Name of the method	Category	Description	Advantages	Limitations
			genetic expression thus serves as an alternative for the genetic testing	and outcomes and also used for personalized treatment options	
4.	Detecting Alzheimer's disease using early mild cognitive impairment	Hybrid biomedical data analysis model	A graph-based SSL technique to assimilate data of multimodal imaging of brain as well as to pick the reasonable predictors based on imaging to optimize the forecast precision	The graph-based SSL approach with data of multimodal imaging of brain	The main challenges are to characterize and authenticate biomarkers of AD progression that leads to an enhanced early diagnosis at early symptomatic and or more specifically presymptomatic stages

System, software based on deep learning, to inevitably obtain and evaluate areas believed to be affected with the virus. Then Silva *et al.* [45] came up with a voting-based approach and a cross-dataset analysis called as Efficient-CovidNet. Here the images from a given patient are categorized as a group in a voting system. The method is examined in the two biggest datasets of COVID-19 CT analysis with a patient-based split. To the best of our knowledge the two datasets are SARS-CoV-2 CT scan dataset and COVID-19 CT dataset. A cross-dataset analysis is also introduced to evaluate the strength of the models in a more accurate scenario in which data come from various divisions. Elaborate discussion on COVID-19 detection patterns using CT images is given in Table 9.7.

9.7 Advent of smart technologies during COVID-19

Ever since the breakout of COVID-19, isolating and distancing have been the two most prevalent practices that we have been made to familiarize. As a COVID-infected patient will be isolated while the therapy still needs to continue, healthcare turning smart was the need of the hour. The current scenario, hence, calls for AI hand in hand with IoT to lead us to a better tomorrow, offering healthcare services to the furthest possible patient. While we were reviewing many studies, we observed that some of the major work has been done in IoT and AI to leverage the

Table 9.7 COVID-19 detection pattern using CT

S. no.	Name of the method	Description	Advantages	Disadvantages
1.	The uAI Intelligent Assistant Analysis System	An aggregate of 2 460 RT-PCR tests were carried on COVID patients and the uAI Intelligent Assistant Analysis System evaluated the CT scans	Post-CT chest the uAI Intelligent Assistant Analysis System could precisely assess the pneumonia in COVID-19 victim	• Movement of patients to undergo CT scan is a limitation • uAI system needs manual adjustment, hence thorough investigation is required for assessing probable effect
2.	Efficient-CovidNet [45], along with a voting-based approach and a cross-dataset analysis	Images from a given patient are categorized as group in a voting system. The method is examined in the two biggest datasets of COVID-19 CT analysis with a patient-based split. A cross-dataset analysis is also introduced to evaluate the strength of the models in a more accurate scenario in which data come from various divisions	• Recommends a superior yet efficient deep-learning model for the testing of COVID-19 in CT scans • Reports various queries regarding the two biggest datasets • Proposes a voting-based estimation method	Lack of good quality datasets, which affects latency
3.	Active contour model	Applies partial differential equation to evaluate initial contour that is applied to 2D lung CT scan to obtain affected portion	Overall performance is good in terms of speed and accuracy	Mainly fails when objects inside images have different intensity values that can be confronted by using multistage segmentation

healthcare service. While the IoT was used mainly used for monitoring a patient remotely, AI, on the other hand, was mainly used to break down healthcare data and used to track and screen patients.

9.7.1 Building ML models to diagnose COVID-19

ML, being a subset of AI, has shown a lot of promise and is immensely used across industries. In healthcare industry, it is primarily used to screen and diagnose diseases. Categorically there are three main stages, the usage of ML has been broken down into. To begin with, the first stage is Assessment followed by Tracing and Projection and then comes Medical Aid. The Assessment is a very crucial stage where in ML applications help a lot by analyzing the medical imaging data, like CT scan of chest. The next stage, Tracing and Projection helps in predicting the number of cases and tracking down the chain of contacts. To Finish, Medical Aid helps in understanding the protein sequences and gene structure of the virus in case a remedy could be found in tackling it either by inoculation or medicine. ML systems can be designed such that it can emulate human intelligence. ML models have been widely trained over datasets that comprise CT scans, MRI, and X-ray images, to detect the irregularities.

We have come across many surveys during the review that has implemented ML and achieved fruitful results. Amongst many studies, there happens to be one such literature by Sandhu *et al.* [46] that demonstrates the way ML model uses cloud computing and GPS technology along with Google Maps to render the COVID-19-infected patients along the selected route and instead propose an alternative route that has relatively less or no infected patients, thus ensuring safety and vindicating the spread of the virus. The model, with time, has enriched itself to reach an accuracy of around 80 percent in proposing an alternative route having minimal infected patients. Another proposal by Choi *et al.* [59] did an analysis of the sentiments of people to deduce the public reaction from social media and other media houses. It mined the feelings from emoticons used in social media, and based on that the ML model supervises this to suggest the actions in order to reduce anxiety and anguish regarding the MERS-CoV.

Debnath *et al.* [47] proposed a way wherein ML can be used to improve the way clinical decisions are made in the ongoing COVID-19 pandemic. Amusingly, in some of the instances, it empowers the scientists to predict the propagation of virus across different regions. In addition to this, ML systems are used to discover the medicine and even at times develop inoculations, thus achieving an antidote for the virus.

9.7.2 Impact of IoT in healthcare

IoT delve into new aspects in patient care using various real-time health monitoring and tracking, thereby allowing seamless communications among the healthcare professionals and patients.

Taiwo *et al.* [60] proposed a smart healthcare support system that can be used being at home. It monitors patients' health and help to fetch the doctor's prescription while at home. From a doctor's perspective, the doctor need not visit the patient instead can use this to diagnose the disease and carry on the prognosis based on the data accumulated remotely. Hence with this, patients can continue to be at their home and get consulted by doctors by sharing their day-to-day health symptoms.

The authors in [49] proposed a technique to track patients and staff and thereby lessen the waiting period. With the usage of smart devices like blood gas analyzers, thermometer, smart bed, glucometer, US, and X-rays, there is a drastic improvement in inpatient care. It builds an integrated information system in a hospital where all events are stowed digitally, and other data analytics are utilized toward problem-solving throughout COVID-19 pandemic. By means of constant examining the health status, it notifies almost every forthcoming ailment and offers a solution for its inhibition. It is beneficial in the exposure of an asthma attack and also as a reminder of on-time medication.

9.8 Conclusion

Hence, in our book chapter, we have provided a comprehensive detailed survey (road map) on various biomedical imaging and array-based sequence data analyses along with their integrated study for different tissue-specific dreadful diseases (such as cancer). We also include a brief review of ML and IoT that helped in paradigm shift in leveraging medical facilities and incorporating smartness of healthcare for COVID-19 treatment.

In this regard, initially, we provided different algorithms on biomedical imaging stated by Bej *et al.* [8] that included multilevel thresholding [9,10], MRF model [11], and clustering algorithms [12]. The advantages, shortcomings, and usages of different algorithms of biomedical imaging are demonstrated here. Second, we yielded different array-based sequence data analysis algorithm that is very much useful for biomedical research. These array-based data might be divided into different categories, viz., single-cell sequencing data, RNA-seq as stated by Shen and Thompson [6] data, microarray data, etc. Various algorithms applied to each category of the sequence data have been notified here. This includes various computational problems such as gene signature discovering, biomarker discovery, disease classification or disease subtype classification, differential expression or differential methylation analysis, prognosis study, gene module detection [13,14], multimodal data integration, etc. For each problem, specific algorithms (or, tools) have been mentioned here for the benevolent of the new researchers in this domain. The advantages, limitations, and overall usages of each category of the algorithms along with the corresponding comparative study of the different categories of algorithms are also described here. As a future work, we will develop a new algorithm using ML and deep learning applied to integrated data consisting of array- and image-based profile together. Moreover, we will also perform some computational work on de novo mutation.

Hence, various algorithms from different backgrounds can be utilized together to solve computational problem in big biological data. Moreover, IoT and ML approaches are used for single RNA-seq data for COVID-19. As a future scope, we will try to comprehensively illustrate the transcriptional changes in peripheral blood mononuclear cells and also the risks of COVID-19 virus on different respiratory system conditions during the recovery stage of COVID-19 by scRNA-seq technique and scRNA data analysis.

References

[1] Jiang S., Zhou D., Wang Y., *et al.* 'Identification of de novo mutations in prenatal neurodevelopment-associated genes in schizophrenia in two Han Chinese patient-sibling family-based cohorts'. *Translational Psychiatry*. 2020.

[2] Geng C., Ning B. and Shi T. 'Single-cell RNA-seq technologies and related computational data analysis'. *Frontiers in Genetics*. 2019.

[3] Kaushal C., Bhat S., Singla A., *et al.* 'Recent trends in computer assisted diagnosis (CAD) system for breast cancer diagnosis using histopathological images'. *IRBM*. 2019; 40: 211–227.

[4] Mann R., Cho N. and Moy L. 'Breast MRI: State of the art'. *RSNA Radiology*. 2019.

[5] Chandrashekar V., Sureshkumar V., Kumar T. S. and Shanmugapriya S. 'Disease prediction based on micro array classification using deep learning techniques'. *Microprocessors and Microsystems*. 2020; 77.

[6] Shen L. and Thompson P. 'Brain imaging genomics: Integrated analysis and machine learning'. *Proceedings of IEEE*. 2019; 108: 125–162.

[7] Sayed E., Dahshan A., Mohsen H., *et al.* 'Computer-aided diagnosis of human brain tumor through MRI: A survey and a new algorithm'. *Expert Systems with Applications*. 2014; 41: 5526–5545.

[8] Bej S., Galow A., David R., *et al.* 'Automated annotation of rare-cell types from single-cell RNA-sequencing data through synthetic oversampling' *BMC Bioinformatics*. 2021; 22: 557.

[9] Bandyopadhyay S. and Mallik S. 'Integrating multiple data sources for combinatorial marker discovery: A study in tumorigenesis'. *IEEE/ACM Transactions on Computational Biology and Bioinformatics*. 2018; 15: 673–687.

[10] Hirotaka M., Kiryu H., Furusawa C., *et al.* 'SCODE: An efficient regulatory network inference algorithm from single-cell RNA-seq during differentiation'. *Bioinformatics*. 2017; 33: 2314–2321.

[11] Kaur R., Juneja M. and Mandal A. 'Computer-aided diagnosis of renal lesions in CT images: A comprehensive survey and future prospects'. *Computers & Electrical Engineering*. 2019; 77: 423–434.

[12] Chaudhuri K., Sharma R. and Halarnker P. 'Kidney and tumor segmentation using U-Net deep learning model'. *5th International Conference on Next Generation Computing Technologies (NGCT-2019)*. SSRN. 2020.

[13] Colaprico A., Olsen C., Matthew H., *et al.* 'Interpreting pathways to discover cancer driver genes with Moonlight'. *Nature Communications*. 2020; 11.

[14] Maulik U., Mallik S., Mukhopadhyay A. and Bandyopadhyay S. 'Analyzing large gene expression and methylation data profiles using StatBicRM: Statistical biclustering-based rule mining'. *PLoS One*. 2015; 10: e0119448.

[15] Mallik S. and Zhao Z. 'Detecting methylation signatures in neurodegenerative disease by density-based clustering of applications with reducing noise'. *Scientific Reports*. 2020; 10.

[16] Baran Y., Bercovich A., Pedros A., *et al.* 'MetaCell: Analysis of single-cell RNA-seq data using *K*-NN graph partitions'. *Genome Biology*. 2019; 20.

[17] Togashi K. 'Ovarian cancer: The clinical role of US, CT, and MRI'. *European Radiology*. 2003; 13: L87–L104.

[18] Bhuyan H. K., Chakraborty C., Shelke Y. and Pani S. K. 'COVID-19 diagnosis system by deep learning approaches'. *Expert Systems*. 2021: e12776. https://doi.org/10.1111/exsy.12776.

[19] Aslam B., Javed A. R., Chakraborty C., Nebhen J., Raqib S. and Rizwan M. 'Blockchain and ANFIS empowered IoMT application for privacy preserved contact tracing in COVID-19 pandemic'. *Personal and Ubiquitous Computing*. 2021: 1–17. 10.1007/s00779-021-01596-3.

[20] Hong H., Sun J. and Cai W. 'Anatomical and molecular imaging of skin cancer'. *Clinical, Cosmetic and Investigational Dermatology*. 2008; 1: 1–17.

[21] Afonso D. P. and Mascarenhas V. V. 'Imaging techniques for the diagnosis of soft tissue tumors'. *Reports in Medical Imaging*. 2015; 8: 63–70.

[22] Mallik S. and Zhao Z. 'Multi-objective optimized fuzzy clustering for detecting cell clusters from single-cell expression profiles'. *Genes*. 2019; 10(8): 611.

[23] Feng C., Liu S., Zhang H., *et al.* 'Dimension reduction and clustering models for single-cell RNA sequencing data: A comparative study'. *International Journal of Molecular Sciences*. 2020; 21(6): 2181.

[24] Ren Q., Ma A., Zou Q. and Ma Q. 'Clustering and classification methods for single-cell RNA-sequencing data'. *Briefings in Bioinformatics*. 2019; 21(4): 1196–1208.

[25] Peng L., Tian X., Tian G., *et al.* 'Single-cell RNA-seq clustering: Datasets, models and algorithms'. *RNA Biology*. 2020; 17(6): 765–783.

[26] Hie B., Peters J., Nyquist S., *et al.* 'Computational methods for single-cell RNA sequencing'. *Annual Review of Biomedical Data Science*. 2020; 3: 339–364.

[27] Zhang H., Zhang J., Zhang H. H., *et al.* 'Automated detection and quantification of COVID-19 pneumonia: CT imaging analysis by a deep learning-based software'. *European Journal of Nuclear Medicine and Molecular Imaging*. 2020; 47: 2525–2532.

[28] Li A., Mallik S., Luo H., Jia P. and Lee D. 'H19, a long non-coding RNA, mediates transcription factors and target genes through interference of microRNAs in pan-cancer'. *Molecular Therapy – Nucleic Acids*. 2020; 21: 180–191.

[29] Mallik S., Seth S., Bhadra T. and Zhao Z. 'A linear regression and deep learning approach for detecting reliable genetic alterations in cancer using DNA methylation and gene expression data'. *Genes*. 2020; 11(8): 931.

[30] Bhadra T., Mallik S. and Bandyopadhyay S. 'Identification of multi-view gene modules using mutual information based hypograph mining'. *IEEE Transaction on Systems*. 2019; 49(6): 1119–1130.

[31] Kandimalla R., Shimura T., Mallik S., *et al.* 'Identification of serum miRNA signature and establishment of a nomogram for risk stratification in patients with pancreatic ductal adenocarcinoma'. *Annals of Surgery*. 2020.

[32] Qin G., Mallik S., Mitra R., Li A., Jia P. and Eischen C. M. 'MicroRNA and transcription factor co-regulatory networks and subtype classification of seminoma and non-seminoma in testicular germ cell tumors'. *Scientific Reports*. 2020; 10: 852.

[33] Mallik S., Odom G., Gao Z., Gomez L., Chen X. and Wang L. 'An evaluation of supervised methods for identifying differentially methylated regions in Illumina methylation arrays'. *Briefings in Bioinformatics*. 2018; 20(6): 2224–2235.

[34] Bandyopadhyay S., Mallik S. and Mukhopadhyay A. 'A survey and comparative study of statistical tests for identifying differential expression from microarray data'. *IEEE/ACM Transactions on Computational Biology and Bioinformatics*. 2014; 11(1): 95–115.

[35] Gomez L., Gabriel J., Young G., *et al.* 'CoMethDMR: Accurate identification of co-methylated and differentially methylated regions in epigenome-wide association studies with continuous phenotypes'. *Nucleic acid Research*. 2019; 14(17): e98.

[36] Li A., Jia P., Mallik S., *et al.* 'Critical microRNAs and regulatory motifs in cleft palate identified by a conserved miRNA-TF-gene network approach in humans and mice'. *Briefings in Bioinformatics*. 2020; 21: 1465–1478.

[37] Mallik S. and Bandyopadhyay S. 'WeCoMXP: Weighted connectivity measure integrating co-methylation, co-expression and protein-protein interactions for gene-module detection'. *IEEE/ACM Transactions on Computational Biology and Bioinformatics*. 2020; 17: 690–703.

[38] Cao B., Zhao J., Yang P., *et al.* 'Multiobjective feature selection for microarray data via distributed parallel algorithms'. *Future Generation Computer System*. 2019; 100: 952–981.

[39] Shukla A. and Tripathi D. 'Detecting biomarkers from microarray data using distributed correlation based gene selection'. *Genes and Genomics*. 2020; 42: 449–465.

[40] Jia L., Peng Q., Chen X. and Sun Z. 'A multi-objective heuristic algorithm for gene expression microarray data classification'. *Expert System with Applications*. 2006; 59: 13–19.

[41] Nikken J. and Krestin G. 'MRI of the kidney—state of the heart'. *European Radiology*. 2007; 17: 2780–2793.

[42] Aguila J., Benitez B. A., Li Z. and Dube U. 'TREM2 brain transcript-specific studies in AD and TREM2 mutation carriers'. *Molecular Neurodegeneration*. 2019; 14.

[43] Arnatkeviciute A., Fulcher B. D. and Fornito A. 'A practical guide to linking brain-wide gene expression and neuroimaging data'. *NeuroImage*. 2019; 189: 353–367.

[44] Gullo R., Daimiel I., Morris E. and Pinker K. 'Combining molecular and imaging metrics in cancer: Radiogenomics'. *Insights into Imaging*. 2020; 11: 1.
[45] Silva P., Luz E. and Getal S. 'COVID-19 detection in CT images with deep learning: A voting-based scheme and cross-datasets analysis'. *Informatics in Medicine Unlocked*. 2020; 20.
[46] Sandhu R., Sood S. K. and Kaur G. 'An intelligent system for predicting and preventing MERS-CoV infection outbreak'. *The Journal of Supercomputing*. 2016; 72: 3033–3056.
[47] Debnath S., Barnaby D. P., Coppa K., *et al.* 'Machine learning to assist clinical decision-making during the COVID-19 pandemic'. *Bioelectronic Medicine*. 2020; 6: 1–8.
[48] Ozkaya U., Ozturk S. and Barstugan M. 'Coronavirus (COVID-19) classification using deep features fusion and ranking technique'. In: Hassanien AE., Dey N. and Elghamrawy S. (eds.), *Big Data Analytics and Artificial Intelligence Against COVID-19: Innovation Vision and Approach*. Studies in Big Data, vol. 78. Springer, Cham; 2020.
[49] Javaid M. and Khan I. 'Internet of Things (IoT) enabled healthcare helps to take the challenges of COVID-19 Pandemic' *Journal of Oral Biology and Craniofacial Research*. 2021; 11(2): 209–214.
[50] Gurcan M., Boucheron L., Can A., *et al.* 'Histopathological image analysis: A review'. *IEEE Reviews in Biomedical Engineering*. 2009; 2: 147–171.
[51] Mallik S. and Zhao Z. 'Identification of gene signatures from RNA-seq data using Pareto-optimal cluster algorithm'. *BMC Systems Biology*. 2018; 12(8): 126.
[52] Mallik S., Qin G., Jia P. and Zhao Z. 'Molecular signatures identified by integrating gene expression and methylation in non-seminoma and seminoma of testicular germ cell tumors'. *Epigenetics*. 2020; 16(2): 1–15.
[53] Akbari Y., Hassen H., Al-Maadeed S. and Zughaier S. M. 'Covid-19 lesion segmentation using lung CT scan images: Comparative study based on active contour models'. *Applied Sciences*. 2021; 11: 8039.
[54] Garg L., Chukwu E., Nasser N., Chakraborty C. and Garg G. 'Anonymity preserving IoT-based COVID-19 and other infectious disease contact tracing model'. *IEEE Access*. 2020; 8: 159402–159414.
[55] Roy S. and Chakraborty C. 'Panic buying situation during COVID-19 global pandemic'. *Journal of Information Technology Management*. 2021; 13(2), 231–244.
[56] Chakraborty C. and Abougreen A. N. 'Intelligent Internet of Things and advanced machine learning techniques for COVID-19'. *EAI Endorsed Transactions on Pervasive Health and Technology*. 2021: 1–14.
[57] Gupta A, Chakraborty C. and Gupta B., 'Secure transmission of EEG data using watermarking algorithm for the detection of epileptical seizures'. *Traitement du Signal*. 2021; 38(2): 473–479. https://doi.org/10.18280/ts.380227.
[58] Shahid O., Nasajpour M., Pouriyeh S., *et al.* 'Machine learning research towards combating COVID-19: Virus detection, spread prevention, and medical assistance'. *Journal of Biomedical Informatics*. 2021; 117.

[59] Choi S., Lee J., Kang M. G., Min H., Chang Y. S. and Yoon S. 'Large-scale Machine Learning of media outlets for understanding public reactions to nation-wide viral infection outbreaks'. *Methods*. 2017; 129: 50–59.

[60] Taiwo O. and Ezugwu A. E. 'Smart healthcare support for remote patient monitoring during COVID-19 quarantine'. *Informatics in Medicine Unlocked*. 2020; 20.

[61] Zhang Y., Ma Y., Huang Y., *et al.* 'Benchmarking algorithms for pathway activity transformation of single-cell RNA-seq data'. *Computational and Structural Biotechnology Journal*. 2020; 18: 2953–2961.

[62] Dash S., Chakraborty C., Giri S. K., Pani S. K. and Frnda J. 'BIFM: Big-data driven intelligent forecasting model for COVID-19'. *IEEE Access*. 2021; 9: 97505–97517. 10.1109/ACCESS.2021.3094658.

[63] Baran Y., Bercovich A., Sebe-Pedros A., *et al.* 'MetaCell: analysis of single-cell RNA-seq data using K-nn graph partitions'. *Genome Biology*. 2019; 20: 206.

Chapter 10

Review of medical imaging with machine learning and deep learning-based approaches for COVID-19

Swapnil Singh[1], *Vidhi Vazirani*[1] *and Deepa Krishnan*[1]

Abstract

COVID-19 came with unprecedented challenges that disrupted activities of government, economies, and societies all around the world. It is caused due to severe acute respiratory syndrome coronavirus 2. We are witnessing how governments and administrations have taken proactive steps to limit the spread of disease. Even though many countries have enforced strict lockdown to curtail its transmission, mortality rates continue to rise. An early detection of COVID-19 is inevitable as it helps in seeking early medical intervention and to minimize community spread. COVID-19 can be diagnosed with the help of gold standard reverse transcription polymerase chain reaction (RT-PCR) tests, quick antigen and antibody tests supplemented with computerized tomography (CT) scan and X-ray imaging. Considering the increase in the number of cases worldwide, there is a need for economical and viable ways to detect COVID-19. RT-PCR tests continue to be dominant; however, there are few concerns related to the sensitivity associated with the test results. Thus, medical community underlines the importance of medical imaging tools like CT scans and chest X-rays (CXRs) and the abnormalities revealed in CXRs and CT scan can help in detecting COVID-19.

Medical imaging and analytic tools that use machine learning and deep learning algorithms can enhance the diagnosis and prediction of COVID-19. There are many effective and proven image recognition techniques in deep learning like convolutional neural networks and transfer learning that can be used to design promising applications for COVID-19 detection. These models can be enhanced using image segmentation and edge detection techniques. In the proposed book chapter, we have reviewed the impact of the COVID-19 pandemic on the global community, the need for reliable, quick, and economical ways to detect it. We have surveyed the existing mechanisms for COVID-19 detection using machine learning

[1]Computer Engineering Department, Mukesh Patel School of Technology, Management, and Engineering, NMIMS University, Mumbai, India

and deep learning algorithms and presented a critical review of the major shortcomings in existing mechanism that could open further research in this area.

Keywords: Machine learning; COVID-19; Deep learning; Medical imaging; Classification

10.1 Introduction

Coronavirus affects distinct species causing varied symptoms and diseases. The latest mutant of the coronavirus family is the novel COVID-19 virus. This mutant has affected millions of people all over the globe. The initial cases of this virus were observed in Wuhan, China in early December 2019. After declaring the virus that had already affected thousands a 'Public Health Emergency Outbreak' on 30 January 2020, the World Health Organization declared the severe acute respiratory syndrome coronavirus 2 a pandemic on 11 March 2020.

With the increase in spread from one country to another, COVID-19 virus has started to show mutations that are more dangerous and hence a cause of concern. These mutations have started to show symptoms which are not displayed by the traditional virus. These symptoms are low-grade fever, dry mouth, non-salivation, gastrointestinal symptoms, and headaches [1]. It is important to detect the virus as it can be easily transmitted from one person to another. Scientists anticipate that the virus can be transmitted via droplets or aerosols released by an infected person. The spread is typically within a 1-m radius [2]. However, some studies suggest that COVID-19 is airborne and can spread to greater distances. This is a cause of great concern. Greenhalgh *et al.* [3] presented 10-fold reasons to support the transmission of COVID-19 being airborne. A reason stated to prove this was the transmission of the virus between people in different rooms. Considering the high transmission rate of the virus, governments all over the world have applied social-distancing restrictions to stop the spread of the virus. But treating a person is difficult considering the social distancing norms. So Rahman *et al.* [4] developed the EdgeSDN-I4COVID, this is a human-less IoT-enabled environment working without interruption. This architecture assures efficient and intelligent management of COVID-19.

Considering the high growth rate of COVID-19, governments were not able to prepare for the pandemic. Dash *et al.* [5] used the Facebook Prophet model to predict the value of cases for the next 90 days, including the peak. They used data from the USA, Brazil, India, France, Russia, and the United Kingdom shows that these are the six most worst hit countries. The model was also able to identify five significant change points and gave a goodness-of-fit as 85% mean absolute percentage error (MAPE).

COVID-19 is curable if it is detected at an early stage and the appropriate medication is given to the patient. Several ways to detect COVID-19 are reverse transcription polymerase chain reaction (RT-PCR), rapid antibody testing (RAT), and imaging techniques like computerized tomography (CT) scan, ultrasound, and chest X-ray (CXR). RAT is the fastest way of detecting COVID-19, and its kits provide results in a few minutes, but it has a lower efficiency than RT-PCR. RAT tests are done by pricking one's finger and putting the blood in the test kit. However, the problem with RAT is that since it tests antibodies and thus gives negative results when the patient is recently infected, indicating a false negative. Another problem is that in case the person has recovered, the person can still have antibodies present in his/her blood, which would give a positive result, indicating a false positive. Scohy *et al.* [6] got an efficiency of 30.2% for RAT tests. Thus, they concluded that even though RAT tests give fast results, they are not reliable.

RT-PCR tests are more accurate than RAT tests, as proved by authors of [6], but they are costly and take a lot of time. Considering a highly populated country like India, RT-PCR test results take days to reach the patient; this creates life-threatening concerns for the patients and people around them. Another concern with RT-PCR test is that it is not able to detect the new mutants of COVID-19. Thus, there is a need to explore other options which are reliable and more efficient. This is where radiology comes into the picture. Pneumonia being the most common symptom of COVID-19 can be detected with the help of CT scans and CXRs. Chendrasekhar *et al.* [7] performed a comparative study on the efficiency of chest CT scans and RT-PCR test. They performed their study on 1,400 individuals out of which 41.6% were males and the average age was 46.28±2.7 years. They represented the results in an odds ratio (OR) with the confidence interval being 95%. They proved that chest CT scan is superior to RT-PCR (OR 3.86, 95% CI), and it is a rapid and more efficient alternative to RT-PCR tests.

Another radiological way of detecting COVID-19 is with the aid of a CXR. CXRs are commonly used to detect pneumonia. CXRs can be obtained easily, as they are cheap, readily available, and give results fast. Yasin and Gouda [8] performed a study on 350 patients who were COVID-19 positive already. Out of these 350 patients, 220 showed baseline abnormalities in the CXRs. Out of the remaining 130 patients, 48 patients showed abnormalities in a follow-up. They concluded that their findings were good for accessing COVID-19.

COVID-19 is spreading and mutating at high pace. Many counties have faced second and third waves of COVID-19. In a country like India which has seen more than 4 lakh positive cases per day, there is a need for an efficient, fast, and cheap way of detecting COVID-19 so that the infected people can be treated on time. RT-PCR tests take a lot of time for giving results and require a lot of workforce and logistics, so it is not an optimal choice, whereas in the case of RAT tests, they have a low efficiency rate. There comes in the field of radiography. As seen earlier, CT scans and CXRs have established their efficiency for detecting COVID-19. CT scans and CXRs provide a fast and efficient way of detecting COVID-19.

Machine learning and deep learning provide us with an opportunity to reduce the burden of doctors and medical professionals. These models when trained properly can give us accurate and efficient detection mechanisms that can help us in an early detection of COVID-19. Training algorithms with the help of CT scans, CXRs, and ultrasound can help us in automating the scanning process for detecting COVID-19. Deep learning algorithms can be used to extract the important features from these radiography images and then be used to train machine learning models. Other feature extraction algorithms can be used to extract features, and then these features can be used to train machine learning models. Image-processing techniques can be used to enhance the radiography images before passing them through the model for training them. These techniques can also be used to localize and pinpoint the infected regions in CT scans, CXRs, and ultrasound images. These applications would not only help in better diagnosis but also in reducing the burden of medical staff, when there is a surge in the number of positive cases.

The major contributions of this survey include the following:

1. Reviewing the machine learning and deep learning architectures that are used by researchers for the detection of COVID-19 giving emphasis to datasets used and contributions by authors.
2. Presented a comparative analysis of the research works reviewed with importance to the challenges addressed by researchers in each work.
3. Identified the research gaps and provided future directions for the same.

This chapter is structured as follows: Section 10.1 consists of the introduction. Section 10.2 talks about the reviewed work. The preliminary discussion gives a brief idea about the various models and techniques discussed in the reviewed work. Further in Section 10.3, a comparative study is done on the work as reviewed in the previous section. Section 10.4 describes the most common research gaps; Section 10.5 as "Conclusion" states the future scope of expanding this study.

10.2 Literature review

10.2.1 Reviewed work

As seen in Figure 10.1, VGG networks were used in maximum research papers reviewed in this book chapter. ResNet, machine learning algorithms, and DenseNet were also frequently used. This chapter also reviews paper which use state-of-the-art algorithms like StackNet, Auxiliary Classifier Generative Adversarial Network, Generalized Regression Neural Network, and Probabilistic Neural Network (PNN) on various datasets and with a different combination of other algorithms and provide promising results.

10.2.1.1 Convolutional neural networks

Convolutional neural networks (CNNs) are in forefront of medical image analysis and have given promising results for disease identification. There are significant studies done using CNN on COVID-19 CXRs and CT scans. In research work [9], authors have proposed a 22-layer CNN model which classifies X-ray images into two class, three class, and four class. The authors created a dataset of 7,390 images. The 22-layer CNN model was tested extensively to select an appropriate number of layers, activation functions, and optimizers. The proposed work has been able to achieve an accuracy of 99.1% for two-class classification, 94.2% for three-class classification, and 91.2% for four-class classification. In comparison with many

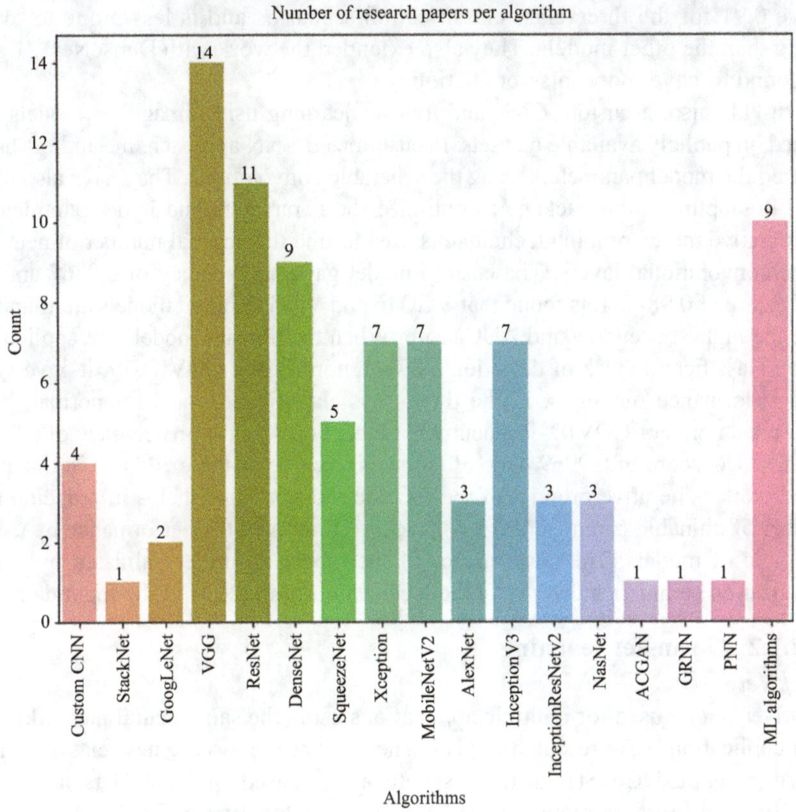

Figure 10.1 Number of research papers per algorithm

related works the authors' research works have attained better score in accuracy, precision, recall, *F*1 score, sensitivity, and specificity. However, the model performed poorly in low-quality X-ray images.

Another research work [10] in the same line is by authors Hernandez *et al.* where they have used CNN with non-COVID-19 pulmonary X-rays and tuning the final layers with COVID-19 X-ray images. The authors have accounted for the data scarcity problem for COVID-19 images through augmentation techniques available in OpenCV. The first approach used by the authors was to train CNN model using pulmonary X-rays from CheXpert. Later final layers were added and trained using CNN with COVID-19 X-ray images. However, the accuracy, precision, recall, and *F*1 score are found to be 0.68, 0.67, 0.63, and 0.65, respectively. The second approach used by authors is with transfer learning using ResNet50, VGG16, and DenseNet121. ResNet50 architecture is found to have better accuracy, precision, recall, and *F*1 score of around 90%. The authors have also extended the work as a multi-classification task with three classes of normal, COVID-19, and pneumonia. The testing accuracy for VGG16 is found to be above 0.91 for the three-class classification scenarios and is less prone to overfitting than the other models. They also extended the work with DenseNet121 and are found to have more false predictions.

In [11] also, a custom CNN and transfer learning using ImageNet models are trained on publicly available datasets. In customized CNN approach, the authors have reduced the model parameters using the separable convolutions. They have also used the Talos optimization package to optimize the parameters and hyper parameters. The iterative model pruning technique is used to find the optimal number of neurons in the convolutional layers. The custom model gave an accuracy of 0.9467 and an AUC score of 0.9842. It is found that VGG16 and VGG19 based models are found to have the highest accuracy and AUC score. When the transfer models are applied on binary classification task of detection between normal and COVID-19, it gave very high-performance measures. In the three-class classification task for normal, bacterial pneumonia or COVID-19 pneumonia InceptionV3 gave an accuracy of 0.9742 and an AUC score of 0.9969. One of the significant contributions made in this proposed work is iterative pruning of the specific models which helps in reducing the number of trainable parameters. They have also improved the performance by using ensemble of models. The performance of the model is further validated by using visualization techniques that verify the localization of the ROI of the input dataset.

10.2.1.2 Transfer learning

StackNet

StackNet can be used for multiple applications using the same neural network; one such application was presented in [12]. The authors proposed a new classification algorithm named CovStacknet. This network is based on StackNets and used VGG16 for feature extraction. After extracting features from CXR images, they used feature engineering to choose the key features for classification. They used a combination of two feature selection methods, the first one was selecting only those features whose variance was greater than a set threshold, the second one was selecting best features using random forest algorithm. Considering the imbalance in all the three datasets considered for this study, they used SMOTE. After these steps, the flatten layer of VGG16 is used to convert the two-dimensional tensors to a vector that could be fed to StackNet. The authors decided to stack logistic regression, extra trees (ET) classifier, support vector machine (SVM), linear discriminant analysis, RF, *K*-nearest neighbours (*K*NN), bagging classifier, decision tree (DT) classifier, adaptive boosting classifier, Gaussian naïve Bayes (GNB), and gradient boosting classifier. They used five estimators in the first layer, three in the next one, and one in the third layer. For the first dataset, labeled OCT (optical coherence tomography), and CXR images for classification, they classified the CXR in two classes, normal and pneumonia, achieving an accuracy of 97%. For the second dataset, COVID-19 CXR dataset consisting of non-COVID-19 X-rays and COVID-19 X-rays, achieving an accuracy of 74%, and for the third dataset, COVID-19 CXR had non-COVID-19 X-rays and COVID-19 X-rays giving an accuracy of 98%. The proposed model was made to first classify normal and pneumonia; thereafter the pneumonia X-ray was classified into COVID-19 and non-COVID-19.

GoogLeNet

GoogLeNet is a state of art algorithm developed by Team GoogLeNet. Mayya *et al.* [13] explained an application of GoogLeNet along with RF to detect COVID-19. Their work consisted of a fusion of image and text classification. For selecting the best combination of features, they used RF and trees on the two cases, first case with two classes which were COVID-19 and non-COVID-19, and the second case with four classes which were COVID-19, H1N1, pneumonia, and normal. Along with RF, they also used RUSboost Trees, Boosted Trees, Medium Trees, Bagged Trees, Coarse Trees, and Fine Trees. The text dataset had 32 attributes, when all of them were taken into consideration, and the accuracy for four-class classification was 77.5% and for two-class classification was 85.8%. Next, they reduced to 28 attributes and achieved an accuracy of 84.2% for four-class classification and 90.8% for two-class classification; finally, they reduced the attribute count to 22 attributes, hence, achieved an accuracy of 83.3% for four-class classification and two-class classification. For the image dataset, it was preprocessed by using a median filter that was used to smooth the intensity of the images, and they used Otsu automatic thresholding to get the target regions and clear borders and hole filling. For image classification, they replaced the fully connected layers for two- and four-class classifications. For the image classification model, the four-class classification gave an accuracy of 95.5% for COVID-19 and 72.43% for other classes, whereas in the case of two-class classification, the COVID-19 accuracy was 80.3% and 75% for non-COVID-19 class. Similarly, for the fusion model, the accuracy of four-class classification is 91.3%, and 91.67% for two-class classification. Since the model is trained on both textual and image data, missing values in the textual data should not affect the performance of the model.

VGG

VGG networks are prominent neural networks that are used in transfer learning. One such work was presented by Panwar *et al.* [14], where they used VGG16 model to produce a new model, named nCoVNet. The images in the dataset were first resized to 224 × 224 × 3. These images were then augmented by rotating the images in the rage of 20 degrees, flipping images horizontally and vertically. The model consisted of an input layer, followed by 18 combinations of convolutional layers with ReLU as activation function and MaxPooling. These layers were part of the VGG16 model. These layers were followed by a flatten layer, an AveragePooling2D layer, a fully connected layer with 64 neurons and ReLU as activation function, a dropout layer with the threshold of 0.5, and then we have an output layer with two neurons. The model was compiled using the Adam optimizer for 80 epochs and 0.0001 as learning rate. After training they got true positives as 41, false negatives as 1, false positives as 9, and true negatives as 33. The training accuracy was in the range of 93%–97% and with the training loss of 0.2%. They tried to solve the problem of data leakage by splitting the dataset using a logical method instead of the traditional train_test_split.

Another such work was presented in [15], they compared VGG16, VGG19, ResNet50V2, InceptionV3, Xception, InceptionResNetV2, NasNetLarge, and

DenseNet121; after comparing these CNN models, the best results were found in the case of VGG19. The fine-tuned VGG19 model was trained and tested using X-ray images, CT-scans, and ultrasounds. Since the dataset was small, data augmentation was performed by flipping images horizontally and vertically. To reduce the effect of sampling bias authors decided to apply N-CLAHE, this method not only normalizes the images but also enhances the minute details in the images. After studying the trends in tuned hyperparameters, five experiments were conducted, each having a separate set of hyperparameters and dataset. The output classes for each of the five experiments were different as well. The highest accuracy observed, using the Ultrasound dataset, was 100%. The parameters were as follows: learning rate was 10^{-5}, dropout rate kept at 0.2, batch size was 2, hidden layer states were set to 64 and 100 epochs. The best accuracy is for the X-ray dataset was 86% and was achieved by tuning the learning rate to 10^{-3} dropout rate at 0.2, batch size and hidden layer state to 8 and 100 epochs. For CT scans, however, the epochs had been set at 70 to avoid overfitting and batch size was reduced to 4 while hidden states were increased to 64. After tuning the learning rate at 10^{-3} and dropout rate at 0.2, an accuracy of 84% was achieved.

Vaid *et al.* [16] presented the work on VGG19 with the main aim being to reduce the false-negative cases as they are a major cause of concern. The model proposed in the study was a modified version of VGG19. A trainable multi-layer perceptron (MLP) was added to the traditional model to increase accuracy. This MLP, consisted of four fully connected layers consisting of 512, 512, 64, and 2 neurons, respectively, the output layer used SoftMax as the activation function. After the architecture was finalized, the hyperparameters were tuned: learning rate was set to 0.001, epochs were 100, and batch size was made 15. Dimensions of the input image was 512×512 and the output was binary classification (COVID-19 vs no COVID-19). The modified VGG19 model gave superior results with an accuracy of 96.3% and 0.151 binary cross entropy loss. The testing data gave 74 true positives, 32 true negatives, 3 false negative, and 1 false positive. However, the study did have some limitations. The number of samples in the dataset was small due to the non-availability of appropriate data. Another limitation stated was that the results were purely based on the X-ray images and did not consider the various external factors that may influence the result.

Brunese *et al.* [17] presented the use of VGG16 with two models to classify the CXRs into healthy and disease classes and other disease classes and COVID-19. Authors proposed a three-step method: first detecting pneumonia from the dataset, second segregating COVID-19 from pneumonia, and third localizing the area where the infection was present in COVID-19 CXRs. They used VGG16 for detecting pneumonia from the dataset and then detecting COVID-19 from the pneumonia samples. They replaced the fully connected layers of VGG16 with average pooling layer, flatten layer, a fully connected layer with 512 neurons, a dropout layer with threshold as 0.5, another fully connected layer with 64 neurons, and finally an output layer with 2 neurons and activation function as SoftMax. After classification, they used Grad-CAM, where a heat map is generated using the gradient information in the last convolutional layer, and then a heat map is created.

This heat map when added with the CXR gives the infected regions. The accuracy for classifying healthy and disease classes was 96% and the time taken by the model was 2.569 s, whereas the model gave an accuracy of 98% for the classification of COVID-19 and other forms of pneumonia and the time taken by the model was 2.498 s. For the future work, the authors aim to use this model over a wider range of pulmonary diseases and find ways to verify the accuracy of the model. A limitation of this chapter was that the dataset was highly biased and not equally distributed; also the authors only restricted their work to VGG16 network and did not explore other transfer learning models.

ResNet

ResNet CNN architectures are based on residual networks. ResNet18, ResNet34, ResNet50, and ResNet101 are popular ResNet architectures. Minaee *et al.* [18] compared ResNet18, ResNet50, SqueezNet, and DenseNet-121. For this purpose, the authors built a custom dataset, COVID-CXR dataset, with CXR of COVID-19 and normal patients. The training set initially had just 84 COVID-19 X-rays and had to be extended to around 420 images using data augmentation. The testing set had 100 COVID-19 and 3,000 normal images. Even after data augmentation, the number of training samples is limited and thus the authors only fine-tune the last layer of each model after performing transfer learning. Each model runs for 100 epochs, has a learning rate of 0.0001, batch size is 20 and uses Adam Optimizer and Cross-Entropy as its loss function. The loss function is minimized using stochastic gradient descent. After training was completed, the models were tested and evaluated using performance metrics like sensitivity and specificity, precision–recall curve, and confusion matrix. The best models were ResNet18 and SqueezeNet. While all models had a sensitivity of approximately 98%, ResNet18 had a specificity of 90.7% while SqueezeNet had a specificity of 92.9%. Both ResNet18 and SqueezeNet had only 2 false negatives, but 321 and 237 false positives, respectively. The authors suggest that the model needs to be trained on larger COVID-19 datasets in order to achieve the desired performance.

More CNN models were compared by Nayak *et al.* [19] who concluded that ResNet50 worked best when performing a binary classification on COVID-19 images. The authors started their study by collecting the right dataset. Images were normalized by dividing the pixels with 255. Data augmentation was performed to increase the number of images. Images were rotated by an angle of 5 degrees (clockwise), horizontally flipped, scaled by 15%, and Gaussian noise (mean = 0 and variance = 0.25) was added to the images. The eight models compared by the study were InceptionV3, MobileNet, AlexNet, GoogLeNet, VGG16, SqueezNet, ResNet34, and ResNet50. Images were resized to 224 × 224 for all models expect for InceptionV3 which has an input size of 299 × 299. Apart from different models, different hyperparameters (optimizer, learning rate, epochs, and batch size) were tested on each model to understand what worked best. For optimizers, Adam, RMSProp, AdaDelta, and SGD were tested. Adam worked best for most models. A batch size of 32 gave the best results for all models expect VGG16 and MobileNet and thus was selected for the study. After comparing all the models using different performance metrics, it was found that ResNet models gave 100% sensitivity. However, ResNet34 outperformed ResNet50 due to its higher accuracy. While ResNet34 gave an accuracy of 98.33%, ResNet50 stood at 97.50%.

Authors of [20] presented a combination of ResNet50 and U-Net for detecting COVID-19 from CT scans, naming the network CoVNet. The ResNet50 model was modified and after all the convolution layers, the final feature maps were fed to a fully connected layer, giving probability for each class. The dataset contained only those CT scan slices of thickness less than 3 mm. From the CT scan images, with the help of U-Net, the lung area, which was the region of interest, was extracted and used for training the model. For COVID-19 class, the sensitivity, specificity, and AUC score were 90%, 96%, and 0.96, respectively, whereas the pneumonia class gave a sensitivity of 87%, specificity of 92%, and the AUC score was 0.95. Similarly, the AUC score for normal class was 0.98, specificity was 96%, and sensitivity was found to be 94%. For better interpretation, the authors used Grad-CAM for highlighting the infected regions in the CT scans. Some limitations stated by the authors about their studies are as follows: (i) since COVID-19 shows symptoms similar to that of pneumonia; (ii) the lugs could be affected by multiple infections at the same time, so it is not possible to differentiate these images just based on the visual appearance; (iii) a large dataset can be used for the study, for creating a better and generalized model; (iv) deep learning models are not interpretable and not transparent.

Ismael *et al.* [21] compared three ways to detect COVID-19 cases using CXRs: deep feature extraction followed by SVM classification, fine-tuning pre-trained CNN models, and building a custom end-to-end trained CNN model. In the first method, the various kernels used in combination with SVM were linear (epsilon = 0.04), quadratic (epsilon = 0.02), cubic (epsilon = 0.01), and Gaussian (epsilon = 0.01). VGG16, VGG19, ResNet18, and ResNet101 were also used for feature extraction; however, the results were not satisfactory enough. ResNet50 gave an average accuracy of 92.6% (all kernels combined). The ResNet50, combined with the linear kernel SVM, gave an accuracy of 94.7%. In the case of fine-tuning, the same CNN models were tuned and tested. Again, ResNet50 gave the highest accuracy of 94.63%, two false negatives, and five false positives. The custom CNN gave an accuracy of 91.83% which was not as good as the previous models. Thus, the best results were obtained using ResNet50 in combination with linear kernel function of SVM.

In a study proposed by Zhong *et al.* [22], ResNet50 was used as base model for feature extraction from CXR images. The authors began by collecting data from three sources: COVIDx, five hospitals from Partners HealthCare system in the United States, and four hospitals in South Korea. There were three classes in this study: COVID-19, non-COVID-19 pneumonia, and control (normal images). After performing essential preprocessing steps, segmentation was performed using an ensemble of five deep neural networks based on the EfficientNet architecture. ResNet50 is used as the backbone of the main model. Features are extracted in two parts of the model. The first part, $F1$ consists of the first 22 layers of the ResNet50 architecture whereas the second part, $F2$ contains the next 18 layers. Between the two parts, there is a special attention module placed that generates a 16 × 16 mask applied on the output of the ResNet50 model. After the two parts and attention model, the features are mapped and passed through the remainder layers of the ResNet50 architecture. To train this model, the Adam optimizer was used along with a learning rate of 3e−5, batch size of 48, 5 epochs, and 2,000 iterations. The aim of the entire model is to learn function f that embeds given image into a d-dimensional space. The next step is to classify the images using the features. To do so, KNN algorithm is used with $k = 10$. The KNN is found using the cosine-similarity measure:

$$S_{i,j} = \langle f(x_i), f(x_j)\rangle / \|f(x_i)\|^2 \|f(x_j)\|^2 \tag{10.1}$$

However, to normalize the embedding, the denominator is set to 1. To calculate the loss in the final paired metric learning stage, the multi-similarity loss function in the following equation is used:

$$\begin{aligned} L = & \frac{1}{m}\sum_{i=1}^{m}\frac{1}{\alpha}\log\left[1+\sum_{j\in P_i} e^{-\alpha(S_{i,j}-\lambda)}\right] \\ & +\frac{1}{\beta}\log\left[1+\sum_{j\in N_i} e^{-\beta(S_{i,j}-\lambda)}\right] \end{aligned} \tag{10.2}$$

where x_i is the anchor image, P_i is the images with same label, N_i is the images with different label, m is the batch size, α, β, λ are the hyperparameters.

To better understand the effectiveness of the proposed architecture, the results were compared with the baseline ResNet50 model. While the proposed model had an accuracy of 83.9%, ResNet50 showed an accuracy of 81.5% on the same data. The proposed model was also more sensitive towards the COVID-19 inputs.

DenseNet

DenseNet or Dense Convolutional Network connects one layer to all the layers in the sequence ahead. Authors of [23] proposed a comparative study wherein CNN models were used for extracting features followed by classification done by machine learning techniques. For the study, the authors custom-made two datasets – Dataset A and Dataset B. The only difference between the two datasets was that they had normal X-ray images from different sources. To increase the size of training samples, data augmentation using the affine transformations was performed. A total of 144 experiments were conducted under this study. Each had a different pair of CNN model and classifier. Since both datasets had different samples, different models worked best for them. For Dataset A, DenseNet121 with MLP worked best. But for Dataset B, DenseNet201 along with MLP worked. Accuracy scores for the two datasets were 98.974% (approx.) and 95.641% (approx.), respectively. However, when data was not augmented, Dataset A gave best results with MobileNet and SVM (linear) and gave the highest accuracy. They took into consideration many performance metrics like confusion matrix, $F1$ score, false-positive rate, and time taken by network for training.

In [24], the authors have proposed a three-step model to detect COVID-19 using CT scan. The process starts with data augmentation. Images were rotated and flipped. The second step is to perform deep feature extraction using the DenseNet201 model as it gave a higher accuracy as compared to other CNN models. The third step is to perform classification. For this purpose, the traditional machine learning models did not give satisfactory results. However, the multi-kernels extreme learning machine-based deep neural networks (MK-ELM-DNN) gave impressive results. The dataset used had two classes (non-COVID-19 and COVID-19). The DenseNet201 model for the current study contains 709 layers, 806 connections, 201 depths, and about 20 million parameters. The extreme learning model (ELM) is a neural network with one hidden layer. It learns at a faster rate and performs better generalization as compared to traditional neural networks. After comparing various functions, the ReLU function was selected alongside ELM model. An accuracy of 98.36% was achieved using the MK-ELM-DNN model. Other metrics were – sensitivity: 98.28%; specificity: 98.44%; precision: 98.22%; *F*1-score: 98.25%; and AUC: 98.36%.

Ohata *et al.* [25] proposed Casecade-SEMEnet which was developed using SEME-ResNet50 and SEME-DenseNet169. There were three datasets used in this study for three different purposes. Dataset 1 was divided into three classes – bacteria, virus, and normal. The ResNet50 model was trained using this dataset and its goal was to categorize the X-ray into one of the three classes. Once it was detected that the X-ray belonged to the virus class, it was passed on to the next CNN model – DenseNet169. To train this model, Dataset 2 was used which had two classes – COVID virus and other viruses. The third dataset, U-Net was used to remove any non-pathological features on the X-ray films. This helped a better classification of X-rays from unknown sources as it performed segmentation. The biggest challenge that the authors faced here was that the size of the image in the ImageNet database which was used to train the CNN models was very small as compared to the training X-ray images. Thus, global average pooling was applied to all input images. SE-Structure was added, and Attention module was used to channel the characteristics. These additions boosted the accuracy. To further enhance results, CLAHE was added to the training set and MoEx structure was used in networks. Dataset 1 gave an accuracy of 85.62% with SEME-ResNet50, and Dataset 2 gave an accuracy of 97.14% on the SE-MoEx-DenseNet169.

SqueezeNet

SqueezeNet provides similar efficiency as AlexNet. Chowdhury *et al.* [26] presented the comparison between SqueezeNet, AlexNet, DenseNet201, and ResNet18 for the detection of COVID-19 with the help of CXRs. These X-rays were collected from various sources and then resized to 224 × 224 for DenseNet201 and ResNet18 and 227 × 227 for AlexNet and SqueezeNet. Since the number of images in the dataset was low, the images were augmented and the normalized. Mini batch gradient decent was chosen as the optimizer, the learning rate was set to 0.0003, momentum as 0.9, and 16 mini-batches. For two-class classification, ResNet18 gave the testing accuracy of 96.7%, AlexNet gave the testing accuracy of 97.5%, whereas the testing accuracy of DenseNet201 was 98%, and the highest testing accuracy was 98.3%. SqueezeNet gave the AUC as 0.998 and *F*1 score as 0.983. For three-class classification, the testing accuracy for ResNet18 was 95%, testing accuracy of AlexNet was 95.4%, whereas DenseNet201 gave the testing accuracy as 96.7%, and again the highest testing accuracy was given by SqueezeNet as 98.3%. The AUC score was 0.99 and *F*1 score was 0.983 for SqueezeNet. The performance of this chapter could be improved by using more images in the dataset, which would help to generalize the models.

Xception

Xception architecture is based on the Inception CNN architecture and is short for 'Extreme Inception'. Khan *et al.* [27] presented the use of Xception architecture to build a model – CoroNet – to detect COVID-19 using CXR images. In addition to the traditional Xception architecture, CoroNet has a dropout layer and two fully connected layers at the end of the model. After finalizing the architecture, three models were prepared. The first and most elaborate set was a four-class classification (COVID-19, Viral Pneumonia, Bacterial Pneumonia, and Normal). The accuracy of this classification was 89.6%, *F*-measure was 89.8%, precision of 90%, recall 89.92%, and specificity 96.4%. The other two models were based on this main multi-class classification model. They were used to perform three-class (COVID-19, normal, pneumonia) and two-class binary (COVID-19, normal) classifications. While the accuracy of the three-class model was 95%, the model made for binary classification gave an accuracy of 99%. Although CoroNet provides a way to detect the deadly virus in a less expensive manner and gives good accuracy especially with binary classification, it needs to be trained and tested using bigger datasets before it can be used practically.

Jain *et al.* [28] after comparing InceptionV3, ResNeXt, and Xception found that the best results were obtained using the Xception model. The dataset used in the comparison was gathered from Kaggle. The model proposed was for a three-class classification (COVID-19, Normal, and Pneumonia). Preprocessing was done using the Keras Data generator. The data was then used to train the model. The CNN models used LeakyReLU for the activation function and SoftMax for the final classification. While the Xception model gave an accuracy of 100% for the training data, the testing data had an accuracy of 97%. The other two models, Inception and ResNet, had a testing accuracy of 96% and 93%, respectively. The biggest limitation of this study, however, was that the dataset was highly imbalanced.

In a more elaborate study as proposed by El Gannour *et al.* [29], six different CNN models were compared – VGG16, VGG19, InceptionV3, Xception, ResNet50V2, and MobileNetV2. The 'COVID-19 Radiography' dataset used for this study was curated by University of Doha and is publicly available on Kaggle. Transfer learning was used to train the model on the COVID-19 dataset. After preprocessing, the images were fed to these models for training. Hyperparameter tuning was performed: learning rate = 0.0001, batch size = 15, and epochs = 50. While most models gave an accuracy of 97%, InceptionV3, and Xception gave an accuracy of 98%. However, Xception proved to be the better model as it had 100% COVID-19 sensitivity compared to the 95% sensitivity displayed by the inception architecture.

MobileNetV2

MobileNetV2 is an improved version of MobileNetV1 and works on the concept of ResNet. Apostolopoulos *et al.* [30] presented the use of MobileNetV2 and other transfer learning algorithms to compare their efficiency in detecting COVID-19 from CXRs. For this purpose, they used two datasets, containing three classes which were normal, pneumonia, and COVID-19. For their study, they used VGG19, MobileNetV2, Inception, Xception, and InceptionResNetV2, and they compared the performance of these models by using ReLU activation function for all layers, a dropout layer between two fully connected layers, Adam optimizer to compile the model, and trained the model for 10 epochs with the batch size 64. VGG19 gave an accuracy of 93.80% on the first dataset whereas the accuracy for MobileNetV2 was 92.85% on the same dataset. Similarly, on the same dataset, Inception, Xception, and InceptionResNetV2 gave an accuracy of 92.85%. The two best performing algorithms, VGG19 and MobileNetV2, were applied on the second dataset. Here MobileNetV2 outperformed VGG19 and gave an accuracy of 94.72%, sensitivity of 98.66%, and specificity of 96.46%. MobileNetV2 is better than VGG19 because it gives a better specificity, thus proving to better for the classification task on a particular dataset. A limitation to the study was that all five algorithms were trained for only 10 epochs, training the models further could increase the efficiency.

An excellent example of MobileNetV2 being deployed in a mobile application was demonstrated by Li *et al.* [31]. Authors used deep learning to build an application that would detect COVID-19 from CXRs. They use a two-stage detection mechanism where DenseNet121 is used as a pretrained attending physician and resident doctor and MobileNetV2 and SqueezeNet are used as medical students. The goal of DenseNet121 is to classify the input X-ray image into normal, pneumonia, and COVID-19. The DenseNet121 acting as the attending physician extracts features from the CXRs, and then this is used to fine-tune the DenseNet121 acting as the Resident Doctors. The tuned DenseNet121 is used to train MobileNetV2 and SqueezeNet using knowledge distillation. MobileNetV2 and SqueezeNet extract features and predict whether the condition of the patient has improved, is stable, or has deteriorated. Authors use probabilistic compact loss for training the MobileNetV2 and SqueezeNet, and the following equation displays the same:

$$L_{pc}(\theta) = \frac{1}{N}\sum_{k=1}^{K}\sum_{i_k \in S_k}\sum_{j=1, j\neq k}^{K} \max\{0, f_j(x_{ik}) + \xi - f_k(x_{ik})\} \tag{10.3}$$

where ξ is the tuning parameter for the network, larger the value, more would be the interclass compactness. MobileNetV2 and SqueezeNet were tested for their resource consumption on six mobile phones. Overall, MobileNetV2 was better than SqueezeNet for high performance phones, whereas SqueezeNet is more suitable for low performance phones.

AlexNet

AlexNet model won ILSVRC10 and had a top-5 error of 17.0%. Maghdid *et al.* [32] presented a comparison between modified AlexNet and a custom CNN by training the model over CT scan and X-ray images. The custom model consists of an input layer, and this was followed by a convolutional layer with 16 filters of size 5×5 and ReLU activation function, following this was batch normalization, two fully connected layers, and finally the output layer with two neurons and SoftMax as activation function. The weights were initialized using Glorot and cross-entropy as loss function. The modified AlexNet network had the input size of $127 \times 127 \times 3$, the batch size was set to 10, trained for 20 epochs, the learning rate was initialized to 0.0003. The accuracy for X-ray was 94% and for CT scan was 94.1% on the custom CNN, whereas an accuracy of CT scan was 82%, and X-ray was 98% for modified AlexNet. A limitation to the work is that the proposed models were only trained for 20 epochs, and further increase in accuracy could be observed.

10.2.1.3 Ensemble

As we have seen, transfer learning models have performed individually well, researchers have tried to combine these models together for even better results. One such work was presented in [33], the authors' ensemble MobileNetV2 and SqueezeNet for feature extraction from the CXR images, and then classified into normal, pneumonia, and COVID-19 using SVM classifier. They preprocessed the image with the help of fuzzy colour technique. Next, these images were given as input to MobileNetV2 and SqueezeNet and features are extracted keeping momentum as 0.9, decay as 0.000001, batch size as 64, using stochastic gradient decent activation function, and learning rate as 0.00001 for both the models. These features were then clubbed using social mimic optimization and given as input to SVM for classification. When MobileNetV2 and SqueezeNet were used individually using the same method, the overall accuracies were 98.54% and 97.81%, respectively, whereas the ensemble model gave an overall accuracy of 99.27% which is clearly better than the individual models. The future work of this model, as stated by the authors, is to use deep learning to find the impact of COVID-19 on other organs to.

Another work was presented in [34] by using DenseNet121 and VGG19 for feature extraction from CXR images and then using SVM for classifying the features into normal, COVID-19, and pneumonia and named this model as CoVNet-19. In the DenseNet121 model the last fully connected layer was removed, the model now gave an output of 32 features in the shape of 32×1, like DenseNet121, VGG19 was also gave an output of 32 features in the shape of 32×1 after the removal of the last fully connected layer. These features were then concatenated to the shape 64×1 and used to train SVM. Before giving input to the model, the images in the COVID-19 class are augmented. For VGG19 and DenseNet121, the Adam optimizer was used to train the model with the learning rate of 0.001 and decay rate of 10 after each epoch, and batch size of 32. Individually the training and testing accuracy for three-class classification of VGG19 and DenseNet121 was 96.17% and 96.08%; and 97.79% and 96.30%, respectively, whereas the CoVNet-19 gave testing and training accuracy as 98.28% and 99.02%. For two-class classification, the training and testing accuracy of VGG19 and DenseNet121 was 98.47% and 99.61%; and 99.87% and 99.60%, respectively, whereas the CoVNet-19 gave testing and training accuracy as 100% and 99.71%. Future work as stated by the authors is to eliminate the limitations to their proposed model, creating a lighter version of the model so that it can be deployed on mobile phones.

10.2.1.4 Generative networks

Generative networks have multiple application areas like generating cartoon, recreating faces, text to image translation, and 3D object generation. Another application area of generative networks is to augment datasets, Waheed *et al.* [36] presented such an application in the case of ACGAN (auxiliary classifier generative adversarial networks) where it was used to produce synthetic X-ray images and predicting COVID-19 and named the model as CovidGAN. Considering the limited size of the dataset, authors realized the need of augmentation; therefore they used the ACGAN approach. The generative network recreated images and the discriminative network labels these images. The generative network took vector-containing noise which was normally distributed and was random in nature, having a standard deviation of 0.02 and the class label as inputs and obtained as single-output image of size $112 \times 112 \times 3$. The class labels were passed through the embedding layer, then through a 7×7 node dense layer, have linear activation function giving an output of $7 \times 7 \times 1$, and the noise tensor with initial shape of $1{,}024 \times 7 \times 7$ gave an output of $7 \times 7 \times 1{,}024$. The class label and the noise tensor are combined and then passed through four convolutional layers, where the output shapes were $14 \times 14 \times 512$ for first layer, $28 \times 28 \times 256$ for second layer, $56 \times 56 \times 128$ for third layer, and finally $112 \times 112 \times 3$ for the fourth and the final layer. The discriminative network took the image of size $112 \times 112 \times 3$ generated by the generative network and the original image then classifies the image as real or face and assigns label of whether it is COVID-19 or normal. Discriminative network had four convolutional layers, each convolutional layer was followed by a batch normalization layer and a Leaky ReLU activation layer; at the end we had a flatten layer and a dropout layer with the threshold being 50%. The output size of the discriminative network is $56 \times 56 \times 64$ for first layer, $28 \times 28 \times 128$ for second layer, $14 \times 14 \times 256$ for third layer, and finally $7 \times 7 \times 512$ for the last convolutional layer. This model was compared with the performance of VGG16. VGG16 used an Adam optimizer for training with a learning rate of 0.001, and the batch size was set to 16. The VGG16 model gave an accuracy of 85%, sensitivity of 69%, and specificity of 95%, whereas the CovidGAN model gave an accuracy of 95%, sensitivity of 90%, and specificity of 97%. As seen from the results, CovidGAN outperformed the VGG16 model. The authors of the paper tend to improve the GAN network of the model and work on a dataset that is big and is from a single source, rather than using multiple sources.

10.2.1.5 Generalized regression neural network and probabilistic neural network

GRNNs are improved neural networks based on nonparametric regression. It is an advanced variant of radial basis neural network. PNN on the other hand is a feed-forward neural network used for classification and is a variant of the Bayesian Network. Ardhya *et al.* [37] proposed a model that combines the two approaches using the AND operator. The proposed model works as a multi-class classifier. It classifies CXR images into four classes – normal, pneumonia viral, pneumonia bacterial, COVID-19. Three sets of experiments are covered in this study – binary classification (COVID-19 vs normal), three-class classification (COVID-19 vs normal vs pneumonia bacterial), and four-class classification (COVID-19 vs normal vs pneumonia bacterial vs pneumonia viral). The dataset used in this study is created by Joseph Cohen. Since the dataset is very small, one-shot learning technique was used. To ensure maximum accuracy, the model is trained using all images, one at a time. However, an optimum number of training iterations is fixed empirically. It derives raw features from the image which are then fed to the GRNN and PNN models. However, it is important to choose the best samples and form a cluster using the enhanced features. Thus, there is a need to combine the results obtained by these models using the ensemble AND operation. Once the clusters are ready, the model can be tested using the testing samples. Raw features are extracted from the testing sample and fed to the ensemble model which classifies it. For experiment 1 (binary classification), 100% accuracy was achieved. In experiment 2 (three-class classification), the highest accuracy of 85.23% was achieved when 13 samples were taken into consideration. Finally, for the last experiment (four-class classification), an accuracy of 74.05% was achieved when a number of samples were 29. Although the model considerably fails for four-class classification, it ensures a 100% accuracy in its binary classification.

10.2.1.6 YOLO

Bhuyan *et al.* [35] used segmentation techniques followed by applying deep learning to detect COVID-19 in CXRs and CT scans. YOLO with full-resolution CNN was used to segment the infected areas in the images. The authors used a dataset consisting of 2,794 images for training and 1,061 images for testing. After segmentation, a CNN is used to classify if it is COVID-19. Classification was performed over 4-fold cross-validation of test dataset. In the fourth cross-fold validation with mass segmentation, the sensitivity was 96.66%, specificity was 99.41%, accuracy was 99%, MCC was 96.07%, and *F*1 score of 96.66%.

10.2.1.7 Machine learning

We have seen how deep learning algorithms were used to detect COVID-19 from CXRs, CT scans, and ultrasounds. Now let us have a look at the application of machine learning algorithms for detecting COVID-19. Authors of [38] have presented us with the used of *F*-tree, iterative neighbourhood component feature selector, and machine learning algorithms like DT, LD, SVM, ensemble, and *K*NN for detecting COVID-19. *F*-transform or fuzzy transform is used for image reduction. Multi-kernel local binary pattern is used to extract features. Next iterative neighbourhood component analysis (INCA) selects the best features. For applying INCA, first min–max normalization is applied on the extracted features, then NCA weights are generated from the normalised features, and finally with the help of *K*NN and

10-fold cross-validation, they extract the top 16 features. Using these features the previously stated group of classifiers were trained. In the DT group, tree fine gave an average accuracy of 83.57% and tree medium gave an average accuracy of 83.56%. Linear discriminant gave an average accuracy of 79.11%, and in the ensemble family, bagged tree gave an accuracy of 90.92%, subspace discriminant gave an average accuracy of 89.87%, and subspace *K*NN gave an average accuracy of 95.58%. For SVM they used different kernels; for cubic kernel, the average accuracy was 96.23%; for quadratic kernel, the average accuracy was 95.84%; for Gaussian kernel, the average accuracy was 95.37%; and the average accuracy for linear kernel was 94.75%. Similarly, different kernels were used for *K*NN also; for fine kernel, the average accuracy was 95.19%; for medium kernel, the average accuracy was 92.25%; for coarse kernel, the average accuracy was 85.84%; for cosine kernel, the average accuracy was 91.70%; for cubic kernel, the average accuracy was 91.79%; and the average accuracy for weighted kernel was 94.78%. As seen from the results, SVM with cubic kernel gave maximum average accuracy which was 96.23%. The limitation to this study is the small size of the dataset. Since they have not used many images, so their model would not be generalized.

Another study was performed in [39] to use local binary patterns and machine learning algorithms to detect COVID-19. Local binary pattern is a method of texture feature extraction of images. The pixel values are compared with that of its neighbours and a binary string is generated using the difference. This binary string is converted to decimal, and this becomes the value of that pixel. The hyperparameter for this is the radius (*R*) and the number of neighbours (*P*). They then applied the extracted features to train naïve GNB, *K*NN, SVM, random tree, and RF; they also used ensemble of RF-RT-SVM, RF-RT-*K*NN, and RF-SVM-*K*NN. They applied different combinations of *R* and *P* on the model are (1,8), (2,16), (3,24), (4,32), (5,40), (6,48), (7,56), (8,64), (9,72), and (10,80); the average accuracies for the models on these combinations are 84.467%, 83.525%, 84.344%, 83.525%, 83.361%, 83.852%, 83.648%, 81.926%, 80.328%, and 80.328%, respectively. It is evidently visible that *R*1 (1,8) gave the best average accuracy, and overall, the ensemble of RT-RF-*K*NN for (6,48) and (7,56) gave the best accuracy as 89.180%. The limitation of this study is the small sample size used for the study.

Thepade *et al.* [40] proposed a way of detecting COVID-19 with the help of global texture feature extraction using colour space. The images are converted from RGB (red green blue) to YCrCB, Kekre-LUV, and CIE-LUV colour spaces, a feature vector is generated considering different combinations of colour space. The first feature vector is the concatenation of CIE-LUV and YCrCb, the second vector is the concatenation of CIE-L, Y, and Kekre-LUV, and the third vector is the concatenation of Kekre-LUV and YCrCb. These feature vectors are given as input to machine learning model for classification; the models used were RF, ET, GNB, and ensemble of ET+RF+SimpleLogistic (SL), ET+RF+GNB, and ET+RF+RT. These models were trained using 10-fold cross-validation. For the first feature vector (Y+CIE-L+Kekre-LUV), GNB gave an accuracy of 65%, ET gave an accuracy of 71.67%, RF gave an accuracy of 82.92%, whereas the ensemble models ET+RF+RT, ET+RF+NB, and ET+RF+SL gave accuracies of 80.83%, 80.83%, and 84.167%, respectively. Clearly, the ensemble of ET+RF+SL performed best for this feature. When the second feature vector (YCrCb+Kekre-LUV) was used, GNB gave an accuracy of 66.67%, ET gave an accuracy of 78.33%, RF gave an accuracy of 82.917%, whereas the accuracies of the ensemble models ET+RF+RT, ET+RF+GNB, and ET+RF+SL were 80.83%, 85.83%, and 87.083%. Again, the ensemble of ET+RF+SL gave the best accuracy for the second feature vector too. For the third feature vector (YCrCb+CIE-LUV), the accuracy for GNB, ET, and RF were 67.5%, 80.83%, and 84.583%, respectively, whereas for the ensemble models of ET+RF+RT, ET+RF+GNB, and ET+RF+SL the accuracies were 83.33%, 85%, and 84.167%, respectively. For the third feature the ensemble of ET+RF+NB gave the best results. Overall, the combination of the feature vector YCrCb+Kekre-LUV and ET+RF+SL gave the best results of 87.083% accuracy, 87% precision, 87.1% recall, 86.9% *F*1 score, and 79.5% Matthews correlation coefficient. Though the proposed model has low computational power, but the data used to train the model is less, due to which the results are not up to the mark.

10.3 Comparative analysis of existing work

In the previous section, we have reviewed major research works in COVID-19 detection and classification using machine learning and deep learning approaches; however, a comparative analysis of these works in the perspective of dataset used, augmentation techniques, major contributions, and challenges will throw light for future research. In Figure 10.2, we have presented the accuracy comparison between the models used in the reviewed works.

In Figure 10.2 we can see the comparison on accuracy between multi-class classification (two class, three class, and four class). For two class, Generative networks [24] give us the best accuracy of 100% and an ensemble of DenseNet and VGG gives an accuracy of 99%. Similarly for three-class classification, the best results are shown by VGG and SqueezeNet, both giving an accuracy of 96%. In the case of four-class classification, GoogLeNet gave an accuracy of 95%, and CNN gave an accuracy of 91%.

In Table 10.1, the major limitations of the research works identified were unavailability of large datasets, imbalanced datasets, and the use of multiple image

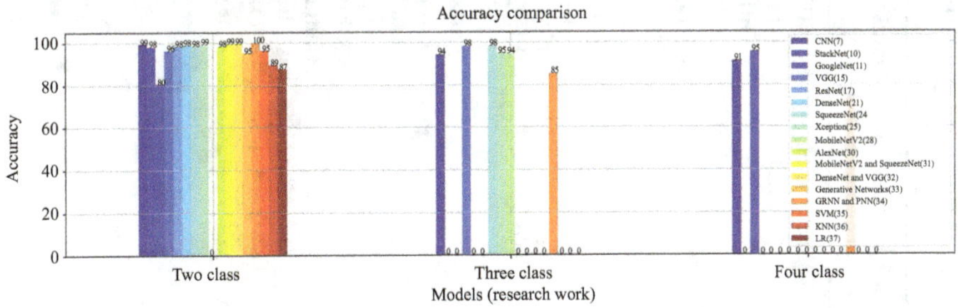

Figure 10.2 Accuracy comparison of state-of-the-art machine learning and deep learning algorithms

Table 10.1 Comparative study of papers reviewed

Research work	Feature extraction	Dataset	Sample size and classes	Data augmentation	Class imbalance	Major contributions	Limitations
[12]	Yes, using VGG16	COVID-19 chest X-ray dataset (GitHub), COVID-19 chest X-ray (Kaggle), and labelled OCT and chest X-ray images for classification (Kaggle)	COVID-19: 634; pneumonia: 4,474; normal: 1,583; 2 combination of classes Normal and pneumonia; COVID-19 and non-COVID-19	Yes, Synthetic minority oversampling technique	Yes, solved using augmentation	Proposed CovStacknet	
[36]	No	IEEE COVID-19 chest X-ray dataset, COVID-19 radiography database, COVID-19 chest X-ray dataset initiative	COVID-19: 403; normal: 721	Yes, using ACGAN	Yes	Proposed a state of art Covid-GAN	GAN architecture can be improved further; small dataset
[37]	Yes, using one shot learning	Joseph Cohen (COVID-19 chest X-ray dataset)	306 (69 COVID-19, 79 in normal, pneumonia viral, pneumonia bacterial); 3 combination of classes COVID-19 and normal; normal, bacterial pneumonia, and COVID-19; normal, bacterial pneumonia, viral pneumonia, and COVID-19	No	No	100% accuracy in binary classification, one-shot learning approach on COVID-19 dataset	Accuracy of four-class classification is very low

[9]	No	COVID-R	2,843 COVID-19 images, 3,108 normal images and 1,439 pneumonia images: a total of 7,390; COVID-19 and normal; normal, bacterial pneumonia, and COVID-19; normal, bacterial pneumonia, viral pneumonia, and COVID-19	No	Yes	Proposed a custom made 22-layer CNN	Model performed poorly in low quality X-ray images
[27]	No	SIRM, Stanford CheXpert	288 samples; normal and COVID-19; normal, COVID-19, and pneumonia	Yes, Python OpenCV	No	Proposed a custom CNN model	Too many false predictions
[11]	No	Paediatric CXR dataset, RSNA CXR dataset, twitter COVID-19 CXR dataset, Montreal COVID-19 CXR dataset	Normal: 7,595; unknown pneumonia: 6,012; bacterial pneumonia: 2,780; COVID-19: 313; normal and COVID-19; normal, bacterial pneumonia, and COVID-19	No	Yes	22	High class imbalance
[13]	No	Italian society of medical and international radiology and other medical resources	240 images out of which 120 were for COVID-19; COVID-19 and non-COVID-19; COVID-19, normal, pneumonia, and H1N1	No	Yes	Proposed a fusion model of GoogLeNet and random forest for image and text classification	There are 120 images for COVID-19 due to which it leads to a bias dataset

(Continues)

Table 10.1 (*Continued*)

Research work	Feature extraction	Dataset	Sample size and classes	Data augmentation	Class imbalance	Major contributions	Limitations
[14]	No	COVID-19 image data collection and Kaggle's chest X-ray images (pneumonia)	142 PA images from 192 images COVID-19 and 142 from the normal class of the Kaggle's chest X-ray images dataset; 2 classes COVID-19 and non-COVID-19	Yes, rotate images, horizontal and vertical flip	No	Proposed a deep learning based neural network called nCoVNet	The dataset is very small in size
[15]	No	CT-scan: COVID-19-CT-dataset; ultrasound: POCOVID-Net: (POCUS); X-rays: COVID-19 image data collection: prospective predictions are the future	X-ray: 729; CT: 746; ultrasound: 911; X-ray classes-normal, COVID-19, and pneumonia; CT classes-normal and COVID-19; ultrasound classes-normal, COVID-19, and pneumonia	Yes	No	Made a comparison between all popular imaging techniques as well as popular CNN models	–
[16]	No	COVID images: publicly available papers/article, normal: NIH clinical centre	181 COVID-19, 364 normal	No	Yes	High accuracy with just 1 false negative	Research based on literature review that may not be peer-reviewed
[17]	No	Dataset collected from various medical facilities	6,523 images out of which 250 were for COVID-19 and 3,520 were normal	Yes (rotation by 15 degrees)	Yes	Highlighting the areas of infection in the chest X-rays	The dataset is highly imbalanced, study was restricted to only one model

[18]	No	COVID chest X-ray dataset for COVID images, GitHub repo chest X-ray 8 dataset for normal	406 images (203 in COVID-19 and normal classes each)	Rotated by an angle of 5 degrees (clockwise), horizontally flipped, scaled by 15% and Gaussian noise (mean = 0 and variance=0.25)	No	Compared most popular models with various tuneable hyperparameters	Models are not tested for multi-class classification
[19]	No	Dataset collected from 6 medical facilities	COVID-19: 1,296; pneumonia: 1,735; normal: 1,325	No	No	Highlighting the infected area using grad-cam	The dataset is small, the model was not analysed over accuracy, precision, and $F1$ score
[20]	Yes, ResNet18, ResNet50, ResNet101, VGG16, and VGG19	COVID-19 X-ray chest and CT – Kaggle; X-ray chest – normal images	180 COVID-19, 200 normal	randomly rotating, shifting, and flipping the training images	No	Proposed and compared three different ways of detecting COVID-19	–
[21]	Yes, ResNet50	COVIDx, 5 hospitals from partners healthcare system in the United States and 4 hospitals in South Korea	4,119 COVID-19, 8,173 control, 5,763 non-COVID-19 pneumonia	No	Yes	Used a combination of deep learning and machine learning	Achieved accuracy not satisfactory for medical based research

(Continues)

Table 10.1 (Continued)

Research work	Feature extraction	Dataset	Sample size and classes	Data augmentation	Class imbalance	Major contributions	Limitations
[22]	No	Custom dataset, COVID-19-X-ray-5k, using COVID-19 chest X-ray dataset and CheXpert	5,184 (5,000 normal, 184 COVID-19)	Yes; Flipping, small rotation, adding small amount of distortions	Yes	Achieved sensitivity of approx. 98% for all models	Data was imbalanced even after augmentation
[23]	Yes, using 12 CNN models	COVID-19 images – JP Cohen, COVID-19-X-rays (Kaggle) Normal (Dataset A) – chestX-ray images (pneumonia)Normal (Dataset B) – NIH chest X-rays	Both datasets: 388 images (194 in COVID-19 and non-COVID-19 classes each)	Yes; Affine transformations	No	Performed a total of 144 experiments using different combinations of CNN models and classifiers	Limited dataset for training DL models
[24]	Yes; DenseNet201 architecture	COVID-19-CT-dataset	746 images (397 non-COVID-19, 349 COVID-19)	Yes; reflection (relative to the x and y axes) rotation (angle values of 90 and 270 degrees)	No	Used extreme learning machine (EML)	Data augmentation was overused (dataset increased from 746 to 3,730)
[25]	Yes; ResNet50, DenseNet169	Dataset 1: chest X-Ray images (pneumonia) Dataset 2: COVID-19 chest X-ray dataset (GitHub) Dataset 3: U-Net	Dataset 1: 5,856 (bacteria, virus, normal) Dataset 2: 441 (COVID-19, other viruses) Dataset 3: 2,000 (1,000 images, 1,000 masks)	Yes; Affine transformation, histogram enhancement	Yes	Model developed gives higher accuracy as compared to base models	Difference in image sizes led to additional steps

[26]	No	Italian society of medical and interventional radiology COVID-19 database, novel corona virus 2019 dataset, COVID-19 positive chest X-ray images from different articles, chest X-ray images	COVID-19: 190; normal: 1,341; viral pneumonia: 1,345	Yes, rotation, scaling, image translation	Yes, solved by image augmentation	Proposed the efficiency of SqueezeNet over DenseNet201, ResNet18, and AlexNet	Lower number of images in the dataset
[27]	Na	COVID-19 images – GitHub repo by Joseph; normal, pneumonia bacterial, pneumonia viral – Kaggle's chest X-ray images (pneumonia)	1,300 (290 COVID-19, 310 normal, 330 bacterial pneumonia, 327 viral pneumonia)	No	No	Proposed model is computationally less expensive and gives 99% accuracy for two-class classification	Proposed model needs further clinical testing
[28]	No	Chest X-ray (COVID-19 and pneumonia)	Total = 6,432; train = 5,467 (COVID-19 = 490; normal = 1,345; pneumonia = 3,632)	Yes, random rotation (range = 10 degrees), flipped horizontally, zoomed in or out (range = 0.4)	Yes	Xception gave 100% training accuracy and 97% testing accuracy	More models could have been compared

(Continues)

Table 10.1 (*Continued*)

Research work	Feature extraction	Dataset	Sample size and classes	Data augmentation	Class imbalance	Major contributions	Limitations
[29]	No	COVID-19 radiography	2,905 images (219 COVID-19, 1,341 normal, 1,345 pneumonia)	No	Yes	100% sensitivity for COVID-19 class using Xception	More popular CNN models could have been compared
[30]	No	(1) GitHub repo by Cohen; (2) Kaggle – RSNA, radiopaedia, SIRM; (3) (Kermany *et al.*)	1,428 (224 COVID-19, 700 pneumonia, 504 normal)	No	Yes	Comparative study of all recent and trending models – best performance by MobileNetV2	Study does not consider other similar virus that may result in similar X-rays
[31]	No	RSNA pneumonia detection challenge (DS1) and COVID-19 image data collection (DS2)	DS1: 179 images for normal, pneumonia, and COVID-19 classes each; DS2: 76 worse, 38 stable, and 45 improves	No	No	Develop a mobile app COVID-MobileXpert	Authors do not consider the traditional performance evaluators like accuracy and loss
[32]	No	Chest X-ray images (pneumonia) (Kaggle), radio helia, COVID-19 chest X-ray dataset (GitHub), BSTI	X-ray: COVID-19: 85 and normal: 85; CT scan: COVID-19: 203 and normal: 153	No	Yes	Comparison of transfer learning and custom CNN	The dataset size is small, authors have not explored other CNNs
[33]	Yes, MobileNetV2 and SqueezeNet	Joseph Paul Cohen dataset, Qatar University (Kaggle – X-ray)	458 (295 COVID-19, 65 normal X-rays, 98 pneumonia)	No	Yes	Proposed an ensemble of MobileNetV2 and SqueezeNet for feature extraction	–

[34]	Yes, VGG19 and DenseNet201	COVID-19 radiography database (Kaggle), chest X-ray images (pneumonia) (Kaggle), COVID-19 chest X-ray dataset (GitHub), COVID-19 chest X-ray dataset initiative (GitHub), and COVID-19 X-ray dataset (Kaggle)	COVID-19: 798; normal: 2,341; pneumonia: 2,345	Yes, width shift, height shift, zooming, shearing, and rotation by a small angle	Yes, tried to solve it using augmentation	Proposed a state of art model called CoVNet-19	The dataset still remains imbalanced after augmentation. Authors should have taken the same number of neutral and pneumonia images and then applied augmentation to the entire dataset
[38]	Yes, using multi-kernel local binary pattern	GitHub, Kaggle	COVID-19: 135; pneumonia: 150; normal: 150	No	No	Proposed the detection of COVID-19 using machine learning and *F*-transform	The dataset used is merely 435 images, this is very less to create a generalised model for practical use
[39]	Local binary patterns (LBP)	COVID-19 image data collection	305 (68 COVID-19, 79 normal, 158 pneumonia)	No	No	Complete machine learning based model	Overall accuracy is higher for DL models

(Continues)

Table 10.1 (*Continued*)

Research work	Feature extraction	Dataset	Sample size and classes	Data augmentation	Class imbalance	Major contributions	Limitations
[40]	Yes, YCbCr, Kekre-LUV, and CIE-LUV	COVID-19 image data collection	60-COVID-19; 60-normal; 60-viral pneumonia; 60-bacterial pneumonia	No	No	Use of luminance Chroma features for COVID-19 classification	Small dataset; maximum accuracy produced is of 84.583% which is low for medical applications, hence model cannot be deployed in real time
[41]	Yes, non-subsampled dual-tree complex contour let transform and grey level co-occurrence	–	COVID-19: 291; influenza A/B: 160; other diseases: 119	No	No	Random forest based model for detection COVID-19 from other pneumonia images	Small dataset, accuracy is not good for medical application

sources. We have tried to address these limitations in the next section and provided a way for working ahead on these challenges.

10.4 Research gaps

Although most papers were successful in designing models that gave a great accuracy score, there were certain common limitations and research gaps. The following are the most important gaps.

10.4.1 Unavailability of large datasets

The sample size of the datasets for most of the research works was very small. The size for the COVID-19 class was even smaller. Since COVID-19 has spread to most of the countries, there have been multiple variants in the COVID-19 virus. There is a need of a bigger dataset, to be able to generalize the model for detecting of COVID-19. A dataset which has samples from different age groups and different locations could help us in developing and training a model that can be generalized and be capable of deployment. For creating such a large dataset, we need the collaboration of local hospitals and the respective state and centre governments, without which collecting data at such a large scale is difficult. In [36] the authors have mentioned about the challenges involved in having a small dataset. They used Generative Adversarial Networks (GAN) to generate synthetic images to increase the sample size. In future, researchers can enhance existing approaches for developing synthetic dataset and can also come up with unique and efficient ways.

10.4.2 Imbalanced datasets

Imbalanced dataset is one of the most prevalent problems that affect the efficient building of machine learning models. In most of research work for COVID-19 detection, authors have addressed the problem of imbalanced datasets. The COVID-R dataset used by researchers in [9] have 3,108 normal images and 4,248 anomalous images out of which 2,843 are COVID-19 images and 1,439 are pneumonia. A similar sample ratio of 1:2 (overall healthy to COVID-19) is maintained in [16] as well. The COVID-CXR dataset that is used in [36] has a total of 1,124 CXR images (403 in COVID class and 721 in normal class). However, the authors have generated synthetic datasets to compensate for the small and imbalanced dataset. In [17] the authors have used the 6,523 CXRs where 250 of them are of COVID-19, 2,753 of patients with other pulmonary diseases and 3,520 healthy patients. In this case the COVID-19 samples are very less compared to other class samples. This case shows a highly imbalanced dataset where the COVID-19 samples are very less in proportion to healthy and other pulmonary diseases. In Table 10.1 the research works that have used imbalanced datasets are mentioned and most of them have used synthetic samples or weighted learning approaches to address this issue. However, the approaches should be verified against all performance measures and real-time diagnosis with radiologists. Furthermore, the computational complexity of these approaches should be tested against the modified samples.

10.4.3 Multiple image sources

In the research works we have analysed; the authors have used datasets from multiple sources. In research work [12], the dataset is developed by combining data from GitHub and Kaggle. The COVID-CXR images are combined from GitHub and labelled OCT and CXR images for classification from Kaggle. In [22] the authors have used COVIDx and data collected from few hospitals in the United States and South Korea. Similarly, from Table 10.1, it is evident that most of the research works have used datasets from varied sources. It is imperative to analyse the extensibility and generalizability of the developed works. The challenges involved in datasets are due to the varying characteristics of demographics, different age-groups, history of medical conditions, lifestyle disorders, and various physiological properties across sex, race, and ethnic groups. Decision-making in medical diagnosis should accommodate all the complexities involved. Hence there is a need for validation of models developed with one dataset to be tested with other datasets.

10.5 Conclusion

With COVID-19 spreading all over the world, it has become vital that we try to detect the virus at the earliest so that the infected person can be isolated and treated. However, the most popular approach to detect the virus is the RT-PCR test that takes hours to give results. The next best shot at detecting the virus is using radiography techniques like CXRs, CT-scans, and ultrasounds. Although the imaging is done within a few minutes, it requires experts and professionals to analyse the obtained images and to detect the virus. Possibility of human errors increases the misinterpretation rates. Thus, it is vital to develop a system that not only makes such predictions in seconds but also yields satisfactory results. In this chapter, we have summarized various research studies based on machine learning and deep learning models. Majority of the models are trained using real-time data and yield good results. Though training these models may be time-consuming, once trained, they take a few milliseconds to test each sample. However, as discussed in many papers, the biggest disadvantage to any COVID-19 related study is that there is very limited amount of reliable data which is not sufficient to train deep learning models. Although the chapter features some papers that give high accuracies, the idea of the model being biased due to imbalanced datasets cannot be completely eliminated. Thus, future research should be done on datasets that have a sufficient number of samples in each class. The best way to tackle the current problem is to merge different models for detecting COVID-19. Merging the X-ray or CT scan method with supervised machine learning models that detect COVID-19 using various parameters like age, sex, diabetic, pneumonia, as discussed in [42], can result in error-free and more accurate results. Apart from clinical methods to limit the spread of the virus, various non-pharmaceutical techniques can be used as well. One such technique as mentioned in [43] is to track the people who were in contact with a positive patient. Thus, the most efficient way to fight the disease is to make a hybrid system that combines various models to detect COVID-19 using radio imaging techniques.

References

[1] Apollo Pulmonologist. New COVID-19 symptoms to look out for [Internet]. Ask Apollo; 2021. [cited 2021 May 5]. Available from: https://healthlibrary.askapollo.com/new-covid-19-symptoms-to-look-out-for/.

[2] World Health Organization. Coronavirus disease (COVID-19): How is it transmitted? [Internet]. World Health Organization. 2020 [cited2021 May 6]. Available from: https://www.who.int/news-room/q-a-detail/coronavirus-disease-covid-19-how-is-it-transmitted.

[3] Greenhalgh T, Jimenez JL, Prather KA, Tufekci Z, Fisman D and Schooley R. Ten scientific reasons in support of airborne transmission of SARS-CoV-2. *Lancet*. 2021; 397(10285): 1603–5.

[4] Rahman A, Chakraborty C, Anwar A, *et al.* SDN–IoT empowered intelligent framework for industry 4.0 applications during COVID-19 pandemic. *Cluster Comput.* 2021; 4. Available from: https://doi.org/10.1007/s10586-021-03367-4.

[5] Dash S, Chakraborty C, Giri SK and Pani SK. Intelligent computing on time-series data analysis and prediction of COVID-19 pandemics. *Pattern Recognit Lett* [Internet]. 2021; 151: 69–75. Available from: https://doi.org/10.1016/j.patrec.2021.07.027.

[6] Scohy A, Anantharajah A, Bodéus M, Kabamba-Mukadi B, Verroken A and Rodriguez-Villalobos H. Low performance of rapid antigen detection test as frontline testing for COVID-19 diagnosis. *J Clin Virol*. 2020; 129.

[7] Chendrasekhar A. Chest CT versus RT-PCR for diagnostic accuracy of COVID-19 detection: a meta-analysis. *J Vasc Med Surg*. 2020; 8(4): 1–4.

[8] Yasin R and Gouda W. Chest X-ray findings monitoring COVID-19 disease course and severity. *Egypt J Radiol Nucl Med*. 2020; 51(1).

[9] Hussain E, Hasan M, Rahman MA, Lee I, Tamanna T and Parvez MZ. CoroDet: A deep learning based classification for COVID-19 detection using chest X-ray images. *Chaos, Solitons Fractals* [Internet]. 2021; 142: 110495. Available from: https://doi.org/10.1016/j.chaos.2020.110495.

[10] Hernandez D, Pereira R and Georgevia P. COVID-19 detection through X-ray chest images. *2020 Int Conf Autom Informatics, ICAI 2020 – Proc*. 2020.

[11] Rajaraman S, Siegelman J, Alderson PO, Folio LS, Folio LR and Antani SK. Iteratively pruned deep learning ensembles for COVID-19 detection in chest X-rays. *IEEE Access*. 2020; 8: 115041–50.

[12] Rabbah J, Ridouani M and Hassouni L. A new classification model based on StackNet and deep learning for fast detection of COVID 19 through X rays images. *4th Int Conf Intell Comput Data Sci ICDS 2020*. 2020.

[13] Mayya A and Khozama S. A novel medical support deep learning fusion model for the diagnosis of COVID-19. *Proc IEEE Int Conf Advent Trends Multidiscip Res Innov ICATMRI 2020*. 2020; 2–7.

[14] Panwar H, Gupta PK, Siddiqui MK, Morales-Menendez R and Singh V. Application of deep learning for fast detection of COVID-19 in X-Rays using nCOVnet. *Chaos, Solitons Fractals* [Internet]. 2020; 138: 109944. Available from: https://doi.org/10.1016/j.chaos.2020.109944.

[15] Horry MJ, Chakraborty S, Paul M, *et al.* COVID-19 detection through transfer learning using multimodal imaging data. *IEEE Access*. 2020; 8: 149808–24.

[16] Vaid S, Kalantar R and Bhandari M. Deep learning COVID-19 detection bias: accuracy through artificial intelligence. *Int Orthop*. 2020; 44(8): 1539–42.

[17] Brunese L, Mercaldo F, Reginelli A and Santone A. Explainable deep learning for pulmonary disease and coronavirus COVID-19 detection from X-rays. *Comput Methods Programs Biomed* [Internet]. 2020; 196: 105608. Available from: https://doi.org/10.1016/j.cmpb.2020.105608.

[18] Minaee S, Kafieh R, Sonka M, Yazdani S and Jamalipour Soufi G. Deep-COVID: Predicting COVID-19 from chest X-ray images using deep transfer learning. *Med Image Anal*. 2020; 65.

[19] Nayak SR, Nayak DR, Sinha U, Arora V and Pachori RB. Application of deep learning techniques for detection of COVID-19 cases using chest X-ray images: A comprehensive study. *Biomed Signal Process Control* [Internet]. 2021; 64: 102365. Available from: https://doi.org/10.1016/j.bspc.2020.102365.

[20] Li L, Qin L, Xu Z, *et al.* Artificial intelligence distinguishes COVID-19 from community acquired pneumonia on chest CT. *Radiology* [Internet]. 2020; Available from: http://arxiv.org/abs/2003.13865.

[21] Ismael AM and Şengür A. Deep learning approaches for COVID-19 detection based on chest X-ray images. *Expert Syst Appl*. 2021; 164.

[22] Zhong A, Li X, Wu D, *et al.* Deep metric learning-based image retrieval system for chest radiograph and its clinical applications in COVID-19. *Med Image Anal* [Internet]. 2021; 70: 101993. Available from: https://doi.org/10.1016/j.media.2021.101993.

[23] Ohata EF, Bezerra GM, das Chagas JVS, *et al.* Automatic detection of COVID-19 infection using chest X-ray images through transfer learning. *IEEE/CAA J Autom Sin*. 2021; 8(1): 239–48.

[24] Turkoglu M. COVID-19 detection system using chest CT images and multiple kernels-extreme learning machine based on deep neural network. *IRBM* [Internet]. 2021; 1: 1–8. Available from: https://doi.org/10.1016/j.irbm.2021.01.004.

[25] Lv D, Qi W, Li Y, Sun L and Wang Y. A cascade network for Detecting COVID-19 using chest x-rays. 2020; 1–22. Available from: http://arxiv.org/abs/2005.01468.

[26] Chowdhury MEH, Rahman T, Khandakar A, *et al.* Can AI help in screening viral and COVID-19 pneumonia? *IEEE Access*, 2020; 8: 132665–132676. doi: 10.1109/ACCESS.2020.3010287

[27] Khan AI, Shah JL and Bhat MM. CoroNet: A deep neural network for detection and diagnosis of COVID-19 from chest x-ray images. *Comput*

Methods Programs Biomed [Internet]. 2020; 196: 105581. Available from: https://doi.org/10.1016/j.cmpb.2020.105581.

[28] Jain R, Gupta M, Taneja S and Hemanth DJ. Deep learning based detection and analysis of COVID-19 on chest X-ray images. *Appl Intell* [Internet]. 2021; 51(3): 1690–700. Available from: http://link.springer.com/10.1007/s10489-020-01902-1.

[29] El Gannour O, Hamida S, Cherradi B, Raihani A and Moujahid H. Performance evaluation of transfer learning technique for automatic detection of patients with COVID-19 on X-ray images. *2020 IEEE 2nd Int Conf Electron Control Optim Comput Sci ICECOCS 2020*. 2020; (1): 1–6.

[30] Apostolopoulos ID and Mpesiana TA. Covid-19: automatic detection from X-ray images utilizing transfer learning with convolutional neural networks. *Phys Eng Sci Med* [Internet]. 2020; 43(2): 635–40. Available from: https://doi.org/10.1007/s13246-020-00865-4.

[31] Li X, Li C and Zhu D. COVID-MobileXpert: On-device COVID-19 patient triage and follow-up using chest X-rays. *Proc – 2020 IEEE Int Conf Bioinforma Biomed BIBM 2020*. 2020; 1063–7.

[32] Maghdid HS, Asaad AT, Ghafoor KZ, Sadiq AS and Khan MK. Diagnosing COVID-19 pneumonia from x-ray and CT images using deep learning and transfer learning algorithms. *arXiv*. 2020; 1–8.

[33] Toğaçar M, Ergen B and Cömert Z. COVID-19 detection using deep learning models to exploit Social Mimic Optimization and structured chest X-ray images using fuzzy color and stacking approaches. *Comput Biol Med*. 2020; 121.

[34] Kedia P, Anjum and Katarya R. CoVNet-19: A deep learning model for the detection and analysis of COVID-19 patients. *Appl Soft Comput* [Internet]. 2021; 104: 107184. Available from: https://doi.org/10.1016/j.asoc.2021.107184.

[35] Bhuyan HK, Chakraborty C, Shelke Y and Pani SK. COVID-19 diagnosis system by deep learning approaches. *Expert Syst*. 2021: 1–18. https://doi.org/10.1111/exsy.12776.

[36] Waheed A, Goyal M, Gupta D, Khanna A, Al-Turjman F and Pinheiro PR. CovidGAN: Data augmentation using auxiliary classifier GAN for improved Covid-19 detection. *IEEE Access*. 2020; 8: 91916–23.

[37] Aradhya VNM, Mahmud M, Guru DS, Agarwal B and Kaiser MS. One-shot cluster-based approach for the detection of COVID-19 from chest X-ray images. *Cognit Comput*. 2021; 1–9.

[38] Tuncer T, Ozyurt F, Dogan S and Subasi A. A novel Covid-19 and pneumonia classification method based on F-transform. *Chemom Intell Lab Syst* [Internet]. 2021; 210: 104256. Available from: https://doi.org/10.1016/j.chemolab.2021.104256.

[39] Thepade SD and Jadhav K. Covid19 identification from chest x-ray images using local binary patterns with assorted machine learning classifiers. *2020 IEEE Bombay Sect Signat Conf IBSSC 2020*. 2020; 46–51.

[40] Thepade SD, Chaudhari PR, Dindorkar MR and Bang SV. Covid-19 identification using machine learning classifiers with histogram of luminance

Chroma features of chest x-ray images. *2020 IEEE Bombay Sect Signat Conf IBSSC 2020*. 2020; 36–41.

[41] Wu Z, Li L, Jin R, *et al.* Texture feature-based machine learning classifier could assist in the diagnosis of COVID-19. *Eur J Radiol*. 2021; 137.

[42] Muhammad LJ, Algehyne EA, Usman SS, Ahmad A, Chakraborty C and Mohammed IA. Supervised machine learning models for prediction of COVID-19 infection using epidemiology dataset. *SN Comput Sci* [Internet]. 2021; 2(1): 1–13. Available from: https://doi.org/10.1007/s42979-020-00394-7.

[43] Garg L, Chukwu E, Nasser N, Chakraborty C and Garg G. Anonymity preserving IoT-based COVID-19 and other infectious disease contact tracing model. *IEEE Access*. 2020; 8: 159402–14.

Chapter 11

Machine-based drug design to inhibit SARS-CoV-2 virus

T. Lurthu Pushparaj[1], *E. Francy Irudaya Rani*[2], *E. Fantin Irudaya Raj*[3] *and M. Appadurai*[4]

Abstract

Researchers worldwide are striving hard to design the best anti-coronavirus drug to overcome the current pandemic situation. Due to the lack of animal and human trials data, the process is still complicating and causing more death worldwide. Since biological testing costs more money and time-consuming, the combination of computerized programs-based evaluation like molecular docking, virtual screening (AutoDock, HEX, Schrodinger, Gaussian, and Glide), and molecular dynamics study serves as a hopeful way in drug developing and studying their effect over severe acute respiratory syndrome (SARS)-coronavirus-causing components like spike (S) protein present around the SARS-coronavirus-2 (SARS-CoV-2), main protease (M-pro), and ribonucleic acid cooperate. The keen analysis of the amino acid sequences in the coronavirus-19 infection-causing proteins will give very important information about the virus transformation and replication cycle. The amino acid sequences and their active sites provided in the 3D crystalline structure of M-pro (PDB ID; 6LU7) afford valuable data to the researchers about the type of inhibitors that corresponds to the SARS-CoV-2 inhibition. Compared to all other deadly viruses like flu, human immunodeficiency virus, and SARS, novel coronavirus SARS-CoV-2 shows superior binding affinity over a human transmembrane protein christened angiotensin-converting enzyme 2, found in human lungs. Since the target is very clear, every scientist aims to design a new drug or check the available prodrug activity through a computer program to defeat the COVID-19 disease. Nowadays, many synthetic and natural drugs have been tested for their suitability against M-pro. Since the coronavirus-19 infection spreads more

[1]PG Chemistry & MRI Research Lab, TDMNS College, Affiliated to MS University, Tirunelveli, India
[2]Department of Electronics and Communication Engineering, Francis Xavier Engineering College, Tirunelveli, Affiliated to Anna University, India
[3]Department of Electrical and Electronics Engineering, Dr. Sivanthi Aditanar College of Engineering, Tiruchendur, Affiliated to Anna University, India
[4]Department of Mechanical Engineering, Dr. Sivanthi Aditanar College of Engineering, Tiruchendur, Affiliated to Anna University, India

vigorously, the traditional real-time PCR test will need more time for infection confirmation, so machine-based imaging studies like MRI, computerized tomography (CT), and X-ray are needed. The MRI and CT need contrast agents (CAs) to give more precise images. The development of image contrast-enhancing agents will give more appropriate outcome image in detecting COVID-19 infection in the early stages. The designing of perfect multimodal CAs is the current research among MRI researchers. It will behave as both targeting and coronavirus-19 killing drug for the current pandemic situation. All the above-said applications can be accomplished only by designing the drug and then studying their binding studies through a computer application.

Keywords: SARS-coronavirus-19; COVID-19 drug; ACE2 enzyme; Main protease; Antiviral docking; Dual-MRI agent

11.1 Introduction

In the fast genetic research world, silicon chip-engineered devices have become a right hand for researchers. Since the application of this is unlimited, a good science researcher can develop a new genetically modified microbe, vaccine, or drug for the deadliest disease. This becomes true on seeing the current pandemic situation rooted by the deadliest beta microbes called severe acute respiratory syndrome coronavirus-2 (SARS-CoV-2), a perfectly laboratory-made virus-containing BAT and PIG genes [1]. Typically, viruses that reason illnesses in people are known to program at least one protease that assumes significant parts in the viral life cycle. Reacting rapidly to obscure microbes is essential to stop the uncontrolled spread of sicknesses that lead to an outbreak, for example, the novel coronavirus. In the past two decades, six coronaviruses, like SARS-coronavirus (fatality rates of 9.6%), MERS-coronavirus (fatality 34%), HCoronavirus-HKU1, HCoronavirus-OC43, HCoronavirus-NL63, and HCoronavirus-229E, have infected the human population in the years 2002 and 2012.

Currently, the new SARS-CoV-2 and a genetically modified SARS-CoV-2 with a high fatality rate >83% identified during December 2019 have killed about 4.8 crore people worldwide. It is hard time for every science researcher to develop a smart vaccine without side effects or a molecular efficient drug in a short time to avoid the current uncontrollable infection. The standard protocols in medicinal research involve defining the exact problem developing or creating a site and design a lead drug or vaccine for genome infections. This methodology will require long periods of innovative work, which requests colossal theory, which cannot execute for the permanent virulent disease. Maybe we need a quick and worthwhile come-up to hinder the viral disease. In silico strategies are a preexamination loom before wet research facility studies, which enjoys the benefit of having the option to make a quick and cost-productive investigation. Also, by selecting suitable algorithms, we can exactly predict the reactive site on the virus from this; we can elucidate the molecular structure of the vaccine candidate and a growth inhibition drug for infected proteins. By choosing the target site, we can synthesize a lead drug for the deadliest virus, which causes coronavirus-19 infection.

The scientists report speculation that inborn traces of coronavirus can incorporate into our cell chromosomes and stick there for a long time even after the disease is cured. They tracked down those undeniable degrees of regular ribonucleic acid (RNA) have created in light of the mix of infection with cell DNA that peruses its grouping and makes a greater amount of it for duplication. It is recommended that in uncommon discovering, individuals can recuperate from coronavirus yet then test positive for coronavirus again months after the fact. The scientists underlined that viral combination did not mean individuals who recuperated from coronavirus-19 stay irresistible. Since the COVID-19 antibodies dependent on messenger RNA (mRNA) may be one way or another change human DNA. The protein, switch transcriptase, is encoded by LINE-1 components, groupings that litter 17% of the human set of chromosomes and address antiques of earlier contaminations by retroviruses.

A genetic laboratory analysis reports that when human cells spike with additional LINE-1 components of coronavirus, DNA adaptation of SARS-CoV-2's groupings settle into the cell chromosomes. The experimental evidence from "National Cancer Institute" supports the original hypothesis that the integrated viral sequences will remain on human cells even after cured of coronavirus. The advanced program that can be incorporated into in silico methods can assist researchers in developing a drug that can target two or more diseases at one time (combination therapy) [2]. In any case, the improvement of the best combos is the most part difficult to make in a brief period span in a prudent and harmless to the ecosystem. To smooth out combos dosing regimens, the improvement of particles with double hindrances abilities against at least two unique classes of the objective would be ideal [3]. It turns out to be more important, if clinically demonstrated FDA-supported antivirus, virus tracking MRI contrast agents (CAs), monoclonal antibody (mAb) drugs are considered for the studies. To develop smart multi-target molecules for the current situation, the researcher needs to pick an appropriate antiviral drug from the drug data bank that is already in use for other viral infections. After that, the researcher can study their limiting linkage with lung TMPRSS2, angiotensin-converting enzyme 2 (ACE2), and RdRc (viral) proteins on SARS-CoV-2.

This chapter will discuss in detail the computer-based designing program used for the designing and pre-synthesis of an antiviral drug for COVID-19 infection. The readers will gain extra knowledge about the process happening in COVID-19 virus replication and the in silico procedure adopted to identify the key amino acid, which is the root cause for the viral replication and structural transmission. The chapter will give in-depth knowledge about the status of antiviral drugs that are under reinvestigation for their ability against COVID-19 infection. In addition, the chapter throws limelight on the importance and application of MRI, dual imaging MRI, and computerized tomography (CT) imaging modalities that are the best among the best than PCR analysis.

The sequence of this chapter is in the following order. First, we have given a detailed introduction based on a literature survey about the in silico methods used in drug designing against COVID-19. Second, we discussed the types of COVID-19 virus and their replication and stereochemical transforming mechanism, followed by the role of antibody and vaccine available against COVID-19. Third, we described the test available for COVID-19 infection. Fourth, we discussed the top-notch in silico methods used in anti-COVID-19 drug research and their working procedure. Fifth, we have given a summary of the previous four portions and the future scope. Finally, we finished the chapter with conclusions followed by references.

11.2 What is SARS-coronavirus-2?

SARS-CoV-2 quite fit with Coronaviridae, a family with huge enveloped RNA. The RNA set of the chromosome of Coronaviridae extends up to 27–32 kb with full of interlinked structural and nonstructural proteins.

The name SARS-CoV-2 is derived from the fact that approximately 82% of the RNA set of the chromosome is identical to the SARS-coronavirus [4], 50% identical with MERS [5], and 79% resemblance with SARS. The X-ray diffracted 3D crystal structure of SARS-CoV-2 has about 88% identical employing a set of coronavirus identified in bats (bat-SLCoronavirus-ZC45 and bat-SLCoronavirus-ZXC21). Coronaviruses are an infectious disease with thousands of thornlike active proteins arranged in a throne pattern mostly on the boundary that could infect pigs, bats, cows, birds, and other mammals. Furthermore, it mutates quickly to one another and humans, causing diseases in the respiratory tract, lung, gastro-intestinal (GI) tract, liver, kidney, and central nervous systems (Figure 11.1).

These infections are competent to be grouped into four typical varieties called alpha COVID, beta COVID, MERS COVID, and SARS-COVID-2 [6]. In the set of COVID-19 chromosomes, the 5′-replicase generates a polyprotein. A frameshift occurs between ORF-1b and ORF-1a, resulting in the formation of two polypeptides: pp1ab and pp1a, which are subdivided into 16 non-underlying proteins (nsp-1 to nsp-10 and nsp-12 to nsp-16) whose mutual mutation is interceded by the main protease (M-pro) (nsp-5, 3CL-pro (3CL protease)/M-pro) and nsp-3, PL-protease

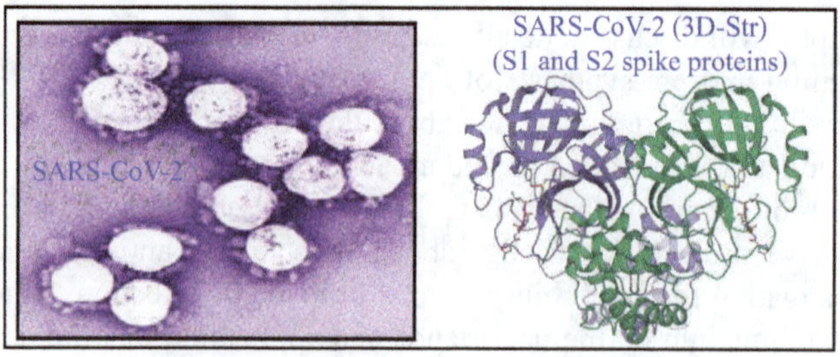

Figure 11.1 Microscopic and 3D molecular image of SARS-coronavirus-2

(PL-pro). The 3′-end modulates multiple core protein molecules that have epithelial layer (M), spike (S) proteins, nucleocapsid (N), envelope (E), hemagglutinin-esterase (HE), as well as eight movable proteins (p6, 3a, 3b, 7a, 7b, 8b, 9b, and orf14). Approximately 29 highly active proteins are involved in SARS-CoV-2 transmission and replication in congregation cells [7]. Every structural protein received the translational pathology from the viral subgenomic messenger called vsgRNAs, which has the RNA cooperate. The crystal structure of RdRc on SARS-CoV-2 revealed that one nsp-12 subunit (cooperate responsive catalytic subunit) contains a nidovirus RdRc-associated nucleotidyltransferase (NiRAN) realm in the nitrogen atom functioned array and anchoring part to connect the C-terminal RdRc with NiRAN domain [8]. The catalytic site has ASP 760, ASP 761 (SDD), and SER 759 residues that lie in the pattern "C" used for the primer binding of RdRc with the congregation. However, the M-pro looks like a calm enzyme but contributes equally to RdRc in the regeneration of SARS-CoV-2. This enzyme consists of about 305 asymmetric amino acid sequences through His41 and Cys145 catalytic divectors and the substrate-binding mark positioned between the sandwiched domains I and II. Tai *et al.* [9] put forward the truth that the amino acid present between 331 and 524 residues of spike protein produces receptor-binding domain (RBD) fragment that helps the SARS-CoV-2 to bind strongly with bat ACE2 (bACE2) and human ACE2 (hACE2) as receptors. Thus, this pointed protein section is accountable for a mutual admission of SARS-CoV-2 and SARS-coronavirus in human lung ACE2-state cells.

Every structural protein received the translational pathology from the viral subgenomic messenger called vsgRNAs, which has the RNA cooperate (RdRc and nsp-12) and the 3′-5′exo-RNA. The crystal structure of RdRc revealed that one nsp-12 subunit contains a nidovirus RdRc-associated nucleotidyltransferase (NiRAN) realm in the nitrogen atom functioned array and anchoring part to connect the C-terminal RdRc with NiRAN domain [8]. The catalytic site has ASP 760, ASP 761 (SDD), and SER 759 residues that lie in the pattern "C" used for the primer binding of RdRc with the congregation. However, the M-pro looks like a calm enzyme but contributes equally to RdRc in the regeneration of SARS-CoV-2. This enzyme consists of about 305 asymmetric amino acid sequences through His41 and Cys145 catalytic divectors and the substrate-binding mark positioned between the sandwiched domains I and II. Tai *et al.* [9] put forward the truth that the amino acid present between 331 and 524 residues of spike protein produces RBD fragment that helps the SARS-CoV-2 to bind strongly with bACE2 and hACE2 as receptors. Thus, this pointed protein section is accountable for a mutual admission of SARS-CoV-2 and SARS-coronavirus in human lung ACE2-state cells.

11.3 Mechanism of SARS-coronavirus-2 infection in human

Coronavirus looks like spherical and has thousands of spike proteins at the periphery. These spike proteins have many amino acid sequences through which they bind over the protease domain congregation cell and undergo replication in humans. Every human has transmembrane proteins, ACE2, in the lungs, GI track, kidney, and brain. Initially, spike proteins attack the ACE2 enzyme through RBD and undergo conformational changes by the fusion of viral molecular RNA with the human congregation cell layer. After the dispersion interaction, the viral ribosome goes into the congregation cell and creates more infections by replicating its arrangement of chromosomes and causes viral contamination. Once tainted, the viral subgenomic messenger, which has nsps, gets collected into multiethnic cooperate composites, to establish a reaction appropriate for recording and replications of the viral arrangement of a chromosome. The viral chromosome sequence on the site will develop virions with primary proteins [10].

11.4 How SARS-coronavirus-2 multiplies?

During the replication cycle inside the congregation, the RNA-subordinate RNA cooperate (RdRc), nitrogen-functioned protein, long-chain ribosome, and modified active ribosomal frameshifting locale of the infection are profoundly associated with connection with RNA of the congregation cell. There are four primary useful destinations installed in the entire ribosome: (a) the mRNA-restricting site; (b) the tRNA-restricting locales that contain the aminoacyl spot, neutral peptide spot, and cleaving function; (c) the peptidyl relocate center (PTP); (d) anchoring center for replication [11]. It demonstrates that ACE2 is set to be a more essential enzyme to recombine SARS-CoV-2 over RdRc. In the spreading stage, the high polar region combined through RdRc, this repeated procedure supports the nonstop Virna RN acid replication. From molecular screening contemplates, it accounted for that the coarticulation of angiotensin-converting and TMPRSS2 enzymes in the lung and stomach-related tracks is a key for SARS-CoV-2 to enter the human tissue anatomy [12]. The report additionally affirmed that amino acid groups like Hi-296, Ar-345, and Se-441 were the reaction performing groups of TMPRSS2, which also contains the highly viral replication supportive amino acids like Ar-435, Se-436, and Gly-464. To help the assertion, the Ar-710 at ACE2 element from 697 to 716 assists the arrangement of the ACE2–TMPRSS2 complex [13]. This connection supports the enzymatic change in ACE2 receptors to make connections with the TMPRSS2 enzyme and Ar-652. This site can be anchored by tracking the presence of the TMPRSS2 enzyme.

From the docking outcome (Figure 11.2), it is affirmed that the Arg652 is situated at the suitable pose toward the protease catalectic group of three amino acids. Also, Arg716 is available at the connection spot of ACE2, and Arg710 offers more in making H-bonds to do appropriate protease-receptor cooperation [14]. The M-pro protein comprises three spaces. A notable β-barrel is mostly taken after chymotrypsin is found in spaces I (deposits 8–101) and II (buildups 102–184). Yet, space III has remnants from 201 to 306 that contain α-helices. The missed remnant from 185 to 200 is utilized to associate spaces II and III individually. It calls attention to space III of M-pro. It is more fundamental for keeping up the proteolytic modification, which occurs by holding the space II and the long circle remnant

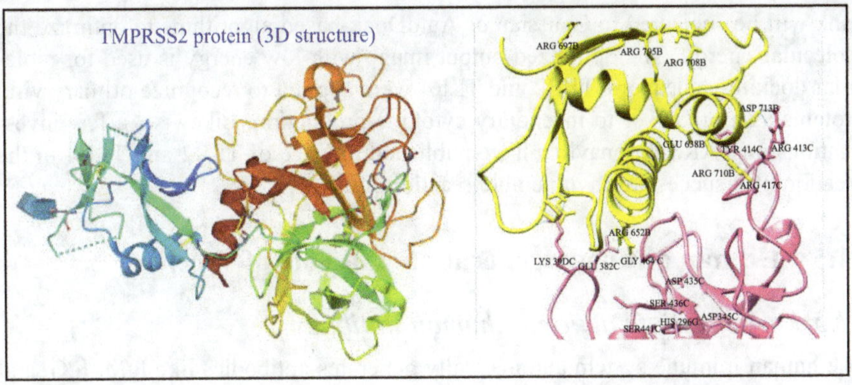

Figure 11.2 The boundary of ACE2 enzyme in lung and TMPRSS2 proteins

185–200 in a chemically positive orientation or potentially situating the N-terminal remnant that assumes a significant part for the reactant action of the enzyme. Any medicament that ideally ties the anchor site of the M-pro pocket may restrain the SARS-CoV-2's replication.

As indicated by in silico crystallographic results, 26 key proteins from 29 other proteins were anticipating as plausible antigens. Among these 26 key proteins, spike "S" protein was chosen as the best immunization competitor as a result of having a flag peptide, one transmembrane helix, negative GRAVY esteem, a major subatomic weight, moderate aliphatic file, beta wrap themes just as having steady, dissolvable, and non-hypersensitive highlights with a remarkable half-life period. This element is a significant boundary that demonstrates that the protein can be foreordained toward the secretory pathway. In addition, nsp-10, orf8, and orf7a proteins with flag peptides were deliberate as probable antibody competitors. The computer-designed antibody can have a polar binding functional group which can buried in the curl-like protein sequence in the virus protein [15]. More contrast to the conventional crystalline structure, the new sterically transformed apo architecture of its M-pro (PDB: 6Y2E) did lack an N3 ligand that is covalently connected to a central protease in the old structure. The RMSD calculated against this most recent M-pro 3D molecular structure with no binding ligand shows the lowest mean rate, when a binding ligand is present. This research is crucial since the M-pro's pocket is inextricably linked to the edge of Glu166, implying that the salty scaffold plays a significant role in the pocket's eternal stability. The medication must link with target invulnerable receptor molecules to produce a continual resistant reaction. These receptors play an important role in detecting the saved microorganism-related subatomic instances (PAMPs) on various organisms, similar to infections, triggering natural resistant commencement, and coordination of the diverse invulnerable comeback. The antibody or drug must link with these receptor molecules to produce a continual resistant reaction. For such application, subatomic level docking procedure will be adopted to find the binding capability of the drugs with toll-like receptors (TLRs). The 3D structure of 'TLRs' collected from the PDB bank will be subjected to Gaussian or AutoDock-based algorithms to optimize the molecular energy. The optimized output image with low energy is used for molecular docking endeavors. TLR2 and TLR4 were applied to recognize primary viral proteins as a precursor to incendiary cytokine production. Likewise, a few investigations on SARS-coronavirus have published the size of TLR2 and TLR4 in the creation of a successful invulnerable reaction [16].

11.5 Human antibody generation and role of vaccine

11.5.1 Immediate action of human antibody

The human immune system automatically generates antibodies like IgM, IgG, and IgA against SARS-CoV-2 when it recognized the presence of a viral set of chromosomes. Half of the affected tissues will receive the self-generated neutralizing antibodies in 7 days. In 14 days, almost all the infected ones will receive the antibody for them [17]. Initially, IgM antibody secretion level increases for the opening week of SARS-coronavirus-2 infection; after consequent weeks it becomes maxima and comes back to normal level in most healthy individuals [18,19]. We can see the self-generated antibody IgG after 1 week of viral infection and it will reach a higher level for 48 days and even until the reinfection happens. Another self-generated antibody IgA will be seen from 4 to 10 days of infection. So the presence of IgM, IgG, and IgA antibodies level will indicate the nature of the virus that causes infection. Multiplex immunoassay study on SARS-CoV-2 antibody confirms the presence of self-generated antibody in sera and saliva.

11.5.2 Role of synthetic vaccine on COVID-19

Natural medicine or computer-based synthesized chemicals could be given as a vaccine for the current pandemic. Once the body gets vaccinated, it will be distinguished by the gathering's inborn invulnerable framework through designing acknowledgment receptors to sort the pathogen-associated molecular model, PAMMs. This PAMM represented in vaccine antigen catches the attention of neutrophils, monocytes, and dendritic cells, which are patrolling throughout the body for 365 days. With the help of the pattern-recognition receptors, the congregation cells will identify the probable danger and turn it into action when they spot the pathogen. They change the appearance of the surface particles and augment favorable to incendiary cytokines. Chemokines bring about the extravasations and fascination of granulocytes, monocytes, and habitual executioner T cells. This results in creating a provocative aggravation microenvironment, in which monoecious segregates into monocytes, and the immature dendritic unit enacts. It activates the growth of the dendrite unit, preceded by the activation of T and B lymphocytes concerning the lymph nodes, by changing the expression of migration receptors on the cell membrane.

Once the T cells get activated, they will distinguish into regulatory CD4+ cells to sustain resistant tolerance. More and more of the immature dendritic cells will migrate toward the lymph nodes when it identifies the protein vaccine

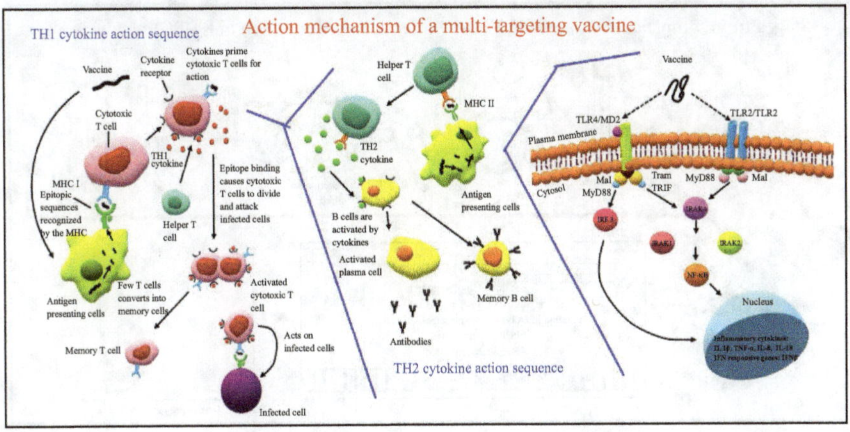

Figure 11.3 Interactions mechanism of TLR with multi-epitope vaccine

antiques. Simultaneously, management of antiques into less significant sections occurs, resulting in the wrinkling of human leukocyte antiques (HLA) in human MHC atoms on the cell surface. Class I major histocompatibility complex (MHC)-clustered atoms make peptides from the antiques formed in the cytoskeleton of debased cells realistic. The phagocyte antiques are fundamentally shown on class II MHC particles [20]. CD4+ T cells respond to antigenic peptides displayed by MHC class II atomic groups, but CD8+ T cells respond to antigenic peptides displayed by MHC class I peptide structures. Animated CD4+ T cells release cytokines that cause an increase in B-cell production, which is required for optimal antique formation (Figure 11.3).

11.6 Real-time COVID-19 identification test (RT-PCR)

Nuclear chain antiques and protein-based findings are used in current analytic studies intended for the SARS-CoV-2 outbreak; nonetheless, popular nuclear chain identification by rRT-PCR remains the highest quality level. In comparison to the currently available serological tests, nucleic analyses have enhanced affectability and explicitness for the viral site. The acknowledgment of SARS-CoV-2 in the internal nose and throat depends upon rRT-PCR filling in as delicate, accurate, and specific virus identification. The technique begins with sample collection and segregation of viral RNA and its transformation into matching DNA. The matching DNA gets enlarged by using Taq DNA collaboration. The rRT-PCR measures the viral burden in 2 days, which has given in Figure 11.4.

Isothermal enhancement is applied to warm cycling-based nucleic corrosive amplification [21]. Worked-on real-time PCR (RT-PCR) is currently accessible to identify assorted locales of the SARS-CoV-2 arrangement of the chromosome [22]. It will identify the SARS-CoV-2's RNA-subordinate S and RNA, which was

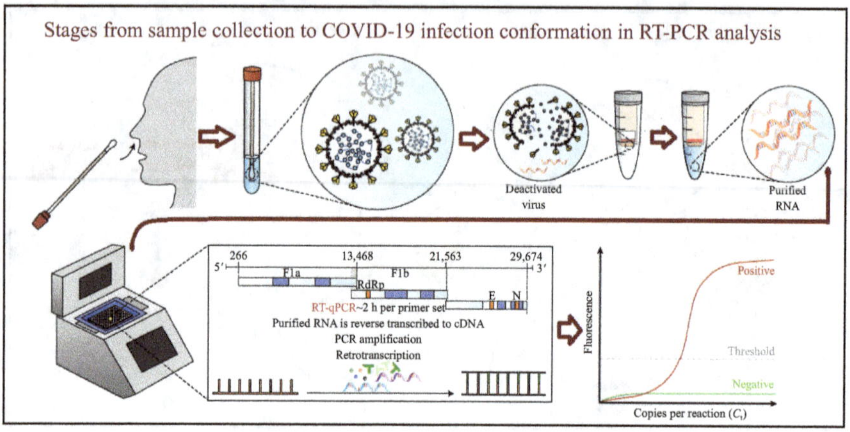

Figure 11.4 COVID-19 infection test procedure using rRT-PCR analyzer

participated in (RdRc)/helicase (Hel) proteins as well as in nucleocapsid (N). The RdRc/Hel measurements are extremely sensitive approaches for detecting viruses.

11.6.1 Limitations of RT-PCR tool

Even though in silico technologies may examine large quantities of proteins for vaccine formulation, researchers need several constraints to be aware of. In silico investigations have acknowledged disadvantages, such as insufficient information in databases, inadequacies in specialized software, including the use of inaccurate inventory tools. As a result, it is critical to pick the ideal method of analysis and experiment with different parameters to get the finest findings for in silico investigations. COVID-19 is now diagnosing using a combo of CT scans and rRT-PCR data. Because RT-PCR examination is so common, it is crucial to look into the data it provides to clinicians and policymakers. The requirement for experienced laboratory personnel and long waited times for results may make nucleic acid amplification more difficult. The global benchmark real-time quantitative PCR (RT-qPCR) takes 4–6 h to complete, not adding the time it takes to transfer the samples to the lab, which could take several days. Variation in viral RNA patterns can alter actual RT-PCR results by targeting various viral genome regions. Furthermore, due to viral evolution, falsified outcomes may occur [23]. Sample storage, minimal nucleic acid filtration, and financial cost and waiting periods are all disadvantages of RT-PCR tests [24]. The rate of PCR sample screening varies depending on the sample type: stool (29%), nasopharyngeal scrub (63%), sputum (72%–76%), bronchoalveolar lavage fluid (79–93%), and oropharyngeal scrub (32%–48%).

Lack of specificity in immunodiagnostic techniques is associated with antigens that are highly conserved to kill coronavirus with autoantibodies in autoimmune conditions. Antibody-based methods are most effective in 7–11 days after exposure, making them less useful for diagnosing an acute infection [25]. Although RT-qPCR involves the current gold standard intended for nucleic acid recognition, novel approaches such as pulse-controlled multiplication are being investigated. Pulse-controlled multiplication requires no RNA excavation and can be completed in 10 min using a tiny device. In the years ahead, S- and N-based antigen detection systems will be used in conjunction with nucleic acid amplification tests to improve COVID-19 diagnostic accuracy at a low cost. Upcoming years, efforts to build new therapeutic platforms could pay off if the analyses are exact, original, and uncomplicated to execute, deliver results promptly, and are inexpensive to produce in mass [26].

11.7 Discussion on in silico methods in COVID-19 drug research

In silico methods aid both scientists and physicians in developing molecular structures for various protein sequences in SARS-CoV-2, locating a suitable target on the virus surface to kill, and designing a drug suit for the anti-bio war against this most lethal virus. It will provide a detailed antimicrobial summary of the new or repurposed drug for other deadly diseases.

11.7.1 In silico-assisted anchoring site analysis

Several PC-assisted programs, such as Glide, AutoDock Vina, MOE DOCK, ClusPro, GOLD, and rDOCK, have been developed in recent years for both corporate and academic purposes to predict the inhibiting mechanism and segregation of a ligand in comparison to a protein.

11.7.1.1 AutoDock Vina

An automatic docking tool is an expansion for "AutoDock." It is a user-friendly procedure available in the free version to predict how molecules bind to a known 3D receptor [27]. AutoDock is the most generally acknowledged atomic group docking apparatus that is comprehensively utilized for the survey of mixtures lined up with likely targets. It is used in multidisciplinary approaches like X-ray crystallography, structure-based medicine designing, lead molecule generation, combinatorics topology archive planning, proteinase-proteinaceous docking, virtual screening (high-throughput screening [HTS]), and synthetic system consideration. Right now, the AutoDock, 4.2 renditions are utilized for a molecular anchor examination of ACE2, TMPRSS2, and RdRc protein against every one of the early announced antiviral physic. AutoDock 4.2 is quicker than AutoDock, and it grants side chains in the macromolecule to be flexible. The functioning proficiency is more than the previous rendition, and firm anchoring is blindingly expedient, and premium quality adaptable anchoring should be possible in 60 s. Of course, up to 40,000 unbending anchoring can be made in 24 h on one CPU. The improved 4.2 rendition of AutoDock has a free-energy scoring task dependent on a direct relapse examination, the AMBER power field, and a significantly greater arrangement of changed protein–ligand buildings with known save constants that could be recognized. The best model was consistently cross-approved with a different arrangement of human immunodeficiency virus (HIV)-1 protease buildings and affirmed that the standard deviation from the original value was lesser than 2.5 kcal/mol. This is an adequate sum to separate between leads with nanomolar, miniature, and milli-hindrance constants. Here some of the new highlights from AutoDock 4.0 are added to the 4.2 renditions. The process gives the Monte Carlo reproduced strengthening (SA) strategy for 2.4 and prior. The Lamarckian genetic algorithm is a major enhancement for the genetic algorithm, and both hereditary techniques are considerably more productive and powerful than SA. For its information and yield, Vina utilizes a similar PDBQT subatomic construction document design via AutoDock. PDBQT records can be created from Open Babel GUI programming and observed by using MGL tools. The yield records with restricting energy esteem can be seen through the Python program.

11.7.1.2 Molecular dynamics

It is a method for splitting down the correct activities of particles and molecules on a computer. The host molecule and the newly designed antiviral drug molecules are allowed to link with one another for a set amount of time, providing insight into the application's dynamic "growth" [28]. It is a Python library to dissect directions from molecule to atom elements (MD) recreations in numerous famous organizations. It can compose the majority of these arrangements, as well, along with iota determinations reasonable for representation or local investigation devices. This analytical procedure permits anyone to peruse molecule-based directions and access the nuclear is arranged through NumPy exhibits. It gives an adaptable and generally quick system for complex investigation assignments. Directions can likewise be controlled and worked out. The MD works on well-known simulation programs like NAMD-10, Amber, Gromacs, and with a series of preparation and analysis tools, joined together in a common interface. To discover the communications of physic with anchoring site Newton's condition of movement shall be applied to this MD framework until the molecules are allowed to connect for a while at a given temperature that observes the law of traditional mechanics. Also, in a constant test, the proportion of trial upsides of tests is performed through estimating instruments regarding time. In the wake of playing out the harmony of the framework, direction investigation and estimation is done, which is equivalent to the examination of the example estimations like factual investigation of estimated perusing. The complete protein structure will be obtained by dissolving it in a water box with parameters LWH of 97.42 Å in the physic evaluation. The addition of neutralizing counter ions like $K+$ and $Cl-$ to the protein molecular structure nullifies the protein surface charges and it is tuned roughly to 0.15 M. The van der Waals (vdW) energy can then be calculated using a smooth cutoff (10–12 Å).

11.7.1.3 The DockThor-VS platform

The DockThor docking program was engineered to administer fundamentally 1D and 2D ligands with zero steric factors that have excellent peptide binding or docking efficiency than the other regular branched ligands with restricted movement. The running program utilizes a phenotypic gathering subject to different strategy solid-state hereditary calculations as solicitation method [29]. Here, the parental substitution system works based on dynamic modified restricted match selection. It provides an unrivaled evaluation that awards perceiving diverse simple planning in a single run by assessing the hyper-surface energy and obtaining everyone grouping of the conveyed structures. These scoring cutoff points will take the going with big data terms for protein–ligand limiting: (a) a curved continuous disorder term that repels the "steric or static" rotatable protections, (b) intermolecular affiliations terms, (c) an ionic active site that has adequate polar joint initiating the process of binding togetherness of the newly designed ligand over the anchoring site on the M-pro, (d) a positive no polar solvation term that is relative just to the dissolvable open surface, and (e) a protein–ligand lipophilic correspondence term.

As far as possible, it will be prepared and endeavored in an immense set (>2,900) of top-of-the-line 3D improvements related to gathered physicochemical profiles and huge recuperating fixations for drug plans. The docking algorithm works on the request of the definite file format, usually a geography doc. will be preferred for the drug molecule, for cofactors, top format will be preferred, and for recording any protein of our interest, in form containing the iota types and inadequate charges from the MMFF94S49 power field will be the required format. The entire atomic power field limits performed by implying assignments without the clients' need intercession. The pursuit space tended to as an association box where the potential results are dealt with at the construction communities, fundamentally lessening the computational expense. The hidden individual group is abstractly conveyed inside the lattice box utilizing erratic qualities for the rotational, translational, and conformational levels of the possibility of the ligand. For every SARS-CoV-2 strong objective, DockThor-VS platform gives a proposed put-down of places to pause for the association box that the client can utilize or change as demonstrated by the protests of his docking test.

11.7.2 Machine-assisted designing and evaluation of COVID-19 drug

Computational screening is currently becoming the primary emphasis for resolving the SARS-CoV-2 infection outbreak. Silicon-based intelligent processors with powerful viral evaluation algorithms have emerged as dominating tools in the pharmaceutical industry and have been utilized in vitro [30] for more than a couple of decades to identify protein blockers and understand protein–protein and protein interactions. Although millions of antiviral medications are available online, numerous experimental, clinical, and computational drug research efforts have been launched to quickly prioritize compounds to recognize them as potential therapeutic drugs for the SARS-CoV-2 disease outbreak. This strategy discloses lucid pathways for the researchers to design and develop similar effective smart drugs in less time. To restudy the efficiency of the drug for the current situation, the researchers can use the data available at the antiviral drug library. From Selleckchem Inc., Kyoto Encyclopedia of Genes, Genomes, and DrugBank databases, the researcher can retrieve the US-approved drug library and Europe-based FDA drugs. Reinvestigating existing antiviral drugs as a potential drug candidate will assist scientists in exploring a proposal for medicines that have well-established pharmacological and safety profiles [31]. Chloroquine and hydroxychloroquine are the two evergreen antiviral drugs that are used for several decades to treat a variety of diseases that have been thoroughly researched and approved for long-term use. Antiviral drug reevaluation using a computational program could be undertaken at any stage of pharmaceutical research along with any number of drug sets (Chen *et al.* [32] used about 7,173 for screening). The target protein and its matching 3D crystalline structure of protein databases such as PDBe, PDBj, RCSB, and BMRB will be the next and perhaps most crucial steps. After selecting the 3D structure using platforms like molecular docking, molecular mechanics calculations, and a combination of quantum mechanics, the investigator can uncover a wide range of active compounds and spot possible molecular mechanisms for the target sites of these well-practiced pharmacologic agents [33]. To do molecular dynamics simulations on the protein targets, the researcher should select the drugs through scoring methods, followed by validations [34]. The following are the most trusted methodologies that are in use to find the protein target and to find the exact antiviral drug for COVID-19 treatment.

11.7.2.1 Molecular docking program

Molecular docking and chemical binding techniques were used to evaluate the pharmaceutical efficacy of antiviral medicines and evaluate them toward enzyme systems of the SARS-CoV-2.

For SARS-CoV-2 treatment, most of the binding studies focus on vital proteases like 3CLpro, S spike, E envelope, methyltransferase proteins, and RNA polymerase [35]. To determine the affinities over 3CLpro, by molecular modeling, the previously approved drug molecules were subjected to molecular docking study. The study shows that lopinavir, nelfinavir, ritonavir drug are best binding at 23.8%, remdesivir binds at 19.0%, and darunavir binds at 14.3% of the total number of the drug studied (Table 11.1). Also, the author insists that the majority of the drugs show no binding over the SARS-CoV-2 virus.

Based on the results received, most of the drugs are now in clinical trials. The 19 virus–transcribed proteins are screened by Wu *et al.* [36]. The drugs were foreseeing for specific proteins, and for chloroquine drugs, the 3CLpro and PLpro were fixed as a target. And for remdesivir drug, proteases like 3CLpro and RdRc have been fixed. The docking simulations show that remdesivir displays better bind affinity than chloroquine drug over the 3CL-pro M-pro. Another study used AutoDock Vina to evaluate 19 drugs against the M-pro site of SARS-CoV-2. The drugs are O6K, chloroquine, hydroxychloroquine, remdesivir, favipiravir, umifenovir, bromhexine, ambroxol, montelukast, dipyridamole, nelfinavir, cinaserin, GS-441524, curcumin, quercetin, kaempferol, lopinavir, entecavir, and N3. O6K and N3 have outstanding binding affinity values of 7.12 and 7.40 kcal/mol, correspondingly. The docking images show that the molecule has the best docking scores and hence anchors the M-pro's niche throughout the crystalline structure. Quinoline

Table 11.1 List of approved natural and synthetic drugs that are in trials against COVID-19 outbreak

S. no.	Targeted proteins under study	Antiviral and other chemical drugs	Studies in progress
1	3CL-pro	Lopinavir	9
2	3CL-pro	Ritonavir	9
3	3CL-pro	Nelfinavir	7
4	3CL-pro	Remdesivir	9
5	3CL-pro	Darunavir	6
6	3CL-pro	Atazanavir	5
7	3CL-pro	Ledipasvir	5
8	3CL-pro	Oseltamivir	5
9	RdRc	Galidesivir	4
10	RdRc	Remdesivir	6
11	RdRc	Ribavirin	4
12	3CL-pro	Captopril	4
13	3CL-pro	Chloroquine	6
14	3CL-pro	Etoposide	4
15	3CL-pro	Hesperidin	3
16	3CL-pro	Hydroxychloroquine	6
17	3CL-pro	Imatinib	2
18	PL-pro	Chloroquine	3
19	PL-pro	Darunavir	2
20	PL-pro	Levamisole	2
21	PL-pro	Lopinavir	4
22	PL-pro	Ritonavir	4
23	RdRc	Favipiravir	5
24	RdRc	Sofosbuvir	2
25	RdRc	Tenofovir	2
26	"S" spike +ACE complex interface	Tazobactam	2

N-oxide (QO) and Quinoline (Q) nitro compounds were analytically explored (Figure 11.5).

The medication candidates are associated well with the M-pro active site, with binding energies ranging from −4.31 to −5.04 kcal/mol. In addition, some of the nitro-QO compound inhibitors, such as N9-QO, N8-QO, and N4-QO, showed slightly higher stabilizing binding energy values than their nitro-quinoline counterparts. Docking tests were done with the commercialized medications CQ and HCQ, which are presently used to treat SARS-CoV-2 contamination, to test the possibility of such discoveries, in addition to their binding, energy conditions were determined to be −2.33 and −2.80 kcal/mol, correspondingly (Table 11.2).

The hydrogen-bonded relation of the N4-Q molecule with Cys44 at 2.78 Å and hydrophobic interactions with other amino acid sequences like Cys145, Gln189, Glu166, Gly143, His41, His163, His164, Met49, Met165, Ser46, Ser144, Thr45, and Val42, respectively, are given in Figure 11.6 (MD-1). These linkages are

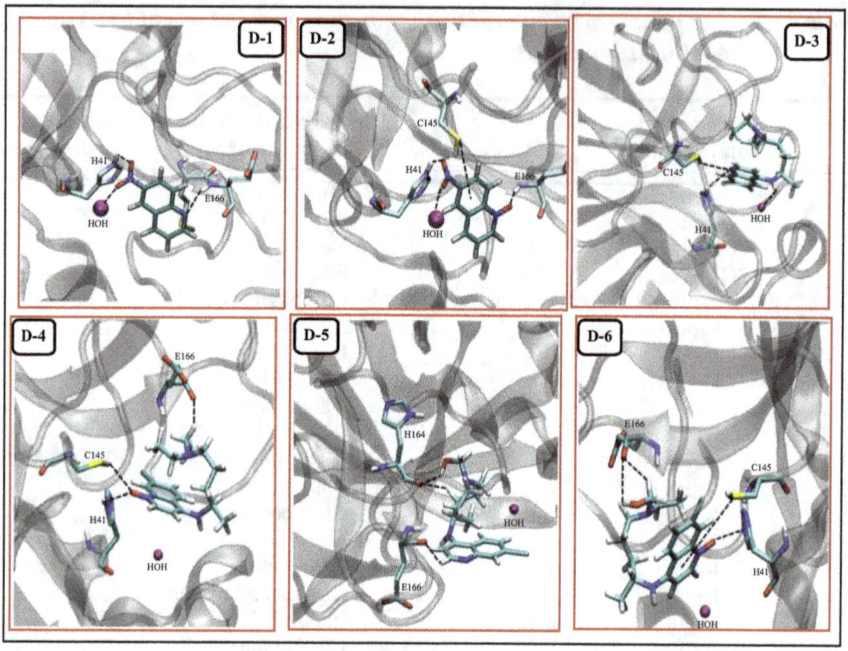

Figure 11.5 *Binding structure of (**D-1**) N4-Q, (**D-2**) N4-QO, (**D-3**) CQ, (**D-4**) CQO, (**D-5**) HCQ, and (**D-6**) HCQO in the M-pro active site*

Table 11.2 *Binding sites and their affinity energy for the antiviral drugs chloroquine and hydroxychloroquine*

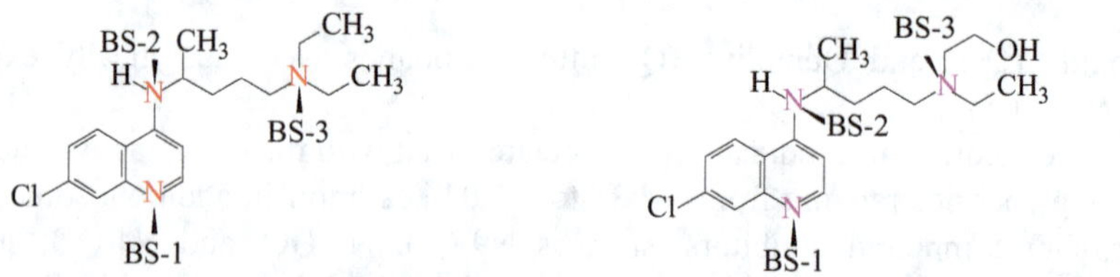

Protein-binding sites (BS)	Affinity energy in kcal/mol	Protein-binding sites (BS)	Affinity energy in kcal/mol
BS 1,2	−2.93	BS 1,2	−3.22
BS 1,3	−2.42	BS 1,3	−2.93
BS 1,2,3	−2.61	BS 1,2,3	−2.84
BS 2	−3.03	BS 2	−3.45
BS 2,3	−3.02	BS 2,3	−3.34
BS 3	−2.94	BS 3	−3.31

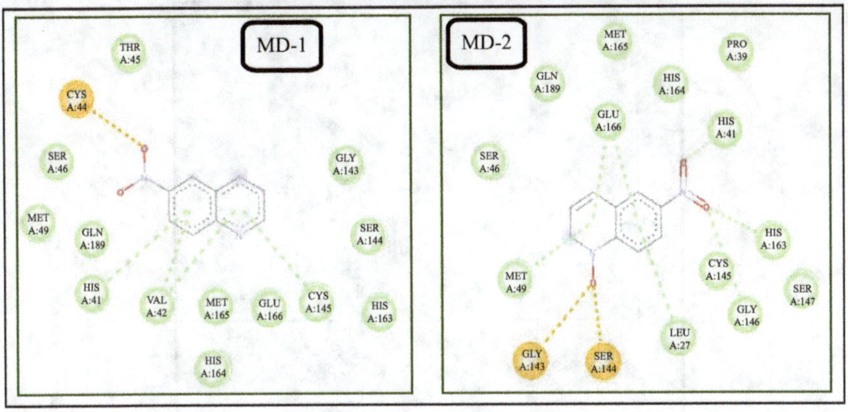

Figure 11.6 Image of molecular dynamics analysis done for N4-Q and N4-QO with M-pro

necessary for decreasing M-pro's enzyme reactions, and they are consistent with the findings of earlier docking studies [37]. The N4-QO molecule, on the other hand, binds to the M-pro was stabilized by four H-bonds such as Ser144 (3.04 Å), Gly143 (3.01 Å), His41 (2.93 Å), and His163 (2.72 Å), and hydrophobic affinity with Cys145, Glu166, Gly146, Gln189, His164, Met49, Met165, Leu27, Pro39, Ser46, and Ser147, respectively, Figure 11.6 (MD-2). Interestingly, the binding affinity of HCQO gets raised to 1 kcal/mol, which confirms their stability than any other derivatives of CQ. Possible variations of HCQO and CQO compounds could be used for evaluating the weight of the N-oxide group at different sites. Every medication nominee's molecular modeling position suggested that they can anchor precisely within the membrane chamber. According to molecular docking and binding energy calculations, viral proteases that are responsible for hewing the viral polypeptides and maintaining the viral regeneration process could be ideal therapeutic targets for viral illnesses. In cases where the virus generated confrontation by transmutation, protease inhibitors have been employed in combination medication therapy. Since the M-pro enzyme contains two polyproteins, pp1a and pp1ab act as the most important foundation for virus duplication. HTVS, SP, and XP-based gliding scores are used to create hit molecules using a docking-based molecular modeling approach, while ADMET can then be used to depict the pharmacologic and physicochemical properties of the suggested lead compounds.

To investigate the affinities of the lead compounds, molecular concept modeling might be used. When comparing the binding affinity of the molecule ABBV-744 to M-pro (G-bind 45.43 kcal/mol), it is discovered that the combination is more stable than other protein–ligand complexes. It is a hypothesis that remdesivir attaches to targets, RdRc and 3CLpro on SARS-CoV-2 with high interaction score. According to the results of a molecular docking study, remdesivir and its enzyme (GS-441524) have excellent binding scores of −6.4 and −7.0 kcal/mol, respectively, and stability that with M-pro (Figure 11.7), indicating supplemental

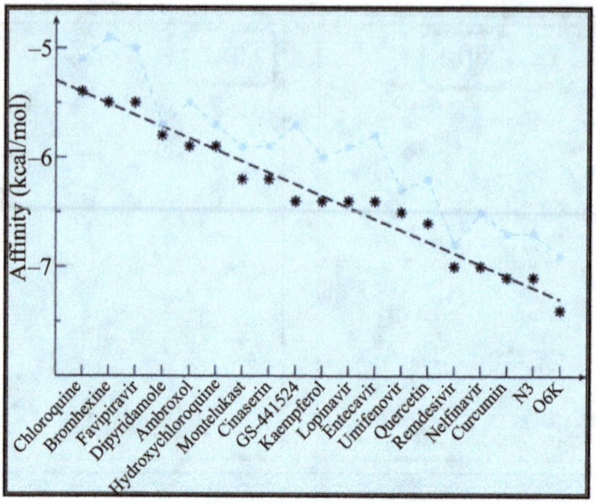

Figure 11.7 Graphical image showing anchoring efficiency of various antiviral drugs in the main protease-anchoring site

stimulatory activity in furthermore to its RdRc inhibition impacts. Remdesivir's binding index is one of the highest therapies, making it an excellent choice designed for the initial treatment of COVID-19 patients for antiviral therapy.

Favipiravir, a tiny viral growth restrictor compound for RdRc produced by Fujifilm Corp. in Japan, did not demonstrate notable interaction with the primary proteolytic. Entecavir has a similar molecular chain just like the remdesivir's metabolite (GS-441524) that is abundantly available at a low price, which can be a better alternative as a potential RdRc and primary target proteins. The properly suited interaction value for entecavir, according to docking study data, is −6.41 kcal/mol. Murugan *et al.* [38] used structure-based quantitative diagnostic criteria (SBCSA) on the drugs such as dihydroergotamine, phthalocyanine, lonafarnib, nilotinib, R-428, tadalafil, and baloxavir marboxil extracted from DBD to evaluate molecules against some of the most prevalent infectious targets, such as 3CL-pro, PL-pro, RdRc, and the spike protein. For the prevention of the COVID-19 virus, baloxavir marboxil is now undergoing drug trials. They claim that drugs like dihydroergotamine, phthalocyanine, R-428, nilotinib, tadalafil, lonafarnib can bind to all three targets in a single attempt making them multi-targeting medicines.

Curcumin has a low absorption (1%) that could limit its use in treating persistent viral illness. Curcumin taken orally, on the other hand, may accumulate in large concentrations in the liver and GI system. It protects the GI from the SARS-CoV-2 virus. It is proved that curcumin is an effective medicine for preventing viral infections in the GI system during medication administration and can continue to play a role even after the respiratory infection has spread to the lungs. Besides these critical functions, this instinctual drug has an adaptable feature in curing swelling, including IL-6, IL-1β, and TNF-α. Also known for preventing liver and digestive tract or GI tract injury, it would be considered for wide-spreading COVID-19 pathological circumstance and was also widely acknowledged to prevent liver and

GI tract rupture, which causes diarrhea. Curcumin stabilizes the interaction with SARS-CoV-2 major protease, according to molecular modeling experiments, with better interaction energy of −7.1 kcal/mol. When it creates stable compounds with the M-pro, the other antimicrobial drugs quercetin and kaempferol, which seem to be abundant in fruits and vegetables, have greater docking studies values of −6.45 and −6.62 kcal/mol, correspondingly (Figure 11.7).

Nelfinavir is used to treat HIV, and a molecular modeling investigation of such an antiviral drug revealed a kind of approaches, a score of −7.01 kcal/mol with the SARS-CoV-2, major proteases. The higher bonding strength indicates their therapeutic implications for inhibiting M-pro in COVID-19 illness. It is currently being tested in clinical trials as an antiretroviral to prevent SARS-CoV-2 replication. Umifenovir is an antimicrobial agent available in Russia and China that has been experimentally used in China to manage COVID-19. In vitro, umifenovir reduces SARS-CoV-2 with an IC50 of 30 M [39]. It has also demonstrated significant benefits as COVID-19 distributed postexposure prophylaxis. According to a molecular modeling study, the M-pro site of SARS-CoV-2 can engage with the major enzyme and limit replicating with an interactive score of −6.51 kcal/mol. An asthma inhibitor molecular drug, montelukast, shows excellent suppression of M-pro, as evidenced by the interaction affinity −6.2 kcal/mol acquired via docking studies. Montelukast has also been shown to be effective as an anti-inflammatory agent in the SARS-CoV-2. Another medication drug dipyridamole has a wide range of antiviral properties and has been clinically demonstrated to be an excellent anti-COVID-19 drug [40]. Dipyridamole's antiviral mechanism includes the inhibition of the M-pro, as demonstrated by an in vitro surface plasmon resonance experiment. The binding energy score is −5.8 kcal/mol.

11.7.2.2 High ambiguity–driven protein–protein DOCKing

Protein–proteins, protein–nucleic acid, and protein–ligand complexes are among the many types of modeling challenges it can handle. High ambiguity–driven protein–protein DOCKing (HADDOCK) found 80 frameworks in 11 tools, including the receptors-2 (TLR2) clusters (s), accounting for 40.0% of the water refined HADDOCK models [41]. The negative HADDOCK score of -112.0 ± 2.850 indicated the vaccine's high binding affinity with the receptors. On human TLR2 receptors, the CTL-1 and CTL-5 epitopes are bounded on SARS-CoV-2 infection. TLR2's interactions with the legend activate the immune system's supervisor and cause interferon and interleukin to combat the infection. According to the well-known Ramachandran design inspection, 68.9% of TLR2 structural residues are found in the positive zone, 31.13% in the allowed zone, and none in the outlier region. The binding results revealed that CTL-5 (WTA GAA AYY) connected posteriorly with the TLR2 receptor's docking groove. The binding score reflects roughly 16.5% of the water-refined HADDOCK generated models. HADDOCK program clustered 33 structures in 7 TLR4 cluster(s) and shows negative gain. The HADDOCK score of -130.9 ± 10.1 indicates good binding energy between the vaccine and the receptor. Here the vaccine masked nearly $2{,}204.4 \pm 22.4$ surface area on the target protein which is less exposed to water (hydrophobic protein surface).

The docked complex with low RMSD score (Table 11.3) implies a high-quality model. HADDOCK grouped 120 structures into 12 MHC class I clusters, accounting for 60.0% of the water-sophisticated HADDOCK mock-up. The low HADDOCK score of -214.7 ± 4.1 shows that the antibody and MHC class I receptor has significant affinities, and the reduced RMSD indicates that the docked complex is stable. HADDOCK groups 64 structures into nine MHC class II clusters, accounting for 32% of the water-refined HADDOCK stimulate models. The stable and strong molecular interaction between the virus active spot and vaccine is proved by the low HADDOCK score. The human MHC class I cell surface receptor HLA-A*0201 is one of the most common ones. HLA-A*0201 has a three-dimensional shape found in the RCSB protein database under the PDB ID 1I4F (Figure 11.8). Chain-A with 275 amino acids and the beta-2 microglobulin chain, which has 100 amino acids, make up HLA-A*0201 [42].

Table 11.3 HADDOCK binding values for TLR-2, TLR-4, MHC-I, and MHC-II with M-protease

No.	Docking parameters	TLR-2	TLR-4	MHC-I	MHC-II
1	HADDOCK value (a.u.)	−112.0	−130.9	−214.7	−212.1
2	Cluster size	20	20	20	20
3	RMSD (Å)	0.3	0.3	0.3	0.3
4	Van der Waals energy (kcal/mol)	−73.2	−72.4	−138.5	−132.5
5	Electrostatic energy (kcal/mol)	−319.7	−238.9	−156.3	−394.9
6	Desolvation energy (kcal/mol)	25.1	−10.9	−45	−0.6
7	Restraints violation energy (kcal/mol)	0.01	1.1	0.0	0.2
8	Buried surface area (Å^2)	2,094.7	2,204.4	3,585.9	4,276.9

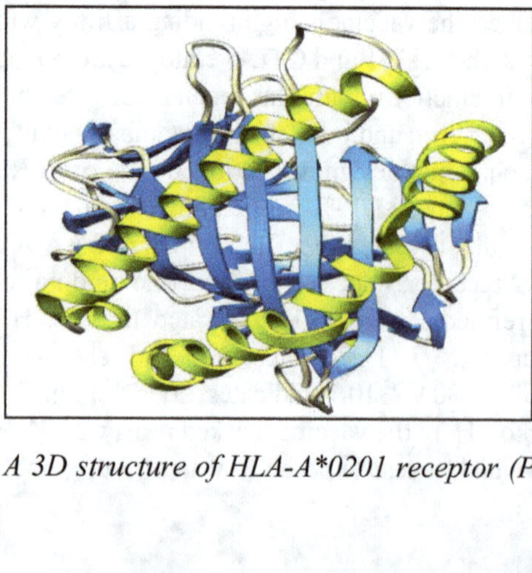

*Figure 11.8 A 3D structure of HLA-A*0201 receptor (PDB ID: 1I4F)*

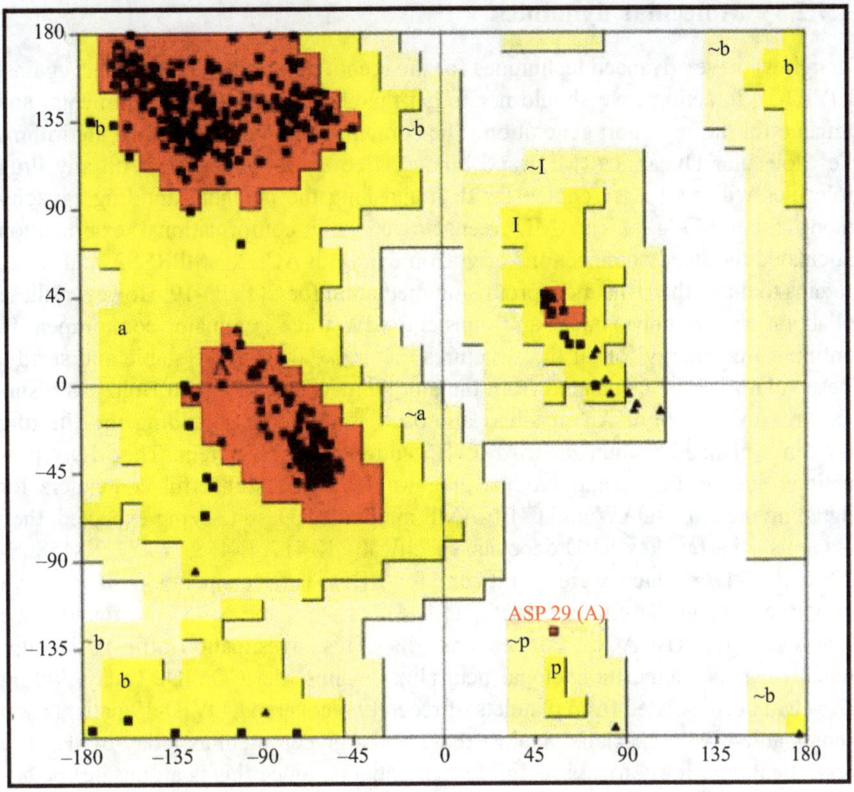

*Figure 11.9 The image showing the Phi (degree) vs Psi (degree) for HLA-A*0201 (Ramachandran plot)*

The Ramachandran plot is adopted to examine the HLA-A*0201 structure for stereochemical characteristics. It shows an increase that approximately 93.72% of the receptor residues are in good agreement, 6.3% of the receptors are all in strong agreement that cannot be vomited from consideration, and therefore most importantly, no antibody residue seems to be in the out-of-limit region (Figure 11.9).

Furthermore, verification of a 3D server demonstrated high structural quality, with over 97.1% of proteins having average 3D–1D scores of 0.2. The HPEPDock server is adopted to analyze the binding of chosen epitopes using the optimized HLA-A*0201 structure. The PepFold administration is adopted to control the 3D designs of chosen epitopes. The energy of planned 3D constructions of CTL epitopes was diminished and upgraded for subatomic docking concentrates with the HLA-A*0201 got. As indicated by the information, CTL-1 and CTL-5 epitopes show good adsorption quantum scores of 251.779 and 246.834 kcal/mol, separately.

11.7.2.3 Molecular dynamics

Though we have advanced techniques for the identification of suitable drugs against COVID-19 infections, we should not forget the chance of getting instrumental and human error during report generation. The combination of computational algorithms like Molecular Dynamics (MD) and bindery free energy assessment on any drug molecules will be a wise choice for distinguishing the potential antidrug capacity among them [43–45]. The MD reenactments and conformational examination anticipated the steady connections of grazoprevir with ACE2, TMPRSS2, and RdRc proteins to make them the most promising mediation for COVID-19. However, these collaborations are noncovalent and transient. vdW force is a major commitment in confining free energy for all the structures that make them more stable and steady. These values can be calculated from the atomic mechanics-Poisson Boltzmann surface area examination. An in silico approach is used for upgrading the limiting between a planned immunizer mAb C-B6 and RBD of S protein. The MD reproductions, just as FEP computations, give way to various cheerful contenders for upgrading the C-B6-DAW and C-B6-AME antibodies. Despite being expected, they distinguished a few key RBD deposits, specifically K-417, L-455, N-487, K-458, S-477, and G-476, which were significant for RBD–FAB cooperation. It is worth noting that among these microstructures, K-417, L-455, and N-487 are found to be more suited for RBDACE2 connections [46]. This investigation affirms the hindrance capacity of the monoclonal neutralizer against the COVID. Today, killing mAbs had been isolated from platelets of recently recovered COVID-19 patients and used as an antiviral specialist against the S spike glycoprotein as a day-by-day life strong treatment for coronavirus-influenced patients. Since this is an unsafe methodology, the specialists adjusted the methodology with known mAb with S-protein. Using the in silico strategy, the scientist examines the atomic system of mAb's limiting with S-protein and plans more powerful mAbs through protein mutagenesis considers. For MD examination of independent apo M-pro just as the ligand-bound particle, the IBM Power-bunch fused with NAMD-10 adaptation was performed. The TIP-3P model for water, the standard particle power field, and the CHARMM-36 power field for the protein are adopted. Before executing the exam, each molecule in the M-pro in the SARS-CoV-2 3D crystal structure in the biochemical and physiological environment was homogenized.

Molecular dimensional analysis is adopted to find the structural stability of the molecule when it binds to the target protein at least for 100 ns. As given in the previous discussion, the repurposing of mitoxantrone and leucovorin drug from the FDA library is adopted for analysis against COVID-19 treatment. Likewise, two more antiviral drugs, birinapant and dynasore, were selected for analysis against the SARS-CoV-2 M-pro site. The chemical structure of the molecules in the antiviral molecule and their steric energy study for a minimum of 100 ns adopted on these antiviral drugs shows an RMSD value of 2.25 Å. These unexpected superior values are due to the improved steric and hydrophobic nature surrounded in the compact cavity when the drug binds over the viral protein. Glutamic acid head (Glu-166) of the principle protease is a critical buildup to hold and frame a steady unpredictablity of revealed lead compounds by shaping hydrogen bonds and salt scaffolds. Additionally, the hydrogen bonding probability of MM/GBSA and its free energy computations confirm the steady and firm binding of the drug molecules with SARS-CoV-2 M-pro protein.

Lycorine, a characteristic alkaloid, accounted for to have various organic properties, like an anti-infection, against the tumor, hostile to the parasite, and bacteria. Emetine, a natural drug molecule has capacities, including prophylactic exercises, and hostile to infection, and against malignancy. The counter SARS-CoV-2 exercises of lycorine and emetine report a similar result. Lycorine destroy SARS-CoV-2 with EC50 = 0.312 μM and emetine with EC50 = 0.463 μM [47]. The revealed hostile to infection movement of lycorine resembles our own (EC50 = 0.437 μM). The computational recreations demonstrate that these decidedly charged mixtures could capably join with mono negative RPF of SARS-CoV-2, adding to weakening the scattering of the infection. Furthermore, it accounts for that the SARS-CoV-2 infection can spread its disease on the cerebrum tissues [48]. Lycorine is less harmful and can cross the blood–cerebrum boundary and fix brain contamination. Vinifera, nympholide A, myricitrin, hesperidin, afzelin, phyllaemblicin B, and biorobin are naturally occurring antiviral and antibiotic drug molecules with high binding affinity on the main proteins and amino acids with nitrogen function proteins on SARA-coronavirus-2. But antiviral drug treatment over ACE2 and RdRc protein target are suppose to have less effect when compare to other targets. So more focused and target cum sequence specific antidrug binding practice is yet to perform and each and every proof against these targets should be noted with utmost care.

Few medications that can hinder the replication cycle of the infection have been proposed and tried with atomic docking that concentrates as a component of the most recent clinical treatment draws near. These medications incorporate chloroquine and hydroxychloroquine. Hydroxychloroquine is more dissolvable than chloroquine and delivers a lesser measure of destructive metabolites. Although chloroquine and hydroxychloroquine, which have been in clinical practice throughout the previous 70 years, are drugs for the treatment of immune system illness, they are utilized similarly as antimalarial drugs. These mixtures have been accounted for as potential expansive range antiviral medications for COVID-19; in any case, their advantages against COVID-19 are questionable, with no obvious impact on hospitalized patients. From an atomic perspective, these drugs are thought to inhibit viral transformation. While increasing the endosomal pH, the drug infection, cell fusion, interfered with the glycosylation of SARS-coronavirus cell receptors, are raised. They also play an important role in the resistance adjusting process, which has a synergistic antiviral effect in vivo. The QM/MM-enhanced molecular dynamics study on the main antiviral drug remdesivir in its monophosphate is adopted to discover the chance of joining with the preliminary strand mRNA connecting with RdRc (PDB; 7BV2) molecule as given in Figure 11.10.

The molecular surface binding investigation of remdesivir mono-phosphate over RdRc shows striking communications that incorporate alluring vdW, $\pi-\pi$ stacking, π-cation, π-alkyl, and covalent just as appalling electrostatic collaborations with RdRc practical gatherings.

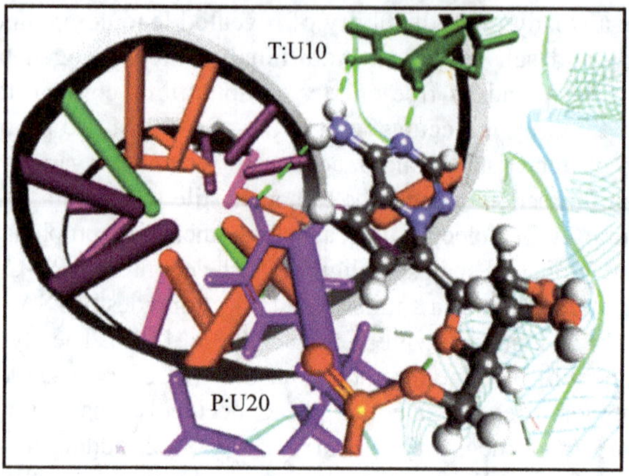

Figure 11.10 QM/MM output image showing the anchoring of remdesivir on helical mRNA genome present in RdRc protease

11.8 Machine-integrated advanced techniques for COVID-19

From the in silico algorithm, the scientists can acquire in-depth knowledge about the newly designed or existing drug properties like binding efficiency on M-pro, antimicrobial property, virus replications inhibition efficiency, and multi-targeting nature. The challenge is to study the in vivo effect of drugs on humans. For this, the most promising techniques like CT and MRI scans are adopted to find the viral infection and the curing ratio of the disease. Nowadays, due to the research in machine learning methods, AI, IoT, etc., these imaging techniques are adopted to get more promising results than the classical ones. Almost every physician, irrespective of their specializations, is dependent on these techniques and based on the computerized output, they are deciding the treatment protocols.

11.8.1 Computerized tomography in COVID-19 detection

To create cross-sectional images of the body, a CT screening uses computers and rotating X-beam machines. Such image provides more information than standard X-beam images. A CT sweep may give 3D pictures of the inner organs just like the clinician envisioning the head, delicate tissues, veins, bones, shoulders, spine, heart, midsection, knee, and chest. During a CT analysis, the machine turns and takes an arrangement of X-beams from different points. The PC-based program will assist us with consolidating the posture to make cross-segments pictures of the body. The region of interest (ROI) on any human internal organ is collected as a 3D picture under CT. A CT check typically exhibits a "switched radiance" model and cryptogram of septal thickening [49]. COVID-19 CT images clearly show the corresponding pneumonic parenchymal surface along with integrated pneumonic opacities having flattened morphology and little lung dissipation. Both MERS-coronavirus and

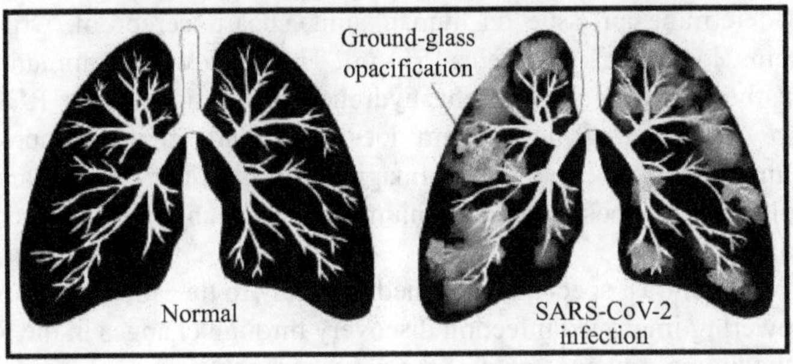

Figure 11.11 Coronavirus-infected lung image obtained on CT scan

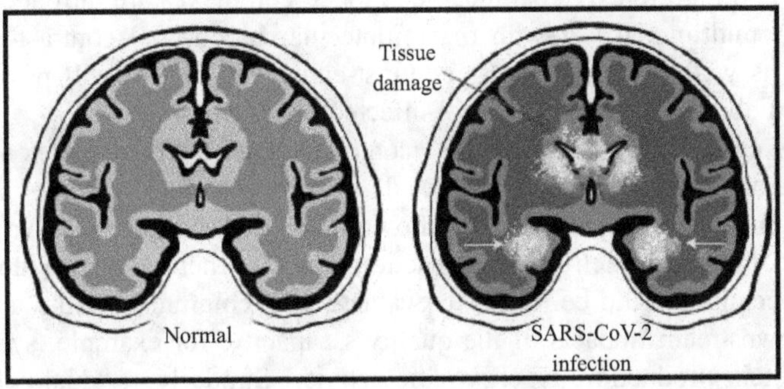

Figure 11.12 Coronavirus-infected brain image obtained on MRI scan

SARS-coronavirus patients have lung fixation with periphery predominance [50]. People with negative rRT-PCR test results for SARS-CoV-2 can have chest infection when tested under CT scan and without further determination to have COVID-19. Subsequently, rising evidence ropes the utilization of chest imaging assessment mostly as positive intended for COVID-19 sickness when people contain negative rRT-PCR tests. Various investigations have examined chest pictures of people tainted by SARS-CoV-2, taking into account that irregularities may likewise be because of different reasons of pneumonia, prompting bogus positive outcomes (Figure 11.11).

In cutting-edge cases, SARS-CoV-2 disease can cause lung tissue harmed with diminished oxygen take-up in contaminated people. The insusceptible reaction to SARS-CoV-2 prompts the release of cytokines and chemokines, as often as possible, the fiery cells that show in CT in the presence of yellow staining. Nevertheless, MRI sweeps of the cerebrum of a patient contaminated with COVID-19 give a lot of top to bottom detail in the delicate tissue than CT (Figure 11.12).

11.8.2 Advanced MRI for COVID-19 treatment

Using electromagnetic field and radiofrequency energy, an MRI test is adopted to visualize the hydrogen atom density inside the human body. Generally, MRIs are adopted to determine an issue on human joints, heart, cerebrum, wrists, ovary, breast, bosoms, lower legs, and veins [51–56]. The radio wave communicated to a collector in the machine converts the hydrogen population in our ROI to a 3D picture. X-ray for imaging bloodstream does not include contrast-improving specialists; in any case, for the more exact imaging of organs that need a paramagnetic metal complex, for the most part, gadolinium-based, which might be given orally or intra-articularly.

These MRI contrast specialists planned remotely to tie especially in pathologic tissue empowering improved infection discovery through changes in the R1 and R2 attractive unwinding rate constants of the neighborhood tissue.

The mix of at least two different upgrading specialists in a solitary MRI output could give top-to-bottom analytic and prognostic data. Two different MRI contrast-enhancing and high relaxive paramagnetic metal complexes are introduced for the analysis. A multimodal CA with macromolecular blood-pool contrast-enhancing properties as well as extravascular contrast-enhancing ability will provide more information about the tumor and viral-infected cells [57].

In this case, a "theranostic" MRI contrast-enhancement complex is used to explore the arrival of a beneficial molecule to the infection site, while the other is used to audit restorative viability by providing a joint simultaneous voxel canny evaluation of remedial delivery and reaction. On the other hand, two atomic MRI contrast specialists could be joined to evaluate both columnist quality articulation and the downstream impacts of the quality's capacity, for example, synapse discharge, protein production, or enzymatic activity. Similarly, a "dual-color image enhancing" MRI strategy is adopted routinely to show a multi-viral specialist imaging through fundamental fluorescence imaging experiments (Figure 11.13).

Additionally, this system will give more point-by-point data with a high spatial goal, limitless imaging profundity, and 3D imaging abilities fundamental for non-intrusive imaging of viral contamination, particularly in delicate tissues. Among the enormous antiviral medications, coming up next are the examined ones for next levels investigation. They chose to repurpose antiviral drugs chloroquine, hydroxychloroquine, ritonavir, lopinavir, and favipiravir. Twist hyperpolarization may open new open doors in the biomedical conclusion of COVID-19 protein connection through MRI filtering methodology. Moreover, even if these medications up-and-comers, which are under clinical examination, may not be helpful for the COVID-19 conclusion [58]. This SABER-based hyperpolarization analysis has been performed with high molecular weight protein and macro enzymes for early diagnosing of "S" spike protein contamination in human organs and is given in Figures 11.14 and 11.15.

The high molecular dimension CA is chosen from the viral database where the drug has remarkable antiviral activity with fewer side effects. The antiviral drug must be in current clinical application. This antiviral specialist drug was successfully analyzed with SABER-based hyperpolarization. The polarization over significant distances was identified and tracked, implying that the advanced imaging methodology can be adopted for other clinical analytic issues. By enhancing each of the components adopted in this technique can be adapted to screen for the

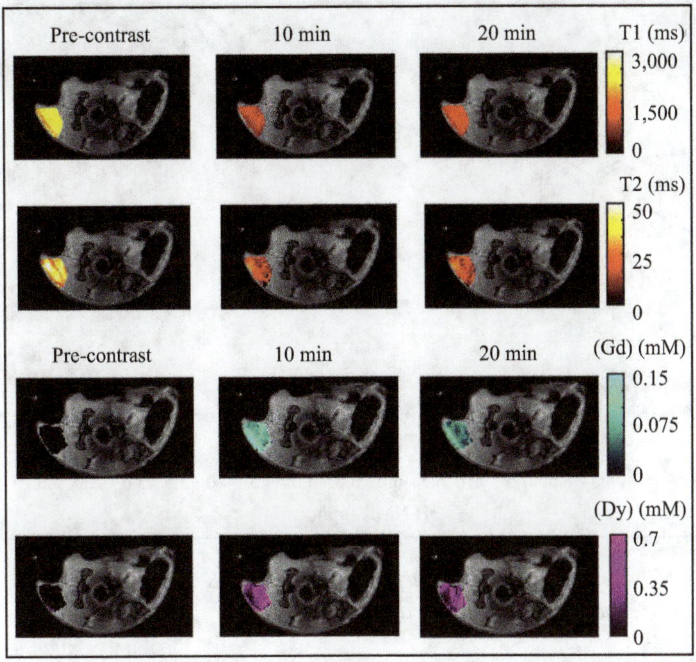

Figure 11.13 Dual contrast agent [Gd(III) and Dy(III)] administered tumor image from fluorescence MRI analysis

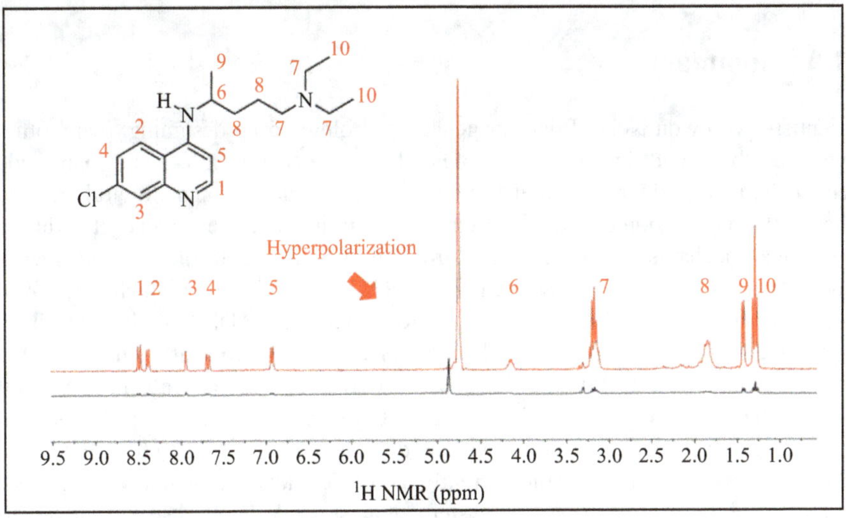

Figure 11.14 SABRE-treated hyperpolarized ¹H NMR image of chloroquine drug

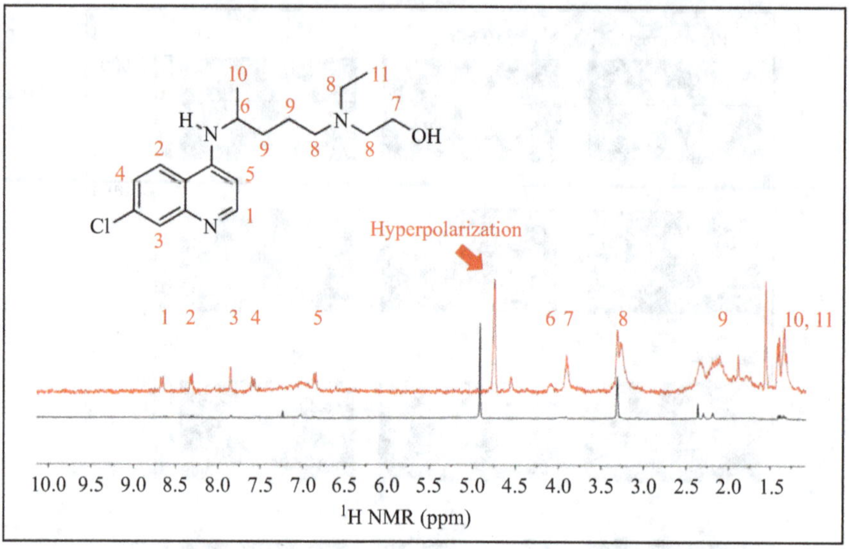

Figure 11.15 SABRE-treated hyperpolarized ^1H NMR image of hydroxychloroquine drug

dispersion and action of the repurposed antiviral medication, hereditarily planned medication, or any new medication in vivo by MRI. It very well might be tackled to additionally explore the subatomic correspondence of extra medication applicants with mooring proteins and uncover unidentified activity on COVID-19, including pharmacokinetics conduct.

11.9 Summary

Scientists, who won Nobel Prize for genetics, virology, drug designing, many other live researchers, and doctors have confessed that the SARS-CoV-2 is a man-made genetically modified virus. Scientists create numerous vaccines and antiviral drugs to prevent the progression of the whole virus, but still it cannot be stopped. It is due to the critical mechanism used in the construction of a viral molecule. The geneticists who designed COVID-19 used three types of RNA, the majority of which came from bats and pigs. Since RNA is important for constructing DNA in living things, aggressive treatment on the virus-affected patient will lead to death. Therefore, the only procedure we can do is to hide the RNA from coronavirus infection. Several vaccines have been reported in the literature, but these are all accepted for medical practices under pandemic situations without doing human trials. Therefore, the future ill effect or the side effect of the currently available vaccine is unknown. Vaccines will activate the human immune system against COVID-19 disease. However, according to the WHO analysis and another medical report, there is widespread concern that patients are dying as a result of SARS-CoV-2 virus infection even after vaccination. On the other hand, it is recognized that the changeover in the protein sequences from normal to high critical version on the coronavirus happens only because of the vaccinated patient who got a COVID-19 infection.

Based on the discussion, it is concluded that each version of COVID-19 requires ACE2 enzyme for multiplication in the respiratory system, GI, kidney, and brain, making it an important enzyme to recombine SARS-CoV-2 over RdRc. In the spreading stage, the high polar region on the virus combined through RdRc, this repeated procedure supports the nonstop viral RN acid replication. Furthermore, the coarticulation of angiotensin-converting and TMPRSS2 proteins within the respiratory system and stomach-related pathways have just been attributed as a key for SARS-CoV-2 to enter the human tissue anatomy. The virus cannot generate energy for its replication like cancer microbes. COVID-19 requires a huge amount of sugars for their survival. This thirst for energy is satisfied by the presence of key amino acids like Hi-296, Ar-345, Se-441, Ar-435, Se-436, Gly-464, and Ar-710 at ACE2, and virus spike proteins. Therefore, if we need to stop the replication, we need a target specific or amino acid-binding or anchoring antiviral drug. These drugs can be newly designed or an already existing one. The requirement is the high water solubility, long stay on the target, less steric strain, and zero side effects. Currently, no antiviral drug has the abovesaid criteria. It is hoped that using in silico methods, we will be able to design a new drug. Researchers can use in silico methods to help them design new efficient drugs, find the anchoring spot over coronaviruses, and test their antimicrobial properties. Researchers can use computer programs such as Biorod, ChemSketch, and ACD labs to design drugs.

For evaluation, the molecular docking and molecular dynamics procedures are addressed to be more user-friendly than the other algorithms. This computerized algorithm will provide detailed amino acid sequences in viruses, enzymes, and any complicated proteins, as well as additional information about the drug's binding efficiency and binding site on the coronavirus and other enzymes and proteins involved in virus replication. For virtual screening, the AutoDock Vina and structural mechanics are found to be more reliable. The catalytic breaking interaction of 3CL-pro at distinct subsists of the polyproteins releases different polypeptides. As discussed earlier, nearly 29 highly active proteins are involved in SARS-CoV-2 transmission and replication in the human lungs cell. 3CL-pro has been identified as a potential-targeted therapy for COVID-19 diagnosis due to its vital role in disease progression and indeed the lack of a near-human counterpart. According to this molecular analysis of the M-pro, the Arg652 moiety is in the proper position to form a link with Arg716 and Arg710, which are present over the ACE2 enzyme in the human lung, brain, kidney, and GI tract. Any drug molecule that can disrupt the linkage of these three amino acids will be the most effective anti-COVID drug. In addition, it has been established that the M-pro protein is responsible for viral replication as well as gene conversion or transmission. As a result, any drug molecule that ideally ties the M-pro pocket may inhibit SARS-CoV-2 replication.

It is claimed that designing and developing a new chemical molecule with these binding properties takes more time. Furthermore, their medicinal trial studies on living organisms will take longer time. As a result, reanalyzing, reusing, or restudying antibacterial and antiviral drugs against COVID infection will be a better option in the current pandemic situation. These, too, require in silico methods for evaluation. For this, many researchers select HIV, cancer, malarial, asthma, and fungal drugs from FDA-approved viral drug data bank and antiviral databases. Antiviral drugs, such as remdesivir, chloroquine, hydroxychloroquine, nitro-derivatives of chloroquine, mitoxantrone, leucovorin, birinapant, and dynasore, have been investigated utilizing docking and molecular modeling to identify potential inhibitors of SARS-CoV-2 M-pro. According to the PCA results, the unique σ-profile-based attribute set "I" connects the primary COVID-19 drugs remdesivir. In any case, the EIDD-2801 in monophosphate structures shows a more vulnerable relationship with drugs that accounts for giving indications against SARS-CoV-2 transmission. Alternatively, dual active drugs for COVID 19 and other deadliest cancer drugs are also under animal trial study. This dual-model drug is used in the most sophisticated CT and MRI scanning procedures. This advanced research will provide information about infection sites, infection area or depth, and live color image monitoring of drug movement inside the human body.

11.10 Conclusion and future scopes

Our discussion highlights the applicability of machine-based strategies to find the target site on SARS-CoV-2 that involves viral replication and to select an appropriate drug to anchor the reactive site followed by the inhibition of viral replication with the most accuracy and low cost. The current pandemic has not given much time to undergo human trials I, II, and III, so we must rely on the existing drug whose efficiency in both ends is known. The problem is still in the selection of antigens to inhibit viral replication. To set right the pandemic in a fast and furious manner, we hope on in silico methods. Every day, the researchers are giving additional instructions regarding the viral protein structure, ACE2 cleavage pattern in lungs, GI tract, kidneys, and brain, DNA contamination in human cells after COVID-19 infection, and the updated activity of drugs under clinical trials. According to the study, in silico methods played a significant role in detecting anchor sites on the SARS-main CoV-2's protease and another key amino acid that supports viral replication. The binding affinity and the drug stability data from molecular docking and molecular dynamics study gives more description about the drug synthesized so far and the various possible reactive sites for drug targeting. Also, it is confirmed that a better potent drug must have the hydrophobic bulky group that can bind on the "anchor" site. The in silico predictions trigger the researchers to discover multimodal inhibitors that can track the infection and kill the target. The discussions also serve as a wake-up call to patients and clinicians to conduct routine COVID-19 infection screenings even after the disease has been cured. Finding the correct and efficient drug is the only way to eradicate this disease.

11.10.1 Future scope

Since there are more parallel computing techniques developed, the selection of an appropriate procedure will be based on its suitability for analysis, result accuracy, and time required. The ever-green PCR test itself makes the wrong decision on COVID infection analysis. The PCR tool can be upgraded with a live gene replicating algorithm to detect coronavirus infections and their structurally changed virus molecule. Once the infection is confirmed, the next step is to locate the virus. This information is critical for patients who have other chronic diseases as well as a coronavirus infection. CT and MRI are the most promising treatments. The advancement in the design of image-enhancing CAs with dual color-producing properties will identify the locations where the virus spreads and the concentration of the virus in the location. From this, the physician can understand the severity of the organ, which got an infection. The biomolecular elemental analysis will give information about the amino acid sequences, enzyme present, and tissue pH. Basic information about the molecular sequence on the ROI is available in the Protein Data bank. Next, it is in the researcher's hand to analyze the chemical bonding sequence through molecular imaging (*AutoDock Vina-4.2*) and analyzing program (*Gaussian algorithm integrated python module*). For instance, the researcher can select antiviral drugs like chloroquine, remdesivir, leucovorin, nelfinavir, and curcumin from viral data bank and perform the docking and molecular dynamics study to find the antiviral efficiency against SARS-CoV-2. Other synthetic scientists can do their research in designing and evaluating drug molecules by using the previously discussed in silico procedures. Once the design is finished through this algorithm, the binding energy and the viral inhibition efficiency can be calculated. This will reduce the laboratory time and the cost of invention. The in vivo study can be performed on animals and human samples using advanced MRI instruments. The live monitoring of the drug action using CT scans and dual-color-based multimodal MRI scanning agents will be the future scope of this study.

References

[1] Rome B. N. and Avorn J. 'Drug evaluation during the Covid-19 pandemic'. *New English Journal of Medicine*. 2020; 382(24): 2282–2284.

[2] Bang S., Son S., Kim S. *et al.* 'Disease pathway cut for multi-target drugs'. *BMC Bioinformatics*. 2019; 20(74): 1–12.

[3] Zhou J., Jiang X., He S., *et al.* 'Rational design of multitarget-directed ligands: Strategies and emerging paradigms'. *Journal of Medicinal Chemistry*. 2019; 62(20): 8881–8914.

[4] Zhang L., Lin D., Sun X., *et al.* 'Crystal structure of SARS-CoV-2 main protease provides a basis for design of improved α-ketoamide inhibitors'. *Science*. 2020; 368(6489): 409–412.

[5] Park M., Thwaites R. S., and Openshaw P. J. M. 'COVID-19: Lessons from SARS and MERS'. *European Journal of Immunology*. 2020; 50(3): 308–311.

[6] Rabaan A. A., Al-Ahmed S. H., Haque S., *et al.* 'SARS-CoV-2, SARS-CoV, and MERS-COV: A comparative overview'. *Le Infezioni in Medicina*. 2020; 28(2): 174–184.

[7] Shanmugaraj B., Siriwattananon K., Wangkanont K., and Phoolcharoen W. 'Perspectives on monoclonal antibody therapy as potential therapeutic

intervention for Coronavirus disease-19 (COVID-19)'. *Asian Pacific Journal of Allergy and Immunology*. 2020; 38(1): 10–18.

[8] Gao Y., Yan L., Huang Y., *et al.* 'Structure of the RNA-dependent RNA polymerase from COVID-19 virus'. *Science*. 2020; 368(6492): 779–782.

[9] Tai W., He L., Zhang X., *et al.* 'Characterization of the receptor-binding domain (RBD) of 2019 novel coronavirus: Implication for development of RBD protein as a viral attachment inhibitor and vaccine'. *Cellular & Molecular Immunology*. 2020; 17: 613–620.

[10] Basu A., Sarkar A., and Maulik U. 'Molecular docking study of potential phytochemicals and their effects on the complex of SARS-CoV2 spike protein and human ACE2'. *Scientific Reports*. 2020; 10: 17699.

[11] Wu C. I. and Wen H. 'Heightened protein-translation activities in mammalian cells and the disease/treatment implications'. *National Science Review*. 2020; 7: 1847–1851.

[12] Hoffmann M., Kleine-Weber H., Schroeder S., *et al.* 'SARS-CoV-2 cell entry depends on ACE2 and TMPRSS2 and is blocked by a clinically proven protease inhibitor'. *Cell*. 2020; 181: 271–280.

[13] Lanjanian H., Moazzam-Jazi M., Hedayati M., *et al.* 'SARS-CoV-2 infection susceptibility influenced by ACE2 genetic polymorphisms: Insights from Tehran Cardio-Metabolic Genetic Study'. *Scientific Reports*. 2021; 11: 1529.

[14] Can H., Koseoglu A. E., Erkunt Alak S., *et al.* 'In silico discovery of antigenic proteins and epitopes of SARS-CoV-2 for the development of a vaccine or a diagnostic approach for COVID-19'. *Scientific Reports*. 2020; 10: 22387.

[15] Shaddel M., Ebrahimi M., and Tabandeh M. R. 'Bioinformatics analysis of single and multi-hybrid epitopes of GRA-1, GRA-4, GRA-6 and GRA-7 proteins to improve DNA vaccine design against *Toxoplasma gondii*'. *Journal of Parasitic Diseases*. 2018; 42(2): 269–276.

[16] Zheng M., Karki R., Williams E. P. *et al.* 'TLR2 senses the SARS-CoV-2 envelope protein to produce inflammatory cytokines'. *Nature Immunology*. 2021; 22: 829–838.

[17] Hou H., Wang T., Zhang B., *et al.* 'Detection of IgM and IgG antibodies in patients with coronavirus disease 2019'. *Clinical & Translational Immunology*. 2020; 9(5): e01136.

[18] Chakraborty C. 'Performance analysis of compression techniques for chronic wound image transmission under smartphone-enabled tele-wound network'. *International Journal of E-Health and Medical Communications (IJEHMC)*. 2019; 10(2): 1–15, 10.4018/IJEHMC.2019040101.

[19] Chakraborty C. 'Chronic wound image analysis by particle swarm optimization technique for tele-wound network'. *International Journal of Wireless Personal Communications*. 2017; 96(3): 3655–3671, ISSN: 0929-6212, 10.1007/s11277-017-4281-5.

[20] Joffre O. P., Segura E., Savina A., and Amigorena S. 'Cross-presentation by dendritic cells'. *Nature Reviews Immunology*. 2012; 12(8): 557–569.

[21] Zhu X., Wang X., Han L., *et al.* 'Multiplex reverse transcription loop-mediated isothermal amplification combined with nanoparticle-based lateral flow biosensor for the diagnosis of COVID-19'. *Biosensors and Bioelectronics*. 2020; 166: 112437.

[22] Corman V. M., Landt O., Kaiser M., *et al.* 'Detection of 2019 novel coronavirus (2019-nCoV) by real-time RT-PCR'. *Eurosurveillance*. 2020; 25 (3): p2000045.

[23] Shen Z., Xiao Y., Kang L., *et al.* 'Genomic diversity of severe acute respiratory syndrome coronavirus 2 in patients with coronavirus disease'. *Clinical Infectious Diseases*. 2020; 71(15): 713–720.

[24] Smyrlaki I., Ekman M., Lentini A., *et al.* 'Massive and rapid COVID-19 testing is feasible by extraction-free SARS-CoV-2 RT-PCR'. *Nature Communications*. 2020; 11: 4812.

[25] Abduljalil J. M. 'Laboratory diagnosis of SARS-CoV-2: Available approaches and limitations'. *New Microbes and New Infections*. 2020; 36: 100713.

[26] Kevadiya B. D., Machhi J., Herskovitz J., *et al.* 'Diagnostics for SARS-CoV-2 infections'. *Nature Materials*. 2021; 20: 593–605.

[27] Trott O. and Olson A. J. 'AutoDock Vina: Improving the speed and accuracy of docking with a new scoring function, efficient optimization and multi-threading'. *Journal of Computational Chemistry*. 2010; 31(2): 455–461.

[28] Tien H., Haoran W., and Binquan L. 'In silico exploration of the molecular mechanism of clinically oriented drugs for possibly inhibiting SARS-CoV-2's main protease'. *The Journal of Physical Chemistry Letters*. 2020; 11(11): 4413–4420.

[29] Guedes I. A., Costa L. S. C., dos Santos K. B., *et al.* 'Drug design and repurposing with DockThor-VS web server focusing on SARS-CoV-2 therapeutic targets and their non-synonym variants'. *Scientific Reports*. 2021; 11 (1): 5543.

[30] Keretsu S., Bhujbal S. P., and Cho S. J. 'Molecular modeling studies of pyrrolo [2, 3-d] pyrimidin-4-amine derivatives as JAK1 inhibitors based on 3D-QSAR, molecular docking, molecular dynamics (MD) and MM-PBSA calculations'. *Journal of Biomolecular Structure and Dynamics*. 2021; 39(3): 753–765.

[31] Pushpakom S., Iorio F., Eyers P. A., *et al.* 'Drug repurposing: Progress, challenges and recommendations'. *Nature Reviews Drug Discovery*. 2019; 18(1): 41–58.

[32] Chen Y. W., Yiu C. P. B., and Wong K. Y. 'Prediction of the SARS-CoV-2 (2019-nCoV) 3C-like protease (3CL pro) structure: Virtual screening reveals velpatasvir, ledipasvir, and other drug repurposing candidates'. *F1000Research*. 2020; 9: 129.

[33] Muralidharan N., Sakthivel R., Velmurugan D., and Gromiha M. M. 'Computational studies of drug repurposing and synergism of lopinavir, oseltamivir and ritonavir binding with SARS-CoV-2 protease against COVID-19'. *Journal of Biomolecular Structure and Dynamics*. 2021; 39(7): 2673–2678.

[34] Muhammad L. J., Algehyne E. A., Usman S. S., Ahmad A., Chakraborty C., and Mohammed I. A. 'Supervised machine learning models for prediction of COVID-19 infection using epidemiology dataset'. *SN Computer Science*. 2021; 2(11): 1–13.

[35] Elfiky A. A. 'Ribavirin remdesivir, sofosbuvir, galidesivir, and tenofovir against SARS-CoV-2 RNA dependent RNA polymerase (RdRp): A molecular docking study'. *Life Sciences*. 2020; 253: 117592.

[36] Wu C., Liu Y., Yang Y., *et al.* 'Analysis of therapeutic targets for SARS-CoV-2 and discovery of potential drugs by computational methods'. *Acta Pharmaceutica Sinica B*. 2020; 10(5): 766–788.

[37] Assis L. C., de Castro A. A., de Jesus J. P. A., *et al.* 'Computational evidence for nitro derivatives of quinoline and quinoline N-oxide as low-cost alternative for the treatment of SARS-CoV-2 infection'. *Scientific Reports*. 2021; 11: 6397.

[38] Murugan N. A., Kumar S., Jeyakanthan J., and Srivastava V. 'Searching for target-specific and multi-targeting organics for Covid-19 in the Drug bank database with a double scoring approach'. *Scientific Reports*. 2020; 10: 19125.

[39] Lu H. 'Drug treatment options for the 2019-new coronavirus (2019-nCoV)'. *BioScience Trends*. 2020; 14(1): 69–71.

[40] Liu X., Li Z., Liu S., *et al.* 'Therapeutic effects of dipyridamole on COVID-19 patients with coagulation dysfunction'. *Acta Pharmaceutica Sinica B*. 2020; 10(7): 1205–1215.

[41] Van Zundert G. C. P., Rodrigues J. P. G. L. M., Trellet M., *et al.* 'The HADDOCK 2.2 webserver: User-friendly integrative modeling of biomolecular complexes'. *Journal of Molecular Biology*. 2016; 428(4): 720–725.

[42] Kumar N. 'Cytotoxic T-lymphocyte elicited vaccine against SARS-CoV-2 employing immunoinformatics framework'. *Scientific Reports*. 2021; 11: 7653.

[43] Elmezayen A. D., Al-Obaidi A., Şahin A. T., and Yelekçi K. 'Drug repurposing for coronavirus (COVID-19): In silico screening of known drugs against coronavirus 3CL hydrolase and protease enzymes'. *Journal of Biomolecular Structure and Dynamics*. 2020: 1–13.

[44] Garg L., Chukwu E., Nasser N., Chakraborty C., and Garg G. 'Anonymity preserving IoT-based COVID-19 and other infectious disease contact tracing model'. *IEEE Access*. 2020; 8: 159402–159414.

[45] Chakraborty C., and Abougreen A. N. 'Intelligent Internet of Things and advanced machine learning techniques for COVID-19'. *EAI Endorsed Transactions on Pervasive Health and Technology*. 2021: 1–14.

[46] Taka E., Yilmaz S. Z., Golcuk M., *et al.* 'Critical interactions between the SARS-CoV-2 spike glycoprotein and the human ACE2 receptor'. *The Journal of Physical Chemistry B*. 2021; 125(21): 5537–5548.

[47] Choy K. T., Wong A. Y., Kaewpreedee P., *et al.* 'Remdesivir, lopinavir, emetine, and homoharringtonine inhibit SARS-CoV-2 replication in vitro'. *Antiviral Research*. 2020; 178: 104786.

[48] Bullen C. K., Hogberg H. T., Bahadirli-Talbott A., *et al.* 'Infectability of human BrainSphere neurons suggests neurotropism of SARS-CoV-2'. *Altex*. 2020; 37(4): 665–671.

[49] Bernheim A., Mei X., Huang M., *et al.* 'Chest CT findings in coronavirus disease-19 (COVID-19): Relationship to duration of infection'. *Radiology*. 2020; 295(3): 200463.

[50] Zhou Z., Guo D., Li C., *et al.* 'Coronavirus disease 2019: Initial chest CT findings'. *European Radiology*. 2020; 30(8): 4398–4406.

[51] Pushparaj L. T. and Alexander V. 'Trinuclear Gd(III) metal complex with amide core display remarkable enhancement in relaxivity'. *Applied Magnetic Resonance*. 2017; 48(8): 813–825.

[52] Salarian M., Turaga R. C., Xue S., *et al.* 'Early detection and staging of chronic liver diseases with a protein MRI contrast agent'. *Nature Communications*. 2019; 10: 4777.

[53] Pushparaj L. T., Francy I. R. E., and Uma D. M. 'HSA and CA-125 binding study of [Pr-(DO3-Ch-Ph-Am-Gd(III))2Pt(IV)] complex as M-MRI contrast agent for ovarian cancer treatment'. *Journal for Innovative Development in Pharmaceutical and Technical Science*. 2021; 4: 1–8.

[54] Anderson C. E., Donnola S. B., Jiang Y., *et al.* 'Dual contrast – Magnetic resonance fingerprinting (DC-MRF): A platform for simultaneous quantification of multiple MRI contrast agents'. *Scientific Reports*. 2017; 7: 8431.

[55] Lindeman L. R., Jones K. M., High R. A., *et al.* 'Differentiating lung cancer and infection based on measurements of extracellular pH with acidoCEST MRI'. *Scientific Reports*. 2019; 9: 13002.

[56] Abbasi A., Javed A. R., Chakraborty C., Nebhen J., Zehra W., and Jalil Z. 'ElStream: An ensemble learning approach for concept drift detection in dynamic social big data stream learning'. *IEEE Access*. 2021: 1–12.

[57] Kevadiya D., Machhi J., Herskovitz J., *et al.* 'Diagnostics for SARS-CoV-2 infections Bhavesh'. *Nature Materials*. 2021; 20:593–605.

[58] Anderson C. E., Johansen M., Erokwu B. O., *et al.* 'Dynamic, simultaneous concentration mapping of multiple MRI contrast agents with dual contrast – Magnetic resonance fingerprinting'. *Scientific Reports*. 2019; 9(1): 19888.

Chapter 12

Stress detection for cognitive rehabilitation in COVID-19 scenario

Ahona Ghosh[1], *Sima Das*[1] *and Sriparna Saha*[1]

Abstract

Due to the current demand for emerging technologies like the Internet of Things integrated with machine learning in industry and academics, brain–computer interface tools like electroencephalogram in healthcare have drawn worldwide attention. As has been noticed that during recent times, mobile phone exposure to people increased in at least 2-fold way, so games have been used as stimuli for detecting how our brain becomes overburdened with increased exposure. After the data acquisition from 14 channels of an electroencephalogram, the activated regions were identified. Features were extracted from the most activated ten electrode channels using discrete wavelet transform. To reduce the dimensions of the feature space for enhancing the performance, principal component analysis was used. The mental state classification was performed using a support vector machine based on the detected stress. The proposed system has outperformed the existing ones for its effectiveness and efficiency in a broad application area of cognitive rehabilitation. Classification accuracy was obtained as 92.79% and different other metrics proved that the combination of channel selection, feature extraction, and classification methods in our proposed approach has outperformed the others. Privacy is maintained, and it is flexible to the user as per his/her convenient time.

Keywords: Electroencephalogram; Stress detection; COVID-19 pandemic; Discrete wavelet transform; Dimensionality reduction; Support vector machine; Cognitive rehabilitation

12.1 Introduction

In this era, stress is a common event that happens to everyone. Machine learning (ML) is set as a benchmark in emerging technology, and EEG is connected with the

[1]Department of Computer Science and Engineering, Maulana Abul Kalam Azad University of Technology, West Bengal, India

brain–computer interface for collecting electrical signals and converts it into a numerical dataset to measure human brain activity. The recent pandemic due to COVID-19 had a tremendous impact on human psychological health [1,2]. In our daily life, many of us are facing challenges during the COVID-19 pandemic era. The challenges are as follows: physical health issues and mental stress. The undertaken research on previous outbreaks caused by Middle Eastern respiratory syndrome [3], severe acute respiratory syndrome [4], and Ebola [5] showed different consequences of a burden on mental health, like depression, panic, anxiety, and stress pandemics [6,7].

Mental stress increases by overwhelming, feeling of fear, chronic health problems, feeling lonely, and isolated from family members. It is natural to feel stressed in a pandemic era, but it is injurious for mental as well as physical health also. The recent pandemic due to COVID-19 has impacted the quality of our lifestyle and well-being with multiple risk factors [8]. While most of the recent studies have focused on the psychological effects of pandemics only on students and academic staff, this chapter has attempted to detect the stress among ordinary people by detecting abnormality or degradation in the brain activities recorded by electroencephalogram.

Artificial intelligence and intelligent systems in smart healthcare especially during the pandemic are experiencing an increasing demand [9] to read and act on complex data, such as photos, speech, text, video, or other signals, to achieve a required goal. Blockchain also has been widely used to trace private contacts of Internet of Medical Things framework users digitally, instead of physical contact in the COVID-19 scenario [10]. Using computed tomography datasets and chest X-ray images, CNN-based pretrained models have been widely employed for COVID-19 detection. However, for training, validation, and testing, most of the approaches utilized a smaller number of data samples for both CT and CXR datasets. As a result, while the model may have performed well during testing, it will not be more effective in the long run [11]. The importance of diagnostics as a cornerstone for making life-saving decisions was demonstrated in this dramatic case [12,13].

Our proposed work can be used to detect human stress in a pandemic. We have discussed how psychological interventions affect the human mind during the increased game-playing habit of the pandemic. We have used electroencephalography to collect datasets from the human brain and generate a brain map to detect which lobe is more active. After identifying the lobe positions, AF3, AF4, T8, T7, P8, P7, O2, O1, FC6, and FC5 channels are selected from the brain map generated by sLORETA software. Based on this, feature extraction is carried out using discrete wavelet transform (DWT). After that, classification is performed using a support vector machine (SVM) for the recognition of the subject's mental state as stressed or not stressed. Performance evaluation metrics, namely recall, error rate, precision, $F1$ score, and accuracy, have been used to assess the efficiency and applicability of our proposed approach to detect stress among game players in real-time scenarios.

There have been several attempts toward cognitive rehabilitation using ML techniques. The gaps found in state of the art have motivated us to consider this area for further exploration. The motivations behind taking up this research challenge include the following:

1. to study the presence of stress in players based on android games;
2. to overcome the shortcoming present in state-of-the-art literature and to gradually improve the performance of stress detection;
3. to detect the three factors of game-based regulating mental state, i.e., relatedness (the capability of gamers to other people in society), the competence of completing necessary game levels, and autonomy.

The contributions of our proposed framework for the detection of stress levels in ordinary people during the pandemic era can be briefed as per the following:

1. It has been able to detect whether the subject is stressed or not stressed.
2. Haar as the wavelet basis function in the DWT used as the feature extractor in our proposed approach has outperformed the other wavelet basis functions used in the state-of-the-art literature.
3. The training set size is larger than the existing benchmarks in the related area as per our knowledge. So, the classification accuracy of the SVM model has been achieved as 92.79%, which outperforms the state-of-the-art literature in its concerned domain. Also, hyperparameter tuning has been carried out to choose the best parameters for achieving the highest accuracy.

The remaining of the chapter is as follows: in Section 12.2, we have discussed related works of stress level detection and cognitive load; in Section 12.3, we have proposed our system and algorithm of the system also be discussed; experimental outcomes are discussed in Section 12.4; last but not the least, concluding statements regarding the proposed approach are given in Section 12.5.

12.2 Related works

Rehabilitation is the art of restoring someone from damages or disorders from mental and physical aspects. Two therapeutic seal robots have been used in [14] to achieve rehabilitation for dementia patients by recording patient's EEG data 20 min before and after the therapy. Patients who liked the seal robots and interacted with them freely were observed to improve cortical neurons activity. However, the durability and repeatability of the positive effects are to be investigated further to find the efficacy of the model in a real-world scenario. Excited, happy, pleased, relaxed, calm, distressed, frightened, angry, depressed, and sad are the emotions considered by Ali *et al.* while recognizing sentiments by EEG [15]. Statistical features, wavelet entropy, modified energy, and wavelet energy features are the determining factor of these emotions, and the average accuracy obtained from three classifiers, namely SVM, *k*-nearest neighbor (*k*NN), and quadratic discriminant analysis, was 83.87%. A minimum number of electrodes, i.e., only four were used to collect data from the EEG device that proves the vital role of the prefrontal cortex in regulating and identifying emotions based on the requirement.

Alpha, beta, gamma1, gamma2, delta, theta band power, corresponding asymmetry, and paired symmetry are the linear features, and detrended fluctuation analysis, sample entropy are the nonlinear features considered by Mahato and Paul in depression detection and severity-scaling application of a six-channel EEG [16]. After selecting features by ReliefF, bagging of SVM was used along with three kernel functions, namely sigmoidal, Gaussian, and polynomial to classify the depression intensity among which Gaussian kernel achieved the highest accuracy and temporal region was proved to be responsible and affected for depressing emotions generated in our brain. Data acquisition from only six channels of the electrode made the framework easier to use and more convenient for common people diagnosing depression. Linear discriminant analysis, genetic algorithm, and decision tree (DT) have been applied to extract and select the most relevant EEG features and differentiate between depressive and non-depressive subjects in [17]. Classification accuracy and optimality remarkably increased during the analysis of the combined and complete set of features rather than separate analysis of individual bands. EEG-based antidepressant response index has been used to detect the treatment response from depressed subjects.

Kernel eigen-filter-bank common spatial pattern has been applied in feature extraction and frequencies ranging between gamma and theta bands have been selected in [18], after which, principal component analysis (PCA) has reduced the feature vector dimension. Single-trial classification accuracy was achieved as 81%. The participant-independent accuracy of the nonlinear SVM classifier was also tested by a condition of leaving one participant based on voting in every iteration throughout the classification process. The experimental setup consisted of only eight electrodes, designing which is less time-consuming and the experiment lasted only for 6 s which also indicates no exhaustion experience during the test data collection. However, the system got tested with only 24 participants, which needs an increase in training size to validate it further in real-time scenarios. Moreover, the other regions apart from the temporal lobe can be tested further during channel selection with methods like mutual information, Fisher's separability criterion. After providing a questionnaire on their previous experience of depression and treatment with antidepressant medication to 21 subjects in [19], Niemiec and Lithgow have identified that people having depression experience in past tend to get a frontal brain asymmetry ratio lying near the distribution boundaries, and the clear alpha peak helped to make the assessment procedure more consistent and robust. After the noise removal using finite impulse response method along with adaptive predictor filter, discrete wavelet transformation, and Kalman derivation, the minimal redundancy maximal relevance method got applied to select features in Cai *et al.*'s depression identification approach using a three-electrode pervasive EEG [20]. Ten-fold cross-validation was applied to test the performance of SVM, artificial neural network, *k*NN, and classification tree that resulted in the highest accuracy of *k*NN as 79%. The theta wave absolute power worked most efficiently in the learning process of discriminating depressed subjects from the normal ones.

Interhemispheric asymmetry and band power as linear features alone, wavelet entropy and relative wavelet energy as nonlinear features alone, and a combination of both got considered to classify healthy and depressed subjects using quadratic and linear discriminant analysis, multilayer perceptron, and radial basis function (RBF) network in [21]. The alpha band as the linear feature and both of the nonlinear features achieved the highest accuracy with a multilayer perceptron, RBF, and linear discriminant analysis, respectively. The combined linear and nonlinear feature set performed best with the RBF in terms of specificity, sensitivity, and accuracy. However, a more generalized outcome can be achieved by testing the framework with a greater number of patients in the future. Among the five layers of CNN, the first four max-pooling layers were used in feature selection and the last one, i.e., fully connected layer was applied in a classification where batch normalization and dropout also took place to reduce the chance of overfitting in [22]. Here EEG data obtained from only two electrodes achieved satisfactory accuracy since the training sample size of the PhysioNet database was also effective for such a motor imagery task and CNN alone has extracted and selected features; thus, the complexity of employing other artificial methods to preprocess, and feature extraction was avoided also.

Artificial intelligence has been widely applied in different COVID-19-based research works [23]. The existing literature on COVID-19 somewhere has attempted to model the lockdown decision-making [24] and somewhere has attempted to detect respiratory distress due to virus attack [25]. Additionally, the convolutional network has verified its efficiency in various fields, including sentiment analysis [26], gesture recognition [27], sign language detection [28]. Table 12.1 presents a comparative study among state-of-the-art works from where it is clear that existing literature lacks suitable infrastructure for stress detection and recovery systems and as per our understanding, the proposed framework has addressed the gaps found in those. The impact of playing different games and beating the other player's scores on human emotion has been analyzed in [29] using EEG. A deep learning-based type 2 fuzzy set has been applied to classify the emotion changes during game playing. Facial expression as well as brain signals were monitored parallelly, and the games for which the negative emotions dominated the positive ones can be avoided for a better quality of life in the future [30]. A bidirectional long short-term memory (LSTM) has been used based on the player's attention while engaged in game playing, and the dimensionality-based scarcity has been handled using feature augmentation technique before feeding it in the LSTM for emotion classification in [31]. The system was validated with some combined five-by-two paired *t*-test and Friedman test. Based on the rating of adversarial effects, the spreading of damaging computer and android games may be controlled by the parents.

12.3 Proposed framework

Here we discuss the different aspects of our proposed methodology. After the description of data acquisition techniques, the working mechanisms of feature extraction and selection [42] are described at first, then the mental state

Table 12.1 A comparative study among state-of-the-art literature

Ref. detail	Motivation	EEG device	Subject	Preprocessing	Feature extraction	Classification/ Clustering	Contribution	Shortcoming found (if any)
Asif *et al.* [32]	Stress level detection in response to the music track	Four-channel MUSE head-band	A total of 13 females and 14 males	Notch band stop filter rejecting frequency between 45 and 64 Hz	Absolute power, relative power, coherence, phase lag, and amplitude asymmetry	Sequential minimal optimization, stochastic gradient descent, logistic regression, multilayer perceptron	The highest accuracy (98.76% for two-level and 95.06% for three-level) was obtained from logistic regression	The training sample can be increased in the number of subjects and features in the future to get higher accuracy using deep learning
Saeed *et al.* [33]	Long-term stress recognition in resting-state by PSS-10 questionnaire	EMOTIV Xavier testbench version 3.1.21 headset	A total of 13 females and 20 males	DC offset removal using fast Fourier transform and minimal eyeblink in closed eye state	Power spectral density of five channels, alpha and beta asymmetry, and feature selection using *t*-test	Support vector machine, naïve Bayes, *k* nearest neighbor, multilayer perceptron, logistic regression	Involvement of psychology experts to label the stress intensity and highest accuracy achieved by SVM and LR having alpha symmetry feature	The training sample can be increased in several subjects and features in the future to get higher accuracy using deep learning models
Ahn *et al.* [34]	Stress assessment using mental arithmetic, Stroop color–word test	Two-channel EEG and one channel ECG	14 male subjects only	EOG signal removal using fast Fourier transform	Right and left normalized alpha and beta band power, and each band's power asymmetry	Analysis of variance to confirm the statistical significance and support vector machine to classify stress situations	The combination of EEG and heart rate variability improved the stress assessing classifier performance	The convenience to put on such a device can be increased by replacing the wet electrode with dry ones and the training sample size can

								be increased for better accuracy
Kalas and Momin [35]	Stress level estimation and reduction	RMS MAXIMUS 24 channel EEG	Ten subjects only	Noise reduction using discrete wavelet transform	Features from two stages, i.e., baseline and task-load got extracted	Calculation of stress indices and grouping into high stress and low stress based on a threshold using *K* means clustering	Helpful in stress management and takes less time and human resource	Sensitivity analysis and intervention can be considered a future extension to check stress reduction
Priya *et al.* [36]	Stress detection during serial subtraction task	EEG having a 10–20 electrode location system	A total of 36 subjects	Artifact-free EEG signal was considered containing 182 s of relaxed state and 62 s of a stressed state	A total of 64 power ratio feature extraction by power spectral density using fast Fourier transform	SVM and *k*-nearest neighbor as a classifier and *k*-fold cross-validation to check the generalized and unbiased performance	Gaussian SVM having KS>2.5 performed better. *k*NN with one neighbor performed well in that work	More evaluation on higher order polynomial SVM can be done in the future as it could achieve good performance but takes more time
Liao *et al.* [37]	Stress prediction by listening to music and calm the mind down	NeuroSky Mind-wave Mobile	Seven subjects only	Not mentioned	EEG frequency using Fast Fourier Transform	Binary classification into two classes, i.e., meditation and attention using deep learning model with ReLU activation function	The highest validation accuracy is 80.13%. High precision for meditation class, better *F*1-score, and high recall for attention class.	Click button addition can be done in the future to control the action where higher attention means higher button click accuracy

(Continues)

Table 12.1 (Continued)

Ref. detail	Motivation	EEG device	Subject	Preprocessing	Feature extraction	Classification/ Clustering	Contribution	Shortcoming found (if any)
						and fully connected layers	Small MSE loss of 0.0882	
Sharma and Chopra [38]	Stress identification during the aptitude test	Not mentioned	Not mentioned	Fifth-order Butterworth filter has outperformed the combined 45-Hz finite impulseResponse (FIR) filter and 0.75 Hz high pass filter	EEG signal decomposition into intrinsic mode function and frequency feature extraction using Hilbert–Huang transform	Support vector machine used in the proposed model has outperformed *k* nearest neighbor, quadratic discriminant analysis, and linear discriminant analysis	The highest accuracy in the alpha frequency band is 94% and the average is 90%. The accuracy of SVM is the highest	The training sample size is not mentioned and integration of deep learning method can be incorporated in the future for greater performance
Peng *et al.* [39]	Chronic stress detection and monitoring	EEG of a 10–20 electrode location system	11	Artifact removal using low pass filter of 40 Hz cut off frequency and EOG removal using wavelet method	A total of 20 features namely max power, absolute power, relative power, center frequency, entropy, correlation dimension, alpha asymmetry	Statistical analysis using Analysis of variance in SPSS 17.0 and paired sample *t*-test to analyze and differentiate between left and right hemisphere activities of the brain	Features had a significant difference for the control and stressed groups in nonlinear EEG analysis. The only relative power of alpha-band was significantly different for control and stressed in	The number of control and experimental group is not the same, thus, more samples should be added. Sensitivity and specificity should be used to evaluate the performance

							linear EEG analysis	
Virmani *et al.* [40]	Stress recognition using ECG and EEG for audio and visual stimuli	10–20 electrode placement system EEG	23	Not mentioned	Two emotional features, namely arousal and valence using power spectral density	Russell's circumplex model-based *k* nearest neighbor and decision tree to classify between stressed and non-stressed subjects	The overall accuracy of *k* nearest neighbor—68% and decision tree—75%	Accuracy is not up to the mark which can be increased by having more training sample size and other models can be tested for better performance
Al-Shargie *et al.* [41]	Stress quantification during three levels of arithmetic task	BrainMaster 24E system	A total of 12 subjects only	Third-order Butterworth filter in passband frequency 0.5–30 Hz and artifact removal using independent component analysis	Wavelet transform for five decomposition levels and one approximation level ranging between 0 and 30 Hz	Two-sample *t*-test having mean *p*-values as 0.03, 0.042, and 0.05 for level one, two, and three, respectively	Accuracy of SVM decreased with increasing level of the given arithmetic task	The right prefrontal cortex has been identified as the responsible brain region for stress; however, the result can be improved further by considering a larger training size

classification using SVM's workflow has been presented. The functionality of our entire system has been pictorially presented in Figure 12.1.

12.3.1 Introduction to EEG

Electroencephalogram abbreviated as EEG has been used as the data acquisition device in our proposed framework [43]. Different regions of the human brain responsible for different activities and the electrode placement based on the international 10–20 system have been depicted in Figure 12.2. Here the 10 and 20 mean the distance between adjacent nodes is 10% or 20% of the entire scalp. Every electrode is represented by a letter followed by a digit where the letters F, P, O, C, and T stand for the frontal, posterior, occipital, central, and temporal region, respectively, and the digit is odd representing the left hemisphere and even representing the right one. N and I denote Nasion and Inion, respectively [44].

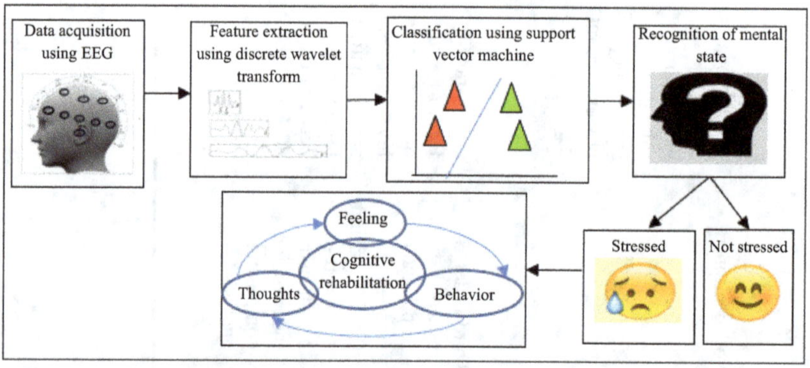

Figure 12.1 Illustration of our proposed framework applied in rehabilitation

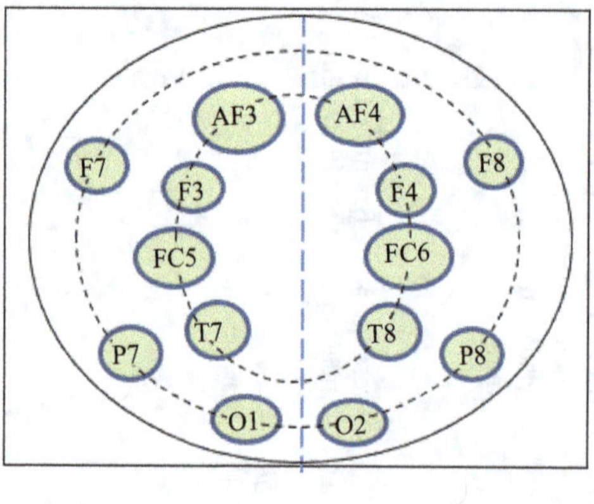

Figure 12.2 EEG electrodes used to acquire data in the proposed approach

12.3.2 Feature extraction using DWT

The wavelet transform concept is the representation or approximation of functions or signals using a function group, called a wavelet function system. Wavelets show two elementary properties: scale and location. The first one, also called dilation, defines the stretch or squish of a wavelet, which is related to the frequency of waves. Location describes the position of the wavelet-based on time or space [45]. Among the two types of the wavelet transform techniques, the continuous wavelet transform (CWT) considers all the probable wavelets over an unlimited number of scales and locations, whereas the DWT makes use of a limited set of wavelets, which are distinct at certain scales and locations. Here lies the main distinction between these two versions. A wavelet can be represented by the first-order derivative of Gaussian function $-(s-n)e^{\left((s-n)^2/2m^2\right)}/\sqrt{2\Pi m^3}$ where the wavelet scale and location are represented by a and b, respectively. The CWT of signal $s(t)$ can be defined by

$$T_c(m,n) = \int_{-\infty}^{+\infty} s(t)\gamma^*_{(m,n)}(t)dt \tag{12.1}$$

where the continuous wavelet basis function is

$$\gamma(t)_{m,n} = \frac{1}{\sqrt{m}}\gamma\frac{(t-n)}{m} \tag{12.2}$$

for which the categories are Haar, db series, coiflet, and so on. Since the EEG signals are discrete, thus DWT has been used in our proposed approach to extract features from it. Compared with the CWT, the DWT limits the m and n of the wavelet basis function $\gamma(m, n)$ to discrete points, which is called the scale discretization and displacement. The DWT of signal $s(t)$ is defined by

$$T_d(t) = \frac{1}{\sqrt{m}}\sum_k W_x(p_0,q)x_{p_0,q}(t) + \frac{1}{\sqrt{m}}\sum_{p=p_0}^{\infty}\sum_k W_y(p,q)y_{p,q}(t) \tag{12.3}$$

where the approximate or scaling coefficient is

$$W_x(p_0,q) = \frac{1}{\sqrt{m}}\sum_{t=0}^{m-1} T_d(t)\tilde{x}_{p_0,q}(t). \tag{12.4}$$

The detailed coefficient is

$$W_y(p,q) = \frac{1}{\sqrt{m}}\sum_{t=0}^{m-1} T_d(t)\tilde{y}_{p,q}(t) \tag{12.5}$$

and p_0 is the arbitrary initial scale. Figure 12.3 has shown the mechanism of wavelet decomposition of a signal $s(t)$ by considering three layers of decomposition for an instance [46] where x and y have been used for the approximate and detail coefficient, respectively.

12.3.3 Feature selection using principal component analysis

Noise regarding eyeblinking artifacts has been removed in our proposed architecture using PCA that is a popular dimension reduction method in ML. The working mechanism of PCA in noise removal has been shown in Figure 12.4. PCA can be described as an orthogonal linear transformation that translates data into a new coordinate system so that the largest variance by some scalar projection of the data falls on the first coordinate (named PC1), the second major variance on the second coordinate (named PC2), etc. [47].

If we consider a *D*-dimensional data matrix *M* of r and $(c+1)$ number of rows and columns where every column among *c* number of columns agrees to an independent variable of matrix *X* and the remaining one column corresponds to a dependent variable denoted by *Y*, the step-by-step procedure to perform PCA in this matrix to obtain reduced dimensionality *d* where $d \leq D$ is shown in the following algorithm.

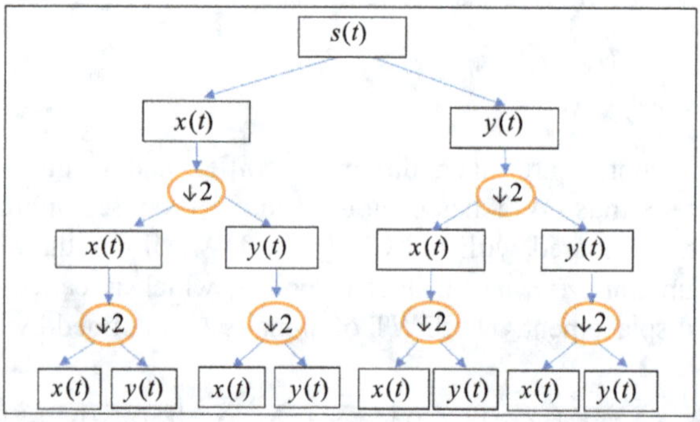

Figure 12.3 Three-layer wavelet decomposition in our proposed framework

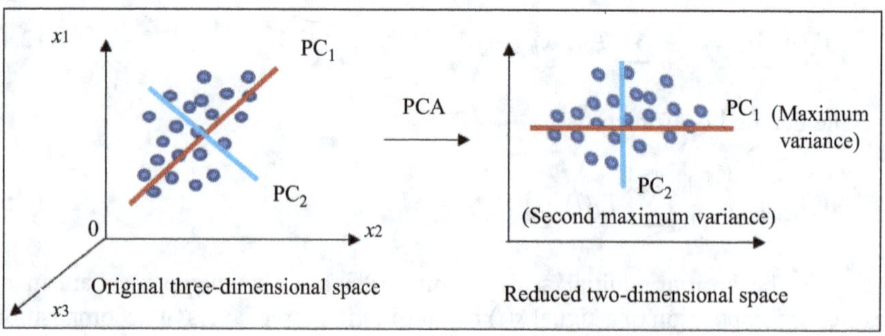

Figure 12.4 The working mechanism of principal component analysis

Algorithm: Principal component analysis

Input: $M = \{m_1, m_2, m_3, \ldots, m_N\}$ and d

Step 1: Calculate the mean $\tilde{m} = \frac{1}{N}\sum_{j=1}^{N} m_j$

Step 2: Calculate the covariance matrix $\mathrm{Cov}(m) = \frac{1}{N}\sum_{j=1}^{N} (m_j - \tilde{m}_j)(m_j - \tilde{m}_j)^T$

Step 3: Decompose the spectral of Cov(m) generating Eigenvectors $V_1, V_2, \ldots, V_D$ and corresponding Eigenvalues $E_1, E_2, \ldots, E_D$ sorted in descending order $E_1 \geq E_2 \geq \ldots \geq E_D \geq 0$

Step 4: For any $m \epsilon \mathbb{R}^D$, the output with the reduced dimension will be

$$Y = \{V_1^T(m - \tilde{m}), \quad V_2^T(m - \tilde{m}), \quad \ldots, \quad V_d^T(m - \tilde{m})\}^T \quad \epsilon \mathbb{R}^D$$

and the approximated value of original m *may be denoted by*

$$m \approx \tilde{m} + (V_1^T(m - \tilde{m}))V_1 + (V_2^T(m - \tilde{m}))V_2 + \ldots + (V_d^T(m - \tilde{m}))V_d$$

12.3.4 Classification using support vector machine

Classification plays a vital role in understanding human behavior and emotions. SVM is one of the popular methods applied in emotion classification [48]. It is often used to classify human emotional states [49], that are captured by EEG [50,51]. In maintaining the accuracy and execution time trade-off, we can trust hierarchical SVM classifiers [52]. SVM in existing literature is also used to classify context-based music emotion recognition and classification [53], speech emotion recognition [54], privacy-preserving [55,56], vision based on paste detection [57], classification of agricultural crops [58], hyperspectral remote sensing images [59], pattern classification [60,61], identification of brain structure [62], hybrid image denoising [63], gesture identification in sign language applications [64], hand gesture recognition, gesture recognition during dance [65], tweet act classification [66,67], etc.

SVM creates a decision boundary between classes in multidimensional space so that testing data points can be easily classified in the correct category according to the requirement [68]. The best decision boundary is called the hyperplane, to design which, some extreme data points in the form of vectors get selected and called as support vector. It is a binary classifier that classifies data points into two classes. In classification problems, where data points need to get classified in more than two classes, SVM applies a one versus all or one versus rest approach which splits the classification problem having multi-class into one binary classifier for every class. SVM can be of two types, i.e., linear SVM and nonlinear SVM applied to linearly separable and nonlinearly separable data, respectively.

Figure 12.5 shows the working mechanism of SVM as a classifier. In the concerned two-dimensional space, two classes can be easily separated using straight lines. But there may be more than one straight line that correctly separates

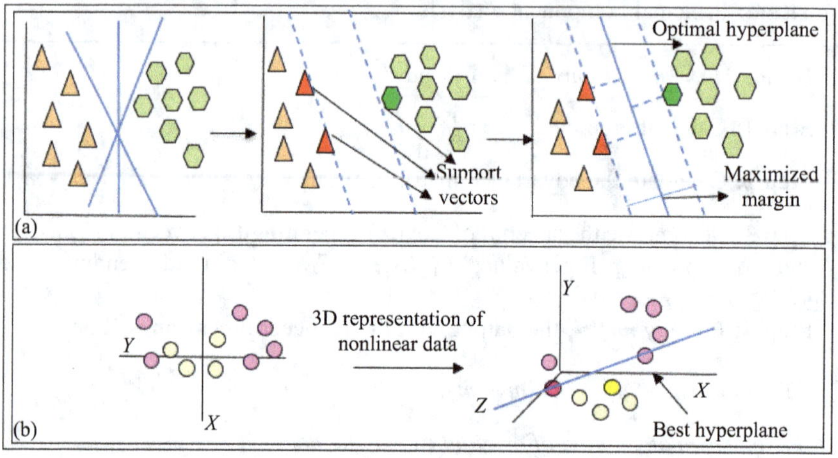

Figure 12.5 The general working mechanism of support vector machine as a classifier: (a) linear support vector machine and (b) nonlinear support vector machine

the classes as shown in the blue line. Hence SVM aims to create a decision boundary, and the best decision boundary among several possible boundaries gets called a hyperplane. The distances between the hyperplane and the support vectors are called margins, and the hyperplane having maximum margin between support vectors is called the optimal hyperplane. For nonlinear data, one more dimension z has to be added since no single straight line can act as the boundary between the classes and it can be calculated by

$$z = x^2 + y^2. \tag{12.6}$$

In three-dimensional space, the hyperplane looks like a parallel to the x-axis whereas in two-dimensional space, considering z=1, the circumference can be obtained with radius as 1 unit.

12.4 Experimental outcomes and discussions

The experimental outcomes are described here, and the classification performance is evaluated using some performance metrics, namely accuracy, precision, error rate, and recall. Python 3.7 and MATLAB® R2015A have been used to simulate the system.

12.4.1 Dataset preparation

A publicly available dataset, named GAMEEMO [69], has been used in our proposed framework to process and analyze EEG signals for the detection of stress or anxiety present in the subject's mind. Four different android games, namely Slender: The Arrival, Goat Simulator, Unravel, and Train Sim World, have been played by 28 different subjects with a total duration of 20 min (each game for 5 min). The games are of horror, fun, cool, and boring genre, respectively. Fourteen electrode channels were considered to collect the data, namely AF3, AF4, T8, T7, P8, P7, O2, O1, FC6, F8, F7, F4, F3, and FC5.

12.4.2 sLORETA-based activated brain region selection

The selection of activated brain regions is performed by assessing electrical actions of the intracortical circulation of the EEG signal collected during game playing using the sLORETA 2.0 platform [70]. We identify that prefrontal, occipital, parietal, and temporal cortices have the peak activation for the two mental states considered by us, i.e., stressed and not stressed. sLORETA solutions of the right, left, back, front, bottom, and top views for the two mental states: stressed and not stressed are illustrated in Figures 12.6 and 12.7.

12.4.3 Discrete wavelet transform–based feature extraction outcome

Based on the sLORETA activation result, in the proposed framework, features got extracted from the brain's prefrontal, frontal and temporal region using ten electrode channels, i.e., AF3, AF4, O1, O2, P7, P8, FC5, FC6, T7, and T8 by DWT resulting in 38 $252\times10\times28\times4$-dimensional feature space for 28 different subjects and 4 games. Haar has been considered the wavelet basis function in the proposed approach since it has performed better than the sym5, db1, and coiflet basis function applied in the existing literature concerning EEG feature extraction. Approximate and detailed coefficients obtained from one subject and one game-

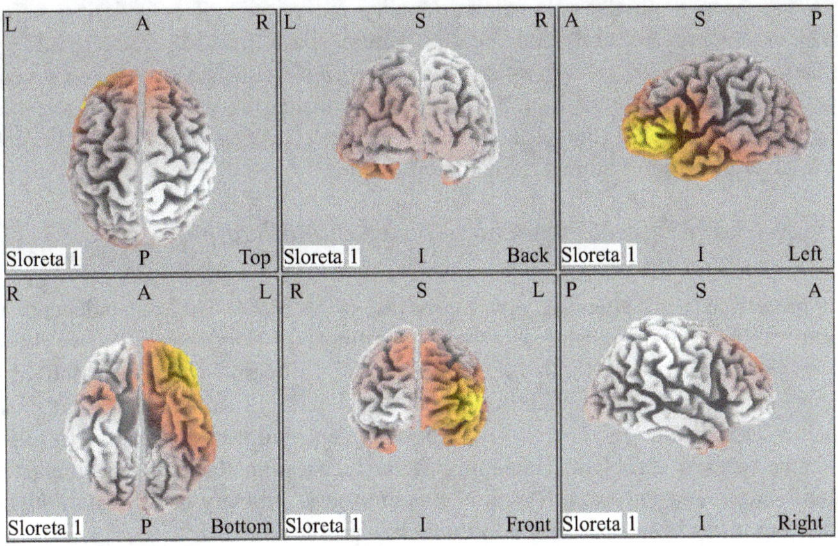

Figure 12.6 sLORETA-based brain activation for the class: not stressed

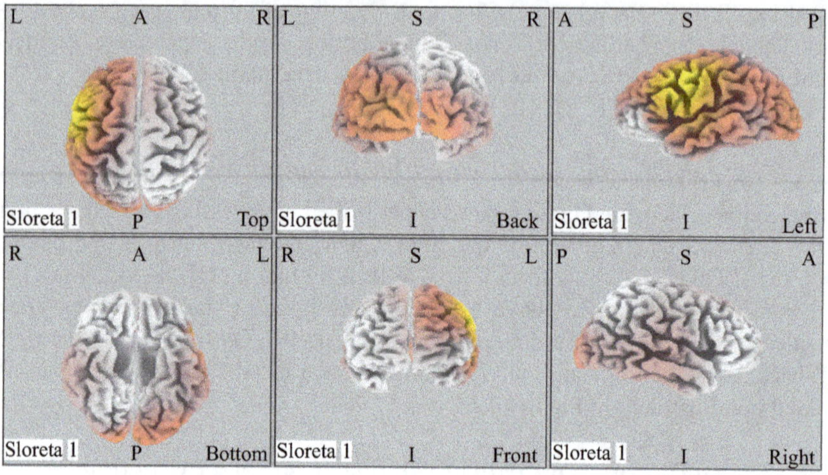

Figure 12.7 sLORETA-based brain activation for the class: stressed

based EEG data for four wavelet functions, namely Haar, db1, sym5, and db5, have been shown in Figure 12.8. From the results, it can be said that the Haar wavelet function is the best choice for the proposed work.

12.4.4 Principal component analysis–based dimensionality reduction outcome

For reducing the number of features leading to the enhancement of performance, PCA has been applied as the dimensionality reduction tool considering seven principal components and reducing the feature space from 38 $252\times10\times28\times4$ dimensions into 38 $252\times7\times28\times4$ dimensions. As it is not feasible to show a seven-dimensional PCA outcome in a 2D space, only considering the two most relevant principal components detected from extracted features by DWT for the GAMEEMO dataset, Figure 12.9 is drawn.

12.4.5 Support vector machine–based classification outcome

The mental state classification was performed using SVM. The user-independent classification got trained using data from all participants. For two reasons, we chose SVM over alternative methods for categorization. To begin with, it has good generalization and accuracy capability with a short training sample. It is the most reliable classification method for real-world settings, and it has been used to solve different types of problems, including facial recognition, handwriting character identification, and intrusion detection. It is created as a binary classification algorithm, but it has been improvised to multiclass problems.

We have used SVM for stress detection in our proposed framework. To train the classifier, the instantaneous frequency value obtained for all five EEG cycles is

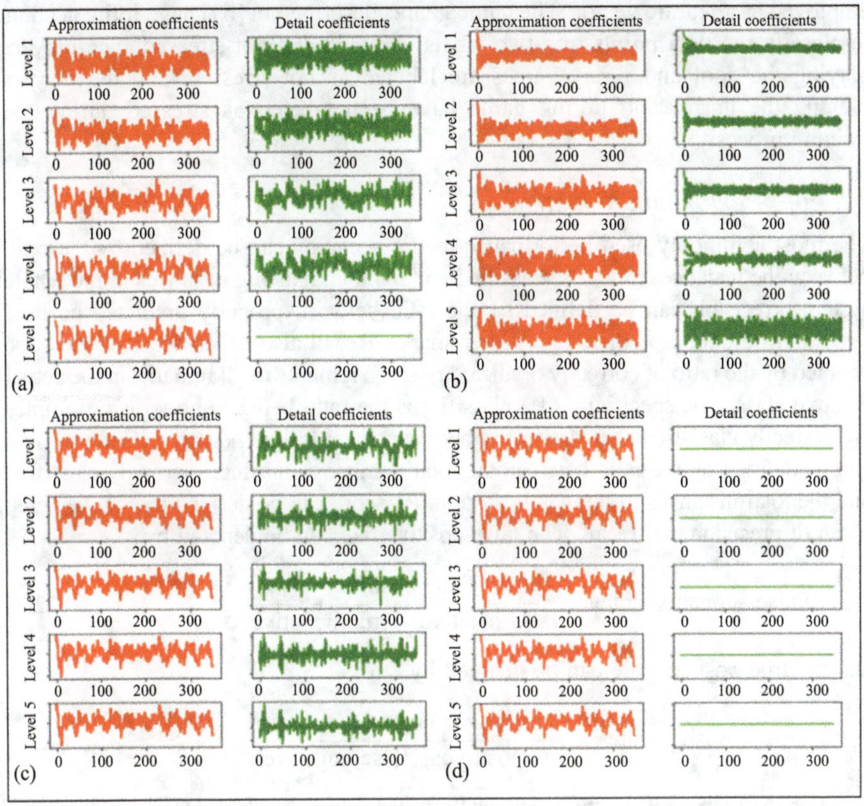

Figure 12.8 Approximation and detailed coefficients (for five levels) applied on GAMEEMO dataset [69]: (a) Haar function, (b) sym5 function, (c) db5 function, and (d) db1 function

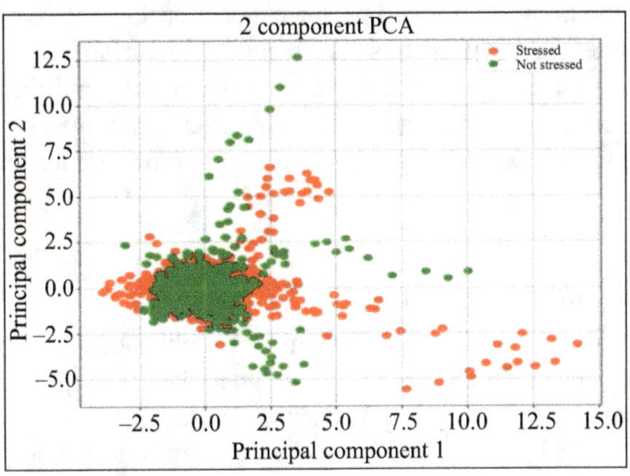

Figure 12.9 PCA-based dimensionality reduction outcome

employed as a feature vector. The game genres described in [69] have influenced us to classify the data points into two labels: stressed and not stressed. The players playing the cool and funny games are labeled as not stressed, and the players playing the horror and boring game have been labeled as stressed during the training process.

12.4.6 Performance metrics

The most commonly used performance metric accuracy can be defined by the ratio between the instances properly classified and the total existing instances in the whole system. Precision can be defined by the ratio between properly predicted positive remarks to the total predicted positive remarks. Recall also called sensitivity can be denoted by the ratio of correctly predicted positive remarks to all remarks in the actual positive class. The specificity of a classifier is the ratio between how many samples are correctly classified as negative to how many samples are negative. The error rate can be defined by the ratio between the total number of instances wrongly classified and the total instances in the whole system. $F1$ score can be defined by the weighted mean of precision and recall. The false-positive rate can be denoted by

$$\text{False} - \text{positive rate} = \frac{\text{false positive}}{\text{false positive} + \text{true negative}} \tag{12.7}$$

and the true positive rate can be denoted by

$$\text{True} - \text{positve rate} = \frac{\text{true positive}}{\text{true positive} + \text{false negative}}. \tag{12.8}$$

For the comparative study, other classifiers, namely kNN, DT, random forest (RF), and naïve Bayes (NB), have been compared with our proposed SVM in terms of accuracy. For SVM, four types of kernel parameter values have been considered here, i.e., linear, sigmoid, RBF, and polynomial, among which, RBF has outperformed the others during the hyperparameter tuning phase.

Apart from the abovementioned performance metrics, we have also taken into consideration some other parameters like receiver-operating characteristic (ROC) which is a proof of identity of the classifier system [71] and the discrimination threshold has been varied with the binary classifier's parameter changes. In our approach, along with ROC, we have also considered area under the curve (AUC) values.

12.4.7 Performance evaluation

Performance metrics as described in Section 12.4.6 obtained from the classification result of SVM are depicted in Table 12.2. The other classifier's performance comparison with SVM based on accuracy is illustrated in Figure 12.10 from where it is obvious that the proposed SVM is more promising to detect the stress in a subject during playing four different games. Figure 12.11 shows ROC curves, and AUC values obtained from those four ROC curves are shown in Table 12.3. From the results, it can be said that

Table 12.2 SVM-based classification outcome

Mental state	Precision	Recall	Error	*F*1 score
Not stressed	0.88	0.63	0.08	0.69
Stressed	0.78	0.87	0.07	0.74
Avg.	0.83	0.795	0.075	1.43

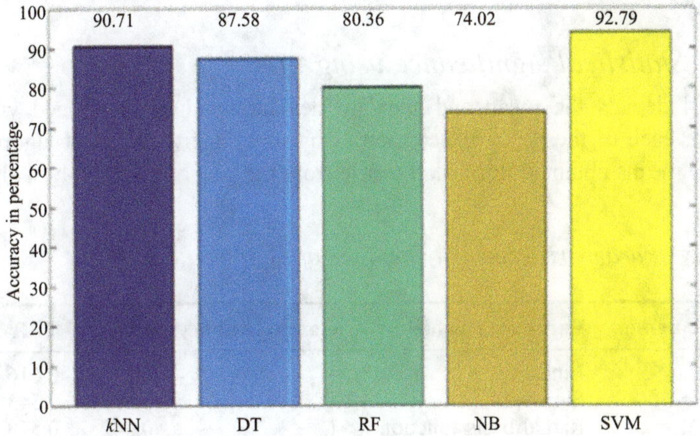

Figure 12.10 Comparison of proposed SVM classifier with other classifiers

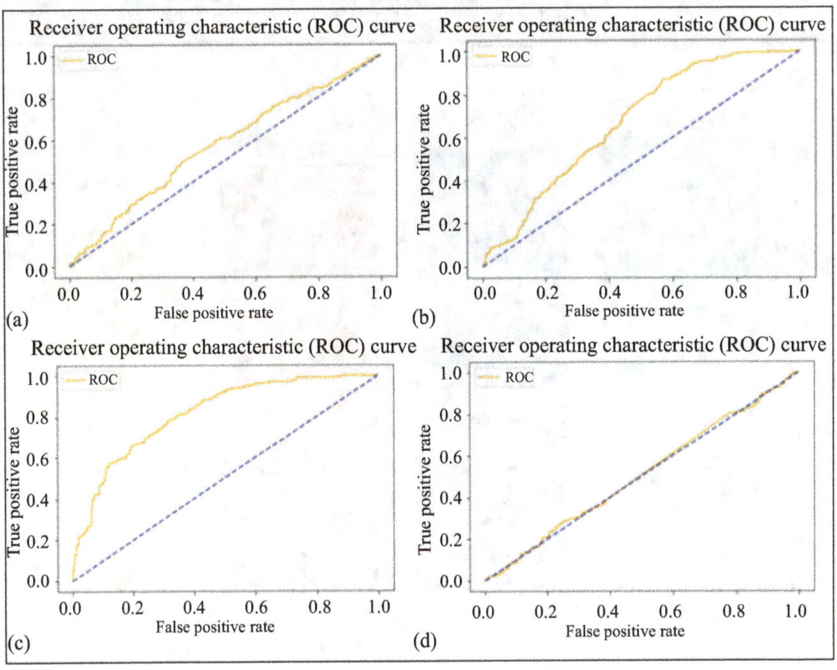

Figure 12.11 Receiver-operating characteristic curve for the four kernels of SVM: (a) for linear, (b) for sigmoid, (c) for RBF, and (d) for polynomial

RBF kernel-based SVM having a gamma value of 0.01 (marked as bold) is the best choice for the current research work [72].

The comparison of our SVM classification result has been carried out by considering accuracy as the metric with the existing related works [29,31,32] in Figure 12.12. From the evaluation of effectiveness and applicability [73] of the proposed approach, it is seen that the proposed framework works better than the related ones.

12.4.8 *Statistical significance using* t-*test*

Table 12.4 depicts the mean and standard deviation values mentioned within the bracket for each of the performance metrics by running five different algorithms 25 times. The means obtained from each metric from the best and second-best algorithms

Table 12.3 Parametric sensitivity analysis of SVM as a classifier

Parameter name	Parameter value	Gamma value	FPR	TPR	AUC
Kernel	Linear	–	0.512	0.616	0.569
	Sigmoid	–	0.498	0.543	0.501
	Radial basis function	1	0.342	0.578	0.657
		0.1	0.231	0.763	0.564
		0.01	**0.152**	**0.912**	**0.89**
		0.001	0.165	0.769	0.745
	Polynomial	–	0.340	0.712	0.672

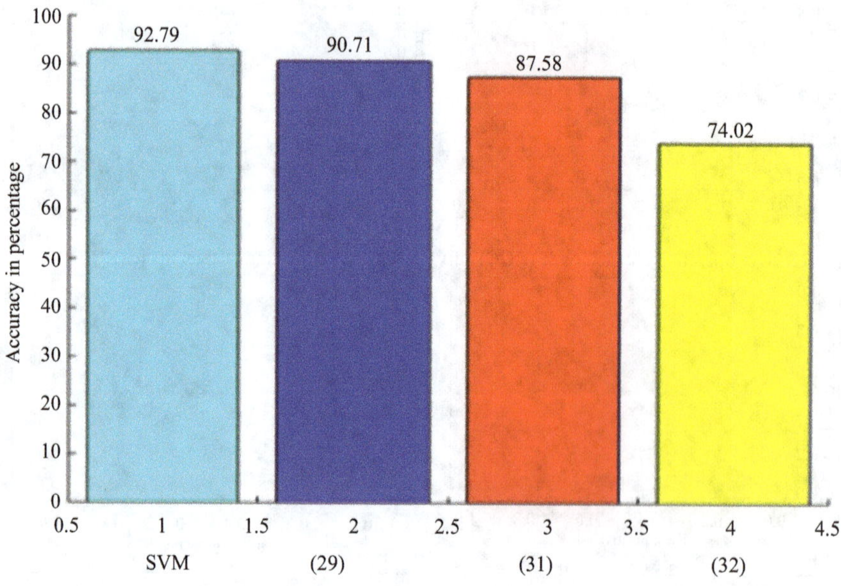

Figure 12.12 Comparison with state-of-the-art literature

Table 12.4 Comparison of different game emotion recognition algorithms for 25 trials

Performance metric	SVM	*k*NN	DT	RF	NB	Statistical significance
Accuracy	**0.93 (0.161)**	0.90 (0.531)	0.87 (0.657)	0.80 (0.645)	0.74 (0.314)	+
Precision	**0.92 (0.134)**	0.87 (0.634)	0.89 (0.453)	0.87 (0.564)	0.75 (0.324)	+
Recall	**0.93 (0.168)**	0.45 (0.324)	0.67 (0.498)	0.78 (0.654)	0.81 (0.134)	+
*F*1 score	**0.86 (0.013)**	0.74 (0.125)	0.67 (0.054)	0.78 (0.435)	0.74 (0.175)	+
Average error rate	**0.07 (0.019)**	0.40 (0.232)	0.25 (0.143)	0.65 (0.435)	0.19 (0.023)	+

have been presented also using the paired *t*-test. The statistical significance level of the difference of the means of the best two algorithms have been presented in Table 12.4's last column, where "+" represents the *t*-value of 49 degrees of freedom that is statistically significant at a 0.05 level of significance by two-tailed test. The sample size for all of the *t*-tests is set as 25. The best ones have been marked with bold.

12.5 Conclusion and future works

Mental state detection using EEG and ML techniques is a rapidly emerging field in this era. Stress affects the mental and physical health of people, and in the modern era, it is a common problem for people belonging to different age groups. To get valid results in detecting human mental pressure during the pandemic era, we need reliable identification of human stress. To identify stress levels, channel selection is also important. The proposed methods are as follows, collection of human brain signals using EEG, feature extraction by DWT, dimensionality reduction by PCA, and the classification by SVM. The current work has classified the mental state of the gamer as not stressed and stressed with an accuracy of 92.79%. Brain maps have also been generated to detect stress levels in the brain's active regions.

The work can be further extended by considering different stimuli apart from the game, like movie watching, music listening, social media posts for detecting stress, and possible rehabilitative measure during the pandemic.

Acknowledgment

The first author (i.e., Ahona Ghosh) is grateful to the university for providing the AICTE Doctoral Fellowship, with appointment letter Ref. No.2.2.1/Regis./Appt. (AG)/Ph.D(ADF)/2021 dated 01.02.2021. The third author (i.e., Sriparna Saha) is grateful to the university for providing research seed money, File No. 9.6/Regis./

SD/Mn.(SS)/2019 dated 19.06.2019 and UGC Start-up Grant under the scheme of Basic Scientific Research, File No. F.30-449/2018(BSR) dated 21.11.2019.

References

[1] Javed B., Sarwer A., Soto E.B. and Mashwani Z.U.R. 'The coronavirus (COVID-19) pandemic's impact on mental health'. *The International Journal of Health Planning and Management*. 2020; 35(5): 993–996.

[2] Xiong J., Lipsitz O., Nasri F., *et al.* 'Impact of COVID-19 pandemic on mental health in the general population: A systematic review'. *Journal of Affective Disorders*. 2020; 277: 55–64.

[3] Willman M., Kobasa D. and Kindrachuk J. 'A comparative analysis of factors influencing two outbreaks of Middle Eastern respiratory syndrome (MERS) in Saudi Arabia and South Korea'. *Viruses*. 2019; 11(12): 1119.

[4] Hasöksüz M., Kiliç S. and Saraç F. 'Coronaviruses and SARS-CoV-2'. *Turkish Journal of Medical Sciences*. 2020; 50(SI-1): 549–556.

[5] Baize S., Pannetier D., Oestereich L., *et al.* 'Emergence of *Zaire Ebolavirus* disease in Guinea'. *New England Journal of Medicine*. 2014; 371(15): 1418–1425.

[6] Buheji M., Jahrami H. and Dhahi A. 'Minimising stress exposure during pandemics similar to COVID-19'. *International Journal of Psychology and Behavioral Sciences*. 2020; 10(1): 9–16.

[7] Elbay R.Y., Kurtulmuş A., Arpacıoğlu S. and Karadere E. 'Depression, anxiety, stress levels of physicians and associated factors in Covid-19 pandemics'. *Psychiatry Research*. 2020; 290: 113–130.

[8] Schoenfeld J. 'The Invisible Risk: Pandemics and the Financial Markets.' In *Tuck School of Business Working Paper No. 3567249*; 2020.

[9] Dash S., Chakraborty C., Giri S.K., Pani S.K. and Frnda J. 'BIFM: Big-data driven intelligent forecasting model for COVID-19'. *IEEE Access*. 2021; 9: 97505–97517.

[10] Aslam B., Javed A.R., Chakraborty C., Nebhen J., Raqib S. and Rizwan M. 'Blockchain and ANFIS empowered IoMT application for privacy preserved contact tracing in COVID-19 pandemic'. *Personal and Ubiquitous Computing*. 2021: 1–17.

[11] Ravi V., Narasimhan H., Chakraborty C. and Pham T.D. 'Deep learning based meta-classifier approach for COVID-19 classification using CT scan and chest X-ray images'. *Multimedia Systems*. 2021: 1–15.

[12] Chakraborty C., Banerjee A., Garg L. and Coelho Rodrigues J.J.P. *Internet of Medical Things for Smart Healthcare – COVID-19 Pandemic*, Big data series. Singapore: Springer Nature; 2020.

[13] Garg L., Chakraborty C., Mahmoudi S. and Sohmen V.S. *Healthcare Informatics for Fighting COVID-19 and Future Epidemics*. EAI/Springer Innovations in Communication and Computing. Cham: Springer Nature; 2021.

[14] Wada K., Shibata T., Musha T. and Kimura S. 'Effects of robot therapy for demented patients evaluated by EEG.' In *IEEE/RSJ International Conference on Intelligent Robots and Systems*. IEEE; 2005. pp. 1552–1557.

[15] Ali M., Mosa A.H., Al Machot F. and Kyamakya K. 'EEG-based emotion recognition approach for e-healthcare applications.' In *2016 Eighth International Conference on Ubiquitous and Future Networks (ICUFN)*; 2016. pp. 946–950.

[16] Mahato S. and Paul S. 'Electroencephalogram (EEG) Signal Analysis for Diagnosis of Major Depressive Disorder (MDD): A Review.' In Nath V. and Mandal J. (eds.) *Nanoelectronics, Circuits and Communication Systems, Lecture Notes in Electrical Engineering*. Springer, Singapore, vol. 511; 2019. pp. 323–336.

[17] Mohammadi M., Al-Azab F., Raahemi B., *et al.* 'Data mining EEG signals in depression for their diagnostic value'. *BMC Medical Informatics and Decision Making*. 2015; 15(1): 1–14.

[18] Liao S.C., Wu C.T., Huang H.C., Cheng W.T. and Liu Y.H. 'Major depression detection from EEG signals using kernel Eigen-filter Bank common spatial patterns'. *Sensors*. 2017; 17(6): 1385.

[19] Niemiec A.J. and Lithgow B.J. 'Alpha-band characteristics in EEG spectrum indicate reliability of frontal brain asymmetry measures in diagnosis of depression.' In *IEEE Engineering in Medicine and Biology 27th Annual Conference*, Shanghai, China, 2005. IEEE; 2005. pp. 7517–7520.

[20] Cai H., Sha X., Han X., Wei S. and Hu S. 'A pervasive approach to EEG-based depression detection'. *Complexity*. 2018; 2018: 1–13.

[21] Mahato S. and Paul S. 'Detection of major depressive disorder using linear and non-linear features from EEG signals'. *Microsystem Technologies*. 2019; 25(3): 1065–1076.

[22] Lun X., Yu Z., Chen T., Wang F. and Hou Y. 'A simplified CNN classification method for MI-EEG via the electrode pairs signals'. *Frontiers in Human Neuroscience*. 2020; 14.

[23] Fong S.J., Dey N. and Chaki J. *Artificial Intelligence for Coronavirus Outbreak*. 1st edn. Springer, Singapore, vol. 74; 2020. p. XI.

[24] Ghosh A., Roy S., Mondal H., Biswas S. and Bose R. 'Mathematical modelling for decision making of lockdown during COVID-19'. *Applied Intelligence*. 2021: 1–17.

[25] Dutta P.K., Ghosh A., De P. and Soltani M. 'A proposed model of a semi-automated sensor actuator resposcopy analyzer for 'covid-19' patients for respiratory distress detection.' In *11th International Conference on Cloud Computing, Data Science & Engineering (Confluence)*, India, 2021. IEEE; 2021. pp. 618–623.

[26] Adhikary S., Ghosh A., Das P., Roy S. and Bose R. 'Scope of sentiment analysis on news articles regarding stock market and GDP in struggling economic condition'. *International Journal of Emerging Trends in Engineering Research*. 2020; 8(7).

[27] Sagayam K.M., Andrushia A.D., Ghosh A., Deperlioglu O. and Elngar A.A. 'Recognition of hand gesture image using deep convolutional neural network'. *International Journal of Image and Graphics*. 2021: 2140008.

[28] Datta P.K., Biswas A., Ghosh A. and Chaudhury N. 'Creation of image segmentation classifiers for sign language processing for deaf and dumb.' In *2020 8th International Conference on Reliability, Infocom Technologies and Optimization (Trends and Future Directions)* (ICRITO). IEEE; 2020. pp. 772–775.

[29] Ghosh L., Saha S. and Konar A. 'Decoding emotional changes of android-gamers using a fused Type-2 fuzzy deep neural network'. *Computers in Human Behavior*. 2021; 116: 106640.

[30] Hajian-Tilaki K. 'Receiver operating characteristic (ROC) curve analysis for medical diagnostic test evaluation'. *Caspian Journal of Internal Medicine*. 2013; 4(2): 627.

[31] Ghosh L., Saha S. and Konar A. 'Bi-directional long short-term memory model to analyze psychological effects on gamers'. *Applied Soft Computing*. 2020; 95: 106573.

[32] Asif A., Majid M. and Anwar S.M. 'Human stress classification using EEG signals in response to music tracks'. *Computers in Biology and Medicine*. 2019; 107: 182–196.

[33] Saeed S.M.U., Anwar S.M., Khalid H., Majid M. and Bagci U. 'EEG based classification of long-term stress using psychological labeling'. *Sensors*. 2020; 20(7): 1886.

[34] Ahn J.W., Ku Y. and Kim H.C. 'A novel wearable EEG and ECG recording system for stress assessment'. *Sensors*. 2019; 19(9): 1991.

[35] Kalas M.S. and Momin B.F. 'Stress detection and reduction using EEG signals.' In *2016 International Conference on Electrical, Electronics, and Optimization Techniques (ICEEOT)*. IEEE; 2016. pp. 471–475.

[36] Priya T.H., Mahalakshmi P., Naidu V.P.S. and Srinivas M. 'Stress detection from EEG using power ratio.' In *2020 International Conference on Emerging Trends in Information Technology and Engineering (IC-ETITE)*. IEEE; 2020. pp. 1–6.

[37] Liao C.Y., Chen R.C. and Tai S.K. 'Emotion stress detection using EEG signal and deep learning technologies.' In *2018 IEEE International Conference on Applied System Invention (ICASI)*. IEEE; 2018. pp. 90–93.

[38] Sharma R. and Chopra K. 'EEG signal analysis and detection of stress using classification techniques'. *Journal of Information and Optimization Sciences*. 2020; 41(1): 229–238.

[39] Peng H., Hu B., Zheng F., *et al.* 'A method of identifying chronic stress by EEG'. *Personal and Ubiquitous Computing*. 2013; 17(7): 1341–1347.

[40] Virmani D., Minocha A., Goyal L., Malhotra M. and Gupta M. 'Se. Re. Ne.: Stress detection using EEG and ECG.' In *Proceedings of 3rd International Conference on Computing Informatics and Networks: ICCIN 2020*. Springer Singapore; 2021. pp. 189–198.

[41] Al-Shargie F.M., Tang T.B., Badruddin N. and Kiguchi M. 'Mental stress quantification using EEG signals.' In *International Conference for Innovation in Biomedical Engineering and Life Sciences*. Springer, Singapore; 2015. pp. 15–19.

[42] Al-Fahoum A.S. and Al-Fraihat A.A. 'Methods of EEG signal features extraction using linear analysis in frequency and time-frequency domains'. *International Scholarly Research Notices*, 2014.

[43] Evans J.R. and Abarbanel A. (eds.). *Introduction to Quantitative EEG and Neurofeedback*. London: Elsevier; 1999. p. XVIII.

[44] Teplan M. 'Fundamentals of EEG measurement'. *Measurement Science Review*. 2002; 2(2): 1–11.

[45] Al-Haj A. 'Combined DWT-DCT digital image watermarking'. *Journal of Computer Science*. 2007; 3(9): 740–746.

[46] Wu Y.L., Agrawal D. and El Abbadi A. 'A comparison of DFT and DWT based similarity search in time-series databases.' In *Proceedings of the Ninth International Conference on Information and Knowledge Management*; 2000. pp. 488–495.

[47] Turnip A. and Siahaan M. 'Adaptive principal component analysis based recursive least squares for artifact removal of EEG signals'. *Advanced Science Letters*. 2014; 20(10–11): 2034–2037.

[48] Yang N., Yuan J., Zhou Y., *et al.* 'Enhanced multiclass SVM with thresholding fusion for speech-based emotion classification'. *International Journal of Speech Technology*. 2017; 20: 27–41.

[49] Nguyen T., Bass I., Li M. and Sethi I.K. 'Investigation of combining SVM and decision tree for emotion classification.' In *Seventh IEEE International Symposium on Multimedia (ISM'05)*, Irvine, CA, USA; 2005. p. 5.

[50] Mehmood R.M. and Lee H.J. 'Emotion classification of EEG brain signal using SVM and KNN.' In *2015 IEEE International Conference on Multimedia & Expo Workshops (ICMEW)*; 2015. pp. 1–5.

[51] Guo K., Candra H., Yu H., Li H., Nguyen H.T. and Su S.W. 'EEG-based emotion classification using innovative features and combined SVM and HMM classifier.' In *2017 39th Annual International Conference of the IEEE Engineering in Medicine and Biology Society (EMBC)*; 2017. pp. 489–492.

[52] Datta S., Sen D. and Balasubramanian R. 'Integrating geometric and textural features for facial emotion classification using SVM frameworks.' In Raman B., Kumar S., Roy P., Sen D. (eds.) *Proceedings of International Conference on Computer Vision and Image Processing. Advances in Intelligent Systems and Computing*, Springer, Singapore; 2017. vol. 459, pp. 619–628.

[53] Han B.J., Rho S., Jun S., *et al.* 'Music emotion classification and context-based music recommendation'. *Multimedia Tools and Applications*. 2010; 47: 433–460.

[54] Yi-Lin L. and Gang W. 'Speech emotion recognition based on HMM and SVM.' In *International Conference on Machine Learning and Cybernetics*; 2005. vol. 8, pp. 4898–4901.

[55] Vaidya J., Yu H. and Jiang X. 'Privacy-preserving SVM classification'. *Knowledge Information Systems*. 2008; 14: 161–178.

[56] Yu H., Vaidya J. and Jiang X. 'Privacy-Preserving SVM Classification on Vertically Partitioned Data.' In Ng W.K., Kitsuregawa M., Li J. and Chang K. (eds.) *Advances in Knowledge Discovery and Data Mining. PAKDD*

2006. Lecture Notes in Computer Science. Springer, Berlin, Heidelberg, vol. 3918; 2006.

[57] Ebrahimi M.A., Khoshtaghaza M.H., Minaei S. and Jamshidi B., 'Vision-based pest detection based on SVM classification method'. *Computers and Electronics in Agriculture*. 2017; 137: 52–59.

[58] Foody G.M. and Mathur A. 'Toward intelligent training of supervised image classifications: Directing training data acquisition for SVM classification'. *Remote Sensing of Environment*. 2004; 93(1–2): 107–117.

[59] Bazi Y. and Melgani F. 'Toward an optimal SVM classification system for hyperspectral remote sensing images'. *IEEE Transactions on Geoscience and Remote Sensing*. 2006; 44(11): 3374–3385.

[60] Niaf É., Flamary R., Lartizien C. and Canu S. 'Handling uncertainties in SVM classification.' In *2011 IEEE Statistical Signal Processing Workshop (SSP)*; 2011. pp. 757–760.

[61] Chakraborty C., Gupta B. and Ghosh S.K. 'Chronic wound characterization using Bayesian classifier under telemedicine framework'. *International Journal of E-Health and Medical Communications*. 2016; 7(1): 78–96. 10.4018/IJEHMC.2016010105.

[62] Akselrod-Ballin A., Galun M., Gomori M.J., Basri R. and Brandt A. 'Atlas Guided Identification of Brain Structures by Combining 3D Segmentation and SVM Classification.' In Larsen R., Nielsen M. and Sporring J. (eds.) *Medical Image Computing and Computer-Assisted Intervention – MICCAI 2006*. Lecture Notes in Computer Science. Springer, Berlin, Heidelberg, vol. 4191; 2006.

[63] Routray S., Ray A.K., Mishra C. and Palai G. 'Efficient hybrid image denoising scheme based on SVM classification'. *Optik*. 2018; 157: 503–511.

[64] Saha S., Bhattacharya S. and Konar A. 'A Novel Approach to Gesture Recognition in Sign Language Applications Using AVL Tree and SVM.' In Sa P., Sahoo M., Murugappan M., Wu Y. and Majhi B. (eds.) *Progress in Intelligent Computing Techniques: Theory, Practice, and Applications*. Advances in Intelligent Systems and Computing. Springer, Singapore, vol. 518; 2018.

[65] Saha S., Konar A. and Roy J. 'Single Person Hand Gesture Recognition Using Support Vector Machine.' In Maharatna K., Dalapati G., Banerjee P., Mallick A. and Mukherjee M. (eds.) *Computational Advancement in Communication Circuits and Systems*. Lecture Notes in Electrical Engineering. Springer, New Delhi, vol. 335; 2015.

[66] Saha S., Ghosh A., Konar A. and Nagar A.K. 'Gesture recognition from Indian classical dance using Kinect sensor.' In *2013 Fifth International Conference on Computational Intelligence, Communication Systems and Networks*; 2013. pp. 3–8.

[67] Chakraborty C., Gupta B., Ghosh S.K., Das D. and Chakraborty C., 'Telemedicine supported chronic wound tissue prediction using different classification approach'. *Journal of Medical Systems*. 2016; 40(3): 1–12. 10.1007/s10916-015-0424-y.

[68] Noble W.S. 'What is a support vector machine?'. *Nature Biotechnology*. 2006; 24(12): 1565–1567.

[69] Alakus T.B., Gonen M. and Turkoglu I. 'Database for an emotion recognition system based on EEG signals and various computer games–GAMEEMO'. *Biomedical Signal Processing and Control*. 2020; 60 (101951).

[70] Jatoi M.A., Kamel N., Malik A.S. and Faye I. 'EEG based brain source localization comparison of sLORETA and eLORETA'. *Australasian Physical & Engineering Sciences in Medicine*. 2014; 37(4): 713–721.

[71] Kharshiing K.D., Kashyap D., Gupta K., *et al.* 'Quality of life in the COVID-19 pandemic in India: Exploring the role of individual and group variables'. *Community Mental Health Journal*. 2021; 57(1): 70–78.

[72] Hussain M., Wajid S.K., Elzaart A. and Berbar M. 'A comparison of SVM kernel functions for breast cancer detection.' In *2011 Eighth International Conference Computer Graphics, Imaging and Visualization*. IEEE; 2011. pp. 145–150.

[73] Ranawana R. and Palade V. 'Optimized precision-a new measure for classifier performance evaluation.' In *2006 IEEE International Conference on Evolutionary Computation*. IEEE; 2006. pp. 2254–2261.

Chapter 13

Arduino-based robot for purification of COVID-19 using far UVC light

C.N. Sujatha[1], B. Sri Charan[1] and K. Himabindu[1]

Abstract

The proposed work elaborates the necessity of sterilisation especially during COVID-19 period. In this chapter, we will discuss about the development and construction of an 'Arduino-based robot for the purification of COVID-19 using far UVC light'. Throughout history, the outgrowing technology has solved major problems. Technology has made everything possible, from making knowledge more available to more people and bringing group of people associated, to making our planet cleaner and even saving lives. But the current circumstance of COVID-19 is threat to human lives as there are high chances of getting sick in no time, so in order to fight with this novel virus. There is necessity to keep our surroundings clean and tidy. Cleanliness is the most important factor to keep ourselves away from diseases. The objective of the current work is to discuss various inventions made during the pandemic scenario and to contribute to the battle against COVID-19 propagation, a novel human corona virus in hospitals, public transports, airlines, and any enclosed areas with an approach, which is a basically a bot named 'Arduino-based robot' which uses ultraviolet (UV) sterilisation method to kill and eliminate all the germs and viruses present in the surroundings and sanitises the entire surroundings by cleaning and disinfecting the environment. Far-UVC (ultraviolet C) radiation has a wavelength range of 207–222 nm. The decontaminating efficiency of far UVC light was previously tested by exposing bacteria that were irradiated on a surface or in suspension. We have developed a UV-based sterilisation method that uses single-wavelength far-UVC light produced by filtered exclaims to selectively inactivate microorganisms while causing no biological damage to exposed cells and tissues. The method is based on biophysical principles, as far-UVC light can penetrate and thus inactivate bacteria and viruses with dimensions in micrometre or smaller, while far-UVC light cannot penetrate even the outer dead-cell layers of human skin, nor the outer tear layer of an eye, due to its high absorbance in biological materials. The far-UVC lamp plays a major role in

[1]Department of Electronics and Communication Engineering, Sreenidhi Institute of Science and Technology, Hyderabad, India

a disinfection robot. This bot will disinfect the virus and clean the areas; it will travel autonomously and sterilise the areas without the need for human intervention. In the discussion section, a demonstration of the bot's implementation and presentation was shown. This robot can also be used as a vacuum cleaner, eliminating the need for and expense of cleaning by humans.

Keywords: COVID-19; Sterilisation; Far-UVC lamp; Diseases; Bacteria; UV and UVC lamp; UV sterilisation

13.1 Introduction

This chapter gives information about an Arduino-based far UVC (ultraviolet C) sterilisation disinfection robot. It is a robot made by using ultrasonic sensor, far-UVC lamp, accelerometer sensor, Arduino Uno. Arduino IDE (integrated development environment) is the software used in building this robot for writing the code that is been dumped in the Arduino Uno. The main purpose of this robot is to sanitise surroundings and to make them free from harmful germs by using UV (ultraviolet) rays. UV sterilisation is the method used to kill the microorganisms using UV lamps [1]. In present days, UV, UVC, and far-UVC lamp are being used for sterilisation process. The UV rays and UVC lamp may affect the tissues in human body, so it cannot be used for sterilisation of surroundings in public places and households. Under extreme conditions, they can be used in public places only in the absence of all living organisms. The better way to solve the previous issue is using a far-UVC lamp. Far-UVC lamps will not affect human tissues and give more powerful and effective results when compared to the other lamps. Far-UVC lamps make use of tiny wavelength far-UV light to eradicate or inactivate microorganisms such as germs, bacteria, and viruses by exterminating their nucleic acids and disrupting their DNA (deoxyribonucleic acid), preventing them from multiplying in large numbers and rendering them incapable of performing essential cellular functions. Our robot makes use of the far-UV excimer lamps [2]. This method is based on the principle that very little penetration from the far UV lamp can cover and kills the germs and viruses, and most importantly the far-UV light can neither penetrate through the outer dead cell layers of human skin nor the outer surface of the human eye. So, the far-UV light does not cause any harm to humans [3]. We can also use few robotic vacuum cleaner components to make its function as a robotic vacuum cleaner. With single robot, we can perform both cleaning and sterilisation of surroundings.

13.1.1 Arduino

Arduino is an open-source platform which enables the users to use in software and hardware projects easily. Arduino project began at Interaction Design Institute Ivrea, Ivrea, Italy in the year 2005. The major goal of Arduino was to give a low-cost and simple solution for students from all disciplines to create projects using numerous sensors and actuators. The Arduino was named after the bar 'Arduino of Ivrea', the place where the founders of the Arduino usually encountered.

Creative Commons attribution share-Alike 2.5 is responsible for hardware designs and distribution of Arduino. Although the Arduino hardware and software designs are accessible for free under copyleft licences, the developer has requested that the name not be changed. ATmega8 AVR (Alf-Egil Bogen, Vegard Wollan, RISC) microcontroller [4] is widely used in Arduino boards with various ranges of flash memory, pins, and features. In 2012, 32-bit Arduino Due with Atmel SAM3X8E was introduced. Single or double row pins or female headers are used to make connections for programming the circuit as well as for incorporating into other circuits. Arduino offers the capacity to link with 'shields', which are add-on modules. For power supply, Arduino board manufactures mostly 5-V linear regulators and 16-MHz crystal oscillators, or ceramic resonators to generate clock pulses. For the simplification of uploading programmes to on-chip flash memory, Arduino microcontrollers are pre-programmed with a boot loader. Programmes are loaded onto board via serial connections to another computer. But currently USBs (universal serial buses) are being used to upload the programmes onto the board for this purpose. USB-to-serial adapter chip-like FTDI (Future Technology Devices International Limited) FT232 is being used. AVR chip with USB-to-serial firmware is used in Arduino Uno model boards. It can re-programme itself by using its own ICSP (in-circuit serial programming) header. Other boards, such as the Arduino mini, rely on a separate USB-to-serial adaptor or Bluetooth.

Arduino board microcontroller has several I/O pins which help in connecting various other circuits. The number of pins will differ from one version to another. Arduino Uno board has 13 digital I/O pins and six analogue pins to provide analogue output in the range of 0–1,023. It has ATMEGA328P had microcontroller in Arduino [5]. Along with these pins, there are several other pins as follows: Tx pin, used for transmission of data; Rx pin, used to receive data; Vin pin, helps in providing input voltage; and 5 and 3.3-V pins are used to supply voltage to external devices.

Analogue pins act as an interface in order to convert analogue data into digital format. With the help of these pins the code written in human understandable language (English language) is converted into a hex file using compiler and stored in memory of microcontroller.

There are several versions of Arduino boards. Some of them are as follows:

- Arduino RS (recommended standard) 232 (male pins)
- Arduino Diecimila
- Arduino Duemilanove (rev 2009b)
- Arduino UNO R2
- Arduino UNO SMD (surface-mounted device) R3
- Arduino Leonardo
- Arduino micro (ATmega32U4)
- Arduino Pro Micro (ATmega32U4)
- Arduino Pro (no USB)

- Arduino Mega
- Arduino Nano (DIO-30 footprint)
- Arduino LilyPad 00 (rev 2007) – no USB
- Arduino robot
- Arduino Esplora
- Arduino Ethernet (AVR+W5100)
- Arduino Yun (AVR+AR9331)
- Arduino Due (ARM (advanced RISC machines/Acron RISC machine) Cortex-M3 core)

For the functioning of Arduino hardware, one has to dump the code in Arduino board. The code for Arduino board can be written in any of other programming languages like Java, C, C++ with their suitable compilers. The Arduino-integrated development environment (IDE) is a Java-based cross-platform development environment that runs on Windows, Linux, and macOS. This software is licensed under the GNU Lesser General Public License (LGPL) or the GNU General Public License (GPL). This software is initiated from IDE for handling and writing of languages. Many code editing features like text copying, cutting and pasting, searching and replacing, highlighting syntax, automatic indenting, and brace matching are included in this software. This software is easy to use because the user can compile and upload programmes using one-click mechanisms. With special rules of code structuring, Arduino IDE supports C and C++. It has software library which contains many commonly used inputs and functions. The application AVRdude is used to convert executable code into a hexadecimal-encoded text file.

Arduino Pro IDE (alpha version) was released on 18 October 2019. Although this version still uses command line interface (CLI), there are improvements like autocompletion support, git integration, and more professional development environment. Eclipse Theia Open Source IDE is a base for front-end of this application. Some main features of alpha release are fully modernised and featured environment. Three modes are classic (similar to classic Arduino IDE), dual, and pro (file system view).

- New board manager
- New library manager
- Board list
- Basic auto completion (Arm targets only)
- Integration with Git
- Serial monitor
- Dark mode

Though many microcontrollers and microcontroller platforms like Parallax BASIC stamp, MIT's (Massachusetts Institute of Technology) Handy Board, Phidgets, Netmedia's BX-24 are available for physical computing, but most of us prefer Arduino for its easy to use nature.

Code is written as a block of statements in Arduino IDE software dump it in Arduino board with USB portal. Later the power supply is given to the board through power sources like power bank, power jack, or supply voltage to vin pin. The code writer can check the functioning of code using serial monitor. The following are the steps involved in writing code in Arduino IDE and dumping:

- Write the code
- Save the file
- Compile the code to find errors
- Uploading of code into a board
- Checking values in a serial monitor

While writing the code, read and write statements are used in order to make the Arduino board to take input values and give output based on the code. DigitalRead command helps in scanning values at the pins. Digital write command is used to print the values. In void setup (), one has to declare the usage of pins. There are three phases in Arduino programme such as declaring of variables, Void setup () and Void loop (). Sinking-0 is set when Arduino is receiving values and Sourcing-1 is set when giving current values out. In this, we used Arduino UNO board for completing the task of microcontroller.

13.1.2 Far-UVC lamp

With a sudden outbreak of coronavirus, people are very keen to keep environment clean and sterile by cleaning at regular interval of times. Chemical disinfectants are used in many areas to clean the environment, but it can have negative effects on humans and they are ineffective against the virus. In current time, there is no proper sterilising equipment. At the moment, there is no safe method to eliminate virus completely. Public areas like hospitals have to sterilised perfectly in order to stop virus transmission. Generally, all of us use germicidal UVC (GUVC) light (254 nm) that is made by phosphor coating and fused quartz rather than a borosilicate glass bulb to eliminate viruses. Due to its longer wavelength, UVC light can cause damage to eye and skin. So, one has to use another lamp which is used for sterilisation and it should not cause any effect to humans. A far-UVC light is a disinfection device which is safe for humans and can be used for sterilisation method. It does not cause any harm to humans because its wavelength is too small to penetrate human skin but can still inactivate virus. Far-UVC light has 99.9% sterilisation efficiency and is safe for non-target organisms. A far-UVC light has 222-nm wavelength and a frequency of 1.4E9 MHz at 539 kJ/mole [6]. Both GUVC light and far-UVC light have strength to penetrate through cells and have energy to disrupt them. This may cause damage to DNA. Thus, radiations of their light can be used as disinfectant or for sterilisation process. A far-UVC light is safe and alternative for GUVC light. There have been two studies performed with far-UVC to prove that it has the same efficiency as GUVC light. Columbia Medical Centre of Research was the first to study the effectiveness of far-UVC. They tested far-UVC light effect on two corona strains like HCoV (human corona virus)-229E (VR-740) and HCoV-OC43 (VR-1558) using human lung cells infected with the virus. After experiment, the results were like HCoV-OC43 and HCoV-229E were eliminated by

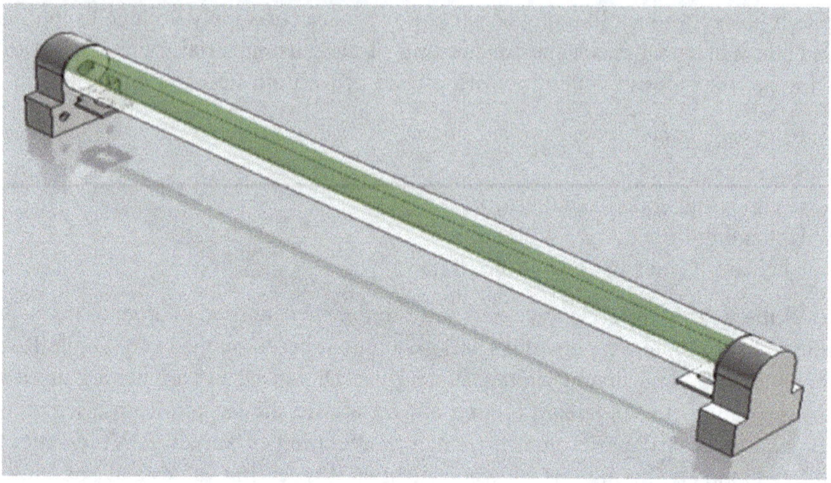

Figure 13.1 A 222-nm far-UV lamp

95% in 11 min, 99% in 16 min, and 99.9% inactivation in 25 min. They concluded that virus is high sensitivity to a far-UVC light. It can also eliminate the SARS-CoV-2 (severe acute respiratory syndrome-coronavirus-2) virus as it is similar to HCoV-OC43 and HCoV-229E [7]. The other study was done by Hiroshima University and included SARS-CoV-2 containing solutions. They placed 100-μL solution containing the virus spread onto a 9-cm sterile polystyrene plate [8]. They placed far-UVC lamp near to that plate. After 30 s of exposure to far-UVC radiation, 99.7% of the SARS-CoV-2 was eliminated in this experiment.

Mainly, we use a 222-nm excimer lamp with a 120-V power supply and operate at 150 W as shown in Figure 13.1. This device is priced at $1,000. It is high-efficiency germicidal lamp and has strength to prevent regrowth of bacteria [9]. Design of a robot and installation of it in-house determines to observe the working performance.

The main intention of our work is to eradicate germs, bacteria, and viruses from the surroundings by designing a robot and placing it in the house/hall for the following purposes:

- To keep the surroundings and objects clean and tidy by sanitising them timely.
- To reduce human efforts and to make life easier.
- To protect humans from becoming victims of dreadful viruses and diseases.

The remaining part of this chapter is organised as follows. In Section 13.2, we present a review of previous efforts relevant to the proposed work followed by a description of an Arduino-based robot. Section 13.3 gives the working and implementation of a proposed robot. Section 13.4 elaborates the performance of the designed robot and provides discussion on its usages. Section 13.5 provides the conclusion of this chapter with future enhancements.

13.2 Literature survey

Human beings are all living in the world where harmful things or diseases come without a notice, so they have to be prepared to eliminate these harmful germs, bacteria, and viruses for a safe and healthy living. At the moment, the entire world is experiencing a COVID-19 epidemic, in which hazardous viruses are ruining our lives and also lowering the economic levels of a country. Doctors are keeping their great efforts to find a cure and scientists are putting their heart and soul into the invention of the vaccine at the earliest to bring us out of this pandemic situation [10–12]. There are several inventions came into light in this pandemic situation. According to the papers written by various authors, the following is the list of some such inventions.

From the paper written by Petrovic, Nenad, and Đorđe Kocić, there is 'IoT (Internet of Things)-based solution for indoor safety'. This system measures the temperature through thermal camera and also checks the usage of mask and social distancing through computer vision techniques. Previously, there are individual system which performs the task of temperature checking, social distance, and mask monitoring. But in this paper, they discussed about the IoT system which is a combination of all three functions. They used the Python version of open CV for writing algorithms of image detection. MQTT (message queuing telemetry transport) is used to act as a bridge to send messages from sensors to servers about the studied details. Whenever a person stands at the door, the infrared thermometer which is attached to Arduino Uno board reads the temperature. When temperature is greater than normal temperature, MQTT message with temperature and location is sent to the security. Doors will be opened automatically for normal temperature people and can proceed to the next stage checking, i.e. mask. The image captured from camera is converted into grey scale image, and Haar cascade classifier is used to check the position of the mask. If the mask is not placed properly then the MQTT sends message to the security. When a person passes through the two checking stages and enters the hall the camera images are again converted into grey scale images and the Haar cascade classifier is applied to images. When more than one person is appeared within the set, threshold distance message will be sent to security. So, by using the previous system, one can analyse the temperature, mask, and social distance [13].

The paper written by Swapnili Karmore says the information about 'medical diagnosis humanoid (MDH)'. This MDH is a humanoid that helps to diagnose whether the person infected with COVID-19 or not. It is a humanoid which works using artificial intelligence (AI) for data processing. They also help in navigating people in hospital by using various sensors like IR (infrared) sensor, camera module, and automatic navigation. First the person is directed to sanitisation stage and then directed to diagnosis stage. At this stage, diagnosis is done by using E-Health kit, CT (computed tomography) scan for chest, blood sample collection and processed using AI. This project is a cost-effective and helps medical staff to test without contact [14]. The paper of Herbert Wanga, Thobius Joseph, and Mauna Belius Chuma's gives information about 'Designing the low-cost water tap'. One of the precautions to prevent COVID-19 is to frequently wash hands. A low-cost automatic water tap was designed which works by solar power and micro-controllers. It can be of great use in public places and gatherings. An infrared sensor is used to detect the presence of hand or object. When one places their hand under the hand, the infrared sensor detects and gives signals to Arduino. They used ULN2803 transistor to amplify the signal and to send enough current to the aquarium pump. The aquarium pump releases for setting the duration of time. The power requirement of the entire system is fulfilled by the solar panel. The previous IoT-based solution for indoor safety uses Raspberry Pi but in the automatic water tap, they used Arduino Uno as a microcontroller [15].

Gordana Lastovicka-Medin presented a report on a prototype gadget for increasing awareness and monitoring. This device alerts the user by vibrating when the user tries to touches the face. According to this paper, it is studied that a person touches his face for about 24 times in 1 h. But during this pandemic, touching of face is not acceptable. So, the device built by them helps to avoid touching of face. This device is in the form of glasses with ultrasonic sensors and servo motors. The servo motor helps in the rotation of sensor in 180 degrees. A buzzer, connected to Arduino board gives a signal when a person tries to touch his face [16]. The most important precaution during this pandemic is sanitisation. It is necessary to sanitise a person or object whenever he is going into public places. 'Temperature detection and automatic sanitisation and disinfection tunnel – COVID 19', the paper of Goda Vasantharao and S. K. Arifunneesa discusses about system that checks the temperature and sanitises the person. The system designed by them uses temperature sensor like the one that is used IoT-based solution for indoor safety along with buzzer instead MQTT interface to alert the security. When the temperature of the person is normal, the system activates the air blower and spraying gun. They have used PIR (passive infrared) sensor to notice the motion of person in a tunnel, unlike the automatic water tap where the ultrasonic sensor was used [17].

A detailed report on the prototype 'Anonymity preserving IoT-based COVID-19 and other infectious disease contact tracing model' is presented in [18]. In the COVID period, it is very important for contact tracing which reduces the outbreak. Tracing the people and taking measures may control the spreading of infections for many people. There were many software models for contact tracing and had an issue like privacy issues of storing contact details, so it is not used as much in Western countries. The authors came up with hardware solution with RFID (radio frequency identification), and they used blockchain concept to store the data which leads to security, i.e., privacy for the stored information. They have implemented the model in Remix IDE and noted their simulations and done their prototype successful. The RFID is placed for humans, animals, and things and it is connected to blockchain, whenever the infected person is near to them, a notification will be sent. This project tries to control the spread of COVID-19.

In [19], the authors discussed about the 'Panic buying situation during COVID-19 global pandemic'. COVID-19 outbreak created huge impact on people and their livelihood. Due to COVID-19, many people lost their lives and many scientists mentioned importance of keeping homes clean and hygienic to stop the outbreak of

COVID. This made humans to think about cleanliness and they started to buy masks, sanitisers, toilet papers, etc. These items have become their first choice to buy as they are willing to keep their surroundings clean. These items caused a huge business for many people and the cost of these items was increased 10 times the original cost and failed to meet the required demand. People are panic about the situation and urge to keep clean and sanitised surroundings.

Onur Dogan, Sanju Tiwari, M. A. Jabbar, and Shankru Guggari have done a research work on AI/ML (machine learning) techniques used in outbreak of COVID-19. They discussed about those techniques in brief and explained how they were used in detection and extracted the data. Mainly CNN (convolutional neural network), RF (random forest), ResNet (residual network), and SVM (super vector machine) approaches are the most used AI/ML techniques against COVID-19. The main objective of AI/ML techniques in COVID-19 are collection, prediction, and diagnosis [20]. 'A review on telemedicine-based WBAN (wireless body area network) framework for patient monitoring' is the paper written by Chinmay Chakraborty, Bharat Gupta, and Soumya K. Ghosh. This paper is about the research towards issues and challenges that were faced during the development of patient monitoring in telemedicine. Because of the emerging developments in the integration of communications and microelectronics and embedded system technologies, there was a structural change in patient monitoring and health information delivery systems. They used wireless body area network (WBAN) infrastructure to be mounted on the people in hospitals. Various sensors are used to generate ECG (electrocardiography), EMG (electromyography), EEG (electroencephalogram), temperature, and many more. In this paper, they covered the key components of WBAN in terms of information collection, data processing, data storage, and patient monitoring in this post. It also discusses WBAN's scalable architecture for providing real-time patient health data. The QoS (quality of service) requirements for integrating internal and exterior sensors into an autonomous system are defined by this architecture [21].

The paper written by Muhammad *et al.* explained about 'Supervised machine learning model for prediction of COVID-19 infection using epidemiology data test'. This paper discusses about building an ML model by using supervised learning technique to detect the COVID-19 infection using an epidemiology labelled data set. It also includes algorithms like decision tree logistic regression and nail by us support with commission and artificial neural network (ANN). This model takes chest X-rays images as a data set and pre-trained models' inspectionV3 ResNet50 and inspection ResNetV2, an auto waitress net pre-trained model, give the highest accuracy that is 98%. The ResNet pre-trained can be used for frontline workers as it can detect the disease at early stage [22]. Whereas in [23] authors have developed a robot for sterilisation process, they used UVC lamp and ozone light to have double disinfection. They carried out by using MATLAB® (Matrix Laboratory), Arduino IDE, and ANNs. They tested the ANN in MATLAB and they tested the behaviour of a robot in Proteus 8 software. They used three microcontrollers, i.e., Arduino. First, Arduino with ANN will decide the location that to be carried out for disinfection process; second, Arduino for displacement; third,

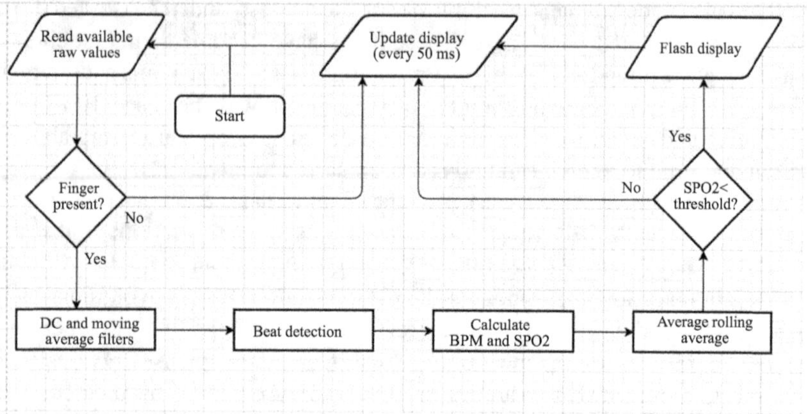

Figure 13.2 Block diagram of a pulse oximeter

Arduino is for obstacle detection. In this way the disinfection process is carried out in their model [23]. Megantoro *et al*. designed a model for disinfection process, it is user controller robot. The disinfection process will be done by using sprayer. It has key components like LoRa (long range) sender/receiver, Arduino Mega 2560, GPS (global positioning system), camera unit, non-contact temperature, accelerometer, and humidity temperatures. They have created one UI integration, where user can see the video streaming, sensors value, etc.; through this, a user controls the robot. The sprayer will spray the disinfection liquid to objects and places and thus disinfection process is done in this model [24].

From the paper of Metcalfe, Benjamin there is 'A cost-effective pulse oximeter designed in response to the COVID-19 pandemic' which works with the help of optical sensors. They designed it by using Arduino Nano microprocessor, MAX3010x pulse oximeter breakout board, and an SSD1306-based display. It is a low-cost optical pulse oximeter that comes with a finger clip. They made a finger clip by using the 3D printing process. This oximeter is convenient for many hours of use as it works on a 9-V battery. Figure 13.2 shows the working of pulse oximeter in the form of block diagram [25].

Social distancing is a must and should be a habit that has to be followed during this pandemic, but there will be times where people forget about it or accidentally violate it. Basil Reji's paper says about the 'smart cap', the device which helps in maintaining the proper social distance. They designed a cap with a PIR sensor which detects the presence of human beings within a radius of 1 m and alerts the person by buzzer sound and also with a message. They used an SIM (subscriber identification module) 808 (GPS–GSM module) module was used to track the location of the person and to send the message when the temperature exceeds the normal range. A face shield was also for additional protection in cases of misplacement of mask. When the person using this cap is tested COVID positive, it is easy to locate the primary contacts because of the SIM 808 (GPS–GSM module).

They used the Arduino Uno as a microcontroller to control the sensors. The entire system works on a 9-V battery with a switch [26]. 'Flexible (portable) COVID-19 detecting device using Arduino and Sensors' was discussed in the paper written by Katha Roy. This a portable device which can be fixed on the mask or wrist. They designed the device based on the principle that the air human exhale is moist, humid in vapour form, and warmer than the surroundings. When person violates the social distance and enters the zone of exhaled gas, this device alerts the person with a buzzer sound. This device will be a great help during this pandemic as the disease is airborne. It is also light in weight unlike the smart cap [27].

Sashmita Raghav's paper discusses about the device 'Suraksha' which helps in maintaining social distance. They made a headgear using a PIR sensor to detect the human. They preferred using of this sensor because of their 120-degree view instead of ultrasonic sensors with a 30-degree view. So, to cover entire 360 degrees, they used three PIR sensors. NodeMCU (node micro controller unit) ESP32, 32-bit microprocessor with on-board Wi-Fi and Bluetooth was used to act as an interface between the buzzer, sensors and to establish connection with a mobile phone to exchange data instead of MQTT and SIM 808 which were used in IoT-based indoor safety and smart cap, respectively. In the case of violating social-distance NodeMCU ESP32 sends the information about duration and closeness of contact and also gives the buzzer sound to alert the user. Figure 13.3 describes about steps involved in working of a Suraksha device [28].

Dr R. Dhaya's paper 'Deep Net Model for Detection of Covid-19 using Radiographs based on ROC (Receiver Operating Characteristics) Analysis' discusses about the CNN models that are developed to find the infected persons using chest X-rays. Their study helps to overcome shortage of test kits due to which spreading of infection is rapid. There are three CNN models ResNet50, ResNetV2, and InceptionV3 out of which ResNet50 is the fastest [29]. The paper of Singh, Sundaram, and Aditya Garg discusses about 'Automatic Door Handle or Knob Sanitiser'. This contraption is powered by an Arduino Nano, an infrared sensor, and a servo motor. It automatically sanitises the door knob that is used in public places. Whenever the IR senses the hand at the door knob, the servo motor pulls the handle of sanitiser bottle to release the liquid to clean the surface of knob and hand [30].

The paper on 'A Review On Smart Health System To Monitor People In Covid-19 Quarantine' of Mr Sushilkumar Thakare and Mahadeo Kokate discusses

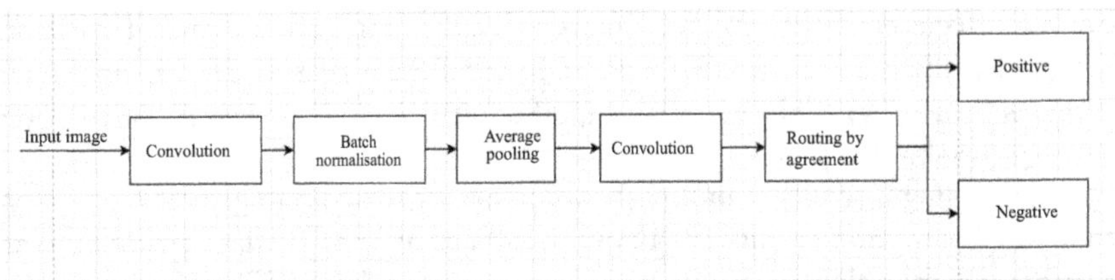

Figure 13.3 Block diagram of the proposed COVID capsule model

about quarantine system. This system is an integration of pulse sensor and breathe sensor. This system is designed by using Arduino Pro mini, the smallest of Arduino series and HC-06 Bluetooth module to establish connection to doctors and family. It helps in monitoring the blood pressure, blood pH (potential of hydrogen), heart rate, body temperature, respiratory rate of the patient who is in home quarantine. If any of the important parameters of the patient falls below the limit, it alerts the family members and doctors through email and twitter messages with the help of Bluetooth module [31]. Bhagwant, Gavade Poonam, and V. V. Purohit discussed about the device used to check the safety regulations at entrance by using IR sensors, temperature sensors. They made a device using three IR sensors, temperature sensor, pulse oximeter interfaced with Arduino Uno microcontroller. Two IR sensors will be placed outside the gate and one sensor inside the gate. When person approaches the gate, temperature was measured by using contactless IR thermometer and the person is asked to place the finger on the pulse oximeter. If the person has normal temperature and blood oxygen levels greater than 90%, then the person is allowed into the hall. Unlike 'IoT-based solution for indoor safety' device which measures the social distance inside the hall, this device allows person to enter the mall only if the sufficient place to maintain is available inside the hall. So, when the person enters the hall, the IR sensor placed inside the gate automatically increases the count [32].

The article in 'The Print' discusses about 'Bag valve masks' that was a low-cost ventilator invented by students of IIT – Hyderabad. These ventilators are made within the cost of Rs. 5,000 which is 100 times less than the conventional machine. These are at present at 3D powered range. At present these are hand powered and can be further developed to be operated with a simple power source like car batteries. They are of a great help in this pandemic period where there is a large requirement of ventilators [33]. The paper 'Far-UVC applications in healthcare' has written by Parker Esswein gives idea about various healthcare devices using far-UVC. This paper tells us about the importance of a far-UV lamp in disinfection and various applications using far-UV in health centres. A far-UVC box sanitiser helps in sanitising objects and far-UVC disinfection wand can be used to sanitise small objects like mobile phones. In these two systems, human support is required and it is limited to few objects. This project is similar to our object but with no human assistance [34]. The paper 'Far UV-C lights and fibre optics-induced selective far-UVC treatment against COVID-19 for fatality-survival trade-off' by Imran Haider, Asad Ali, Tooba Arifeen, and Abdus Sami Hassan gives information about the effectiveness of far-UVC lights in eradicating corona virus. This paper gives an idea about the usage of far-UV light in public places and for the treatment of humans. A far-UVC light with the help of optical fibre can treat a person without damaging the skin [35].

Simply using a sanitiser and mask would be a great help in protecting us from the viruses, but to sanitise our surroundings, there is no such product available. This bot is a product which helps us sanitise our surroundings without any harmful effects. UV is the electromagnetic radiation in the range of 100–400 nm [36] as shown in Figure 13.4. We have three lamps: UV (254 nm), which is harmful to

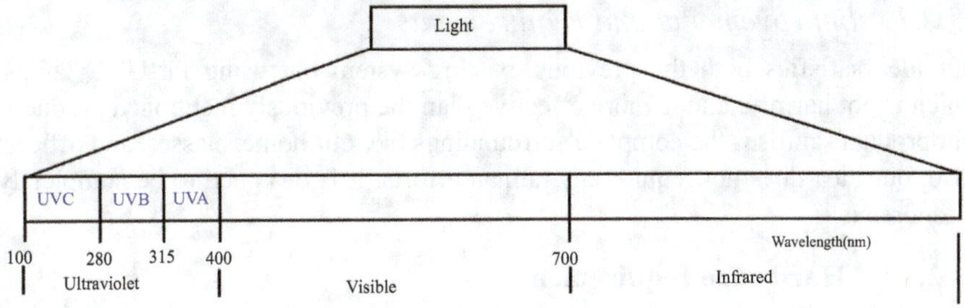

Figure 13.4 Band of spectrum

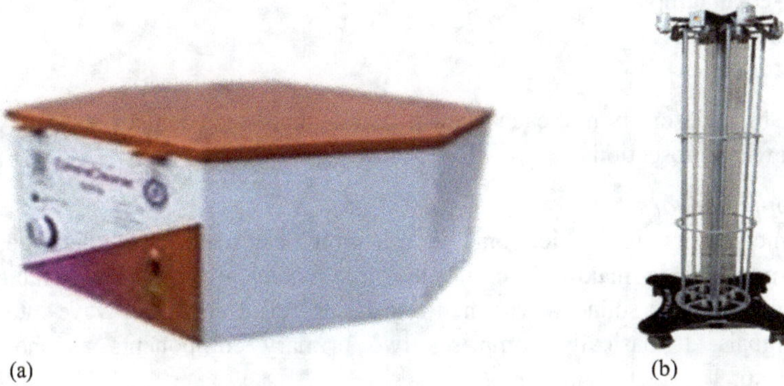

Figure 13.5 (a) Corona cleaner-source and (b) the UV blaster

human skin, UVC lamp which is also dangerous to the human skin and the radiation received from that emitter in surfaces depends on the location where it is present [37]. Far-UVC (222 nm) is the third lamp which is not harmful to human skin and does not contain the traces of mercury [38]. Therefore, it is safe to use in this project, and hence it can be used for sterilisation process.

Existing solutions are displayed in Figure 13.5. Figure 13.5(a) shows a picture of a corona cleaner which uses UVC light to inactivate the RNA (ribonucleic acid) of the viruses thereby not allowing the transfer of viruses and bacteria. This device sanitises all the portable electronic gadgets through UVC lamps. It is portable and easy to use [39]. Figure 13.5(b) shows the picture of the 'the UV blaster', which again uses UVC light to sanitise virus-prone areas. It is used in hotels, restaurants, airports, shopping malls, metros, and factories. This can be operated with a remote using a mobile or laptop using a Wi-Fi link. It includes six UVC lamps, each with a UVC power of 43 W and wavelengths of 254 nm for 360-degree lighting [40].

'The disinfection period for a space of around $12\times12\text{-ft}^2$ size is around 10 min', says the concern, adding that a 400-ft^2 area can be sanitised in 30 min if the device is placed in various locations throughout the room.

13.2.1 Improvements and requirements

Our idea satisfies both the previous existing system but using far-UVC lamps, which is not harmful and is more effective than the previously mentioned products. Our product sanitises the complete surroundings like our home, classes, and offices. Also, our idea does not require any human efforts. It is designed to be completely autonomous.

13.2.1.1 Hardware requirements

In order to build our robot, various hardware components were used. The lists of various components used in this robot are as follows:

- Ultrasonic sensors
- Far-UVC lamps
- Arduino Uno
- Motor driver

The brief description of each of the following hardware components is given in the following subsections.

Ultrasonic sensors

Ultrasonic sensors are the electronic devices which can measure the distance of an object or target in making use of ultrasonic waves. It measures distance by releasing ultrasonic sound waves then translating reflected sound wave into electrical signals. It basically comprises two primary components as shown in Figure 13.6.

- Transmitter: used for emitting sound using Piezoelectric Crystals;
- Receiver: receives the sound after it travels to and from the target or object.

To determine the distance between the ultrasonic sensor and the object, the sensor considers the time taken by the transmitter and the receiver. We know

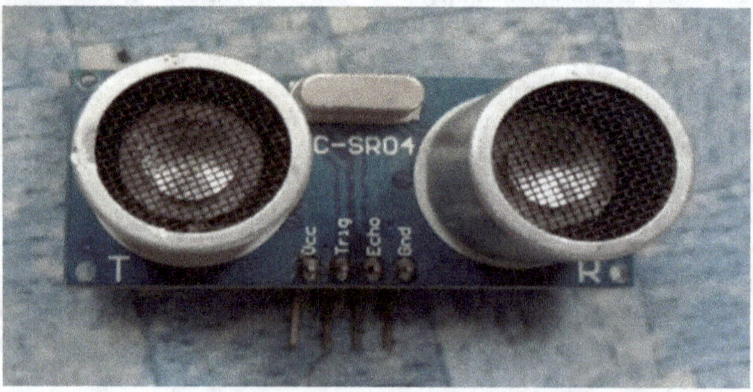

Figure 13.6 Ultrasonic sensor

speed = distance/time. For calculating the distance, we take $D = 1/2T \times C$, where D is the distance, T is the time, and C is the speed of sound, i.e., 343 m/s. As the sensor covers the distance twice, i.e., from transmitter to object and object to receiver so, we will take 1/2 in the formula for calculating distance. Ultrasonic sensors are used as proximity sensors. They are used in automatic self-parking and obstacle detection systems, anti-collision systems, and in manufacturing industry. Ultrasonic sensors have a wide number of applications in the field of robotics. They can also be used as level sensors to monitor, detect, and identify [41]. They are employed in the medical field to create images of inside organs, cancers, and unborn infants.

IR sensors are commonly employed as proximity sensors for obstacle detection, although they have a few flaws, such as low precision when compared to ultrasonic sensors. Obstacle detection is more accurate using ultrasonic sensors. They will work by generating sound waves and waiting for the sound to reflect back. The distance will then be calculated based on the time it takes to reach the object and the time it takes to reflect back [42]. In some of the sensors, they use separate emitter and receiver, but in ultrasonic sensor both are combined in one package and it can be used for many applications where size is at a premium. A radar also works in the same way as an ultrasonic sensor, but most of the people use ultrasonic sensors as it is readily available in the market and these are available at low cost, and they can detect the objects more accurately than radar. As a result, many people prefer to employ ultrasonic sensors instead of radar.

Technical specifications of an ultrasonic sensor: power supply – +5 V DC; quiescent current – <2 mA; working current – 15 mA; effectual angle – <15 degrees; ranging distance – 2–400 cm/1″ to 13 ft; resolution – 0.3 cm; and measuring angle – 30 degrees.

Far-UVC lamps

A method for limiting or stopping viral transmissions in the air and inactivating them in a short period of time is possible. Germicidal UV light would be effective, but when directly used, would be hazardous to the human eye and skin. In contrast to this, far-UV lamps would be effective as they emit far-UVC light which kills pathogens and bacteria efficiently and inactivates their cellular functionality causing no harm to humans [43]. According to researches, it is said that on a continuous exposure of far-UVC light for 25 min, 99.9% germs and bacteria would be eradicated. Therefore, the far-UV lamps form the heart of our project.

Arduino Uno

The Arduino Uno is a microcontroller board which is based on ATmega328p [44]. It has 14 digital input/output pins out of which 6 pins are used as PWM outputs, 6 analogue inputs, a 16-MHz crystal oscillator, 4 hardware serial ports, a power jack, an ICSP header, and a USB connection as shown in Figure 13.7. This board is designed for low-cost projects. It has a flash memory of 32 kb, EEPROM (electrically erasable programmable read-only memory) of 1 kb, and SRAM (static random-access memory) of 2 kb.

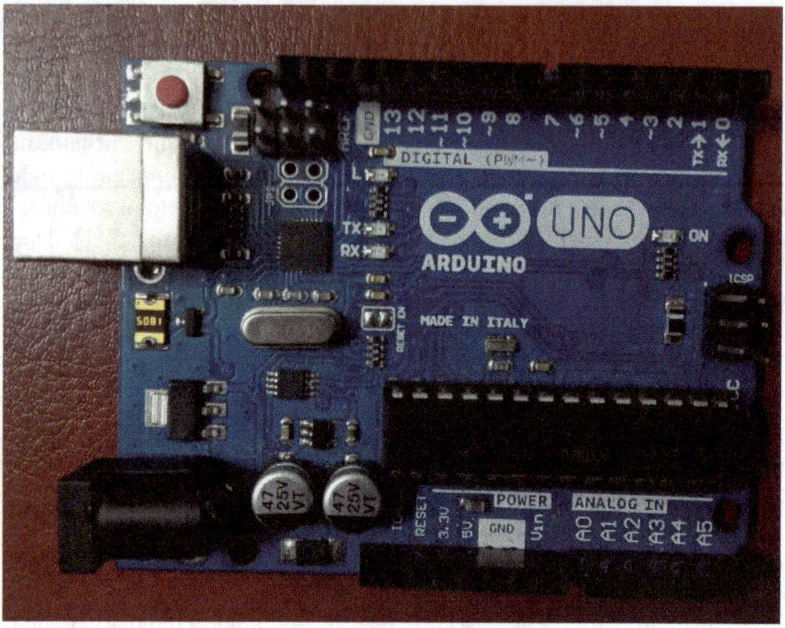

Figure 13.7 Arduino Uno

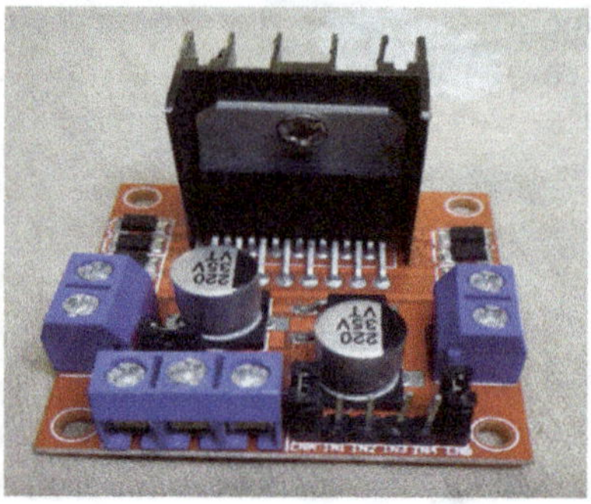

Figure 13.8 Motor driver

Motor driver

Motor drivers form an interface between the motors and control circuits. It has a voltage regulator, a power led, a 5-V jumper ENA, and ENB pins. IN1, IN2, IN3, and IN4 are direction control pins at the edges of motor driver as shown in Figure 13.8. They require a large amount of current whereas low current signals are worked on by the controller. So, the job of a motor driver is to transform a low-current signal into a high-current signal that may be used to drive a motor.

12-V battery
Lead–acid batteries are used in marine industries. In general, it has two 6-V batteries in series, or a single 12-V battery. Batteries are arranged with several single cells in series manner, where each cell produces approximately 2.1 V. In a 12-V battery, six single cells are arranged in series producing an output voltage of 12.6 V. A battery is a mostly used component in projects. In the place of a battery, we can use voltage regulators based on requirement of applications.

13.2.1.2 Software requirements

We need to develop the code for functioning of the bot. We need to dump the code we developed in the Arduino for functioning of the bot. For this purpose, we use the software called Arduino IDE. The Arduino-integrated development environment is software which comprises a text editor in which code is to be written, a text console, a toolbar which has buttons to perform collective functions and a list of menus. It connects to an Arduino and Genuino hardware for uploading programmes and also sets up a mode of communication between them. This is the main text editing programme used for Arduino Programming. First, the IDE interprets, translates, and compiles the sketches into codes that Arduino can understand. After compilation, the Arduino code is dumped into the board's memory.

In Figure 13.9, the circuit diagram of the proposed Arduino-based far-UVC robot is displayed. Figure 13.9 shows the design of the proposed idea using circuit. io software. It is a software tool where we can stimulate and design our model. In this software Arduino is interfaced with ultrasonic sensors and motor driver to get a clear idea about the connections. On stimulating this design in this software, we can know about the errors in our design and rectify them before going for the implementation of it in hardware. The ultrasonic sensors have four pins-Vcc, ground, Tx, and rx pins. The Vcc pin is connected to 5-V Arduino. The Tx pin is connected to digital pin, and rx pin to digital pin. The motor driver is connected to four pins of Arduino. The gear motors will be connected to out pins of motor driver. The far-UVC lamp will be connected to Arduino.

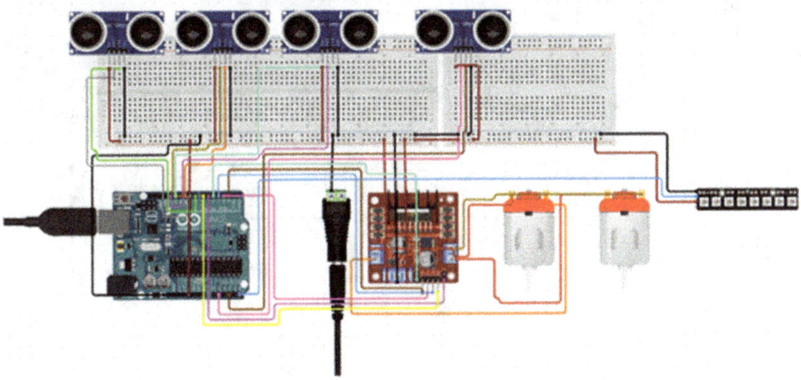

Figure 13.9 Component interfacing circuit diagram

13.3 Working of the proposed robot

First, we make a box out of wood. At the bottom surface of the box, four wheels would be attached at the four corners for the robot to move. Four LED (light-emitting diode) far-UVC lamps would be put in the centre of each edge, on the four sides of the box. These lamps on emitting UV light would kill germs and bacteria and thus sanitise or clean the entire floor by moving on wheels.

Four pole-shaped far-UVC lamps would be positioned at the four corners of the box's top surface, helping to sanitise the entire surroundings and objects around us. To move back and forth, this bot does not require the use of a remote control or an app. It moves on its own like a robotic vacuum cleaner and contains vacuum cleaner components, so it acts as vacuum cleaner as well as a sterilisation robot. Figure 13.10(a) is the block diagram which represents the various steps and devices involved in the design of the bot. Figure 13.10(b) gives the information about step-wise process involved in the function of the bot. From Figure 13.10(a) and (b), it is

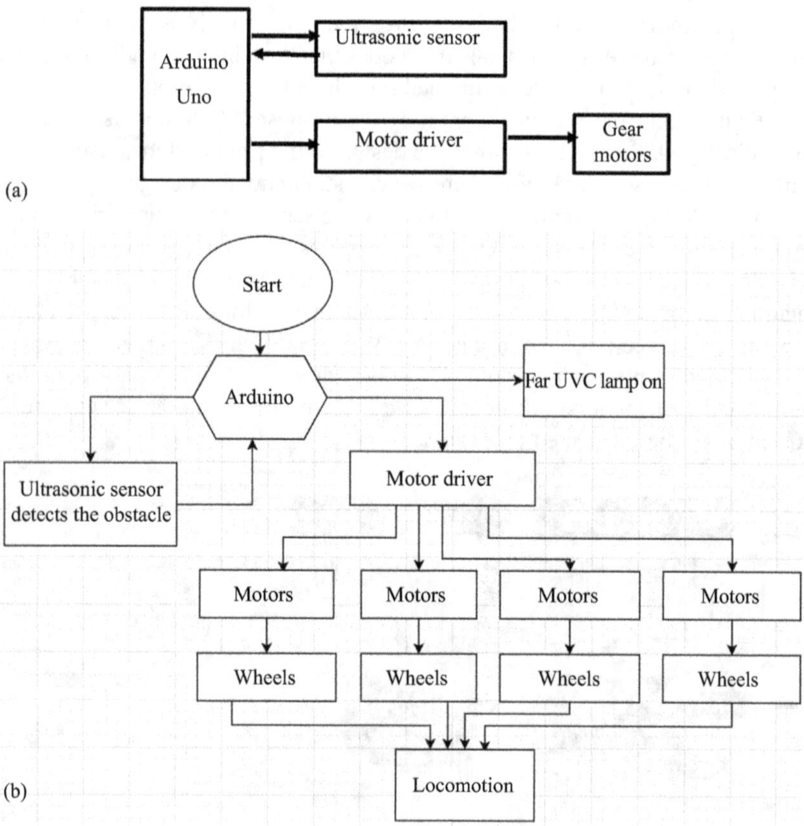

Figure 13.10 (a) Block diagram of the bot and (b) flow chart describing the design flow

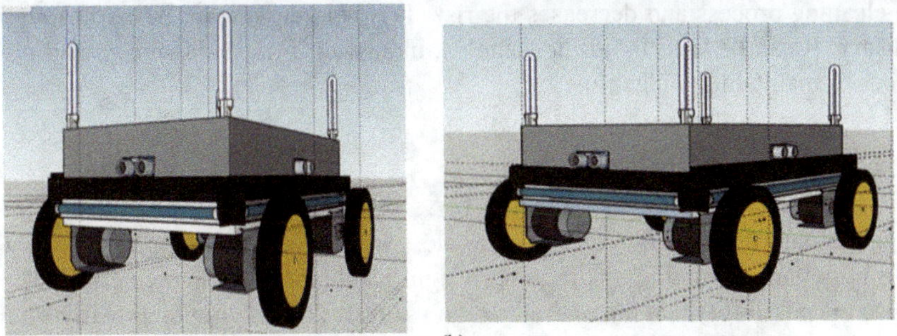

(a) (b)

Figure 13.11 (a) Front and (b) side view of the project

evident that the Arduino Uno is a key component of the proposed work. This is the brain of the proposed work as it controls and sends the information; here the ultrasonic sensor detects the objects and sends the information to Arduino and it decides what operation has to be done. Based on ultrasonic observations, Arduino Uno commands the motor driver to regulate the gear motors.

There are components like ultrasonic sensors which help the bot to detect obstacles in their paths and move forward. This entire set-up can be employed in houses, offices, malls, theatres, and hospitals. This set-up would sanitise the entire place in about 15 min. It would cause no harm to humans and would prove to be a boon to many as it is automatic and needs no human efforts to operate it and also helps us keep our surroundings and objects clean, thereby protecting us from dangerous diseases or viruses and keeping us clean, hygienic, and healthy. CAD (computer-sided design) models of the proposed idea are shown in Figure 13.11.

Figure 13.11(a) and (b) shows the view of a CAD model of our project. The two parts show the box in which ultrasonic sensors, Arduino Uno, and other electrical components are placed internally. On the top of the surface, pole-shaped far-UVC lamps are placed as shown in Figure 13.11 for sanitising the surroundings and at the bottom surface, four LED shaped far-UVC lamps are placed for sanitising the ground.

13.3.1 Value proposition

The prototype of our product might cost as much as Rs. 8,000. We intend to build the robot ourselves to save money. The far-UVC lamp would cost between Rs. 3,000 and Rs. 4,000. However, the cost of mass manufacture of the far-UVC lamp will be lower. The robotic vacuum cleaners have a high demand nowadays, as we combining both cleaning and sanitising in our robot; there will be a high market range for this product. It can also be utilised in hospitals, as hospitals are locations where cleanliness is prioritised. As a result, this sort of solution will be beneficial in sanitising the rooms, cleaning the floors, and reducing the efforts of staff. The cleaning team is at greater risk during COVID; however, this model aids them in the cleaning process and decreases the risk. It is very significant in the hospitality industry. It can be used by all households, industries, offices, hospitals, and other places to maintain the cleanliness.

13.4 Results and discussions

With the outbreak of COVID-19 pandemic, sanitisation of surroundings is given most importance. But this task requires a significant amount of human effort. There is also the possibility that the individual who sanitises our environment will become sick with a virus. This risk is greatly decreased by the use of this bot.

We have done the prototype and placed in our home; it moves throughout the entire house but does not cover the coroner areas. In balcony, it was moving without any errors and showing accurate results. Ultrasonic sensor plays a major role in detecting the objects, and it was spotting the objects as well as sending the values to Arduino, and the locomotion is accurate in the use of ultrasonic sensor. As we have four ultrasonic sensors, it detects the front, sides, and back perfectly and is precise in detecting the objects, and the locomotion of the robot is accurate and autonomous.

Figure 13.12 shows the interfacing of ultrasonic sensor and Arduino. The ultrasonic sensor detects the objects and sends back the information to the Arduino. We have kept ranges for the ultrasonic sensor by using speed–distance formula.

Distance = speed × time/2

Speed of sound is 343 m/s.

Based on the previous two conditions, we decide the range of an ultrasonic sensor (depending on our requirement, we have to give time or distance values).

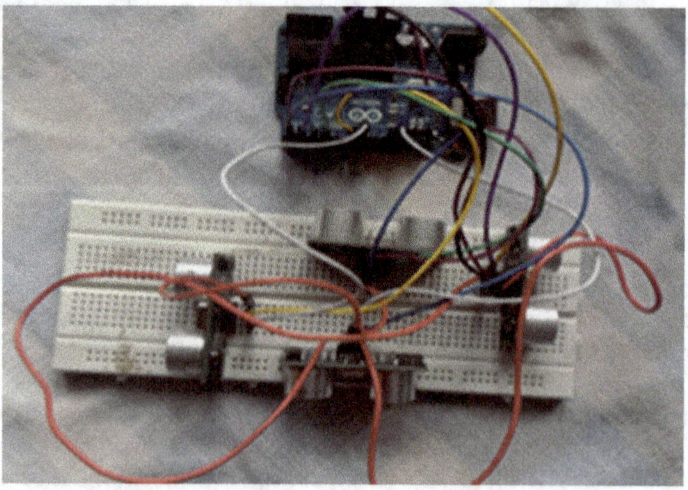

Figure 13.12 Arduino interfaced with ultrasonic sensors

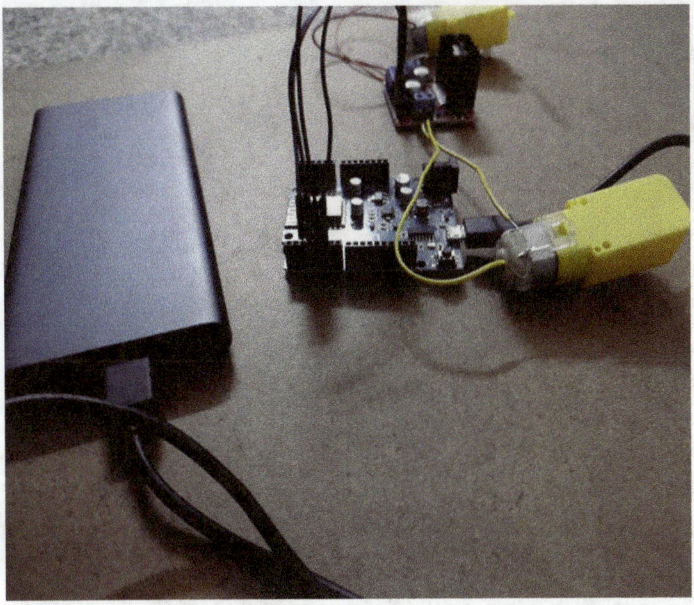

Figure 13.13 Interfacing of Arduino, motor drivers, and gear motors

Interfacing of the Arduino with a motor driver and gear motors is shown in Figure 13.13. Whenever the ultrasonic sensor detects the object, the information is sent to the Arduino. Now Arduino determines and sends the instruction to motor driver regarding the direction of movement. The motor driver regulates the power to move gear motors.

The robot model was successfully created in AutoCAD, and the prototype was completed as shown in Figure 13.14. The ultrasonic sensor is connected to Arduino of 2, 3, 4, 5 pins, and other ultrasonic sensors were connected in the same way. The transmitter pin will send the wave and when it identifies the object, it sends the echo wave to receiver pin of ultrasonic sensor that goes to Arduino; now Arduino decides and sends commands to a motor driver, then the motor driver controls the gear motors. In this way, the robot locomotion works. The far-UVC lamp will be ON while the robot is moving. The lamp will sanitise the room while it was moving and at the same time it will clean the floor.

After implementing this robot steriliser using Arduino and ultrasonic sensors, it has been observed that some difficulty aroused from ultrasonic sensor, like getting trouble while it was moving in corner areas of rooms or halls. To overcome such problems, LIDARs (light detection and ranging) can be used in the place of ultrasonic sensors along with an accelerometer sensor in the future enhancement of the proposed work. LIDAR and accelerometer sensors make the robot into a complete autonomous. A typical remote-sensing method for estimating the exact distance of an object on the earth's surface is LIDAR. It benefits us by sending out pulsed light waves into the environment. These pulses re-enter the sensor after

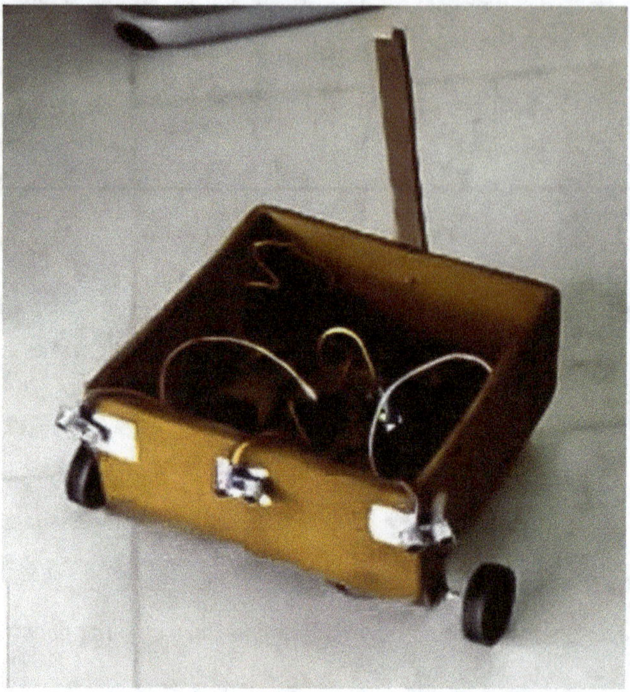

Figure 13.14 Prototype of an Arduino-based far-UVC robot

bouncing off nearby objects. The sensor calculates the distance travelled by using the time it took for each pulse to return to the sensor. So that it can recognise corners and walls in less time, allowing us to do the sanitisation in less time. In addition to that, we can develop an app for the proposed work so that it would be more helpful for the people in controlling the robot remotely. This bot will be a great help in sanitising the surroundings and making them clean and tidy, by eradicating germs and preventing from being infected from dangerous virus. This bot can be used in public places like malls, theatres, parks, and schools to reduce the chance of persons being affected.

We can add a feature to this model like making the robot climbing up the walls and cleaning the walls too. In order to achieve this, we need to change the shape of the model such that it can climb the walls. Then the robot will be capable of cleaning walls and floors. It would be great advantage for the people. The mobile application can also be developed so that we can control it and if needed we can change the option either it is being used for sanitising the floor or walls. In a hospital the patient/staff can also use it if they needed for cleaning. The same robot can be used for monitoring the patient condition in the hospital room using AI/ML techniques. The robot will supply food to patients, it checks the temperature and oxygen level of patients and sends data to store using blockchain technology, and this feature reduces the work of staff and provides comfort for patient too.

13.5 Conclusion and future scope

In this pandemic and post pandemic situation, the proposed target will keep surroundings clean by sanitising and continues the sanitisation process at regular interval of times. Generally, as cleaning of a certain area or surface requires a lot of human effort, this design is employed in order to decrease the human efforts and at the same moment to have instantaneous cleaning. So, our proposal in this chapter is very keen on this factor and made it to use less human effort by making it an autonomous robot and sanitising the surroundings in short interval of time. The cost is also very less which is affordable by all categories of people. Far-UVC lamps have been used in sanitising the surroundings as they do not affect the humans. This product when once released in market would prove to be a boon to the society as it requires no human efforts and is completely automatic. Adding up to this, this robot most importantly safeguards the health of humans by eliminating all the dreadful germs and viruses. In the present COVID time, it is highly preferred for COVID treat hospitals where sanitisation is very essential to protect the doctors, nurses, serving people in the premises. Also, the far-UV light generated from the far-UVC excimer lamps would cause no harm to humans and its cost is quite affordable. It cleans the entire surroundings and objects in very less time and with no requirement of human efforts. This bot would definitely hike up the market levels and would be a great contribution to the society. In future, we can use a LIDAR sensor for accurate automatic locomotion of a robot and an app to control the robot. We can also incorporate features of robotic vacuum cleaners and design the robot to climb the walls such that it cleans and sanitises the walls, floors, and other surfaces; further this robot can be used in hospitals for supplying food, checking temperature and oxygen levels of a patient. The patient and staff can control the robot using mobile application which in turn makes hospitals into smart hospitals.

References

[1] Armani AM, Hurt DE, Hwang D, McCarthy MC, and Scholtz A. ‘Low-tech solutions for the COVID-19 supply chain crisis’. *Nature Reviews Materials*. 2020;5(6):403–6.

[2] Welch D, Buonanno M, Grilj V *et al.* ‘Far-UVC light: A new tool to control the spread of airborne-mediated microbial diseases’. *Scientific Reports*. 2018;8(1):01–07.

[3] Olcay A, Albayrak SB, Akturk IF *et al.* ‘A new Far-UVC based method for germ free hospitals and travel: Initus-V’. medRxiv. 2021.

[4] Louis L. ‘Working principle of Arduino and using it as a tool for study and research’. *International Journal of Control, Automation, Communication, and Systems*. 2016;1(2):21–9.

[5] Badamasi YA. ‘The working principle of an Arduino’. *11th International Conference on Electronics, Computer, and Computation (ICECCO)*, IEEE. 29 September 2018. pp. 1–4.

[6] Department of Public Health, Environmental and Social Determinants of Health. UV radiation, World Health Organization. https://www.who.int/uv/faq/whatisuv/en/index2.html, 9 March 2016.

[7] Buonanno M, Welch D, Shuryak I, and Brenner DJ. 'Far-UVC light (222 nm) efficiently and safely inactivates airborne human coronaviruses'. *Scientific Reports*. 2000;10(1):1–8.

[8] Kitagawa H, Nomura T, Nazmul T *et al.* 'Effectiveness of 222-nm ultraviolet light on disinfecting SARS-CoV-2 surface contamination'. *American Journal of Infection Control*. 2001;49(3):299–301.

[9] ProLampSales. Sailon UVC – 222 nm Far UV Light – 150 W – 455 mm, ProLampSales. https://www.prolampsales.com/products/sailon-uvc-222nm-far-uv-light-150w-455mm, 2021.

[10] Bhuyan HK, Chakraborty C, Shelke Y, and Pani SK. 'COVID-19 diagnosis system by deep learning approaches'. *Expert Systems*. 2021:e12776. https://doi.org/10.1111/exsy.12776.

[11] Dash D, Chakraborty C, Giri SK, Pani SK, and Frnda J. 'BIFM: Big-data driven intelligent forecasting model for COVID-19'. *IEEE Access*. 2021;9:97505–17. 10.1109/ACCESS.2021.3094658.

[12] Aslam B, Javed AR, Chakraborty C, Nebhen J, Raqib S, and Rizwan M. 'Blockchain and ANFIS empowered IoMT application for privacy preserved contact tracing in COVID-19 pandemic'. *Personal and Ubiquitous Computing*. 2021:1–17. 10.1007/s00779-021-01596-3.

[13] Petrovic N and Kocic Đ. 'IoT-based System for COVID-19 Indoor Safety Monitoring (preprint)'. *International Conference on Electrical, Electronic, and Computing Engineering (IcETRAN)*. 2020. pp. 1–6.

[14] Karmore S, Bodhe R, Al-Turjman F, Kumar RL, and Pillai S. 'IoT based humanoid software for identification and diagnosis of Covid-19 suspects'. *IEEE Sensors Journal*. 2020.

[15] Wanga H, Joseph T, and Chuma MB. 'War against coronavirus (COVID–19) in Tanzania: Designing a low cost automatic water tap'. *International Journal of Computer Applications Technology and Research*. 2020;9(04):150–4.

[16] Lastovicka-Medin G. 'Social engineering and prototype awareness enhancing during international coronavirus outbreak'. *9th Mediterranean Conference on Embedded Computing (MECO)*, IEEE. 8 June 2020. pp. 1–4.

[17] Vasantharao G and Arifunneesa SK. 'Temperature detection and automatic sanitization and disinfection tunnel-COVID 19'. *The International Journal of Analytical and Experimental Modal Analysis*. 2020;12:0886–936.

[18] Garg L, Chukwu E, Nasser N, Chakraborty C, and Garg G. 'Anonymity preserving IoT-based COVID-19 and other infectious disease contact tracing model'. *IEEE Access*. 2020;8:159402–14.

[19] Roy S and Chakraborty C. 'Panic buying situation during COVID-19 global pandemic'. *Journal of Information Technology Management*. 2021;13(2):231–44.

[20] Dogan O, Tiwari S, Jabbar MA, and Guggari S. 'A systematic review on AI/ML approaches against COVID-19 outbreak'. *Complex and Intelligent Systems*. 2021:1–24.

[21] Chakraborty C, Gupta B, and Ghosh SK. 'A review on telemedicine-based WBAN framework for patient monitoring'. *Telemedicine and e-Health*. 2013;19(8):619–26.

[22] Muhammad LJ, Algehyne EA, Usman SS, Ahmad A, Chakraborty C, and Mohammed IA. 'Supervised machine learning models for prediction of COVID-19 infection using epidemiology dataset'. *SN Computer Science*. 2021;2(1):1–3.

[23] Ocaña J, Flores E, Naquin E, Pacheco A, and Felix E. 'Smart system model to disinfect SARS-CoV-2 in physical environments'. *Journal of Contemporary Issues in Business and Government*. 2021;27(2).

[24] Megantoro P, Setiadi H, and Aji Pramudita B. 'All-terrain mobile robot disinfectant sprayer to decrease the spread of covid-19 in open area'. *International Journal of Electrical and Computer Engineering (IJECE)*. 2021;11(3):2090–100.

[25] Metcalfe B, Iravani P, Graham-Harper-Cater J, Bowman R, Stirling J, and Wilson P. 'A cost-effective pulse oximeter designed in response to the COVID-19 pandemic'. *Journal of Open Hardware*. 2021;5(1).

[26] Reji B, Rathesh A, Suresh S, Jose N, and Benny J. 'Smart Cap for Prevention of Contagious Diseases and Social Distancing Using Arduino'. *Bangalore Humanitarian Technology Conference (B-HTC)*, IEEE. 8 October 2020. pp. 1–5.

[27] Roy K. 'Flexible (Portable) COVID 19 detecting device using Arduino and sensors'. *International Journal of Engineering Research in Computer Science and Engineering*. 2021;8(3):32–3.

[28] Raghav S, Vijay G, Harika PS *et al.* 'Suraksha: Low Cost Device to Maintain Social Distancing during CoVID-19'. *4th International Conference on Electronics, Communication and Aerospace Technology (ICECA)*, IEEE. 5 November 2020. pp. 1476–80.

[29] Dhaya R. 'Deep net model for detection of covid-19 using radiographs based on roc analysis'. *Journal of Innovative Image Processing (JIIP)*. 2020; 2(03):135–40.

[30] Singh S and Garg A. 'Automatic door handle or knob sanitizer'. *Journal on Today's Ideas-Tomorrow's Technologies*. 2020;8(1):35–40.

[31] Thakare MS and Kokate M. 'A review on smart health system to monitor people in Covid-19 quarantine'. *International Journal of Advance Scientific Research and Technology*. 2020;5:28–33.

[32] Bhagawan GP and Purohit VV. 'Safety regulations checks at entrance for COVID safety'. *International Journal of Research Publication and Reviews*. 2021;2(3):383–6.

[33] Sharma K. 'The ideas and innovations IITs have come up with to help India fight coronavirus'. The print. 1 April 2020.

[34] Peters D, Esswein P, Krugel L, Obrycki V, Marcoux D, and Linderman T. 'Far-UVC Applications in Healthcare'. University of Wisconsin-Madison, Department of Biomedical Engineering BME. 7 October 2020. p. 27.

[35] Haider I, Ali A, Arifeen T, and Hassan AS. 'Far UV-C lights and fiber optics induced and selective far UV-C treatment against COVID-19 for fatality-survival tradeoff'. TechRxiv, Powered by IEEE. 2017, Volume XX. pp. 1–9.

[36] Cole CA, FOrbes PD, and Davies RE. 'An action spectrum for UV photo-carcinogenesis'. *Photochemistry and Photobiology*. 1986;43(3):275–84.

[37] Lindblad M, Tano E, Lindahl C, and Huss F. 'Ultraviolet-C decontamination of a hospital room: Amount of UV light needed'. *Burns*. 2020;46(4):842–9.

[38] Seuylemezian A, Buonanno M, Guan L, Brenner DJ, and Welch D. 'Far-UVC light as a new tool to reduce microbial burden during spacecraft assembly'. *Advances in Space Research*. 2001;67(1):496–503.

[39] Santosh Patnaik. UV-based coronavirus cleaner for gadgets arrives. The Hindu; July 19 2020. https://www.thehindu.com/news/national/andhra-pradesh/uv-based-coronavirus-cleaner-for-gadgets-arrives/article31863658.ece, 10 May 2021.

[40] Raj A. UV Blaster, DRDO new UV Disinfection Equipment[ONLINE]. Infotonline; May 4 2020. https://infotonline.com/uv-blaster-drdo-new-uv-disinfection-equipment/, 10 May 2021.

[41] Dimitrov A and Minchev D. 'Ultrasonic sensor explorer'. *19th International Symposium on Electrical Apparatus and Technologies (SIELA)*, IEEE. 29 May 2016. pp. 1–5.

[42] Prasojo I, Nguyen PT, and Shahu N. 'Design of ultrasonic sensor and ultraviolet sensor implemented on a fire fighter robot using AT89S52'. *Journal of Robotics and Control*. 2020;1(2):59–63.

[43] Buonanno M, Welch D, Shuryak I, and Brenner DJ. 'Far-UVC light (222 nm) efficiently and safely inactivates airborne human coronaviruses'. *Scientific Reports*. 2020;10(1):1–8.

[44] Nayyar A and Puri V. 'A review of Arduino board's, Lilypad's & Arduino shields'. *3rd International Conference on Computing for Sustainable Global Development (INDIACom)*, IEEE. 16 March 2016. pp. 1485–92.

Chapter 14

Effect of COVID-19 pandemic on waste management system and infection control

Ramkrishna Mondal[1] and Chinmay Chakrabarty[2]

Abstract

Late within the year of 2019, the entire world roused by a reality of an epidemic of coronavirus disease (COVID-19). It has become very vital and important to take all possible precaution till the world finds a definite treatment against this disease as there is least information about its behavior and origin. World Health Organization (WHO) informed that proper guidelines need to be followed for COVID-19 waste management as it is extremely infectious and contaminated. Personal protective equipment has become a very vital element to guard from exposure of any infectious materials. It is usually used in healthcare or hospital settings during any outbreak. These enormous challenges are with all stakeholders for avoiding spread through waste. Additionally, to WHO, each country was adopted different safety measures and developed guidelines to control the contamination and manage the waste. The previously mentioned guidelines are very useful for managing the infectious waste and providing protection and security of waste handlers. Not only the spread of COVID-19 is reduced by practicing appropriate technologies to handle wastes, but it generates worth through increasing the recyclability chance of waste. Due to COVID-19, there were lots of social and economic changes happened in the world, which leads to reduction in manufacturing units and various business processes. All these have significantly affected waste management that is a very vivacious step for the health outcomes of the patients as well as caregivers, especially during the COVID-19 pandemic. Among all the issues created by COVID-19, the problem that will create major mess is, not handling biomedical waste properly. If the spreading needs to be controlled, it requires a strict monitoring of the complete cycle starting from the point of generation. However, due to the invaluable service of waste management sector only, it is possible to avoid spread of the COVID-19 and ensure that the weird tons of waste will not be gathered that increases health risks and the spread of disease.

[1]Department of Hospital Administration, All India Institute of Medical Sciences Bhubaneswar, Bhubaneswar, India
[2]Department of ECE, BIT Mesra, Ranchi, India

Keywords: Biomedical waste; Coronavirus disease (COVID-19); Biomedical waste; Municipal solid waste; Waste management; Rethinking; Effective waste management; Personal protective equipment

14.1 Introduction

Improper handling of waste, be it medical waste or healthcare waste or biomedical waste (BMW) or household waste or municipal solid waste (MSW), will lead to severe public health and environmental effects. Proper management of the said wastes is mandatory to avoid any effect in environment and health protection. Coronavirus disease (COVID-19) generates further challenges in waste management, and significance of proper waste management should receive more attention during this pandemic. COVID-19 spread rapidly all over China and it exposed the deficits in BMW management. Subsequently, COVID-19 was declared an International Public Health Emergency on January 31, 2020 by WHO as it rapidly invaded due to high infection rate first in China, followed by other countries of the world [1]. In the Wuhan city, the daily BMW generation ascended by five times, 250 t, from 40 t far exceeding its daily processing capacity of the BMW treatment plant. Till first 2 months of 2020, a major number of new cases and death were from China, whereas adjoining countries like Asia, North America [2], and Europe, remained relatively safe [3] but later on all suffered a lot and now even some of them are in the second wave phase. Both China and the United States during COVID-19 had come up with a similar type of issues regarding BMW management that were timely management of the waste. According to a WHO report, there is hardly any evidence of transmission of COVID while handling BMW by the waste handler who does not protect themselves properly [4]. The Solid Waste Association of North America reported that if the sanitation workers maintain social distances from other people, it will reduce their risk of getting infected with the virus [5]. The need for personal protective equipment (PPE) was hastening worldwide for the protection of doctors, nurses, healthcare workers, and waste handling staff, which leads to a huge production of PPE. Subsequently, waste also increasing, which could be either infected or not infected, due to lockdowns and the introduction of home quarantines to control COVID-19 [6]. Although the pandemic had negative impact on universal economic activities, it has made a lot of positive environmental changes also [7]. The pandemic has made a significant impact not only on BMW generation but also on MSW production and composition. As per the WHO and the US Centers for Disease Control and Prevention (CDC), the waste generated during pandemic may be classified into two categories: (i) within healthcare facilities and (ii) outside healthcare facilities [8]. It can be said that COVID-19 has transformed the waste production dynamic [9] with probable criticality in every step of the waste management starting from the segregation, collection, transport, treatment, and disposal [10]. In the pandemic, maintaining social distancing and other measures to protect from COVID-19 leads to increase in plastic use, a situation that needs policy consequences [11]. This rising plastic use leads to a channel for contamination and increases the chance of spread. To control the pandemic a prohibition of movements was implemented, which affects the countries that depend on external technologies for waste reprocessing and management. As a result, the waste generated in that said period is disposed of rather than recycled. COVID-19 pandemic like emergencies made the sustainable management of BMW problematic and amplified. The hefty waste either needs to be collected for disposing or recycled. Both the processes are compromised because of the shortage of manpower and hard work to implement infection control measures [12,13]. These disrupted services lead to mishandling of waste and it increased up to 300% at few rural communities of the United Kingdom (UK) [14]. Due to this pandemic the UK Environment Agency allowed a temporary storage of waste and incineration ash at sites that further threatens the environment [15]. The waste management system as a whole needs to be considered, from waste generation, to treatment, including resource use, and disposal of extra waste to reduce the socioeconomic and environmental impacts of waste as well as shielding of waste management chains will help to achieve sustainable cities and communities [16]. In the last two decades, COVID-19 pandemic is the third major zoonotic disease episode. First, it was the SARS (severe acute respiratory syndrome) in 2002–03 and the second was MERS (Middle East respiratory syndrome) in 2012. The disease was first reported to WHO by the Chinese Health Officials on December 31, 2019 as atypical pneumonia of unknown reason [17]. According to Van Doremalen *et al.*, the survival period varies from hours to days depending on the materials and environment. Survival phases on copper and cardboard vary from 3 to 4 h, while on plastic, stainless steel varies from 1 to 3 days and some time as high as up to 9 days, even in tap or waste water at 20°C for 2 days [18,19]. This longer survival period can lead to a high danger of communal spread by inappropriate. In this chapter, first various impacts like socioeconomic, environmental and also impacts on waste generation and waste management are discussed. Different subsequent challenges faced due to these impacts on waste management are enumerated. Lastly, it described the new models or rethinking in the processes of waste management during pandemic.

14.2 Socioeconomic and environmental impact

Socioeconomically and demographically it indicates that COVID-19 is distressing every person in a different way [20]. Due to the lack of suitable data, it is very difficult to fully opine that why this COVID-19 affected different groups differently in the society, although poor have been affected most [21]. Moreover, local and global business got disturbed severely by this pandemic [22]. It has been found that even after taking corrective and preventive steps, a very less number of international communications started in China [23]. Different economic institutes and World Bank are very much worried about the pandemic impact on economy. Loss of job and business and go-slow of national transformations must be restored to diminish the socioeconomic impact. After the pandemic started in, stock exchange markets detected the major decline after 2008 economic disaster. The market slide continues as global markets also fell down quite a lot. However, later slowly it gained up after October/November 2020.

As a global pandemic, COVID-19 contributed a lot of environmental issues, especially in BMW management. Wuhan city generates 200 t of BMW, four times greater than the capacity of its waste treatment capabilities [24]. Ocean Asia, a leading NGO, mentioned that BMW generated in Hong Kong spoiled the seaside atmosphere [25]. Due to COVID-19, countries must announce lockdown measures to safeguard their citizens and limit the exposure from COVID-19 [26]. Several air changes were found around the world like air pollutants that came down in New York by 50%, 25% reduction of emission in China due to 40% decrease of coal use and a significant reduction of air pollution during pandemic [27]. Nevertheless, financial influences of COVID-19 were very vital, but they highly contributed toward an ecofriendly decarbonized environment, and air quality improved significantly as reported in the various literature [28,29]. Satellite pictures of NASA in order to analyses air quality show 20%–38% reduced pollutants in Korea, Spain, Germany, and the USA [30].

14.3 Impact of waste generation

With the increasing number of patients, BMW generated from the COVID-19 patient wards are also increasing and becoming a bigger concern for hospital. Thus, we have to ensure that this contaminated trash from hospitals should not cause any harm to the public before they are safely disposed. Changes in BMW characteristics are as follows: BMW includes the waste generated from hospitals, medical institutions, medical laboratories, etc. where there are many patients who are managed [31]. Generally, 75%–90% waste generated from hospital is general, nonhazardous waste and does not require any special management, and only 10%–25% are BMW and require special treatment for disposal. But, in a pandemic situation, all the wastes generated within a facility would be measured as BMW and managed with full precautions. To manage these unusual amount of BMW, the existing waste treatment facilities need to be modified based on the real information of the amount produced and availability of the treatment facilities [32]. A report from UNEP says that hospitals generating waste 0.5 kg/bed/day before pandemic increased the same during pandemic by 3.4 kg/bed/day. In India, waste generation increased from 0.5 to 2.5–4 kg/bed/day as reported by Ramteke and Sahu [33]. Also, in a study at a Chinese hospital by Peng *et al.* [10], it is reported that the average waste generation rate is more than 6 kg/bed/day during pandemic. Asymptomatic infections are caused by the COVID-19 virus [34,35], so that there are obstacles in determining the level of COVID-19 transmission in communities and between countries. A method that is quite effective in detecting and analyzing the spread of virus is COVID-19 surveillance in wastewater as it provides unbiased results and it can be used as an early warning system. Wastewater monitoring is a virus identification system that has contaminated the environment and society;

reducing COVID-19 in wastewater can also be used as a marker of reducing COVID-19 cases in the community or region [36]. A most recent study conducted in the United States adopted a wastewater control approach. It was used to reveal the phylogeny of the COVID-19 strain and to enable to evaluate the efficacy of public health interventions to overcome outbreaks [37]. Waste generations in some countries and regions were decreased due to many factors like lockdowns and travel restrictions, especially in tourist cities like Barcelona by 25%; Macao, China, by 17%–25%; and Catalonia, Spain by 17%. On the contrary, COVID-19 leads to increase waste generation in some areas, like England, more than 90% higher than usual [38]. The social-distancing measures reduced the generation of BMW but shifted part of the BMW toward MSW [39]. Most of the developing countries were facing the issues of poor management of BMW much before pandemic [40]. As per the Asian Development Bank report, Manila, Kuala Lumpur, Hanoi, and Bangkok produced 154–280 t of BMW daily during pandemic [41]. Detailed data of MSW and BMW generation in different countries are shown in Table 14.1.

PPE Waste: Till today PPE is the most dependable and reasonably priced item for defending contamination and spread of any viruses. In starting of the pandemic,

Table 14.1 Waste generation in different regions of the world

<table>
<tr><th colspan="2">Decrease in waste generation</th><th colspan="2">Increase in waste generation</th></tr>
<tr><th>Country</th><th>Waste generation</th><th>Country</th><th>Waste generation</th></tr>
<tr><td>Macao, China
Source: Environmental Protection Bureau Macao SAR</td><td>MSW decreased by 17%–25%</td><td>England [38]</td><td>MSW increases to by 0%–20%</td></tr>
<tr><td>Morocco
Source: Ouhsine O</td><td>MSW generation decreased 2%–10%</td><td>Tehran, Iran [42]</td><td>MSW increased by 34.7% and BMW increased by 18%–62%</td></tr>
<tr><td>Trento, Italy [9]</td><td>MSW decreased by 14% (4,058 t/day)</td><td>South Korea
Source: MoE Korea</td><td>BMW increased by 2,600 t/day</td></tr>
<tr><td>Milan, Italy
Source: AMSA</td><td>Total BMW and MSW decreased by 27.5%</td><td></td><td></td></tr>
<tr><td>Catalonia, Spain
Source: Generalitat de Catalunya and ACR</td><td colspan="3">MSW generation decreased by 17% (242,000 t/day) but BMW increased by 350% (1,200 t/day)</td></tr>
<tr><td>India [8]
Ahmedabad, India
Source: TOI</td><td colspan="3">MSW decreased by about 20%–40% but BMW increased by 67%–82%, (1,000 kg/day)</td></tr>
<tr><td>New York, USA
Source: Waste Advantage</td><td colspan="3">MSW increased to 30% but commercial waste decreased by 50%</td></tr>
<tr><td>Tokyo, Japan
Source: UNEP</td><td colspan="3">Commercial waste reduced by 57% but MSW increased by 110%</td></tr>
</table>

Table 14.2 Masks used by some countries

Country	Mask used data
The Republic of Ireland Source: Farsaci	9 million masks/week
Africa Source: Nzediegwu and Chang	700 million masks/day
Iran [45]	5.5 million masks/day
Italy [9]	40 million masks/day

PPE was used chiefly by healthcare experts only, but as pandemic continues, PPE has been used by general population very widely, which leads to increase the demand of PPE during the pandemic. Almost every country has instructed mandatory facemask use for its citizens. The mask uses of some countries are shown in Table 14.2. A mask or PPE is largely composed of plastic (>80%) [43]. The increase in demand and the mandatory masks use transformed the plastic waste generation dynamics and enhanced intricacies of management of plastic and hindered the hard work to decrease plastic trash [44].

Plastic waste: with the change in lifestyle, the use of plastics also increases for convenience and reassurance. But at the same time concern about the reduction of plastic waste was prevalent among everybody based on the world pollution due to plastic. During this pandemic, there is a shift from concern about environmental pollution of plastic to preferring plastic packaging [46]. Demand has risen abruptly for packaging and transportation during this pandemic [47]. In most countries, to control the spread quarantine caused an increase demand for online shop services [44]. Overall, when compared to pre-pandemic, the online trading has increased in pandemic and post pandemic era (16.6%) [48].

Food waste: COVID-19 has made changes in the life style and in the consumption habits, which stimulate food loss and waste (FLW). In April 2020, a survey of US households found, during pandemic, cooking at home increased by 54% ($n = 1{,}005$) [49], which implies more food waste, whereas 57% conveyed less waste, which means net effect with no change. Individuals waste more food, with an anticipation of shortage of food during crisis, which results in excess food storage [50]. In Spain, consumption data shows increase in food purchases (29.8% and 10.9%) in first and second weeks and then decreased by 20.3% in the third week of lockdown, which indicates that pandemic had very less effect on the FLW by 12% hike that might be due to the socioeconomic crisis [51].

14.4 Impacts on waste management

As per the CDC, hazards of transmission of COVID-19 are high in persons who are in close contact with an already diseased person or by touching a surface or object, which is a less known mode of virus spreads. However, OSHA states that acquaintance chance will be increased for the workers who deal with waste and wastewater management. A WHO report showed that in 2000, 21 million people were infected with hepatitis B, 2 million with hepatitis C, and 260,000 with HIV because of polluted needle [52]. However, the waste thrown by isolated families could lead the waste handler workers as well as cloth pickers to risk. It is furthermore crucial to ensure that waste should not be mixed at regular dumping grounds. A good waste management stratagem denotes the program of a facility for managing produced waste for treatment and disposal. In response to the pandemic, every country has implemented the best suitable management strategies based on their resources [42,53]. There should be appropriate facilities to keep waste in temporary storage in sealed container and in very secure areas, in the case of problem in treatment and disposal methods. Disinfectant must use to avoid probable virus transmission. Mobile incineration and autoclaves can be used to dispose the extra BMW generated in pandemic. Designated vehicles should be used for transferring waste with proper record [41] and special permit to collect healthcare waste for smooth handling. The authorities should strictly oversee the process that regulations are followed properly based on national and local guidelines. Any good management system requires an assessment available options, plans, and clearly defined roles and responsibilities of personnel. There should be a waste management committee that will implement the plan. Strategies should be periodically reviewed, and all staff involved in waste management processes should be updated with the periodic changes [54]. Overall, the optimized use of resources and proper waste segregation minimize the waste significantly [45]. As waste generation cannot be predicted with increasing infections, temporary waste treatment technologies like autoclaves burn incinerators, it is difficult to manage waste effectively [55]. Suitable waste management always helps in raising the quantity of recyclable waste by the use of these alternative technologies during the pandemic [42]. Considering all these options, healthcare waste can be utilized to augment value to the country's economy during the pandemic [11,56].

Various international organizations published many policies or guidelines related to waste management from time to time. Some countries have laws related to BMW and some instantly issued new strategies and plans to overcome the pandemic. Unexpected rise in BMW is a huge challenge for all. India also released policies in time to time on BMW management [44]. In Iran, pandemic causes the clearance of infectious waste to entirely stop for a certain period [45]. The National Institute of Public Health, Romania, includes quarantine home generated waste as infectious waste and implements firm waste management actions [57]. Diverse decontamination and discarding methods and technologies are used based on factors like, quantity, type, and costs, some of them are given in Table 14.3 [29,56]. In all-purpose, an amalgamation of chemical disinfection and incineration, the most widely accepted, safe, simple and effective technology would be adopted [29]. In the case of overloaded BMW treatment facilities, industrial furnaces or cement kilns may be used safely [41]. On-site and mobile treatments are preferred due to their flexibility in retorting to fluctuating demands. Fixed, mobile, coprocessing facilities, and nonlocal disposal methods were all successively used in China,

Table 14.3 Disinfection and disposal techniques for biomedical waste (BMW)

Broad categories	Specific technologies
Chemical	Sodium/calcium hypochlorite, chlorine dioxide
Physical	Microwave
	High-temperature steam
Incineration	Pyrolysis vaporization
	Rotary kiln
	Plasma

although all these are supplementary methods of techniques used in waste management [58].

14.4.1 Waste management adjustments

A survival period of viruses on diverse surfaces may vary going up to 9 days [28], which represents that the waste from COVID patient could be a source of infection and managing it will pose a risk to waste workers [9]. The different countries made different adjustments in their waste management. Few common adjustments are summarized next.

14.4.1.1 Healthcare waste/BMW

Whatever best practices available for safe healthcare waste management should be followed, including enough human and material resources to segregate and dispose the waste safely. All waste produced during patient care, including those with confirmed cases, is infectious and should be collected safely as per the national guideline [59–61]. The waste moved out of hospital should be properly handled and treated accordingly or disposed as per the law of the land. All healthcare waste handlers must wear appropriate PPE and perform hand hygiene accordingly. Considering the outbreak, it is expected that infectious waste volume will increase and so of PPE waste, therefore, to handle this additional waste treatment capacity that needs to be increased. Alternative treatment technologies, like autoclaving or high temperature incinerators, may need to be put in place to ensure their sustained operation. The ratio of waste to infectious virus is much less in MSW compared to BMW, but the risk of infection cannot be overlooked from any of the waste. Most of the countries agreed that the recycling method carried very less risk and, thus, normal waste handling and management can be processed like as before the pandemic. In case the waste is polluted with infectious waste, it needs to be managed properly [62].

14.4.1.2 Household waste/MSW

There is no guideline available for household waste/MSW management by any authorized body, but some basic measures should be followed. A waste bag may be kept in the room for items used by the patient, and care-givers must remove their gloves and masks immediately after use in another bag and should be kept near door during leaving. Waste bags must be closed before being removed and never be emptied in another bag. Strict hand hygiene should be maintained after handling waste bag.

14.4.1.3 PPE waste

In the UK, for quarantine patients, PPE waste needs to be put into a black bag waste bin and can be permitted to store for 72 h. The Portuguese Environment Agency recommends that all PPE waste generated by ordinary citizens must be put in a closed and watertight trash bags and disposed preferably by incineration or landfill as opined by Patrício Silva *et al.* [63]. China did not issue any guidelines related to PPE waste. A survey by OCEANSASIA reported that a huge number of surgical masks were found lying on Soko Islands.

14.4.1.4 Dead bodies

Although the danger of virus spread from dead bodies is very less, workers handling dead bodies must follow standard precautions. The mortuary staff preparing or handling the body must wear proper PPE, including impermeable apron, and PPE must be judiciously removed and disposed as per protocol, and hand hygiene must be performed. The dead body of a confirmed or suspected case should be wrapped properly and transferred to the mortuary area as early as possible.

14.5 Challenges in handling waste

Worldwide, the spread of COVID-19 has amplified the use of PPE manifold, and all these littered PPE waste from healthcare and home might be a vector for COVID virus, due to the potential ability of survival of the virus even up to 7 days on masks, gloves, and fomite. Additionally, a polymer plastic, polypropylene, takes long time to degrade and likely culminate in further plastic pollution as reported by WHO [52]. A COVID-19 patient can generate 3.4-kg waste per day that shows the gradual increasing trend in waste quantity in pandemic [41]. The BMW from the healthcare institution and hospital in India is generating 517 t/day. Out of 517 t/day, only 501 t/day waste could be treated in Common Biomedical Management Waste Treatment Facility over 28 states of India. The rest 16 t/day wastes are accumulated untreated daily. Some states like Goa, Andaman Nicobar, Mizoram, Nagaland, and Sikkim are not having CBWTFs at all [44]. Many other countries are also facing alike challenges to manage the vast quantity of waste [41]. Healthcare solid waste in France increased from 40% to 50% and in the Netherlands, it increased to 50% from 40% similar to India and Iran as reported by Zand and Heir [42] and Prata *et al.* [44]. European administrations are facing challenges in retaining waste management staff, providing them a good atmosphere and space for extra waste generated in pandemic. In many of the developing countries, there are no effective BMW management policies and resources. South Asia is a thickly populated section of the world with 24.89% of the global population. Safe and accurate BMW management is a legitimate necessity for such areas to avoid a further health crisis. Also, the urban–rural inequality in waste management is a great challenge. The

INCLEN Program Evaluation Network Study Group reported that a big section of healthcare system (82% of primary, 60% of secondary, and 54% of tertiary care) is lacking in proper waste-handling system [4]. In rural areas, informal practitioners with no or very little practical knowledge handle BMW, and awareness of BMW segregation and management is more different among staff in urban than in rural areas. Lots of studies recommended that these previously mentioned countries need to formulate comprehensive guidelines to seal knowledge gaps in the BMW handling. Developing countries have neglected BMW management in obedience with rules for a long time. The discussed issue of indiscriminate dumping of waste will pose a severe environmental impact and occupational health risks. Besides, ignorant public conduct will put waste handlers at risk as the quarantined domestic litters are disposed with the regular household MSW. During these pandemics, like India, many countries have come up with some thought-provoking problems that include the following:

- The significantly increasing quantity of hazardous elements led to tricky issues of separate waste collection.
- During pandemic, no formal training was given to sanitary workers on how to handle the waste. Arranging regular training to the operators is also a challenging issue.
- Irregularity in supply of PPEs and disinfectants increase the probabilities of collection staff who are prone to get infected.
- Inappropriate donning and doffing of the PPEs among waste worker may increase spread between them.
- Not keeping the social-distancing measures at collection centers and treatment areas.
- Wastewater of healthcare facilities may contain virus, staff who are handling wastewater treatment plants may at a high risk of infection.
- No door-to-door collecting staff are there from residential areas, and the one-point collection is predominant for increasing the infection risk.
- Use of separate vehicles for infected and noninfected waste transport and lack of disinfectant to clean the vehicles increase the chance of spreading the virus.
- Lack of proper monitoring review and verification systems in towns and villages.
- Challenges in implementing strategies and advisory at the ground level people who handling waste.
- Difficulty to make general public aware within short span of importance and rules of segregating the waste.
- At few places, manual loading or unloading of the waste is required, which raises the probabilities of contaminations.

14.6 Rethinking effective waste management

WHO forecasted that the pandemic will continue for an extended time and it will have a longstanding effect on environmental sustainability. Accordingly, the whole world is focusing on prevention plans and vaccine research. Most of the countries were accustomed with or restructured their strategies of waste management for the COVID-19 outbreak. In this connection, China can offer valued inputs considering their experiences of building an all-inclusive disposal system through a mixture of central disposal as well as on-site emergency disposal of waste (like mobile treatment and industrial kilns). The pandemic not only reformed people's lifestyle but stirred extra contemplation on the human and nature relationship. In addition, there are few critical issues about whether the existing systems of BMW management can quickly restore the waste processing, and ability of general population to focus on waste reduction. These issues need to be discussed and studied for betterment in the future. There is not a solitary resolution available for different countries, which varies in terms of infested cases, health resources; therefore diverse resolutions should be implemented. There are lots of issues in dealing with appropriate and actual waste management as it involves many departments and many individuals, requiring interdepartmental collaboration. For a country to determine whether it can manage a substantial rise in BMW production, it should analyze its existing strategies, rules, structures, and also the present operation status of waste management. The main issue is not how to frame the strategies and policies, rather how successfully can they be implemented. To creating a sustainable waste management system throughout and subsequently the pandemic at national or local levels, both strategy makers and experts need to consider at least seven thematic significance areas as mentioned by UNICEF [4].

14.6.1 Policy, regulatory, and guidelines

Although International principles and strategies to managing BMW are available and widely referred to and followed by countries, this only offers a decent foundation in healthcare waste management during the COVID-19 pandemic. Supplementary rules and guiding principle will always be necessary based on the country-specific need and available resources to control the waste generated from both healthcare and non-healthcare facilities, especially when there is an increased generation of infected wastes. During an emergency or pandemic time, a robust arrangement is required with clearly defined roles and responsibilities assigned for waste management, including exigency plan, preparedness for further improvement through review of existing policies. It is very important to conduct a quick valuation of the existing facility systems of the country or city to detect the gaps and how to increase the usage of available facilities toward maximum capacity.

14.6.2 Handling of infectious waste

It is vital to have knowledge about the huge healthcare waste production in the pandemic, but at the same time, scientific understandings, like the viability of the virus, should also be paid attention to make a sound waste management system [4]. It needs to be ensured for the appropriate segregation, packaging, and storage of possibly contaminated wastes. The collection regularity should be based on priority and the type of waste. A proper use of PPE and hand hygiene along with precautionary practices to protect the health of waste employees should be maintained.

14.6.3 *Suitable disposal methods*

Selection of appropriate treatment choices is relative and required to study numerous aspects. It is not limited to national and international principles only, but also ecological and work-related safety, waste characteristics, suitable technologies expenses, maintenance factors, etc. are very important. In reality, in developing countries, there are many facilities that are lacking most desirable technologies for waste treatment. In this situation, it is suggested that such countries should have at least temporary or interim treatment methods like single-chamber incineration or automated pressure pulsing gravity autoclaves, etc. In emergency pandemic, developing countries can put on these interim treatment options, in harmony with the national and international guiding principles. As a sustainable development concept, coprocessing, open burning, and temporary storage as a momentary measure may be considered [41].

14.6.4 *Information, education, and communication*

Healthcare workers are habitually skilled in handling healthcare waste, but capacity building and awareness program is now very much necessary for households and other nonmedical public. Program using a user-friendly communication channel such as radio, television, and websites with everyday displays can intensify public awareness on safe waste handling.

14.6.5 *Data management and learning*

For planning and policy development, the first step is a collection of data. Thus, the importance of data as is immense. However, the availability of the data is often very difficult, particularly during an emergency as resources are allocated during emergency on urgent responses. Help of academic institutions to gather data is a very useful option. Regular discussion is a good practice and is needed to exchange views and lessons learnt for continuous improvement during any emergency situation, specially in pandemic.

14.6.6 *Monitoring of segregation*

There should be a monitoring of the first and foremost step of the biomedical waste management, i.e. segregation that limits the waste generation as well as the spread of infection. Biomedical waste segregation deficiency index (BMWSD index) may be used to monitor the segregation that could be used for training need and corrective and preventive action as discussed by Mondal and Satyanarayana [64,65]. The study shows how BMWSD index improves over 3 months, depicted in Figure 14.1.

14.6.7 *Basic principles for managing waste*

During pandemic, some basic ideologies and guidelines were followed to manage infectious waste during infectious disease pandemic.

Waste generated through healthcare facilities (BMW) is as follows: these types of waste should be achieved using national and international guidelines. Enhanced

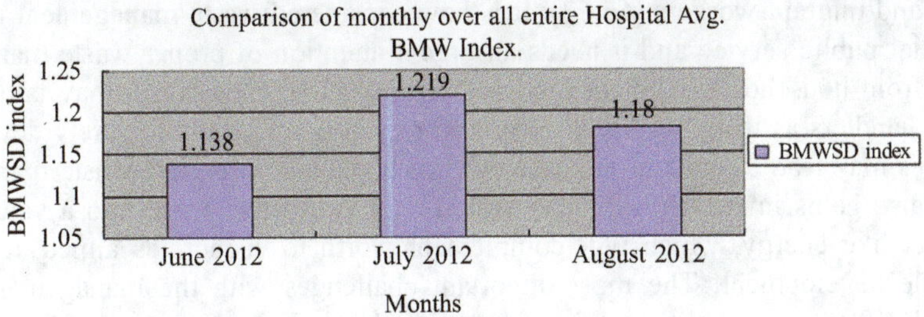

Figure 14.1 Comparison of monthly improvement in average BMWSD index over all entire hospital

treatment and disposal capacities in epidemic areas should be identified based on the analysis of the gaps in capacity for waste, options available, mode of treatment and disposal, local constraints, and considering infection concerns for human health and environmental impacts.

Waste generated through households is as follows: priority should be given to the steadiness of existing waste management services. Contingency planning includes securing availability of necessary human resources and equipment. Special attention is mandatory to alleviate dangers to people doing the waste operations. Reinforce awareness amongst waste management service providers guarantees an adequate supply of materials, and training, and capacity building of the staff.

14.6.8 Fund raising and national and international collaboration

The local government should realize the need of fund-raising activities importance in relation to the BMW management. In future, to tackle such pandemic situation, sufficient fund should be maintained. National and international level collaborations with various agencies are necessary for such abovementioned activities.

The author proposed a new model of waste management during pandemic. First, there should be a detailed assessment or planning of the capacity of the both waste generators and waste handlers. These will help use to plan properly. Out of the three Rs (reduce, reuse, and recycle), first two could not be applicable during COVID-19 pandemic but with suitable technology, recycle must be tried. The main difficulty was the shortage of incinerators. Suggestion for establishment of new incinerators should be thought of to make big hospitals and be self-sufficient with a provision of extra capacity if needed, although the space constrain should be considered and may be relaxed if feasible. More staff training to handle waste keeping all possible precautions is required. Mobile incinerator and industrial incinerators may also be used during pandemic.

14.7 Conclusion and future scopes

COVID-19 made a high impression on economic development and health outcomes. Apart from the economic slowdown, COVID-19 majorly affects the daily wage and migrant workers [66,67]. It is now considered waste management as an essential public service and it needs an urgent attention of proper waste management from households, medical facilities. The contaminated waste may taint the waste handlers as they are directly exposed to waste and use poor safety devices, and this may lead to gradual increase of virus spread. Appropriate waste management also helps in recycling of the waste or renovates the waste into a valuable product like energy, which will complement worth to economies aimed at sustainable development. The most important challenges with the management of COVID-19 are its safe disposal from the point of generation to treatment facilities. There is a great concern on the managing of COVID-19 waste, because the positive cases increase rapidly, and the hospitals are overburdened by such BMW and if precautions do not seem to be ensured then could end in contaminations among sanitary workers. Proper and systematic sanitization practices and adequate PPE for workers involved in handling and collection of BMWs should be mandatory. The staff should be provided with proper and regular training to handle the waste and stop transmission of virus through the waste. Proper segregation in healthcare waste is mandatory for any healthcare organization, which should be monitored in a strict manner. In these, connection matrix methods of monitoring to assess training need assessment with the use of BMWSD index that may be adopted [64,65]. Public awareness for waste segregation at the point of generation at homes before it can harm the other masses should be promoted, which will help to segregate the waste utilized in homes. As PPE is regularly used by everyone, which is made up of plastic, forthcoming research should oriented towards biodegradable environment-friendly protecting items. Regular monitoring is essential, while eliminating COVID-19 waste with the aim that the workers should not get infected by it. The communities at large, who are at home quarantine, must manage their waste properly to make sure the protection of municipal workers and ragpickers. Proper safety kits and training must be used for municipal workers engaged in handling during the outbreak. There are lots of challenges, but suitable strategies and careful handling can alleviate the hazards a lot.

References

[1] Bashir MF, Ma B, and Shahzad L. A brief review of socio-economic and environmental impact of Covid-19. *Air Quality, Atmosphere & Health* 2020; 13:1403–1409. doi:10.1007/s11869-020-00894-8. Epub ahead of print. PMID: 32837620; PMCID: PMC7395801.

[2] Bashir MF, Ma B, Bilal, *et al.* Correlation between climate indicators and COVID-19 pandemic in New York, USA. *Science of the Total Environment* 2020; 728:138835. https://doi.org/10.1016/j.scitotenv.2020.138835.

[3] Chakraborty I and Maity P. COVID-19 outbreak: migration, effects on society, global environment and prevention. *Science of the Total Environment* 2020; 728:138882. https://doi.org/10.1016/j.scitotenv.2020.138882.

[4] WHO and UNICEF. Water, sanitation, hygiene and waste management for the COVID-19 Virus. Interim Guidance, WHO/2019-nCoV/IPC_WASH/2020.2. [Online] April 23, 2020; 1–6. [Cited: April 15, 2021] https://apps.who.int/iris/bitstream/handle/10665/331846/WHO2019-nCoV-IPC_WASH-2020.3-eng.pdf.

[5] Calma J. The COVID-19 pandemic is generating tons of medical waste. [Online] Mar 26, 2020. [Cited: April 15, 2021] https://www.theverge.com/2020/3/26/21194647/the-covid-19-pandemic-is-generating-tons-of-medical-waste.

[6] Lal P, Kumar A, Kumar S, *et al.* The dark cloud with a silver lining: Assessing the impact of the SARS COVID-19 pandemic on the global environment. *Science of the Total Environment* 2020; 732:139297.

[7] Espejo W, Celis JE, Chiang G, and Bahamonde P. Environment and COVID-19: Pollutants, impacts, dissemination, management and recommendations for facing future epidemic threats. *Science of the Total Environment* 2020; 747:141314. doi:10.1016/j.scitotenv.

[8] Somani M, Srivastava AN, Gummadivalli SK, and Sharma A. Indirect implications of COVID-19 towards sustainable environment: An investigation in Indian context. *Bioresource Technology Reports* 2020; 11:100491.

[9] Ragazzi M, Rada EC, and Schiavon M. Municipal solid waste management during the SARS-COV-2 outbreak and lockdown ease: Lessons from Italy. *Science of the Total Environment* 2020; 745:141159.

[10] Peng J, Wu X, Wang R, Li C, Zhang Q, and Wei D. Medical waste management practice during the 2019–2020 novel coronavirus pandemic: Experience in a general hospital. *American Journal of Infection Control* 2020; 48(8):918–921.

[11] Klemeš JJ, Fan YV, Tan RR, and Jiang P. Minimising the present and future plastic waste, energy and environmental footprints related to COVID-19. *Renewable and Sustainable Energy Reviews* 2020; 127:109883. https://doi.org/10.1016/j.rser.202.

[12] European Commission. *Waste Management in the Context of the Coronavirus Crisis*. Brussels: European Commission, 2020.

[13] Association of Cities and Regions for Sustainable Resource Management. Municipal waste management and COVID-19. Municipal waste management and COVID-19. Association of Cities and Regions for Sustainable Resource Management, 2020.

[14] Roberts K, Stringfellow AM, and Williams ID. Rubbish is piling up and recycling has stalled – waste systems must adapt. The Conversation, 2020. Available from: https://theconversation.com/rubbish-is-piling-up-and-recycling-has-stalled-waste-systems-must-adapt-137100.

[15] UK Environment Agency. COVID-19 and storing waste at unpermitted sites due to exceeding your storage limits: RPS C17. UK Environment Agency, 2020.

[16] United Nations. Sustainable development goal 11: Make cities and human settlements inclusive, safe, resilient, and sustainable. United Nations, 2020.

[17] Poon LLM and Peiris M. Emergence of a novel human coronavirus threatening human health. *Nature Medicine* 2020; 26(3):317–319.

[18] van Doremalen N, Bushmaker T, Morris DH, *et al.* Aerosol and surface stability of SARS-CoV-2 as compared with SARS-CoV-1. *The New England Journal of Medicine* 2020; 382(16):1564–1567.

[19] Wang D, Hu B, Hu C, *et al.* Clinical characteristics of 138 hospitalized patients with 2019 novel coronavirus–infected pneumonia in Wuhan, China. *JAMA* 2020; 323(11):1061–1069. https://doi.org/10.1001/jama.

[20] Collivignarelli MC, Abbà A, Bertanza G, Pedrazzani R, Ricciardi P, and Miino MC. Lockdown for CoViD-2019 in Milan: what are the effects on air quality? *Science of the Total Environment* 2020; 732:139280. https://doi.org/10.1016/j.scitotenv.2020.139280.

[21] Messner W. The institutional and cultural context of cross-national variation in COVID-19 outbreaks. medRxiv 2020. https://doi.org/10.1101/2020.03.30.20047589.

[22] Goodell JW and Huynh TLD. Did congress trade ahead? Considering the reaction of U.S. industries to COVID-19. *Finance Research Letters* 2020; 36:101578. https://doi.org/10.1016/j.frl.2020.101578.

[23] Bogoch II, Watts A, Thomas-Bachli A, Huber C, Kraemer MU, and Khan K. Pneumonia of unknown etiology in Wuhan, China: Potential for international spread via commercial air travel. *Journal of Travel Medicine* 2020; 27. https://doi.org/10.1093/jtm/taaa008.

[24] Luan PT and Ching CTS. A reusable mask for coronavirus disease 2019 (COVID-19). *Archives of Medical Research* 2020; 51:455–457. https://doi.org/10.1016/j.arcmed.2020.04.001.

[25] Hellewell J, Abbott S, Gimma A, *et al.* Feasibility of controlling COVID-19 outbreaks by isolation of cases and contacts. *The Lancet Global Health* 2020; 8:e488–e496. https://doi.org/10.1016/S221.

[26] Zambrano-Monserrate MA and Ruano MA. Has air quality improved in Ecuador during the COVID-19 pandemic? A parametric analysis. *Air Quality, Atmosphere & Health* 2020; 13:929–938. https://doi.org/10.1007/s11869-020-00866-y.

[27] Gautam S. COVID-19: air pollution remains low as people stay at home. *Air Quality, Atmosphere & Health* 2020; 13:853–857.https://doi.org/10.1007/s11869-020-00842-6.

[28] Conticini E, Frediani B, and Caro D. Can atmospheric pollution be considered a co-factor in extremely high level of SARS-CoV-2 lethality in northern Italy? *Environmental Pollution* 2020; 261:114465. https://doi.org/10.1016/j.envpol.2020.114465.

[29] Sharif A, Aloui C, and Yarovaya L. COVID-19 pandemic, oil prices, stock market, geopolitical risk and policy uncertainty nexus in the U.S. economy: Fresh evidence from the wavelet-based approach. *The International Review of Financial Analysis* 2020; 70:101496. https://doi.org/10.1016/j.irfa.2020.101496.

[30] Knowland EK, Keller C, Ott L, *et al.* Local to global air quality simulations using the NASA GEOS composition forecast model: GEOS-CF, 2020.

[31] Rupani PF, Nilashi M, Abumalloh RA, Asadi S, Samad S, and Wang S. Coronavirus pandemic (COVID-19) and its natural environmental impacts. *International Journal of Environmental Science and Technology* 2020; 17:4655–466.

[32] Sarkodie SA and Owusu PA. Global assessment of environment, health and economic impact of the novel coronavirus (COVID-19). *Environment, Development and Sustainability* 2020: 1–11.

[33] Ramteke S and Sahu BL. Novel coronavirus disease 2019 (COVID-19) pandemic: Considerations for the biomedical waste sector in India. *Case Studies in Chemical and Environmental Engineering* 2020; 2:100029. doi.org/10.1016/j.cscee.2020.100029.

[34] Nishiura H, Kobayashi T, Suzuki A, *et al.* Estimation of the asymptomatic ratio of novel coronavirus infections (Covid-19). *International Journal of Infectious Diseases* 2020; 94:154–155. https://doi.org/10.1016/j.ijid.20.

[35] Mizumoto K, Kagaya K, Zarebski A, and Chowell G. Estimating the asymptomatic proportion of coronavirus disease 2019 (Covid19) cases on board the diamond princess cruise ship. *Eurosurveillance* 2020; 25(10):1–5. https://doi.org/10.2807/15607917.es.2020.25.10.20.

[36] O'Bannon D., Xagoraraki I, and O'Brien E. Wastewater-based Epidemiology for Early Detection of Viral Outbreaks. *Women in Water Quality*. Springer Nature Switzerland, 2020; 75–79. https://doi.org/10.1007/978-3-030-17819-2.

[37] Nemudryi A, Nemudraia A, Surya K, *et al.* Temporal detection and phylogenetic assessment of SARS-CoV-2 in municipal wastewater. *Cell Reports Medicine* 2020; 1(6):10098. https://doi.org/10.1016/j.xcrm.2020.100098.

[38] ADEPT. COVID 19 – Waste survey results, week commencing 18th May. [Online] ADEPT, 2020. www.adeptnet.org.uk/documents/covid-19-waste-survey-results-wc-18th-may.

[39] Naughton C. Will the COVID-19 pandemic change waste generation and composition? The need for more real-time waste management data and systems thinking. *Resources, Conservation and Recycling* 2020; 162:105050.

[40] Rahman MM, Bodrud-Doza M, Griffiths MD, and Mamun MA. Biomedical waste amid Covid19: Perspectives from Bangladesh. *The Lancet Global Health* 2020; 8(10):e1262. https://www.thelancet.com/journals/langlo/article/PIIS2214-109X(20)30349-1/abstract.

[41] Asian Development Bank (ADB). Managing infectious medical waste during the COVID-19 pandemic. [Online] Asian Development Bank (ADB), 2020. www.adb.org/publications/managing-medical-wastecovid1.

[42] Zand AD and Heir AV. Emerging challenges in urban waste management in Tehran, Iran during the COVID-19 pandemic. *Resources, Conservation and Recycling* 2020; 162:105051.

[43] Prata JC, Silva ALP, Walker TR, Duarte AC, and Rocha-Santos T. COVID-19 pandemic repercussions on the use and management of plastics. *Environmental Science & Technology* 2020; 54(13):7760–7765.

[44] Vanapalli KR, Sharma HB, Ranjan VP, *et al.* Challenges and strategies for effective plastic waste management during and post COVID-19 pandemic. *Science of the Total Environment* 2021; 750:141514.

[45] Rodríguez-Pardo J, Fuentes B, Alonso de Leciñana M, *et al.* Acute stroke care during the COVID-19 pandemic. Ictus Madrid Program recommendations. *Neurologia* 2020; 35:258–263.

[46] Grodzińska-Jurczak M, Krawczyk A, Jurczak A, Strzelecka M, Rechciński M, and Boćkowski M. Environmental choices vs. Covid-19 pandemic fear – Plastic governance re-assessment. *Socialist Register* 2020; 4(2):49–66.

[47] Feber D, Lingqvist O, and Nordigården D. How the packaging industry can navigate the coronavirus pandemic. mckinsey.com. [Online] 2020. www.mckinsey.com/industries/paper-forest-productsand-packaging/our-insights/how-the-packaging-industry-can-n.

[48] Clement J. Coronavirus global online traffic impact as of September 2020. [Online] September 2020. www.statista.com/statistics/1105495/coronavirus-traffic-impact.

[49] Hunter. Food Study Special Report. [Online] slideshare.net, 2020. www.slideshare.net/HUNTERNY/hunter-food-study-special-report-america-gets-cooking-231713331.

[50] Brizi A and Biraglia A. "Do I have enough food?" How need for cognitive closure and gender impact stockpiling and food waste during the COVID-19 pandemic: A cross-national study in India and the United States of America. *Personality and Individual Differences* 2021; 168:110396.

[51] Jribi S, Ben Ismail H, Doggui D, and Debbabi H. COVID-19 virus outbreak lockdown: What impacts on household food wastage?. *Environment, Development and Sustainability* 2020; 22(5):3939–3955.

[52] World Health Organization. Safe Healthcare Waste Management. *Policy Paper*. Department of Protection of the Human Environment Water, Sanitation and Health. Geneva: World Health Organization, 2016.

[53] Singh N, Tang Y, Zhang Z, and Zheng C. Covid19 waste management: Effective and successful measures in Wuhan, China. *Resources, Conservation & Recycling* 2020; 163(105071):1–3. https://doi.org/10.1016/j.resconrec.2020.105071.

[54] Thakur V. Framework for PESTEL dimensions of sustainable healthcare waste management: Learnings from COVID-19 outbreak. *Journal of Cleaner Production* 2021; 287:125562.

[55] Yu H, Sun X, Solvang WD, and Zhao X. Reverse logistics network design for effective management of medical waste in epidemic outbreaks: insights from the coronavirus disease 2019 (COVID-19) outbreak in Wuhan (China). *International Journal of Environmental Research and Public Health* 2020; 17:1770.

[56] Ilyas S, Srivastava RR, and Kim H. Disinfection technology and strategies for COVID-19 hospital and bio-medical waste management. *Science of the Total Environment* 2020; 749:141652.

[57] Mihai FC. Assessment of COVID-19 waste flows during the emergency state in Romania and related public health and environmental concerns. *International Journal of Environmental Research and Public Health* 2020; 17(15):5439.

[58] Yang L, Yu X, Wu X, *et al.* Emergency response to the explosive growth of health care wastes during COVID-19 pandemic in Wuhan, China. *Resources, Conservation and Recycling* 2021; 164:105074.

[59] Bhuyan HK, Chakraborty C, Shelke Y, and Pani SK. COVID-19 diagnosis system by deep learning approaches. *Expert Systems* 2021:e12776. https://doi.org/10.1111/exsy.12776.

[60] Dash S, Chakraborty C, Giri SK, Pani SK and Frnda J. BIFM: big-data driven intelligent forecasting model for COVID-19. *IEEE Access* 2021: 1–13. 10.1109/ACCESS.2021.3094658.

[61] Aslam B, Javed AR, Chakraborty C, Nebhen J, Raqib S, and Rizwan M. Blockchain and ANFIS empowered IoMT application for privacy preserved contact tracing in COVID-19 pandemic. *Personal and Ubiquitous Computing* 2021; 1–17. 10.1007/s00779-021-01596-3.

[62] Ikiz E, Maclaren VW, Alfred E, and Sivanesan S. Impact of COVID-19 on household waste flows, diversion and reuse: The case of multi-residential buildings in Toronto, Canada. *Resources, Conservation and Recycling* 2021; 164:105111.

[63] Patrício Silva AL, Prata JC, Walker TR, *et al.* Increased plastic pollution due to COVID-19 pandemic: Challenges and recommendations. *Chemical Engineering Journal* 2021; 405:126683.

[64] Mondal R and Satyanarayana P. *Bio-Medical Waste Segregation Monitoring in Healthcare Establishment – An Indian Scenario*. LAP LAMBERT Academic Publishing, 2018. ISBN-10: 6139941172; EAN:9786139941179.

[65] Mondal R and Satyanarayana P. A study on bio-medical waste segregation monitoring in a tertiary care hospital at Andhra Pradesh. *Asian Journal of Management* 2017; 8(1):73–77. doi:10.5958/2321-5763.2017.000117.

[66] Roy S and Chakraborty C. Panic buying situation during COVID-19 global pandemic. *Journal of Information Technology Management* 2021; 13 (2):231–244. doi:10.22059/jitm.2021.80625.

[67] Chakraborty C, Roy S, Sharma S, and Tran TA. *Environmental Sustainability for Green Societies: The Impact of the COVID-19 Pandemic*. Springer Nature, 2020. ISBN: 978-3-030-66489-3.

Chapter 15

Natural adjunctive therapies options other than COVID-19 antiviral therapies

Betul Ozdemir[1] *and Zeliha Selamoglu*[2]

Abstract

The coronavirus disease 2019 (COVID-19) pandemic is the largest health problem worldwide. Unfortunately, the lack of an effective and clear treatment causes it to be a major health problem. There are currently no effective antiviral drugs or vaccines. The symptoms and course of the disease differ individually. Symptoms vary from asymptomatic to intensive care, even death. The individual variation of this symptom pattern is related to viral load, individual's current comorbid conditions, age, gender, and most importantly, immune status. Considering the course differences of the disease in all these individual, familial, and demographic distributions, it suggests that genetic and environmental factors play an important role. There is a systemic inflammatory response in COVID-19. High levels of chemokine and proinflammatory cytokines are detected in patients. Nutrition is one of the most important factors for health. With the support of the immune system, people can be protected from COVID-19 and make the process easy when suffering from disease. Apart from the current treatments, some herbal and natural products are used as adjunctive therapy. Key dietary components such as vitamins C, D, E, zinc, selenium, nonflavonoids, flavonoids, polyphenols, and curcumin have been shown to have immunomodulatory properties, which can help with infectious illnesses. Most of these nutrients also have been demonstrated to be useful in the treatment of COVID-19. The importance of such dietary elements in immunity and their particular consequences in COVID-19 patients are discussed in this review.

Keywords: COVID-19; Immunmodulation; Adjunctive therapies; Vitamin D; Vitamin C; Vitamin E; Zinc; Selenium; Nonflavonoids; Flavonoids; Polyphenols; Curcumin

[1]Department of Cardiology, Faculty of Medicine, Niğde Ömer Halisdemir University, Niğde, Turkey
[2]Department of Medical Biology, Faculty of Medicine, Niğde Ömer Halisdemir University, Niğde, Turkey

15.1 Introduction

The 2019 novel coronavirus (2019-nCoV) or it is now referred to as the severe acute respiratory syndrome coronavirus 2 (SARS-CoV-2) that origins in Wuhan City of Hubei Province of China then is rapidly spreading the rest of the world and causes the coronavirus disease 2019 (COVID-19) [1]. In this pandemic period, which affects many individuals, some of the burdens on the health system should be relieved with easy methods [2,3]. Many people with similar symptoms of fever, cough, and shortness of breath applied to health institutions in Wuhan around December 12, 2019 [4]. On March 11, 2020, it was announced to the whole world that COVID-19 was a pandemic. In order to take precautions in pandemics, it is necessary to know the origin of the pathogen, its hosts and evolution. The exact origin of SARS-CoV-2 is still unclear. It has been determined that the genetic structure of SARS-CoV-2 and the genetic structure of the bat SARS-like corona virus are 96% similar. However, new coronavirus genomes have been shown in pangolins showing 85.5%–92.4% similarity to SARS-CoV-2. In the animal kingdom, only bats and pangolins have been found to be infected with SARS-CoV-2-associated coronaviruses [5]. Coronaviruses have a structurally enveloped genetic stalk containing a positive single-stranded RNA [6]. Coronaviruses are divided into four subfamilies: alpha-, beta-, gamma-, and delta-coronaviruses. SARS-CoV-2 is a member of the beta-coronavirus family. Its anatomy has been recognized as spike (S) protein, membranes (M) protein, and envelope (E) protein. The S protein attaches to the cell and allows the parasite to infiltrate the host. The N protein, which is a member of the helix nucleocapsid holding genomic RNA, is just another element of beta-coronavirus [7]. SARS-CoV-2 transmission is known to occur through respiratory droplets and contact pathways. Transmission occurs through droplets from all mucous membranes such as the mouth, nose, and eyes. Contact with surfaces around an infected person causes indirect transmission. Transmission may also occur during the presymptomatic incubation period [8]. Follow-up of contacts is as important for infection control as the diagnosis of infection [9]. After an incubation period of approximately 5.2 days appear the symptoms of COVID-19 infection. The period from the beginning with an average of 14 days is expected for COVID-19 symptoms, and also the patient's immune system response and average of the age of the patient effect on that period are observed. It causes contamination in asymptomatic patients [10]. It has been shown that symptoms generally emerge on the 4th and 5th days after contact [11]. The most common symptoms are fever, cough, fatigue, and shortness of breath. The diagnostic approaches for corona virus diagnosis are basic molecular experiments on respiratory samples (esophagus swab/nasopharyngeal swab/saliva/bronchoalveolar lavage and endotracheal extracts). SARS-CoV-2 RNA, determined by reverse transcription polymerase chain reaction, is collected from the nasopharyngeal swab widely. Apart from the nasopharyngeal swab, virus particles are also detected in the stool and blood. Other laboratory examinations are not specific to the virus and indicate infection. In the measurements made, the white-cell count is normal or low. The platelet count in the whole blood test is usually normal. C-reactive protein (CRP) is elevated due to inflammation. Procalcitonin levels are normal and elevated, which should suggest a bacterial coinfection. Elevated prothrombin time, creatinine, and D-dimer levels indicate the severity of the disease. Chest CT scan presented as an indicator for pneumonia is important clinical assay. SARS-CoV-19 virus predominantly affects the pulmonary system. First, cells in the respiratory system are infected by SARS-CoV-19 and cause inflammation and are observed with some clinical symptom. In pulmonary involvement, a diffuse ground glass appearance is seen on chest tomography. However, the mechanism of the infection pathway is not clear. Angiotensin-converting enzyme 2 (ACE2) receptor for entry into the cells that are abundant in the lower respiratory tract. Importantly, in the brain, heart, intestinal epithelium, vascular endothelium, and the kidneys is expressed ACE2 that makes potential targets capacity for all these organs. In addition, other organ involvement, septic shock, and metabolic acidosis may occur [12]. According to the pathological findings of autopsies and biopsies restriction, in addition to the lung SARS-CoV-19 can inter numerous tissues and organs, as the liver, spleen, heart, brain and kidney [13].

15.2 Immune system and inflammatory responds

Although the physiopathogenesis of SARS-CoV-2 in the body is not known exactly, it is similar to other coronavirus family. SARS-CoV-2 first binds to epithelial cells in the upper respiratory tract, namely the oral and nasal cavities. It then proceeds to the lower respiratory tract and infects alveolar type II pneumocytes. SARS-CoV-2 invades cells using ACE2 receptors [14]. ACE2 is an amino peptidase enzyme that changes angiotensin (Ang) II into Ang (1-7). It is well known that the function of Ang II is a major role in contraction blood vessel, proinflammatory, and pro-fibrotic effects. In contrast, Ang (1-7) is a potent vasodilator, an inhibitor of the apoptotic, and an inhibitor of the proliferative agent. In almost all of the pathological conditions, especially those of the cardiovascular system, ACE enzyme prevents ACE2 enzyme in your body that produces Ang II. Furthermore, the two enzymes ACE/ACE2 play a major role in the renin–angiotensin system homeostasis that regulates blood pressure. In humans, ACE2 receptors are found in many organs. These can be listed as upper respiratory system (nasopharynx, nasal, and oral mucosa), lower respiratory system epithelium, gastrointestinal system (small intestine, colon), kidney, liver, and vascular endothelial cells [15]. The S protein recognizes the ACE2 receptor in the body and provides entry into the cell [16]. After the virus enters the cell, the viral RNA is first copied. Then membrane proteins (S, M, and E) are synthesized. It is transported to the endoplasmic reticulum–Golgi for packaging. Together with genomic RNA, it forms N protein nucleocapsids. The pathogen is transported to the plasma membrane and excreted by exocytosis [17]. SARS-CoV-2 binds to ACE2, causing downregulation of ACE2 receptors, leading to an increase in Ang II. Ang II causes pulmonary vasoconstriction, acute lung injury, and pulmonary edema and fibrosis [18]. Endothelial dysfunction and hypercoagulation may result in pulmonary embolism in

COVID-19 [19]. COVID-19 tries to destroy the respiratory tract and begins to grow quickly in the early stages of infection, though many patients remain asymptomatic [20–22]. Monocytes and macrophages show the first response. Viral replication continues. Vasodilation, endothelial permeability, and leukocyte aggregation are all caused by tissue injury and chronic inflammation. The chronic inflammation in some individuals continues to escalate, leading in systemic inflammation. Several distal organs can be harmed by systemic problems. COVID-19 infection causes cytokine storm and multiple organ damage. The occurrence of cytokine storm is associated with age and gender. In the cytokine storm, proinflammatory cytokines are released uncontrollably and their amounts increase. Excessive cytokine release that occurs causes acute respiratory distress syndrome (ARDS) development in the lungs [23]. When the virus enters macrophages and dendritic cells, it leads to the activation of immunity [24]. It causes cytokine release after CD4+ T cells. Uncontrolled release of cytokines and mediators causes cytokine storm syndrome. The exact mechanism of this syndrome against viral infections is still unknown [25]. Acute lung injury is the result of cytokine storm syndrome. This is seen in patients with SARS-CoV-2 infection, lung disease that can lead to widespread lung damage, inflammation, and ultimately death. High amounts of proinflammatory cytokines and chemokines have been found in the plasma of patients infected with SARS-CoV-2. It has been found that patients with critical illness have higher cytokine concentrations in their plasma [12]. Interleukin 6 (IL-6) plays an important role in cytokine storm syndrome. It has both anti-inflammatory and proinflammatory effects. IL-6 levels have been shown to be associated with the severity of the disease [26]. Whether SARS-CoV-2 releases immunity, and if so, which antibody titers are protective is still a matter of debate. It has been observed that infected patients develop antibody titers 10–15 days after symptom onset. More research is needed to see if antibody titers can predict whether or not a person will recover first from condition.

15.3 Proinflammatory cytokines

During illness in serum IL-1B, IL-6, interferon-gamma (IFNγ), IFNγ-inducible protein-10 (IP10) and monocyte chemotactic protein-1 (MCP1) increase levels of certain inflammatory cytokines. Increasing the amount of proinflammatory cytokine increases the number and function of helper type 1 (Th1) lymphocytes. IL-4 and IL-10 with increasing T-helper type 2 (Th2) are the activation of lymphocytes. At high levels in people is severe disease granulocyte colony stimulating factor, IP10, MCP1, macrophage inflammatory protein 1, and TNFα was determined [9]. In COVID-19, a "cytokine storm" is an important condition that determines the severity of the disease. In the cytokine storm, a large number of immune cells arrive at the infection site, the vascular barrier is damaged, and as a result, multiple organ failure occurs. COVID-19 has been observed to increase the levels of many cytokines. IL-1, TNFα, and IL-6 are the most important proinflammatory cytokines. Increase in IL-6 is associated with higher mortality [27].

15.4 Immunomodulators and adjunctive therapies

The best protection from COVID-10 is to observe social distance, masks, or personal hygiene. However, a healthy lifestyle, exercise, and a healthy diet are also important. Unfortunately, there is no gold standard treatment protocol for COVID-19. This global epidemic must be fought with all available data, including artificial intelligence [28]. Although supporting protocols are recommended, a clear protocol has not been established. Unfortunately, there is currently no vaccine or medical treatment with proven efficacy against SARS-CoV-2 infection. All current studies are conducted with drugs that have previously been shown to be effective in the treatment of SARS-CoV. There is no drug that will directly affect the patient, which will directly affect the virus. For this reason, adjunctive therapies, whose attachments are linked to their previous viral effects, are very valuable. In the treatment of COVID-19, it is necessary to increase immunity and reduce inflammation. In this, it is necessary to reduce the virus–cell relationship and prevent replication. It has been observed that immunomodulators and adjunctive therapies are used to give benefit to COVID-19 patients through antiviral, anti-inflammatory, antioxidant, antithrombotic and immunomodulatory effects.

15.4.1 Phenolic compounds

Phenolic compounds are widely distributed in plants. These compounds are a large group of molecules that have various functions in plant growth, development, and defense, as seconder metabolites in the plants. The compounds include those compounds that can protect the plant against insects, fungi, bacteria, and viruses. Also, there are signal molecules, pigments, and flavors that can attract or repel in phenolic compounds. During this century, there was major changing in trends of consumer preferences toward the natural products owing to the growing knowledge about the health ailment arising due to synthetic additives. Phenolic compounds found in plants are considered to be one of the main stones of the human diet. Many of these phenolic compounds found in natural foods have antioxidant properties. While these compounds are not essential for plant growth, they are essential for human health. Many studies have been conducted on phenolic compounds due to their antioxidant effects.

Phenolic compounds are widely found in nature and have biological and pharmacological activities. There is an aromatic ring attached to the hydroxyl group in their structure. The structure of phenolic compounds varies widely from simple to complex. Phenolic compounds play an important role in the food chain due to their antioxidant effects. These compounds with antioxidant effects are used to extend the shelf life of foods. Unlike synthetic antioxidants, being natural provides additional gain.

There is increasing awareness that these bioactive compounds can have significant positive effects on people's health, physical well-being, and mental states. Prevention and treatment of human diseases in different countries is possible by herbs and plant extracts for medical purposes. The effects of these compounds

Table 15.1 Different classes of flavonoids and dietary sources

Class	Name	Dietary source
Flavones	Chrysin	Fruit skins
	Apigenin	Parsley, celery
Flavonones	Naringin	Citrus, grapefruits
	Eriodictyol	Lemons
	Hesperidin	Oranges
Flavonols	Quercetin	Onion, lettuce, tea, berries, broccoli, tomato, apples, olive oil, cranberry
	Rutin	Buckwheat, tomato skin, citrus, red pepper, red wine
Flavononols	Astilbin	White grape skin
	Genistin	Soybeans
	Taxifolin	Fruits
Isoflavones	Daidzin	Soybeans
	Daidzein	Soybeans
	Genistein	Soybeans
Flavanols	(+)-Catechin	Tea
	(+)-Gallocatechin	Tea
	(−)-Epicatechin	Tea
	(−)-Epigallocatechin	Tea
	(−)-Epicatechin gallate	Tea
	(−)-Epigallocatechin gallate	Tea
Anthocyanidins	Cyanidin	Cherry, grapes, strawberry, raspberry
	Epigenidin	Stored fruits
	Delphinium	Dark fruits
	Pelargonidin	Dark fruits

present in plants show that extensive research is required for drug production. Naturally, occurring antiviral compounds with least toxicity have been found to be the best choice against coronaviruses. Many bioactive compounds are produced as secondary metabolites in plants. The most useful classification of phenolics in two major companies, flavonoids and non-flavonoid polyphenols, is shown in Table 15.1. There are over 6,000 different flavonoids that have been identified, and this number continues to increase. Flavonoids, a large group of phenolic compounds, are found in many fruits and vegetables, giving color and flavor to the foods they are found in. The antioxidant effects of flavonoids are for having three properties. Metal chelating capability, which is significantly influenced by the configuration of hydroxyl and carbonyl groups surrounding the molecule, the availability of hydrogen that is capable of reducing free radicals, and the flavonoid's capacity to delocalize the unpaired electron precursors are all important factors. Flavonoids show their antioxidant effects by chain-breaking reactions. Due to the synergistic effects with other products in plants, instead of taking phenolic compounds as supplements, taking them naturally into foods makes their antioxidant effects stronger. Recently, antioxidants have gained importance due to their role in free radical scavenging to stop the process of oxidation. Nowadays, natural antioxidants importance in human health and nutrition is increased by researching of antioxidants. The Mother Nature's defender can boost up the immune system, lower cholesterol and blood pressure level, many benefits from a compound that comes from many fruits and vegetables. Polyphenolic compounds such as flavonoids have been used since ancient times for their positive effects on health, even before modern medicine was developed. The phenolics are fascinating biologically active compounds that have exhibited great promise in both the inhibition and treatment of many human ailments. Plants create these chemicals in responses to damage or infection by microbial or fungal pathogens. It has antioxidant, anti-inflammatory, antitumor, antimicrobial effects. Biologically, active compounds act by targeting specific sites in cells. It has direct effects on proteins, receptors, and enzymes. They affect the inhibition or activation of enzymes. They provide a modification of proteins. Phenolic compounds are attached to peptides and proteins by hydrogen bonding. As a group effect, it is valuable for human health due to their antioxidation, anti-inflammation, modulation of signal transduction, anti-microbial activity, and anti-proliferation activities. Use of phytochemicals as antiviral agents provides a hope against proliferation of SARS-CoV-2.

15.4.1.1 Resveratrol

Polyphenols, nonflavonoids, and flavonoids are abundant in red wine, grapes, berries, and nuts. These compounds have been shown to have antioxidant, antitumor, and antiviral effects in the organism [29]. Resveratrol (RESV) is a nonflavonoid compound and has anti-inflammatory properties [30]. Besides its anti-inflammatory effect, RESV contributes to antiviral and cellular survival. RESV has been shown to disrupt the SARS-CoV-2 spike protein and to inhibit ACE2 receptor binding [31]. Despite these effects, many studies are needed for effective dosage and safe use.

15.4.1.2 Celastrol

Celastrol has been shown to have anti-inflammatory effects in lung diseases by suppressing NF-κB signaling [32]. It has also been shown to have curative effects in lung diseases by increasing antioxidant defenses by decreasing levels of IL-8, TNFα, and monocyte chemoattractant protein-1 [33]. It has been shown to control ARDS by reducing proinflammatory cytokines and NF-κB activation [34]. Celastrol has been shown to decrease S protein proliferation and cell viral entry [35].

15.4.1.3 Curcumin

Curcumin is a phenolic acid that is found in turmeric. Curcumin possesses anti-inflammatory and immunomodulatory properties, analogous to many other plant phenolic acids [36]. Curcumin protects the cell entrance by binding to the SARS-CoV-2 virus's S protein and the ACE2 receptors protein's viral binding ability [37]. It is known that curcumin's antithrombotic, anti-cytokine, and antifibrotic properties can be used in COVID-19 patients [38]. Despite the known effects of curcumin, more studies are needed because the safety dose in COVID-19 patients is not known.

15.4.1.4 Quercetin

Quercetin may be found in abundance in fruits like apples and citrus, as well as vegetables like onion, broccoli, and tomato. Quercetin functions as an antioxidant that protects bodily tissues from oxidative stress and boosts cell survival rates [39]. Quercetin has high anti-inflammatory activity. It does this by inhibiting the cyclooxygenase enzyme and by inhibiting prostaglandin synthesis [40]. Quercetin decreases viral replication, resulting in decreased viral load.

15.4.1.5 Bee products

Interest in alternative medicine to bee products has increased significantly over the last decade [41]. Propolis has been used from ancient ages due to its useful features in the popular medicine for the treat of various diseases. Most investigators have supported the pharmacological mechanisms as antiseptic, anti-inflammatory, antioxidant features of propolis with their studies [42,43]. Propolis is a gum made by bees from bioactive plant parts. It is currently used as adjuvant therapy in diseases. Anti-inflammatory, immunomodulatory, antitumoral, and antioxidant effects have been proven [44]. While there are many studies proving the antimicrobial activity of propolis, there are limited studies for its antiviral activity. However, it should not be forgotten that bee products contain plenty of phenolic compounds and have predictable antiviral, immune modulatory, and antioxidant effects. The chemical composition of propolis contains many functional compounds. One of the most effective components of propolis is caffeic acid phenethyl ester that is a flavonoid-like compound. Caffeic acid phenethyl ester is an antioxidant component. Pollen, as another honey bee product, is a source of protein, amino acid, mineral, and vitamin for human health. Pollen is collected from many plants by the honey bee. Pollen is a powerful antioxidant and is a polyphenolic compound [45–47]. Phenolic compounds are found in propolis and pollen structure. Due to its antioxidant effects, NF-κB (nuclear factor-κB) regulates the expression and transcription factors of adhesion molecules in endothelial cells. NF-κB is activated with an increase in reactive oxygen species. Anti-inflammatory activities of phenolics may be mediated by transcriptional factor NF-κB in cells [48]. Bee products are known to be potent antioxidants. It was observed that NF-κB activity increased when there was oxidative damage [49–51]. NF-κB is an oxidative stress response factor. Antioxidants can block activate NF-κB [52]. Since there is no clear treatment protocol defined for COVID-19, all therapies that we think can be effective are very valuable.

15.4.2 Melatonin

Melatonin, a pineal gland hormone, has anti-inflammatory and immunomodulatory effects. Melatonin modulates cytokine release by affecting T and B cells with melatonin receptors [53]. One reason for the severe course of COVID-19 in the elderly population may be associated with low melatonin levels [54]. An amount of 2 mg of melatonin taken in the evening is healthy. Administration of COVID-19 melatonin should begin with the contamination of the individual with the sick person.

15.4.3 Zinc

The trace mineral zinc plays an important role in the inflammatory process. Proinflammatory cytokines increase in zinc deficiency. In zinc deficiency, proinflammatory cytokines sensitivity increases in lung epithelial tissues; in addition, cell-barrier functions are impaired. This is why zinc is an essential element in COVID-19 infection [55]. Zinc increases the amount of IL-2, an anti-inflammatory cytokine. In addition, it inhibits the proliferation of coronavirus [56].

15.4.4 Ascorbic acid (vitamin C)

As is known, ascorbic acid in vitamin C is a powerful antioxidant and immune enhancing, especially in high doses. Its powerful antioxidant effect can be used as adjunctive therapy in symptomatic COVID-19 patients to clear cellular toxicity. Vitamin C is effective in infection control. In a study, it was observed that cold attacks decreased with vitamin C support [57]. At the same time, vitamin C has been shown to have an effect on CRP levels [58]. In a study, considering the known benefits of vitamin C, it was applied to COVID-19 patients and a significant decrease in inflammatory markers was detected in patients with severe COVID-19 disease [59]. TNF- and other proinflammatory cytokines are known to be reduced by vitamin C, whereas anti-inflammatory cytokines are increased (IL-10). It has been shown that vitamin C increases the secretion of IL-10. IL-10 operates on the basis of a negative feedback loop with IL-6 so that vitamin C indirectly controls the inflammatory cytokine IL-6 by controlling IL-10 levels [60]. Administration of vitamin C can positively affect COVID-19 patients with ARDS by reducing inflammation, pathogen infectiousness, and virulence, as well as optimizing the immune defense [61]. Cytokine storm, which is a feared situation in patients with COVID-19, can be controlled with vitamin C.

15.4.5 Vitamin D

Vitamin D is a steroid hormone precursor that is fat-soluble. Vitamin D deficiency is a common health problem, and there are many factors that cause it. In the COVID-19 pandemic, vitamin D deficiency was frequently observed in severely ill patients, suggesting the importance of vitamin D supplementation [10]. Vitamin D enhances cellular immunity by increasing the expression of antimicrobial peptides. Vitamin D is known to increase intercellular connections, thereby reducing pulmonary edema caused by viruses [62]. Vitamin D regulates the immune response by modulating the release of proinflammatory cytokines while increasing the release of anti-inflammatory cytokines [63]. Although this has been claimed that vitamin D insufficiency enhances the incidence and severity of COVID-19 infestation, there has been no definitive research to support this theory. Vitamin D intake is indicated to increase immunity versus COVID-19 and prevent human fatalities, according to the theory. Vitamin D deficiency is considered to help defend the respiratory epithelium against bacterial spread [64]. RP, a marker of inflammation, has been correlated with vitamin D deficiency [65]. Vitamin D supplementation increases ACE2 concentrations by decreasing RAS activity in acute lung injury [66]. An increase in ACE2 leads to a decrease in viral activation. Vitamin D levels have been found to be low in severe COVID-19 patients. Vitamin D replacement is still a matter of debate [67].

15.4.6 Vitamin E

Vitamin E is the main component of antioxidant defense. Vitamin E aids immune regulation by regulating immune cells and increasing IL-2 cytokine secretion through its antioxidant effect [68]. In the studies, the protective effect of vitamin E from respiratory tract infections was mentioned. Both immunomodulator and antioxidant effects are important for COVID-19 so vitamin E is one of the essential vitamins for adjunctive therapies.

15.4.7 Selenium

Selenium (Se) is a vital micronutrient for public health. Se deficiency is a common health condition worldwide. Se viral infections are known to be the determinant of the response. Although Se levels are high in seafood, for most foods, the Se content depends on the Se level in the soil. The trace element selenium is the main components of the antioxidant defense. Studies have shown that the immune response changes in Se deficiency. A study conducted in China found that the change in Se levels changed the rate of recovery from COVID-19 [69]. It is important to prevent cytokine storm, which is one of the most important causes of mortality in COVID-19 patients; therefore elements with high antioxidant and immunomodulatory effects such as Se are important [70].

15.4.8 Omega-3 fatty acids

Omega-3 fatty acids are polyunsaturated fatty acids. Severe complications of COVID-19 are seen as a result of cytokine storm. It occurs due to intravascular disseminated coagulation, ARDS, and multiple organ dysfunction syndrome, resulting in death from cytokine storm. For this reason, substances with anti-inflammatory effects are important. They can control the cytokine storm due to the anti-inflammatory, immunomodulatory, and antiviral effects of eicosapentaenoic acid and docosahexaenoic acid, which are omega-3 fatty acids. Omega-3 fatty acids activate macrophages by increasing cytokine release [71]. It reduces the inflammatory process by downregulating the nuclear factor-beta of omega-3 fatty acids. Among lipids, omega-3 fatty acids can inactivate viruses by regulating lipid status. On the other hand, omega-3 fatty acids can help suppress prostaglandin (proinflammatory) production by inhibiting cyclooxygenase enzymes. It also reduces the platelet-activating factor. Thromboembolic events are common in COVID-19, and reducing or inhibiting platelet activation can reduce these events [72]. Because of these effects, omega-3 fatty acids are important in adjunctive natural therapies in COVID-19.

15.5 Dietary ingredients in immunity

There is limited information on nutritional support for COVID-19 patients. However, nutritional therapy has a negligible effect. Foods that have a role on the immune system in patients diagnosed with COVID-19 play an important role. Natural bioactive compounds are valuable in COVID-19 patients for their anti-inflammatory effects and their effects on controlling the disease. As discussed, many natural products can reduce the symptom burden of COVID-19. They have also been shown to have antiviral properties and boost immunological responses. Organic compounds of these minerals and vitamins include fruits, vegetables, meats, fish, chicken, and milk products. Many studies on the effect of nutrition on the immune system have been conducted from past to present. The relationship between COVID-19 and nutrition has just begun to be investigated. The quality and quantity of proteins are an important basis for the immune system. Due to their anti-inflammatory effects, foods containing essential amino acids are in the food group of high biological value. We can sample eggs, meat, fish, and milk [73]. The question is whether dietary vitamins and minerals are adequate for COVID-19. For these substances, the effective dose and duration of use are still unknown.

15.6 Conclusion and future scope for natural antiviral therapies against COVID-19

The distribution of the COVID-19 outbreak differs in all geographic regions. Although the reason for this is not known clearly, it can be associated with eating habits, use of natural medicines, vitamins, or minerals. Since there is no medical antiviral treatment with a net effect, adjunctive therapies come to light. Although there is no clear evidence with these therapies, studies should be increased on these therapies that slow viral spread and increase the response to treatment. When contamination with COVID-19 occurs, it is necessary to protect from the disease by keeping the immune system strong or by reducing its inflammatory reactions in the case of disease. Although there is no mono therapies affecting these conditions, many studies are needed for the use of mono or combined therapies.

References

[1] Wang D., Hu B., Hu C., *et al.* 'Clinical characteristics of 138 hospitalized patients with 2019 novel coronavirus-infected pneumonia in Wuhan, China'. *JAMA*. 2020;323(11):1061–9.

[2] Muhammad L.J., Algehyne E.A., Usman S.S., Ahmad A., Chakraborty C. and Mohammed I.A. 'Supervised machine learning models for prediction of COVID-19 infection using epidemiology dataset'. *SN Computer Science*. 2021;2(11):1–13, 2.

[3] Chakraborty C., Gupta B. and Ghosh S.K. 'Mobile metadata assisted community database of chronic wound images'. *Wound Medicine*. 2014;6:34–42.

[4] Zhu N., Zhang D., Wang W., *et al.* China Novel Coronavirus Investigating and Research Team. 'A novel coronavirus from patients with pneumonia in China, 2019'. *New England Journal of Medicine*. 2020;382(8):727–33.

[5] Zheng J. 'SARS-CoV-2: An emerging coronavirus that causes a global threat'. *International Journal of Biological Sciences*. 2020;16(10):1678–85.

[6] Velavan T.P. and Meyer C.G. 'The COVID-19 epidemic'. *Tropical Medicine & International Health*. 2020;25(3):278–80.

[7] Masters P.S. 'The molecular biology of coronaviruses'. *Advances in Virus Research*. 2006;66:193–292.

[8] Arons M.M., Hatfield K.M., Reddy S.C., *et al.*; Public Health–Seattle and King County and CDC COVID-19 Investigation Team. 'Presymptomatic SARS-CoV-2 infections and transmission in a skilled nursing facility'. *The New England Journal of Medicine*. 2020;382(22):2081–90.

[9] Garg L., Chukwu E., Nasser N., Chakraborty C. and Garg G. 'Anonymity preserving IoT-based COVID-19 and other infectious disease contact tracing model'. *IEEE Access*. 2020;8:159402–14.

[10] Pan X., Chen D., Xia Y., *et al.* 'Asymptomatic cases in a family cluster with SARS-CoV-2 infection'. *The Lancet. Infectious Diseases*. 2020;20(4):410–1.

[11] Guan W.J., Ni Z.Y., Hu Y., *et al.*; China Medical Treatment Expert Group for Covid-19. 'Clinical characteristics of coronavirus disease 2019 in China'. *The New England Journal of Medicine*. 2020;382(18):1708–20.

[12] Huang C., Wang Y., Li X., *et al.* 'Clinical features of patients infected with 2019 novel coronavirus in Wuhan, China'. *The Lancet*. 2020;395 (10223):497–506.

[13] Xu Z., Shi L., Wang Y., *et al.* 'Pathological findings of COVID-19 associated with acute respiratory distress syndrome'. *The Lancet. Respiratory Medicine*. 2020;8(4):420–2.

[14] Zhou P., Yang X.L., Wang X.G., *et al.* 'A pneumonia outbreak associated with a new coronavirus of probable bat origin'. *Nature*. 2020;579 (7798):270–3.

[15] Hamming I., Timens W., Bulthuis M.L., Lely A.T., Navis G. and van Goor H. 'Tissue distribution of ACE2 protein, the functional receptor for SARS coronavirus. A first step in understanding SARS pathogenesis'. *The Journal of Pathology*. 2004;203(2):631–7.

[16] Shereen M.A., Khan S., Kazmi A., Bashir N. and Siddique R. 'COVID-19 infection: Origin, transmission, and characteristics of human coronaviruses'. *Journal of Advanced Research*. 2020;24:91–8.

[17] Li X., Geng M., Peng Y., Meng L. and Lu S. 'Molecular immune pathogenesis and diagnosis of COVID-19'. *Journal of Pharmaceutical Analysis*. 2020;10(2):102–8.

[18] Imai Y., Kuba K., Rao S., *et al.* 'Angiotensin-converting enzyme 2 protects from severe acute lung failure'. *Nature*. 2005;436(7047):112–6.

[19] Wang M., Hao H., Leeper N.J. and Zhu L.; Early Career Committee. 'Thrombotic regulation from the endothelial cell perspectives'. *Arteriosclerosis, Thrombosis, and Vascular Biology*. 2018;38(6):e90–5.

[20] Bhuyan H.K., Chakraborty C., Shelke Y. and Pani S.K. 'COVID-19 diagnosis system by deep learning approaches'. *Expert Systems*. 2021: e12776. https://doi.org/10.1111/exsy.12776.

[21] Dash S., Chakraborty C., Giri S.K., Pani S.K. and Frnda J. 'BIFM: Big-data driven intelligent forecasting model for COVID-19'. *IEEE Access*. 2021:1–13. 10.1109/ACCESS.2021.3094658.

[22] Aslam B., Javed A.R., Chakraborty C., Nebhen J., Raqib S. and Rizwan M. 'Blockchain and ANFIS empowered IoMT application for privacy preserved contact tracing in COVID-19 pandemic'. *Personal and Ubiquitous Computing*. 2021:1–17. 10.1007/s00779-021-01596-3.

[23] Coperchini F., Chiovato L., Croce L., Magri F. and Rotondi M. 'The cytokine storm in COVID-19: An overview of the involvement of the chemokine/chemokine-receptor system'. *Cytokine & Growth Factor Reviews*. 2020;53:25–32.

[24] Li G., Fan Y., Lai Y., *et al.* 'Coronavirus infections and immune responses'. *Journal of Medical Virology*. 2020;92(4):424–32.

[25] Tisoncik J.R., Korth M.J., Simmons C.P., Farrar J., Martin T.R. and Katze M.G. 'Into the eye of the cytokine storm'. *Microbiology and Molecular Biology Reviews*. 2012;76(1):16–32.

[26] Coomes E.A. and Haghbayan H. 'Interleukin-6 in Covid-19: A systematic review and meta-analysis'. *Reviews in Medical Virology*. 2020;30(6):1–9.

[27] Ragab D., Salah Eldin H., Taeimah M., Khattab R. and Salem R. 'The COVID-19 cytokine storm; what we know so far'. *Frontiers in Immunology*. 2020;11:1446.

[28] Chakraborty C. and Abougreen A.N. 'Intelligent Internet of Things and advanced machine learning techniques for COVID-19'. *EAI Endorsed Transactions on Pervasive Health and Technology*. 2021:1–14.

[29] Bravo L. 'Polyphenols: Chemistry, dietary sources, metabolism, and nutritional significance'. *Nutrition Reviews*. 1998;56(11):317–33.

[30] Gao Y., Fu R., Wang J., Yang X., Wen L. and Feng J. 'Resveratrol mitigates the oxidative stress mediated by hypoxic-ischemic brain injury in neonatal rats via Nrf2/HO-1 pathway'. *Pharmaceutical Biology*. 2018;56(1):440–9.

[31] Wahedi H.M., Ahmad S. and Abbasi S.W. 'Stilbene-based natural compounds as promising drug candidates against COVID-19'. *Journal of Biomolecular Structure & Dynamics*. 2021;39(9):3225–34.

[32] Habtemariam S., Nabavi S.F., Berindan-Neagoe I., *et al.* 'Should we try the antiinflammatory natural product, celastrol, for COVID-19?'. *Phytotherapy Research*. 2020;34(6):1189–90.

[33] Shi K., Chen X., Xie B., *et al.* 'Celastrol alleviates chronic obstructive pulmonary disease by inhibiting cellular inflammation induced by cigarette smoke via the Ednrb/Kng1 signaling pathway'. *Frontiers in Pharmacology*. 2018;9:1276.

[34] Wei Y. and Wang Y. 'Celastrol attenuates impairments associated with lipopolysaccharide-induced acute respiratory distress syndrome (ARDS) in rats'. *Journal of Immunotoxicology*. 2017;14(1):228–34.

[35] Iwata-Yoshikawa N., Okamura T., Shimizu Y., Hasegawa H., Takeda M. and Nagata N. 'TMPRSS2 contributes to virus spread and immunopathology in the airways of murine models after coronavirus infection'. *Journal of Virology*. 2019;93(6):e01815–8.

[36] Aggarwal B.B., Gupta S.C. and Sung B. 'Curcumin: An orally bioavailable blocker of TNF and other pro-inflammatory biomarkers'. *British Journal of Pharmacology*. 2013;169(8):1672–92.

[37] Das S., Sarmah S., Lyndem S. and Singha Roy A. 'An investigation into the identification of potential inhibitors of SARS-CoV-2 main protease using molecular docking study'. *Journal of Biomolecular Structure & Dynamics*. 2021;39(9):3347–57.

[38] Lelli D., Sahebkar A., Johnston T.P. and Pedone C. 'Curcumin use in pulmonary diseases: State of the art and future perspectives'. *Pharmacological Research*. 2017;115:133–48.

[39] Xu D., Hu M.J., Wang Y.Q. and Cui Y.L. 'Antioxidant activities of quercetin and its complexes for medicinal application'. *Molecules*. 2019;24(6):1123.

[40] Jan A.T., Kamli M.R., Murtaza I., Singh J.B., Ali A. and Haq Q.M.R. 'Dietary flavonoid quercetin and associated health benefits – An overview'. *Food Reviews International*. 2010;26(3):302–17.

[41] Pasupuleti V.R., Sammugam L., Ramesh N. and Gan S.H. 'Honey, propolis, and royal jelly: A comprehensive review of their biological actions and health benefits'. *Oxidative Medicine and Cellular Longevity*. 2017;2017: 1259510.

[42] Banskota A.H., Tezuka Y. and Kadota S. 'Recent progress in pharmacological research of propolis'. *Phytotherapy Research*. 2001;15(7):561–71.

[43] Burdock G.A. 'Review of the biological properties and toxicity of bee propolis (propolis)'. *Food and Chemical Toxicology*. 1998;36(4):347–63.

[44] Sforcin J.M. 'Biological properties and therapeutic applications of propolis'. *Phytotherapy Research*. 2016;30(6):894–905.

[45] Mărghitas L.A., Stanciu O.G., Dezmirean D.S., *et al.* 'In vitro antioxidant capacity of honeybee-collected pollen of selected floral origin harvested from Romania'. *Food Chemistry*. 2009;115(3):878–83.

[46] Talas Z.S., Ozdemir I., Ciftci O., Cakir O., Gulhan M.F. and Pasaoglu O.M. 'Role of propolis on biochemical parameters in kidney and heart tissues against L-NAME induced oxidative injury in rats'. *Clinical and Experimental Hypertension*. 2014;36(7):492–6.

[47] Selamoglu Z.S., Ozdemir I., Ciftci O., Gulhan M.F. and Savci A. 'Antioxidant effect of ethanolic extract of propolis in liver of L-NAME treated rats'. *Advances in Clinical and Experimental Medicine*. 2015;24 (2):227–32.

[48] Babu P.V. and Liu D. 'Green tea catechins and cardiovascular health: An update'. *Current Medicinal Chemistry*. 2008;15(18):1840–50.

[49] Eckerson H.W., Wyte C.M., and La Du B.N. 'The human serum paraoxonase/arylesterase polymorphism'. *American Journal of Human Genetics*. 1983;35(6):1126–38.

[50] Zheng J.P., Zhang Y., Edvinsson L., Hjalt T. and Xu C.B. 'NF-kappaB signaling mediates vascular smooth muscle endothelin type B receptor expression in resistance arteries'. *European Journal of Pharmacology*. 2010;637(1–3):148–54.

[51] Simão S., Gomes P., Pinto V., *et al.* 'Age-related changes in renal expression of oxidant and antioxidant enzymes and oxidative stress markers in male SHR and WKY rats'. *Experimental Gerontology*. 2011;46(6):468–74.

[52] Xu J., Fan G., Chen S., Wu Y., Xu X.M. and Hsu C.Y. 'Methylprednisolone inhibition of TNF-alpha expression and NF-kB activation after spinal cord injury in rats'. *Brain Research. Molecular Brain Research*. 1998;59(2):135–42.

[53] Srinivasan V., Maestroni G.J., Cardinali D.P., Esquifino A.I., Perumal S.R. and Miller S.C. 'Melatonin, immune function and aging'. *Immunity & Ageing*. 2005;2:17.

[54] Gunn P.J., Middleton B., Davies S.K., Revell V.L. and Skene D.J. 'Sex differences in the circadian profiles of melatonin and cortisol in plasma and urine matrices under constant routine conditions'. *Chronobiology International*. 2016;33(1):39–50.

[55] Skalny A.V., Rink L., Ajsuvakova O.P., *et al.* 'Zinc and respiratory tract infections: Perspectives for COVID-19 (Review)'. *International Journal of Molecular Medicine*. 2020;46(1):17–26.

[56] te Velthuis A.J., van den Worm S.H., Sims A.C., *et al.* 'Zn(2+) inhibits coronavirus and arterivirus RNA polymerase activity in vitro and zinc ionophores block the replication of these viruses in cell culture'. *PLoS Pathogens*. 2010;6(11):e1001176.

[57] Johnston C.S., Barkyoumb G.M. and Schumacher S.S. 'Vitamin C supplementation slightly improves physical activity levels and reduces cold incidence in men with marginal vitamin C status: A randomized controlled trial'. *Nutrients*. 2014;6(7):2572–83.

[58] Jafarnejad S., Boccardi V., Hosseini B., Taghizadeh M. and Hamedifard Z. 'A meta-analysis of randomized control trials: The impact of vitamin C supplementation on serum CRP and serum hs-CRP concentrations'. *Current Pharmaceutical Design*. 2018;24(30):3520–8.

[59] Hiedra R., Lo K.B., Elbashabsheh M., *et al.* 'The use of IV vitamin C for patients with COVID-19: A case series'. *Expert Review of Anti-Infective Therapy*. 2020;18(12):1259–61.

[60] Zhou L. and Xu H. 'A Clinical Study for the Efficacy and Safety of Adalimumab Injection in the Treatment of Patients With Severe Novel Coronavirus Pneumonia (COVID-19)'. 2020. http://www.chictr.org.cn/showprojen.aspx?proj=49889.

[61] Hoang B.X., Shaw G., Fang W. and Han B. 'Possible application of high-dose vitamin C in the prevention and therapy of coronavirus infection'. *Journal of Global Antimicrobial Resistance*. 2020;23:256–62.

[62] Gorman S., Buckley A.G., Ling K.M., *et al.* 'Vitamin D supplementation of initially vitamin D-deficient mice diminishes lung inflammation with limited

effects on pulmonary epithelial integrity'. *Physiological Reports*. 2017;5 (15):e13371.

[63] Jeffery L.E., Burke F., Mura M., *et al.* '1,25-Dihydroxyvitamin D3 and IL-2 combine to inhibit T cell production of inflammatory cytokines and promote development of regulatory T cells expressing CTLA-4 and FoxP3'. *Journal of Immunology*. 2009;183(9):5458–67.

[64] Merzon E., Tworowski D., Gorohovski A., *et al.* 'Low plasma 25(OH) vitamin D level is associated with increased risk of COVID-19 infection: An Israeli population-based study'. *The FEBS Journal*. 2020;287(17):3693–702.

[65] Daneshkhah A., Agrawal V., Eshein A., Subramanian H., Roy H.K. and Backman V. 'Evidence for possible association of vitamin D status with cytokine storm and unregulated inflammation in COVID-19 patients'. *Aging Clinical and Experimental Research*. 2020;32(10):2141–58.

[66] Xu J., Yang J., Chen J., Luo Q., Zhang Q. and Zhang H. 'Vitamin D alleviates lipopolysaccharide-induced acute lung injury via regulation of the renin-angiotensin system'. *Molecular Medicine Reports*. 2017;16(5):7432–8.

[67] Panagiotou G., Tee S.A., Ihsan Y., *et al.* 'Original publication: Low serum 25-hydroxyvitamin D (25[OH]D) levels in patients hospitalized with COVID-19 are associated with greater disease severity'. *Clinical Endocrinology*. 2020;93(5):629–30.

[68] Wu D. and Meydani S.N. 'Vitamin E, immune function, and protection against infection'. In: Weber P., Birringer M.,Blumberg J., Eggersdorfer M., and Frank J. (eds.) *Vitamin E in Human Health. Nutrition and Health*. (pp. 371–384). Cham: Springer; 2019.

[69] Zhang J., Taylor E.W., Bennett K., Saad R. and Rayman M.P. 'Association between regional selenium status and reported outcome of COVID-19 cases in China'. *The American Journal of Clinical Nutrition*. 2020;111(6):1297–9.

[70] Kieliszek M. and Lipinski B. 'Selenium supplementation in the prevention of coronavirus infections (COVID-19)'. *Medical Hypotheses*. 2020;143: 109878.

[71] Albert C.M., Hennekens C.H., O'Donnell C.J., *et al.* 'Fish consumption and risk of sudden cardiac death'. *JAMA*. 1998;279(1):23–8.

[72] Zabetakis I., Lordan R., Norton C. and Tsoupras A. 'COVID-19: The inflammation link and the role of nutrition in potential mitigation'. *Nutrients*. 2020;12(5):1466.

[73] Iddir M., Brito A., Dingeo G., *et al.* 'Strengthening the immune system and reducing inflammation and oxidative stress through diet and nutrition: Considerations during the COVID-19 crisis'. *Nutrients*. 2020;12(6):1562.

Chapter 16

Risk assessment and spread of COVID-19

Challa Sri Gouri[1], D. Ajitha[2], Nikhil Mulaguru[3] and Goteti Rithika[3]

Abstract

COVID-19 has brought tremendous changes in everyone's lifestyle. It also brought awareness among us on how analysis and prediction of situations play a crucial role. These kinds of situations and risk assessments are considered critical factors in reducing the seriousness of the situations. Due to a lack of risk assessment, proper preventive measures cannot be taken. Generally, if an epidemic occurs throughout the world and shows its impact on more people, it is declared a pandemic. In a pandemic situation, the greatest weapon one can use to fight against it is risk assessment and taking measures. The word risk assessment refers to the procedure of identifying, evaluating the factors that cause harm to the environment, and living beings. It also involves making decisions on how to put an end to it. For example, if we consider COVID-19 pandemic, to manage the risk of spreading, analysis was done on understanding the situations that increase the risk of transmission of the virus, identifying the majorly affected people in that situation, coming up with some solution to stop this from happening or to control the situation. In COVID-19, the government provided many practical measures such as wearing masks, sanitizing our surroundings repeatedly, and maintaining a physical distance. This book chapter will have clear discussions on the steps taken to assess the risk and stop the spread of pandemics like COVID-19. We believe that prevention is always better than cure. The chapter presents an analysis of prevention using prediction techniques. Using sentiment analysis in machine learning, weighted density ensembles, forecasting models, and risk assessment can be done. Further, a bot named SAUCHA is proposed for automatic sanitization.

Keywords: Pandemic; Risk assessment; Prediction techniques; Forecasting models; Weighted density ensembles; Sentiment analysis

[1]Department of Electronics and Communication Engineering, Sreenidhi Institute of Science and Technology, Hyderabad, India
[2]School of Computer Science and Engineering (SCOPE), VIT, Vellore, India
[3]Department of Mechanical Engineering, CVR College of Engineering, Hyderabad, India

16.1 Introduction

The novel coronavirus disease 2019 (COVID-19) outbreak rapidly spread worldwide, causing a public health crisis globally [1]. Risk assessment consists of two words: risk and assessment. Risk can be defined as a situation in which the chance of people being harmed due to any hazard is high. Assessment refers to the analysis of factors that can cause harm. The magnitude of the increase in confirmed cases in an influenza pandemic is a proxy for epidemic size and disease transmissibility [2]. This complete process will help us to identify the problem, understand, and analyze the reasons and the risks associated with it. Risk analysis includes two major steps. They are risk evaluation and risk control. Whenever there is an occurrence of any situation that has a negative impact on the health of the people this risk assessment is used. This book chapter will discuss the steps taken to assess the risk of COVID-19 and its spread [3].

Coronavirus belongs to the family of viruses that is capable of causing common cold to severe health issues. The first case of coronavirus was found in the month of December. In the month of February, many countries were affected by this making it an issue of international concern. The name COVID-19 was issued to the coronavirus disease on the February 11, 2020 by the World Health Organization. It is declared as a pandemic in the month of March. The word pandemic in medical terminology can be defined as the condition in which there is a rapid spread of a disease throughout the world, affecting millions of people. This data shows us how rapid the spread of the virus was.

Assessing the risk associated with COVID-19 WHO issued few guidelines to all the countries like maintaining 1-m distance from each other, wearing masks, and sanitizing regularly. Countries also issued guidelines for lockdown to stop the transmission and to break the chain of virus. COVID-19, in our opinion, has become a pandemic, with small chains of transmission in many countries and large chains resulting in widespread infection in a few countries such as Italy, Iran, South Korea, and Japan [3]. The findings revealed that controlling infectious disease transmission is the primary concern in pandemic disease [4]. This chapter gives information about various methods used for risk assessment and different strategies for the management of epidemics.

16.2 Technology and epidemics

Pandemics have a massive impact on our lives, economies, and social orders. A pandemic is characterized as a sickness that quickly spreads in various nations and countries. Pandemics slaughter vast numbers of individuals. In recent years, we have seen three lethal pandemics: the 1918 Spanish Flu, 1957 Influenza, and 1968 Hong Kong Flu [5,6]. The outburst of the 2013 Ebola virus in Africa has affected numerous lives. Effective regulation of this flare-up depends on fast and viable coordination and correspondence. Early location and reaction are fundamental to effective control. However, its utilization in the Ebola outbreak reaction has been restricted. Because of the requirement for the early disclosure of new EVD cases and immediate treatment, colleagues passed information to empower a smooth and fast information stream [7]. A successful regulation of external ventricular drain (EVD) depends on a methodology that includes different intercessions: case the board, observation and contact following, correspondence, and social assembly. In addition, the utilization of active surveillance, comprising close management and collection of vital signs and critical clinical indications, is essential to the strong restraint of EVD.

Gene Xpert was initially designed to detect tuberculosis cases but has since been modified to allow rapid testing of various pathogens, including HIV, malaria, STIs, and Ebola. It is one of the technologies used to detect Ebola in the DRC. For example, technicians at the INRB laboratory in Kinshasa can use Gene Xpert to test for the Zaire strain of Ebola in just 1 h, with the help of USAID, WHO, Canada, the Global Outbreak Alert and Response Network, and the Emerging and Dangerous Pathogens Laboratory Network. If a sample is found to be negative, it is tested again to see if it contains any other Ebola strains, other viral hemorrhagic fevers, or other diseases [8].

OraQuick is a quick diagnostic test developed in collaboration with the US Centers for Disease Control and Prevention (CDC) and GOARN. In less than 30 min, OraQuick will test blood or saliva samples for Ebola [9]. Users can enter the latest data or change the data saved on their phones using the ODK Collect Application. When the data is finalized, it is submitted. During submission, the location is automatically integrated with the data. The form hub technology created forms using the same paper forms that were used to collect data [10]. Whenever new cases are discovered, the contact tracer enters the information into a new case on the phone then sends it directly to the form center server. If for any reason, the phone does not have an Internet connection, the collected data is stored temporarily on the phones. At the end of the day, when they are returned to the control center, the phones are connected to the Internet, and stored data is affixed to the server.

The Dashboard technology mainly focuses on providing information based on proofs to assist the management to make timely decisions. A TV is used to show the live updates of daily contacts, the interviewers. It can also show symptomatic contacts as well as maps displaying the location of contacts that have been traced up in the last 2 days. One of the dashboard segments also shows lab results for speculated and confirmed cases. The detected contacts and cases within the cities were plotted with the help of coordinates that were recorded on the ODK forms and then combined using ArcGIS Mapping software to display the contacts and cases in the cities. These informed areas concentrated on social mobilization, sensitization, and awareness generated by social mobilization teams.

COVID-19 is a global pandemic on par with World War II and the 1918 Spanish Flu. For suppressing the COVID-19 pandemic, physical distancing and self-quarantine are required. To maintain this mandate while preserving the current state of things, various human behaviors, such as entertainment, education, meeting, and working, have transitioned from online to offline. This resulted in the emergence of a variety of digital technologies. There are extensive digital technologies being used in the COVID-19 epidemic. Based on the different types of technology, it is categorized into hardware and software. To tackle COVID-19, roughly 15 hardware and over 50 distinct kinds of software technologies were deployed [11–13]. Compared with the Spanish flu, SARS CoV-2 has spread very quickly across every continent in a matter of months. In addition, the use of hardware and software technology remarkably enhanced the healthcare sectors capability to recognize, track, and contain infected persons.

Hardware technologies, for example, computerized tomography machines in the medical field and computers, phones, and video-based communication platforms in work, education, and daily life, have brought about an unprecedented transformation in our lives.

Hardware: The computerized tomography machine is commonly used for early detection and diagnosis because of the coronavirus's distinct characteristics. It is the most widely suggested technology in healthcare sector. The computerized chest tomography has a higher sensitivity for COVID-19 diagnosis than the RTPCR test [14]. Using chest computerized tomography devices and deep learning technology, coronary artery diseases can also be detected and differentiated from pneumonia and other lung diseases [15]. Various technologies, such as mobile phones, computers, and robots, are indispensable for remote surveillance and diagnosis during the epidemic. The majority of coronavirus patients can be managed remotely, with home quarantine instructions. Though video consultations can often be conducted over the phone, the video provides visuals and a therapeutic presence. Mobile devices and webcam attached computer applications like Zoom and WebEx play a crucial role in providing virtual education, work from home, and everyday life.

Software: In comparison to hardware technology, many software technologies are more widely used. Video-based communication platforms are the most advanced technology in the healthcare domain. COVID-19 patients and those requiring other normal healthcare services can benefit from phones, tablets, computers, and social media. Video-supported communication platforms, such as Zoom, WebEx, and Google, meet are digitally safe and effective conferencing in this particular time. Online video lectures can be carried by using Blackboard, coursera, and other platforms that enable continuous knowledge distribution for education. Digital information is used for virtual services data exchange at work using online surveys, Google Sheets, and other telework tools. Furthermore, social media platforms such as Twitter, WhatsApp, Facebook, Instagram, and YouTube, and technologies such as Google Trends and GIS System track, locate, and analyze outbreaks in real time [16].

Mix use: Aside from hardware and software, there are around five kinds of integrated technologies used to monitor, prevent, and detect outbreaks, such as IoT, artificial intelligence, virtual reality, computerized tomography, and the Internet of Medical Things. The majority of people who use technology are divided into four categories: healthcare, education, work, and others [17]. There are two types of users when it comes to technology: providers and receivers. In the healthcare sector, for example, medical professionals are the suppliers who employ technology to give service. In contrast, patients and infected individuals are the receivers.

Employers and teachers are examples of providers, whereas employees and students are receivers in the education and work sectors. Even though they utilize diverse types of technology in their daily lives, they all employ the same kind.

16.2.1 Healthcare

During the pandemic, medical professionals and patients with various chronic diseases are the most frequent consumers of digital technology. On the front lines, radiologists, surgeons, and nurses are diagnosing and treating patients. The radiologists play a critical role in diagnosing computerized CT scan for a patient either positive or negative for COVID-19 disease and describing primary CT characteristics and lesion distribution. In addition, patients with various chronic conditions, particularly those who have already been infected with the coronavirus, get services and treatment from healthcare experts via technology during the same time. Patients with many immune suppressed or chronic diseases, for example, will have to choose between risking iatrogenic COVID-19 exposure at the time of a doctor visit and delaying required treatments. In addition, patients must deal with the unavoidable utilization of technology, for example, the computerized tomography equipment, video communication platforms to acquire advice and directions from a healthcare expert, whether they choose a direct appointment, postpone a visit, or use virtual healthcare [18]. As a result, the main groups of technology users at COVID-19 are healthcare professionals and their patients.

16.2.2 Education

Because of COVID-19, a considerable portion of the population was forced to study from home to comply with the quarantine obligation. The teachers quickly adapted to online teaching and put significant effort into preparing for online classes and engaging the students. The majority of the education sector uses video-based communication devices and platforms. During this epidemic, students and teachers have surpassed the general public as the second most frequent consumers of digital technology [19].

16.2.3 Work

Work professionals have emerged as a significant segment of technology users during the pandemic. During COVID-19, researchers, scientists, and employees continue to work remotely using digital technologies. From the work standpoint, regardless of the technology employed, most work professionals serve as contributors and receivers. An employee, for instance, receives guidance from their boss while also having to report their work via Zoom.

16.2.4 Others

Apart from the two primary users listed before, health authorities, government officials, and the public all use technology. To deal with this global spread, individuals worldwide are becoming more familiar with the technology they use daily. Public health experts and government officials, for example, employ mobile-based monitoring technologies to follow the spread of an epidemic or big data technologies to assess outbreaks and devise policies. At the same time, the general population receives information via digital devices from all over the world.

16.3 Prediction techniques

After the outbreak of COVID-19, many techniques were used to control its transmission. The control measures taken by various governments include three stages: screening, suppression, and mitigation. Screening refers to checking the body temperatures of a person using a thermometer to analyze whether he/she is affected by the fever caused by the virus. Suppression and mitigation are considered integrated steps that are carried out based on the results of screening. In case he/she has abnormal temperatures, they can isolate themselves, which helps in avoiding the transmission of virus. This isolation will also help them in reducing the effect of viruses on their health that is known as mitigation. Prevention is better than cure. If we are able to predict the conditions, managing the situation becomes a piece of cake for us. There are various prediction techniques proposed, which can be effectively implemented. Various improvements are possible in the existing analysis, which can help us in the prediction of epidemics.

The three major points we need to consider while discussing the epidemics caused by animals or other organisms are their toxicity, means of spread, and measures to be taken. As we are a part of the food chain, toxicity at any level can have an everlasting impact on us. It can also cause the spread of microbial diseases. Many microbial diseases or epidemics in the past were also spread due to various organisms and animals. As per the statistical data, it is very clear that 60% of all human diseases originate in animals.

Let us have a look at the data indicating reasons for various epidemics:

Rabies—mammals
Anthrax—spore-forming bacteria and infected animals
Arbovirus—arthropod-borne virus
Avian influenza—poultry, animals
B virus—macaque monkeys
Brucellosis—goats, sheep, cow
Cat scratch disease—young cats and kittens

To stop the spread of these kinds of diseases, it is essential to monitor toxicity at each level. These kinds of diseases caused by animals are known as zoonotic diseases. These diseases can be airborne, vectors (transmitting infected agents from animals), close proximity to animals, and foodborne. The motto of discussing these points in prediction techniques is that when we analyze the past data, we can take some measures that can help us be ready to face any epidemics in the future.

Few other prediction techniques are as follows:

1. Data analysis
2. Mathematical prediction models
3. Recursive-based prediction model

4. Beesham's prediction model
5. Boltzmann function-based prediction model
6. Performance evaluation criteria

Data analysis: In prediction techniques, data analysis is considered the major step. In this step, we collect the data from the past epidemic experiences and start working on it using various techniques and models. The experts majorly do this data analysis in that field to give the best results in preventive measures. Working on data related to epidemics can help us to be prepared for any future situation.

Mathematical model: A mathematical model can be defined as the diagrammatic representation through which we can analyze the reasons behind a particular aspect. It has a set of variables and equations that are satisfied by the system.

Recursion-based prediction model: We can analyze the relation between the number of cases confirmed in a day and the number of cases confirmed on a previous day. It helps us in relating death and recovery cases [15].

Beesham's prediction model: Due to the increase in the number of corona cases, several models were recommended for predicting the COVID-19 outbreak in the literature using exponential function. In the similar manner, Beesham's mathematical model, which was recommended for considering the confirmed cases of the COVID-19 in South Africa [20], was also using an exponential function.

A Boltzmann function-based prediction model: The Boltzmann function helped us by providing a prediction model for the COVID-19 outbreak. The derived relation, which is represented by an Equation, is related to the sigmoid function. The exception is linear transform [21].

Another common technique used for prediction is analyzing the condition of the person affected by the virus. This study helps us in understanding the factors and taking preventive measures as per the requirement. Wearable devices also play a crucial rule in monitoring and detecting cases of COVID-19. Devices such as smart watches can be used to track the health condition of a person. Many of the papers also suggest that these wearable devices can analyze and predict the virus attack even before seeing the symptoms analyses modern trends of Internet-based surveillance, taking advantage of computational science methods: Web queries, Google Trends [22]. We can clearly understand that various techniques can be implemented to predict epidemics even before they occur. The major tool for prediction is data. If we successfully gather enough data from past situations, analysis and prediction are quite simple tasks.

16.4 General methods followed for risk assessment

In the previous sections of this book chapter, we had an elaborate discussion of risk assessment. In this section, let us discuss various methods used for risk assessment in detail with their specifications, advantages, and disadvantages.

In general, risk assessment includes the following steps:

1. Identification of the problem
2. Analysis of its effects

3. Assessment of risks
4. Preparing report
5. Reviewing and implementing the measures

While working on risk assessment, we consider the following factors. Risks generally include health, environment, finance, technology, safety. In general assessment, we also use 10Ps principle. Risk assessment can be performed in two ways: individual and group. Individual risk assessment is carried out by considering each and every individual. This helps us to understand the risk at the root level. This assessment majorly focuses on the psychological and ideological factors of individuals. Most of the individuals feel there is no risk for them and their situation is in control. This type of analysis is considered essential during pandemics. Group risk assessment is generally performed in a group or large scale where individual's conditions are not given much priority. For example, risk assessment during a cyclone comes under this category. We also name this as system risk assessment. As we are aware, a system can be linear or nonlinear. When a system is linear, assessment is easier. In the case of nonlinear as data changes frequently, probabilistic analysis can only be possible.

In organizations, a concept called risk register is used to access the risks. This register will store all the information related to the risks, which helps that organization monitor, analyze, and manage the risks. The fisheries science and management practitioners at a recent time have begun to carry out formal risk management processes for fishing activities [23]. A personal perspective and lessons learnt through risk assessments applied to the management of numerous significant species and ecosystems are presented. The significance of engaging and empowering stakeholders through more intuitive risk assessment methodologies so that they can actively comprehend and participate in the risk assessment process is one of the key lessons gained [24]. The development of the "Risk Society," in which governments, communities, organizations, and individuals spend much of their day-to-day efforts managing risk and, where possible, transferring risk to others, has been linked to the modernization of many nations over the last century, according to prominent sociologist Ulrich Beck [25].

The health sector's policies and regulations are becoming increasingly risk-based. As a result, indicators that focus on the risk to life expectancy, or the average number of years foregone or added as a result of a proposed policy instrument, are increasingly routinely used to evaluate health policy [26].

To understand risk assessment in detail, let us discuss the following methods:

1. What-if analysis
2. Fault-tree analysis (FTA)

16.4.1 What-if analysis

As the name suggests, what-if analysis is the process in which a person with the knowledge on that particular aspect will ask questions to analyze what happens if some undesired event occurs. To assess the risks associated with a particular undesirable event that may cause health hazards, one must be aware of its origin, causes, and consequences and should have complete information about that aspect.

In this analysis technique, people with expertise in that particular topic will sit together. They start with identifying the problematic situation, its effects, and methods that can be used to tackle them. They discuss existing solutions, their disadvantages, and the improvements that are needed. Through this thorough discussion, they discover opportunities for new methods to be successfully implemented [27]. The steps that are followed by them are as follows:

1. Presenting detailed diagrams and guidelines
2. Prepare questions
3. Analysis and assessment of risk
4. Discussion
5. Summary of the major points
6. Preparation of plan of action

Limitations of this method:

1. Majorly depends on the questions that are framed.
2. Active participation of members is essential.
3. This method is considered introspective.
4. Reviewer plays a major role.

Advantages of this method:

1. Simple and easy
2. No requirement of specialized tools

16.4.2 Fault-tree analysis

This is a method in which we understand the reason for a failure due to which we get undesired outcomes or events. In FTA, Boolean logic is used. This system is mainly used in various engineering streams to detect the reasons behind systems failure and decrement the chances of risks associated with that. Aerospace engineers majorly employ this technique during designing [28]. FTA technique was developed in the year 1962 in Bell laboratories. At present, it is used in reliability systems for risk assessment. In this analysis, by creating a logic diagram, we will be able to figure out the relation between fault, subsystem, and safety design elements.

The system's failure is considered the root of the tree, which represents the outcome that is undesired. While we are working on top-down analysis, this failure may happen due to two reasons. They are mistakes during normal operation or errors in the maintenance operation. Any error among these two will result in failure. So it is considered OR logic. Again considering the normal operation, it has two branches, which leads to another OR logic. To overcome the failure, improvements must be made in the design that is considered logical AND. By programming these logics, we can get the probabilities of failure using the FTA technique.

Early on, we have seen human errors and negligence causing disasters [29]. There are few algorithms and analysis that help in predicting the probability of errors occurring. One such analysis is the FTA [30]. FTA is an analysis tool that helps identify faulty events and would result in damages and disasters if not corrected on time [31]. It can be said that FTA is a hierarchical model defining the topmost columns—the ones that are the most important operations, which include various fields of production, distribution, maintenance based on the implementation area [32]. Thus, making the FTA defined events as a set of true or false assertions, cutting down all the undesirable conditions using the logic gates [33].

It would be a good practice to implement FTA before initiating any projects or activities to overcome hurdles later on and can avoid great tragedies. Some of the applications of FTA are reliable power systems [34]. Gas leaks from the industrial sites can be halted [35]. Usage of hazardous methods in the production can be seized in its initial stage [36]. Implementations of both Environmental Impact Assessment (EIA) and FTA together bring awareness in the public about the environment and help in detecting the areas of errors and prevent it from happening, ensuring a secure environment [8].

To represent these logics in FTA symbols like basic event, external event, undeveloped event, conditioning event, intermediate event, let us have a brief discussion on the steps included in FTA:

1. Identification of undesired event
2. Understanding the working of system
3. Designing the fault tree
4. Analyzing the fault tree
5. Assessing the risks

Advantages of FTA:

1. It is suitable for computer programs.
2. Capable of finding faults in different paths.
3. Effective in analyzing the reasons for faults.

Let us also discuss the guidelines that are issued by the World Health Organization to control this situation.

16.4.3 Guidelines issued by World Health Organization

WHO issued the guidelines based on the phase in which they are. The phases are as follows:

1. Providing information to the people and bringing awareness to them.
2. Developing proper understanding of people, which makes them ready to face any situation.
3. Taking proper measures so that people can adapt themselves to the situation.
4. Measures to be taken and steps to be followed.
5. How to handle activities after and during the epidemic.

Hand hygiene, respiratory hygiene, and basic food safety procedures are among the WHO's basic recommendations to the general population to avoid exposure to and transmitting a variety of diseases [37]. Furthermore, providing supportive care to infected individuals can be pretty helpful [38].

The chance of contracting COVID-19 is determined mainly by age, gender, and other conditions (obesity, diabetes, lung disease, kidney disease, and heart disease) [39].

The key points of the mentioned guidelines are as follows:

1. Avoiding social gatherings
2. Maintaining social distance
3. Wearing masks
4. Sanitizing regularly and repeatedly
5. Providing accurate and regular updates to people.

16.5 Prevention and management of epidemics

Prevention can be defined as the steps that we take to stop or prevent something from happening. Management with respect to epidemics can be defined as the measures that we take to control the spread and transmission of disease. In the epidemics, subject prevention and management are considered key factors. Prevention is the step that we take to avoid the disease from occurring. Management is the step that we take to control the effect or impact of the epidemics after it occurs. In this section, we will have an elaborate discussion on various preventive measures and management techniques. The strategies proposed in this regard are focused on one of the best analysis techniques of machine learning, that is, sentimental analysis.

During the ferocious outburst, clinical specialists have been attempting to develop novel treatments and vaccines, and scientists were working in the fields of data science and technology have been attempting to discover the infectious agent and aid in its control through the use of information-based methods [40].

Despite advances in medical research in treatment, pathogen discovery, and diagnostics, infections can still spread widely and cause serious health consequences. Modern technology, on the other hand, has introduced new approaches and tools [41].

The general preventive measures that can be taken to protect ourselves from COVID-19 are as follows:

1. Do not touch your face.
2. Sanitize your hands regularly and repeatedly.
3. Maintain distance from others. Do not shake hands.
4. Use a napkin while sneezing or coughing to cover your mouth and nose.
5. Never use other's belongings.
6. Avoid going to crowdie places and social gatherings.
7. Wash everything before using.
8. Wear a mask.
9. Self-isolation can be considered the best measure in case if you feel you are sick.

Management of epidemics: If we can predict the epidemics through the techniques that we discussed in the previous section, like what-if analysis and fault-tree analysis, management becomes very easy as we can understand and analyze the situation very easily. Management completely concentrates on stopping the spread of virus and reducing the number of people affected by it. Epidemic preparedness is very crucial in this regard. Another crucial factor to be considered is the management of epidemics that comprises combination of various sectors like public and health. Active involvement and response from all the sectors are also important. Coordination and cooperation between various sectors is crucial in effective management.

The causes of epidemics may be different but most of the effects are almost similar. Even during this COVID-19, one of the countries was able to effectively manage the situation. As a result, the rate of transmission and number of corona deaths were very low when compared to all other countries. The reason behind this is that particular already faced this kind of situation which helped them in predicting and taking measures as per the requirement.

Various strategies are employed for the effective management of epidemics. Let us explore them.

16.5.1 Strategies proposed

When compared to all other countries, Africa is the country that is least affected by COVID-19. The main reason behind this is the steps taken for the early detection of cases and self-isolation. When we are discussing the strategies for effective management following points must be considered:

1. Health and public sector workers must be provided support and their safety must be considered a major priority.
2. Proper maintenance of hospitals.
3. Developing strategies that will help us in making our health system strong.
4. Strategies must be framed considering individual case studies.
5. Active response and communication between various departments for effective management of the situation.
6. Food, water, and health facilities must be properly provided.

Strategies of various countries

Japan: In Japan, they have followed the strategy of identifying the contaminant zones. In these zones, they doubled the rate of tests. Strict rules were made to stop the travelers from other places to these contaminant zones. The major point is the cost of treatment that is completely covered by the government [42].

South Korea: They employed a screening strategy in huge number for the individuals with symptoms. They were successful in bringing awareness to people about thermal screening and sanitization. Strict rules were imposed and social gatherings were banned.

By considering various strategies implemented by different countries effective strategies are listed as follows:

1. Maintaining physical distance
2. Tracing the infected person and his contacts
3. Performing corona tests

4. Improvement facilities and staff in hospitals
5. Pre-supply of PPE kits
6. Proper communication and coordination
7. Immediate response

16.5.2 Sentimental analysis using machine learning

The term sentimental analysis refers to a tool used to analyze the emotions in text. Using these machines can analyze feelings and emotions without human interference. The models are trained to understand the feelings hidden behind the text, such as anger and sarcasm.

The prominence of rapidly growing online social networks and media-based societies has impacted young researchers to work on sentiment analysis. These days, most businesses depend on customers or people's opinions regarding their products from social media [43]. Due to the lack of opinion text present in the digital form, there was very less working interest on computational linguistics in the end decade of the twentieth century was noticed [44].

Working of this technique: Various techniques and algorithms are used to train the models to perform sentimental analysis. The Bayes theorem of probability can be used to check whether a word is given in positive or negative context:

$$P\left(\frac{A}{B}\right) = P\left(\frac{B}{A}\right) \times \frac{P(A)}{P(B)}$$

In this, words can generally be calculated against each other. Using the trained models, we can analyze whether the word is positive or negative.

Apart from the Bayes theorem of probability, the other algorithms used in the analysis are as follows:

1. linear regression,
2. support vector machines.

Deep learning can also be used when multiple algorithms are used at the same time.

For example, if you type "I am so sad," using the sentimental analysis datasets, the machine will understand that sad is a word that describes negative emotion.

- **Use of sentimental analysis in management of COVID-19**

In the present situation, social media is playing a vital role. This sentimental analysis can be performed on any social media handles like Twitter, Instagram, and Facebook [45]. For this analysis, we require two stages as follows:

1. Dataset preparation stage
2. Analysis stage

Using this, we can analyze the intensity of words and the polarity of words, which helps to know the condition of a person. This method can help us to reduce his/her fear and make them mentally strong when they are affected by COVID-19.

This method will help us in fighting effectively with the coronavirus. Using this analysis, public statement can be analyzed and we can take measures according to that to strengthen them. In this analysis process, first social media platforms are tracked. Then data is collected through them. Once the collection of data is processed, data analysis is performed to analyze the sentiments behind the statements.

16.6 Protecting the living beings from the impact of epidemics

The epidemics have different kinds of impacts on various fields. In the case of COVID-19 pandemic, it affected the lives of teachers, students, migration workers and laborers. It has a negative impact on each and every field. It has affected the economy very badly. Apart from these things, people's mental health is also getting disturbed as they are restricted to their houses. In terms of economy every family is facing problems as they are unable to get their salaries on time, prices of essential commodities and vegetables increased suddenly. Most of the people are suffering from food scarcity.

The impacts of COVID-19 are much more when compared to the two world wars. In the two world wars only few countries participated but almost all the countries were affected due to this COVID-19. In Italy and the United States, the numbers of deaths due to coronavirus were very high. Let us discuss the impacts on each field in a detailed manner.

16.6.1 Impact of COVID-19 on agriculture sector

This pandemic has had a devastating effect on the agriculture sector. It affected the production and marketing of food items. This also affected the prices of commodities. The increase in the prices of commodities has a severe impact on the consumption of food. We also know that many of the states were affected by locust attacks during this crisis period, which can also be considered one of the major reasons affecting the production rate. Even though relaxations were given to the agriculture sector due to labor scarcity, good harvest was not possible. Due to restrictions imposed on transportation and marketing of products during the lockdown, many food products were damaged as per the government reports [35].

16.6.2 Impact of COVID-19 on economy

COVID-19 majorly impacted the economy of several countries. Pandemic showed its impact on GDP, stock market, oil prices, global expenses, etc. It was wreaking havoc on financial markets. It was a threat and can be compared to the phase of the Great Depression that occurred after the two world wars. Many countries suffered in different ways. If we consider Japan, its main stock index saw the lowest mark since 2016. In the case of Spain, the main stock exchange drastically dropped. It was 10,000 points before. Due to the pandemic situation, it is only under 7,000 points. Boeing lost 18% of its value that can be considered very high [46].

16.6.3 Impact of COVID-19 on educational sector

The most severely affected is the educational sector. Due to the pandemic, the system of education is entirely changed. It is shifted to complete online mode. This has its own pros and cons. Majorly, the children in villages with issues related to the Internet, PCs, and laptops lose interest in classes, resulting in an increase in dropouts. Most of the schools are not taking these online classes too. This way of learning completely depends on the dedication and self-motivation of the students. Promoting the students to next classes without exams would completely affect the standards of education they are pursuing. This will cause a lack of seriousness among students [47]. Recovery from these impacts will take much time. It needs many efforts. This pandemic leads to the digitalization of the world. Even post-pandemic, there will be many changes in the existing systems. We need to adapt ourselves to these situations and accept the changes. We must implement the leanings of these epidemics and analyze the situation to tackle future situations effectively. We must not neglect them after the pandemic. We must work on them. Technologies must be used effectively to come up with the best solutions.

16.7 Our contribution

The major problem to everyone after the COVID-19 is fear of bacteria, germs, and viruses. The extreme places for germs, bacteria, and virus are through the floor. Even though in the major places like hospitals and malls they clean regularly, there will be germs and bacteria on the floor itself as there will be many different people visiting there. Some of them become airborne and spread. So, when they touch our feet or shoes and when we kick up that can spread to the air we breathe and can cause illness to us.

16.7.1 Proposed method and its working

Health is considered wealth, and to ensure safe health, we have come up with a bot that detects germs, bacteria, and viruses and sanitizes a person before entering a place like a hospital or shopping mall. The working of the bot is when a person stands on it, his legs/shoes will be completely sanitized by ultraviolet rays and shown on the LCD placed on the bot. Once the feet/shoes are completely sanitized using ultraviolet rays directly, a person will get sanitizer to sanitize his hands perfectly. We are attaching an automatic stand for our bot, which can be closed or closed opened based on the algorithm. So, the person's hands and legs will be virus-free and ensure no germs spread through floors. Our bot also has an add-on feature that is it can even sanitize the floor of hospitals as we are attaching freely movable tyres to it. These tyres can even be closed once they are done with cleaning the floor. The functionality of SAUCHA is clearly indicated in Figure 16.1.

The major problem to everyone after the COVID-19 is fear of bacteria, germs, and viruses. The extreme place for the germs, bacteria, and virus are through floor. Even though in the major places like hospitals, malls they clean regularly there will

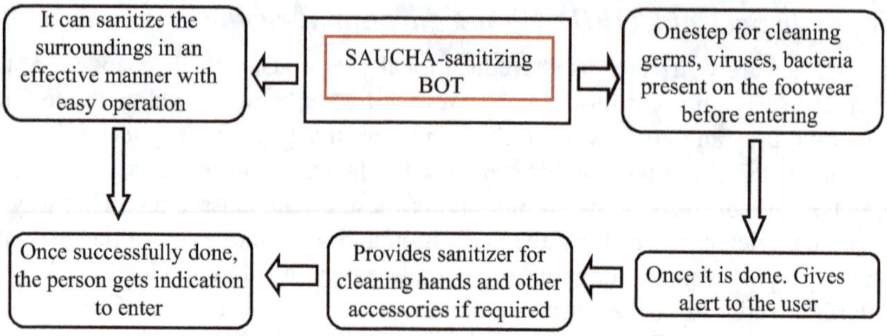

Figure 16.1 Functionality of SAUCHA

be germs and bacteria on the floor itself as there will be many different people visiting there.

UVC radiation is a known disinfectant for air, water, and nonporous surfaces. This radiation has effectively been used for decades to reduce the spread of bacteria, such as tuberculosis. For this reason, UVC lamps are often called "germicidal" lamps. This UVC LED plays a vital role in killing the germs and bacteria on the surfaces. Nowadays, people show a great interest toward technology and every human-made things can be achieved through technology. So a robot controlled through Bluetooth will have a great impact on attracting the people as well as its very convenient to the user.

As we know that even after COVID-19 sanitization plays a vital role, most of the people think about it, so this UVC sanitization had an effective sanitization and helps in killing germs and bacteria, and an autonomous hand sanitizer is also very important to avoid common contact, which helps in preventing the spread of the virus.

16.7.2 Components required

1. Arduino Uno
2. UV-LED
3. Ultrasonic sensor (hcsr04)
4. LCD display (16×2)
5. IR sensor
6. Servo motor
7. Bluetooth module
8. Relay module
9. 12-V batteries
10. Wheels
11. Dummy motors
12. Side shaft motors
13. L298n motor driver
14. On/off switch

15. L-clamps
16. Jumper wires

These components are connected together for the implementation of SAUCHA as shown in Figure 16.2.

16.7.3 Software required and simulation

1. Arduino IDE
2. Proteus

To clearly observe the structure of bot, the CAD model of the proposed method is shown in Figure 16.3.

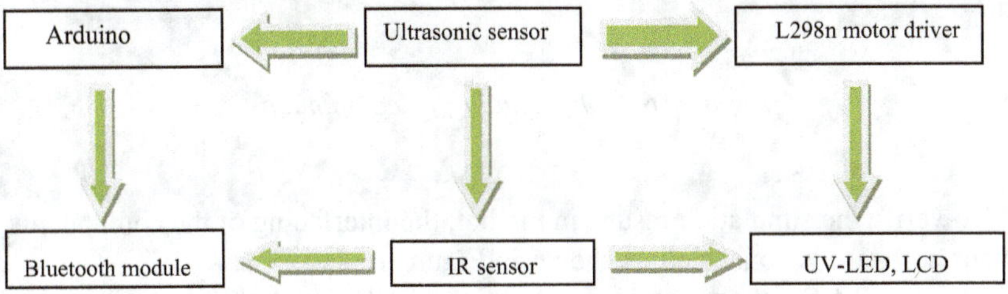

Figure 16.2 Block diagram of SAUCHA

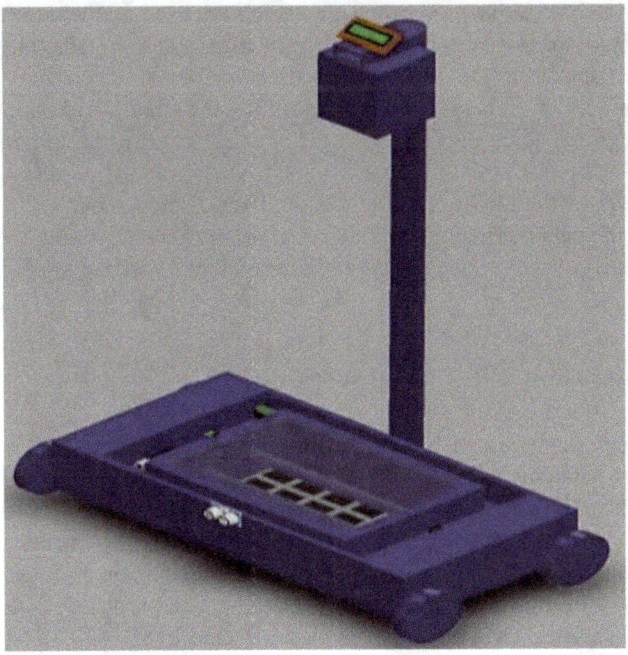

Figure 16.3 3D model of SAUCHA

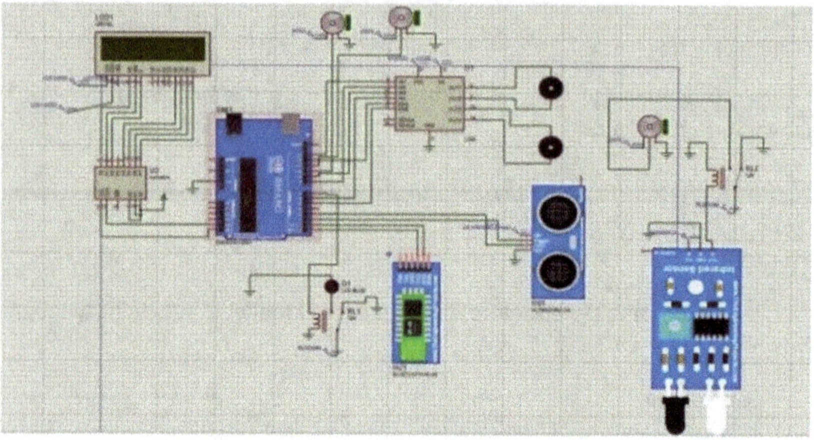

Figure 16.4 Interfacing of components

To verify the simulation results in the bot, the interfacing of the components in Proteus software is connected as shown in Figure 16.4.

The bot LCD is connected to Arduino. LCD is used for displaying the instructions and information. An ultrasonic sensor is used to measure the distance between the person and the bot. UV-LED is used to disinfect the person. A motor driver is used to control the motors and the wheels are used for the movement of the bot. The servomotor is used for flipping UVC LEDs, and a servomotor is also used in a sanitizer dispenser. An IR sensor is used for obstacle detection during the movement of our bot. Relay is used for controlling the circuit. Arduino IDE is used for writing and uploading the code in to the board. Proteus is the software used for the simulation of our circuit. When a person is detected, the ultrasonic sensor detects and drives the motor to rotate the sanitizer dispenser that will open and it will sanitize the person. Bluetooth module that is connected to Arduino can be used to transfer data which can be an add-on feature for future scope to access the data from bot.

16.8 Conclusion and future scope

This pandemic as discussed brought many changes in various fields. With the occurrence of pandemics, people start realizing the importance of health, hygiene, and well-being. The bot proposed in this chapter can be installed in various places where more people are moving and interacting to sanitize their hands and foot to avoid the spread of COVID. In future the per capita income on health sector would increase. Apart from that the individual expenditure on products related to health sector also increases. The sector that is least affected by the COVID-19 is health sector. Apart from that tremendous changes occur in different sectors. Mainly educational sector will witness many changes that will majorly concentrate on development of skills. Pandemic helped many innovators to come up with their wonderful innovations. In this year itself under the MSME, many start-ups were registered. Many industries used this crisis time as an opportunity to analyze themselves and bring changes as per the requirement. This also helps different countries analyze their mistakes and work on prediction, epidemic management techniques, and the improvements that need to be done in the health sector. Preparation and proper planning can be implemented to have preparedness to face any epidemics in future. There is also scope for new technologies in epidemic management.

Epidemics have much impact on society when compared with the world wars that occurred in the past. The major key to successfully facing these epidemics is exact data about that particular disease, effective management strategies, and improvement in the field of technology that can help us work much on prediction and prevention. The major reason behind failure in effectively managing the situation during epidemics is lack of proper information, neglecting the measures to be taken, no proper awareness among people.

Various machine learning techniques provide us help in analyzing the situation, mental health of people. During times of epidemics, the government must make sure that fake news is not spread on social media. Even it should restrict the news channels. The media must provide exact information to people, but it should not panic them. When we analyze the death reports of people, we understand that the major reason was their fear and psychological conditions rather than the effect of the virus. During such times, situations must be dealt with sensitively. Researchers have been developing signaling for very low power consumption [48]. Furthermore, introducing the IoT models allows identifying flagged, probable, or proven infected cases or a flagged area or object [49], to take precautionary steps. COVID-19 or 2019-nCoV is no longer pandemic, but rather endemic, with more than 651,247 people around world who have lost their lives after contracting the disease [50]. On the economic front, the major foreseen impact of AR/VR in intraoperative navigation would be reducing time of operative procedures, infection rates, revision rates, and length of stay [51]. Contact tracing was one of the important strategies used for reducing, halting, and reversing deaths and infections caused due to COVID-19 [52].

References

[1] Wu Z and McGoogan JM. Characteristics of and important lessons from the corona virus disease 2019 (COVID-19) outbreak in China: Summary of a report of 72314 cases from the Chinese center for disease control and prevention. *JAMA*. 2020; 323: 1239–42 10.1001/jama.2020.2648.

[2] Chong KC, Zee BCY and Wang MH. Approximate Bayesian algorithm to estimate the basic reproduction number in an influenza pandemic using arrival times of imported cases. *Travel Medicine and Infectious Disease*. 2018; 23: 80–6.

[3] WHO Coronavirus disease 2019 (COVID-19) situation report—44. Pandemic Influenza Risk Management Guidance, 2020. https://www.who.int/docs/default-source/coronaviruse/situation-reports/20200304-sitrep-44-covid-19.pdf?sfvrsn=783b4c9d_2.

[4] Adhikari SP, Meng S, Wu Y-J, *et al.* Epidemiology, causes, clinical manifestation and diagnosis, prevention and control of coronavirus disease (COVID-19) during the early outbreak period: A scoping review. *Infectious Diseases of Poverty*. 2020; 9(1): 29.

[5] Qiu W, Rutherford S, Mao A and Chu C. The pandemic and its impacts. *Health, Culture and Society*. 2017; 9: 1–11. 10.5195/HCS.2017.221.

[6] Ahn I, Jeong B-J, Bae S-E, Jung J and Son HS. Genomic analysis of influenza A viruses, including avian flu (H5N1) strains. *European Journal of Epidemiology*. 2006; 21: 511–9.

[7] Bempong NE, De Castañeda RR, Schütte S, *et al.* Precision global health – The case of Ebola: A scoping review. *Journal of Global Health*. 2019; 9(1).

[8] World Health Organization. New technology allows for rapid diagnosis of Ebola in the Democratic Republic of the Congo. 2017.

[9] Ahn I, Jeong BJ, Bae SE, Jung J and Son HS. Genomic analysis of influenza A viruses, including avian flu (H5N1) strains. *European journal of epidemiology*. 2006; 21(7): 511–9.

[10] Tom-Aba D, Olaleye A, Olayinka AT, *et al.* Innovative technological approach to Ebola virus disease outbreak response in Nigeria using the open data kit and form hub technology. *PLoS One*. 2015; 10(6): e0131000.

[11] Bhuyan HK, Chakraborty C, Shelke Y and Pani SK. COVID-19 diagnosis system by deep learning approaches. *Expert Systems*. 2021: e12776. https://doi.org/10.1111/exsy.12776.

[12] Dash S, Chakraborty C, Giri SK, Pani SK and Frnda J. BIFM: Big-data driven intelligent forecasting model for COVID-19. *IEEE Access*. 2021: 1–13. 10.1109/ACCESS.2021.3094658.

[13] Aslam B, Javed AR, Chakraborty C, Nebhen J, Raqib S and Rizwan M. Blockchain and ANFIS empowered IoMT application for privacy preserved contact tracing in COVID-19 pandemic. *Personal and Ubiquitous Computing*. 2021: 1–17. 10.1007/s00779-021-01596-3.

[14] Geldsetzer P. Use of rapid online surveys to assess people's perceptions during infectious disease outbreaks: A cross-sectional survey on COVID-19. *Journal of Medical Internet Research*. 2020; 22(4): e18790.

[15] Fanelli D and Piazza F. Analysis and forecast of COVID-19 spreading in China, Italy and France. *Chaos, Solitons and Fractals*. 2020; 134. article 109761.

[16] Vargo D, Zhu L, Benwell B and Yan Z. Digital technology use during COVID-19 pandemic: A rapid review. *Human Behavior and Emerging Technologies*. 2021; 3(1): 13–24.

[17] Bempong N-E, De Castañeda RR, Schütte S, *et al.* Precision Global Health – The case of Ebola: A scoping review. *Journal of Global Health*. 2019; 9(1).

[18] Greenhalgh T, Koh GC and Car J. Covid-19: A remote assessment in primary care. *BMJ*. 2020; 368.

[19] Dhawan S. Online learning: A panacea in the time of COVID-19 crisis. *Journal of Educational Technology Systems*. 2020; 49: 5–22.

[20] Beesham A. Mathematical modelling of COVID-19 in South Africa. *Asian Pacific Journal of Tropical Medicine*. 2020; 13(5): 235.

[21] Fu X, Ying Q, Zeng T, Long T and Wang Y. Simulating and forecasting the cumulative confirmed cases of SARS-CoV-2 in China by Boltzmann function-based regression analyses. *Journal of Infection*. 2020; 80(5): 578–606.

[22] Google. Google Trends. 2018. https://trends.google.com/trend (Accessed 11 Nov 2018).

[23] Hobday AJ, Smith ADM, Stobutzki IC, *et al.* Ecological risk assessment for the effects of fishing. *Fisheries Research*. 2011; 108(2–3): 372–84.

[24] Fletcher WJ. Review and refinement of an existing qualitative risk assessment method for application within an ecosystem-based management framework. *ICES Journal of Marine Science*. 2015; 72: 1043–56.

[25] Beck U. *Risk Society: Towards a New Modernity*, 1992, Sage, New Delhi.

[26] Yokota F and Thompson KM. Value of information analysis in environmental health risk management decisions: Past, present, and future. *Risk Analysis*. 2004; 24: 635–50.

[27] Golfarelli M, Rizzi S and Proli A. Designing what-if analysis: Towards a methodology. *DOLAP: Proceedings of the ACM International Workshop on Data Warehousing and OLAP*. 51–58. 2006. 10.1145/1183512.1183523.

[28] Patil R. An overview of fault tree analysis (FTA) method for reliability analysis. *Journal of Engineering Research and Studies*. 2013; 4: 6–8.

[29] Aini MS and Fakhru'l-Razi A. Latent errors of socio-technical disasters: A Malaysian case study. *Safety Science*. 2013; 51(1): 284–92.

[30] Shalev DM and Tiran J. Condition-based fault tree analysis (CBFTA): A new method for improved fault tree analysis (FTA), reliability and safety calculations. *Reliability Engineering & System Safety*, 2007; 92(9): 1231–41.

[31] Ericson II CA. Fault tree analysis. *System Safety Conference*, Orlando, Florida. vol. 1. 1999.

[32] Khan FI and Haddara MR. Risk-based maintenance of ethylene oxide production facilities. *Journal of Hazardous Materials*. 2004; 108(3): 147–59.

[33] Guth MAS. A probabilistic foundation for vagueness and imprecision in fault-tree analysis. *IEEE Transactions on Reliability*. 1991; 40(5): 563–71.

[34] Volkanovski A, Čepin M and Mavko B. Application of the fault tree analysis for assessment of power system reliability. *Reliability Engineering & System Safety*. 2009; 94(6): 1116–27.

[35] Cariappa AGA, Acharya KK and Adhav CA. Impact of COVID-19 on the Indian agricultural system: A 10-point strategy for post-pandemic recovery. *Outlook on Agriculture*. 2021. https://doi.org/10.1177/0030727021989060.

[36] Hamka MA. Safety risks assessment on container terminal using hazard identification and risk assessment and fault tree analysis methods. *Procedia Engineering*. 2017; 194: 307–14.

[37] World Health Organization, "Q and A on coronaviruses." https://www.who.int/fr/news-room/q-a-detail/q-acoronaviruses.

[38] D'Antiga L. Coronaviruses and immunosuppressed patients: The facts during the third epidemic. *Liver Transplantation*. 2020; 26(6): 832–4.
[39] Fanelli D and Piazza F. Analysis and forecast of COVID-19 spreading in China, Italy and France. *Chaos, Solitons and Fractals*. 2020; 134. article 109761.
[40] Atif I, Cawood FT and Mahboob MA. The role of digital technologies that could be applied for prescreening in the mining industry during the COVID-19 pandemic. *Transactions of the Indian National Academy of Engineering*. 2020: 1–12.
[41] Johnson HA, Wagner MM, Hogan WR, *et al.* Analysis of web access logs for surveillance of influenza. *Medinfo*. 2004; 11(Pt 2): 1202–26.
[42] Sayeed UB and Hossain A. How Japan managed to curb the pandemic early on: Lessons learned from the first eight months of COVID-19. *Journal of Global Health*. 2020; 10: 020390. PMCID: PMC7688188 PMID: 33282218.
[43] Parvathy G and Bindhu JS. A probabilistic generative model for mining cybercriminal network from online social media: A review. *International Journal of Computers and Applications*. 2016; 134(14): 1–4. doi:10.5120/ijca2016908121.
[44] Cambria E and White B. Jumping NLP curves: A review of natural language processing research. *IEEE Computational Intelligence Magazine*. 2014; 9 (2): 48–57. doi:10.1109/mci.2014.2307227.
[45] Alamoodi AH, Zaidan BB, Zaidan AA, *et al.* Sentiment analysis and its applications in fighting COVID-19 and infectious diseases: A systematic review. *Expert Systems with Applications*. 2021; 167: 114155. PMCID: PMC759187 PMID: 33139966.
[46] Verma P, Dumka A, Bhardwaj A, Ashok A, Kestwal MC and Kumar P. A statistical analysis of impact of COVID19 on the global economy and stock index returns. *SN Computer Science*. 2021; 2.
[47] Pokhrel S and Chhetri R. A literature review on impact of COVID-19 pandemic on teaching and learning. *Higher Education for the Future*. 2021; 8. https://doi.org/10.1177/2347631120983481.
[48] Chakraborty C, Gupta B and Ghosh SK. A review on telemedicine-based WBAN framework for patient monitoring. *Telemedicine Journal and e-Health*. 2013; 19(8): 619–26. ISSN: 1530-5627, 10.1089/tmj.2012.0215.
[49] Garg L, Chukwu E, Nasser N, Chakraborty C and Garg G. Anonymity preserving IoT-based COVID-19 and other infectious disease contact tracing model. *IEEE Access*. 2020; 8: 159402–14. 10.1109/ACCESS.2020.3020513, ISSN: 2169-3536.
[50] Muhammad LJ, Algehyne EA, Usman SS, Ahmad A, Chakraborty C and Mohammed IA. Supervised machine learning models for prediction of COVID-19 infection using epidemiology dataset. *SN Computer Science*. 2021; 2(11): 1–13.
[51] Shelke Y and Chakraborty C. Augmented reality and virtual reality transforming spinal imaging landscape: A feasibility study. *IEEE Computer Graphics and Applications*. 2021; 41(3): 124–38. 10.1109/MCG.2020.300035.
[52] Roy S and Chakraborty C. Panic buying situation during COVID-19 global pandemic. *Journal of Information Technology Management*. 2021; 13(2): 231–44. doi:10.22059/jitm.2021.80625.

Index

www.ingramcontent.com/pod-product-compliance
Lightning Source LLC
LaVergne TN
LVHW011554200926
848484LV00001B/314